THIRD EDITION

GLOBAL
HEALTH CARE

ISSUES AND POLICIES

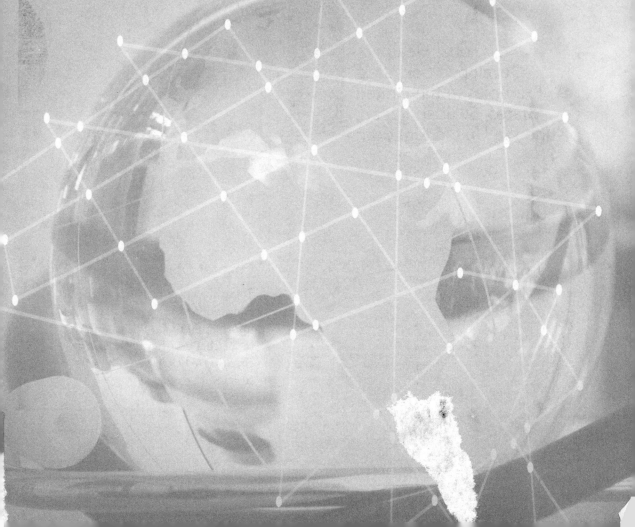

The Pedagogy

Global Health Care: Issues and Policies, Third Edition drives comprehension through various strategies that meet the learning needs of students while also generating enthusiasm about the topic. This interactive approach addresses different learning styles, making this the ideal text to ensure mastery of key concepts. The pedagogical aids that appear in most chapters include the following:

Global Health in Developed Societies: Examples in the United States, Sweden, Japan, and the United Kingdom

Carol Holtz

Objectives

After completing this chapter, the reader will be able to:

1. Compare and contrast population health statistics for the United States, Sweden, Japan, and the United Kingdom.
2. Compare and contrast the major health issues and healthcare systems of the United States, Sweden, Japan, and the United Kingdom.
3. Relate healthcare disparities within and among the countries of the United States, Sweden, Japan, and the United Kingdom.
4. Discuss the high rates of longevity for residents of Japan and Sweden.

INTRODUCTION

This chapter gives examples of developed countries and their major health issues and trends. These countries were chosen because they vary in terms of their healthcare systems, population health statistics, and geographic areas. We will review many of the health issues in greater detail in other chapters of this text.

Chapter Objectives

These objectives provide instructors and students with a snapshot of key information they will encounter in the chapter. They serve as a checklist to help guide and focus study.

This chapter has examined the health and health care of the countries of the United States, Sweden, Japan, and the United Kingdom. Included in this comparison were population statistics, types of government healthcare programs, economics and healthcare spending, and healthcare personnel.

Study Questions

1. Why do you think the United States has the world's highest rate of obesity? How does this problem relate to chronic health diseases such as cardiovascular disease, hypertension, and diabetes?
2. In spite of the country having the highest level of per capita expenditures, why does the United States still have a relatively high rate of infant mortality as compared to other developed countries?
3. What are some reasons that contribute to Japan and Sweden having the world's best longevity rates? Even though it spends the most dollars per capita on health care, why is the United States so far behind in terms of longevity?
4. What are some health disparities within the United Kingdom, and how might they be solved?

Case Study: Addressing U.S. American Indians (Native Americans)/Alaskan Natives and Diabetes

The mortality rate for American Indians, which includes Alaskan Natives (Native Americans), has increased primarily due to the effects of type 2 diabetes. The U.S. Department of Indian Health Service has provided a Special Diabetes Program for Indians resulting in increased spending for health care; however, the rate for age-adjusted deaths has increased as compared to white Americans.

Infectious diseases are decreasing while chronic diseases, such as type 2 diabetes, are increasing in this population. Data collected were mainly from Navaho Indians living in the western part of the United States. Other major health issues include obesity, cardiovascular diseases, smoking, and hypertension. Also discussed was the high rate of sedentary lifestyles as compared to historically much greater daily physical activities.

Case Study Questions

1. Create a culturally congruent plan for reduction of exceptionally high levels of type 2 diabetes among American Indians/Alaskan Natives.
2. Why do American Indians have higher levels of increased smoking, obesity, and sedentary life styles, which contribute to the type 2 diabetes rates than whites?
3. Why is the Indian Health Service an important part of health care that is historically "owed" to American Indians/Alaskan Natives?

Data from Kunitz, S. (2008). Changing patterns of mortality among American Indians. *American Journal of Public Health, 98*(3), 404–411.

Study Questions

Review key concepts using these end of chapter questions.

Case Studies

Read and analyze real-life global health situations and apply knowledge from the chapter to answer critical thinking questions.

THIRD EDITION

GLOBAL
HEALTH CARE

ISSUES AND POLICIES

EDITED BY

CAROL HOLTZ, PHD, RN
Professor of Nursing
WellStar School of Nursing
Kennesaw State University
Kennesaw, Georgia

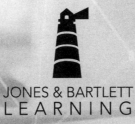

JONES & BARTLETT
LEARNING

World Headquarters
Jones & Bartlett Learning
5 Wall Street
Burlington, MA 01803
978-443-5000
info@jblearning.com
www.jblearning.com

Jones & Bartlett Learning books and products are available through most bookstores and online booksellers. To contact Jones & Bartlett Learning directly, call 800-832-0034, fax 978-443-8000, or visit our website, www.jblearning.com.

Substantial discounts on bulk quantities of Jones & Bartlett Learning publications are available to corporations, professional associations, and other qualified organizations. For details and specific discount information, contact the special sales department at Jones & Bartlett Learning via the above contact information or send an email to specialsales@jblearning.com.

The content, statements, views, and opinions herein are the sole expression of the respective authors and not that of Jones & Bartlett Learning, LLC. Reference herein to any specific commercial product, process, or service by trade name, trademark, manufacturer, or otherwise does not constitute or imply its endorsement or recommendation by Jones & Bartlett Learning, LLC and such reference shall not be used for advertising or product endorsement purposes. All trademarks displayed are the trademarks of the parties noted herein. *Global Health Care: Issues and Policies, Third Edition* is an independent publication and has not been authorized, sponsored, or otherwise approved by the owners of the trademarks or service marks referenced in this product.

There may be images in this book that feature models; these models do not necessarily endorse, represent, or participate in the activities represented in the images. Any screenshots in this product are for educational and instructive purposes only. Any individuals and scenarios featured in the case studies throughout this product may be real or fictitious, but are used for instructional purposes only.

The authors, editor, and publisher have made every effort to provide accurate information. However, they are not responsible for errors, omissions, or for any outcomes related to the use of the contents of this book and take no responsibility for the use of the products and procedures described. Treatments and side effects described in this book may not be applicable to all people; likewise, some people may require a dose or experience a side effect that is not described herein. Drugs and medical devices are discussed that may have limited availability controlled by the Food and Drug Administration (FDA) for use only in a research study or clinical trial. Research, clinical practice, and government regulations often change the accepted standard in this field. When consideration is being given to use of any drug in the clinical setting, the health care provider or reader is responsible for determining FDA status of the drug, reading the package insert, and reviewing prescribing information for the most up-to-date recommendations on dose, precautions, and contraindications, and determining the appropriate usage for the product. This is especially important in the case of drugs that are new or seldom used.

13283-0

Production Credits

VP, Executive Publisher: David D. Cella
Executive Editor: Amanda Martin
Associate Editor: Danielle Bessette
Associate Production Editor: Juna Abrams
Senior Marketing Manager: Jennifer Scherzay
Product Fulfillment Manager: Wendy Kilborn
Composition: S4Carlisle Publishing Services
Cover Design: Kristin E. Parker
Rights & Media Specialist: Wes DeShano

Media Development Editor: Troy Liston
Cover Images: © Rawpixel/Shutterstock; © Sascha Burkard/Shutterstock; © Kuzma/Shutterstock; © szefei/Shutterstock; © Aman Ahmed Khan/Shutterstock; © De Visu/Shutterstock; © Lucian Coman/Shutterstock; © Guschenkova/Shutterstock; © DONOT6_STUDIO/Shutterstock;
Printing and Binding: Edwards Brothers Malloy
Cover Printing: Edwards Brothers Malloy

Library of Congress Cataloging-in-Publication Data
Names: Holtz, Carol, editor.
Title: Global health care : issues and policies / [edited by] Carol Sue Holtz.
Description: Third edition. | Burlington : Jones & Bartlett Learning, [2017]
   | Includes bibliographical references and index.
Identifiers: LCCN 2016003859 | ISBN 9781284070668 (pbk.)
Subjects: | MESH: Global Health | Cross-Cultural Comparison | Delivery of
   Health Care | Health Policy
Classification: LCC RA441 | NLM WA 530.1 | DDC 362.1--dc23 LC record available
   at http://lccn.loc.gov/2016003859

6048

Printed in the United States of America
20 19 18 17 16   10 9 8 7 6 5 4 3 2

Contents

Chapter 14   Global Perspectives on Nutrition   381
Carol Holtz, Marvin A. Friedman, and Emily Peoples

Chapter 18   Global Health of Children   497
Kathie Aduddell

Chapter 19   Global Health of the Older Adult   517
David B. Mitchell

Preface

The main purpose of this text is to provide knowledge and a better understanding of global health and health care with its related policies and issues. As stated by the Institute of Medicine in *America's Vital Interest in Global Health* (2012, p. 1), "The failure to engage in the fight to anticipate, prevent and ameliorate global health problems would diminish America's stature in the realm of health and jeopardize our own health, economy, and national security." One cannot argue the need to have a global perspective and many have stated this need eloquently. As Kofi Annan, Ghanaian diplomat, seventh secretary-general of the United Nations, and 2001 Nobel Peace Prize recipient noted, "It has been said that arguing against globalization is like arguing against the law of gravity." He also related, "[W]e have different religions, different languages, different colored skin, but we all belong to one human race."

WHAT IS GLOBAL HEALTH?

Global health is an area of study, research, and practice that places a priority on improving health and achieving equity in health for all people worldwide. It refers to such health problems as infectious and insect-borne diseases that transcend national borders and spread from one country to another. It also includes health problems that have a global, political, and economic impact. Global health problems are best addressed by cooperative actions and whose solutions involve more than one country. Because global health problems can cross national borders, countries can learn from one another's experiences, such as how certain diseases are spread, treated, and controlled. International cooperation is essential to address and treat health problems that transcend borders. Approximately 90% of the world's resources are spent on diseases that affect only 10% of the world's population. Working to solve global health problems will help ensure that money and resources are distributed more fairly across the globe.*

---

*Institute of Medicine. (2012). *America's vital interest in global health.* Retrieved from http://www.familiesusa .org/issues/global-health/matters/

Acknowledgments

This text represents the combined efforts of numerous well-educated, very dedicated, experienced, and hard-working contributors in addition to my own work. The administrators of Kennesaw State University in greater Atlanta, Georgia, USA, have given me tremendous support and encouragement to complete this textbook. I wish to thank the outstanding editors of Jones & Bartlett Learning for supporting my ideas, and for their help in organizing, writing, and editing this textbook.

I wish to thank my husband of 47 years, Dr. Noel Holtz, a neurologist and employee of the WellStar Health System, Marietta, Georgia, for his love, devotion, and consistent support. I dedicate this book to my husband, Noel Holtz; my children, Pamela Poulos and David Poulos, Aaron Holtz, and Daniel and Maggie Holtz; and to my grandchildren, Andrew, Brandon, Caroline, Ben, Eva, and William Holtz;, Sarah and Meryl Gilmore, and David Jr. and Jeremy Poulos. I give all of my children and grandchildren this legacy of scholarship, hard work, and perseverance that I learned from my grandparents and parents, as well as my in-laws and many teachers, who always believed in me and encouraged me to achieve my scholarly pursuits.

Contributors

Kathie Aduddell, EdD, MSN, RN
Director/Professor of Nursing
Texas Lutheran University
Seguin, Texas

Barbara J. Blake, PhD, ACRN, FAAN
Professor of Nursing
Kennesaw State University
Kennesaw, Georgia

Mary Ann Camann, PhD, RN
Associate Professor of Nursing (In Memoriam)
Kennesaw State University
Kennesaw, Georgia

Mary de Chesnay, PhD, RN, FAAN
Professor of Nursing
Kennesaw State University
Kennesaw, Georgia

Bowman O. Davis Jr., PhD
Professor Emeritus of Biology
Kennesaw State University
Kennesaw, Georgia

Ibrahim Elsawy, PhD
Regional Director of Arab World Projects
Institute for Global Initiatives
Associate Professor
Kennesaw State University
Kennesaw, Georgia

Marvin A. Friedman, PhD, DABT, DATS, SNF
Scientific Advisor
Oviedo, Florida

T. Mark Haney, MBA, MHA, FACHE
Senior Vice President, WellStar Hospital System,
    President of WellStar Paulding Hospital
Marietta, Georgia

Govind Hariharan, PHD
Professor of Economics, Finance, and Quantitative
    Analysis
Kennesaw State University
Kennesaw, Georgia

Carol Holtz, PhD, RN
Professor of Nursing
Kennesaw State University
Kennesaw, Georgia

Ping Hu Johnson, MD, PHD
Associate Professor of Health, Physical Education,
 and Sport Science
Kennesaw State University
Kennesaw, Georgia

Michal Lipschuetz, RN, MPH, MSc
Nursing Administration
Hadassah Medical Center
Jerusalem, Israel

Janice Long, PhD, RN
Professor of Nursing (retired)
Kennesaw State University
Kennesaw, Georgia

David B. Mitchell, PhD
Associate Dean, College of Health and Human
 Services
Distinguished Scholar in Gerontology and
 Professor of Health, Physical Education,
 and Sport Science
Kennesaw State University
Kennesaw, Georgia

Monica Nandan, PhD
Acting Dean, College of Health and Human
 Services
Kennesaw State University
Kennesaw, Georgia

Dula F. Pacquiao, EdD, RN, CTN-A, TNS
Consultant
Transcultural Nursing Education, Research
 and Practice
Adjunct Lecturer, University of Hawai'i
Hilo School of Nursing and Rutgers University
 School of Nursing

Emily Peoples

Kenneth D. Phillips, PhD, RN
Professor and Associate Dean for Research
 and Evaluation
College of Nursing
University of Tennessee
Knoxville, Tennessee

Larry Purnell, PhD, RN, FAAN
Professor Emeritus, University of Delaware;
 Adjunct Professor, Florida International
 University
Consulting Faculty, Excelsior College, Professor,
 Universita de Moderna, Italy, Newark, Delaware

Richard L. Sowell, PhD, RN, FAAN
Professor of Nursing
Kennesaw State University
Kennesaw, Georgia

Gloria A. Taylor, DNS, RN
Professor of Nursing
Kennesaw State University
Kennesaw, Georgia

Orly Toren, PhD, RN
Associate Director for Development Research
 in Nursing
Hadassah Medical Center
Jerusalem, Israel

Astrid H. Wilson, DNS, RN
Professor of Nursing
Kennesaw State University
Kennesaw, Georgia

Anelise Zamarripa-Zoucha, BSN, RN
Pittsburg, Pennsylvania

Rick D. Zoucha, PhD, APRN-BC, CT, FAAN
Associate Professor of Nursing
Duquesne University
Pittsburgh, Pennsylvania

SECTION I

GLOBAL HEALTH ISSUES, POLICY, AND HEALTHCARE DELIVERY

Global Health: An Introduction

Carol Holtz

Objectives

After completing this chapter, the reader will be able to:

1. Define global health.
2. Identify global health terminology, agencies, and significant historical events.
3. Relate the state of the world's population growth and relevance to world health.
4. Discuss the Millennium Developmental Goals and the latest progress made toward their attainment.
5. Relate reasons for health and healthcare disparities worldwide.
6. Define indices of health.
7. Compare and contrast the universal "right to health care" and realistic global healthcare access.
8. Relate global health and healthcare priorities.
9. Discuss the issues related to global migration of healthcare workers.

WHAT IS GLOBAL HEALTH?

Global health is an area of study, research, and practice that places a priority on improving health and achieving equity in health for all people worldwide. It is determined by problems, issues, and concerns that transcend national boundaries. These problems, issues, and concerns emphasize transnational health issues, determinants, and solutions, and involve many disciplines within and beyond the health sciences and promote interdisciplinary collaboration (Beaglehole & Bonita, 2010; De Cock, Simone, Davison, & Slutsker, 2013; Koplan et al., 2009; Macfarlane, Jacobs, & Kaaya, 2008).

Globalization

Globalization is the increased interconnectedness and interdependence of people and countries (WHO, 2014a). In the 1960s, the World Bank first advocated global thinking in regard to health issues with the phrase, "Think globally and act locally" (Beaglehole & Yach, 2003). There are negative aspects to globalization, which include global warming, cross-border pollution, financial crises, international crime, and the spread of human immunodeficiency virus (HIV)/acquired immune deficiency syndrome (AIDS) and the Ebola virus.

The globalization of disease began with the European explorers and conquerors who came to the Americas and spread smallpox, measles, and yellow fever among the various indigenous populations. They also brought typhus, influenza, and the plague. The poorest were the most vulnerable, whereas the small group of elite, wealthy groups had better nutrition, better health care, and better sanitary (hygienic) conditions. More recently, the spread of HIV/AIDS, tuberculosis (TB), severe acute respiratory syndrome (SARS), West Nile virus, Ebola virus, and other infectious diseases have emerged as a global concern. The rapid movement of people and food products as a result of travel has also resulted in new health problems such as mad cow disease (bovine spongiform encephalopathy or BSE) and avian influenza. Globalization has recently changed the lifestyles of developing countries resulting in new chronic diseases from the importation of high-sodium, high-fat fast foods, along with the more sedentary lifestyles promoted by technologies (e.g., TV, appliances). Moreover, in developing countries today, populations are rapidly acquiring chronic diseases (such as heart disease, cancer, stroke, and obesity leading to diabetes), which are adding a *double burden of disease* given the still challenging acute infectious diseases (Beaglehole & Yach, 2003).

HISTORY OF GLOBAL HEALTH

World Health Organization

The **World Health Organization (WHO)** was established just after World War II as an intergovernmental agency for the purpose of leading and coordinating worldwide health activities. Its activities are initiated when consensus regarding world health priorities is reached. Today's world health is elevated when the economic development of nations is improved via the cooperation of governmental and nongovernmental agencies. In the last decade, numerous efforts directed at global health have been initiated, including the Global Alliance for Vaccines and Immunizations, the Global Tuberculosis Partnership, and the Global Fund on HIV/AIDS (Ruger, 2005).

The World Bank began operations in 1946. Although it was originally established to finance European reconstruction after World War II, today it serves as a major resource for the health, nutrition, and population (HNP) of developing countries. A few examples of the historical activities of the World Bank include the 1968 appointment of Robert McNamara as president of the organization. His term as president resulted in the initiation of a population control program, which provided funding for family planning. In 1971, McNamara emphasized the need to combat malnutrition. Additionally, in 1974, the Onchocerciasis Control Program was developed in cooperation with the United Nations Development Program, the Food and Agriculture Organization, and WHO. This program was created to eliminate river blindness in West Africa. After 30 years, the onchocerciasis program has protected an estimated 34 million people and also has cleared an estimated 25 million hectares of land for agricultural use (Ruger, 2005).

In 1985, WHO gave $3 million in grants for the World Food Program for emergency food supplies to Sub-Saharan Africa. This effort was followed in 1987 by WHO and the United Nations cosponsoring a Safe Motherhood Project in the same region—the first of a series of global initiatives for this area. In addition, in 1998, WHO lent $300 million to India's Women and Child Development Program (Ruger, 2005).

At present, the World Bank is the largest financial contributor to health projects throughout the world. When making loans, it allows repayment periods up to 35 to 40 years and gives a 10-year grace period. Although one of the main purposes of the World Bank is to generate and disseminate knowledge, its main advantage over other global healthcare agencies is its ability to generate and mobilize healthcare resources. One of the criticisms of the World Bank is its reliance on user fees, which are said to cause a disproportionate burden on the poor and sick people of the world. For the poorest developing countries the bank's assistance plans are based on poverty reduction strategies. The World Bank develops a strategy pertaining uniquely to the country in question. The government then identifies the country's priorities and targets for the reduction of poverty, and the World Bank aligns its aid efforts correspondingly (The World Bank, 2014).

Alma-Ata

In 1978, in Alma-Ata, Kazakhstan (formerly part of the Soviet Union), leaders within the world community assembled to discuss and solve the issue of primary care for all world inhabitants. The Alma-Ata Declaration stated that governments have the responsibility for the health of their people, which can be fulfilled only by the provision of adequate health and social measures. According to this document, a main social target of governments, international organizations, and the whole world community in coming decades was to be the attainment by all peoples of the world, by the year 2000, of a level of health care that would permit them to lead a socially and economically productive life. Primary health care is the key to attaining this target as part of the development of social justice (Hixon & Maskarinec, 2008). The Alma-Ata Declaration states that citizens cannot always provide primary health care by themselves, so governments must include everyone, not just those who can afford health care, in their health-related programs. This document urges member states:

1. To ensure political commitment at all levels to the values and principles of the Declaration of Alma-Ata, keep the issue of strengthening health systems based on the primary healthcare approach high on the international political agenda, and take advantage, as appropriate, of health-related partnerships and initiatives relating to this issue, particularly to support achievement of the Millennium Development Goals (MDGs).

2. To accelerate action toward universal access to primary health care by developing comprehensive health services and by developing national equitable and sustainable financing mechanisms, mindful of the need to ensure social protection and protect health budgets in the context of the current international financial crisis.

3. To put people at the center of health care by adopting, as appropriate, delivery models focused on the local and district levels that provide comprehensive primary healthcare services, including health promotion, disease prevention, curative care and end-of-life services that are integrated and coordinated according to need.[1]

In 2005, WHO established a commission on Social Determinants of Health: A Renewal of the Alma-Ata Declaration. In 2008, this commission completed its report recommending a renewal of the goal of primary health care for all and new attention to the need for addressing health disparities worldwide. The Renewal of the Alma-Ata Declaration addressed the following issues:

1. The aging of the world population
2. The plight of indigenous populations
3. Food and nutrition
4. The impact of conflicts and violence
5. The environment and health
6. Global and national inequalities
7. The impact of health on the global economy, social standing, and hierarchy
8. Health disparities among and within nations
9. Best practices and country studies
10. The importance of expanding social determinants of health studies (Hixon & Maskarinec, 2008)

The principles of the Alma-Ata Declaration and Primary Health Care remain at the heart of the global discussions on the post-2015 agenda. These focus on several concepts and priorities, such as *sustainable well-being* for all, *maximizing healthy lives*, and *accelerating progress* on the health MDG's agenda, particularly on the unfinished business of the burden of major National Coverage Determinations and universal health coverage (Thirty-fifth Anniversary of the Alma-Ata Primary Health Care Declaration Conference).

Access to Health Care

A continuing goal is access to health care to achieve health equity and increase the quality of life for all people worldwide. Access to healthcare impacts:

1. Overall physical, mental, and social health status
2. Prevention of disease and disability
3. Detection and treatment of health issues
4. Quality of life
5. Preventable death
6. Life expectancy (Access to Health Services: Healthy People, 2014)

---

[1]Reprinted from Landscape Analysis of Barriers to Developing or Adapting Technologies for Global Health Purposes, World Health Organization, p. 40. Copyright 2010. http://apps.who.int/medicinedocs/documents/ s17778en/s17778en.pdf

STATE OF THE WORLD'S POPULATION

Worldwide, a child born in 1955 had an average life expectancy at birth of only 48 years. By 2000, the average life expectancy at birth had increased to 66 years and, if past trends continue, the global life expectancy at birth is projected to rise to 73 years by 2025. These improvements in longevity have resulted from improved living conditions overall, advances in medical science, and a number of population-level interventions. However, major disparities persist. During the past decade, in low-income countries, average life expectancy at birth increased from 55 to 57 years (3.6%), while increasing from 78 to 80 years (2.6%) in high-income countries. The world's population as of October 31, 2011, reached 7 billion. Although women on average are having fewer children than they were in the 1960s, the world population continues to rise. At present, there are more people who are younger and also more people who are older than ever before. In some of the poorest countries, high fertility rates hamper the infrastructure development and perpetuate poverty, while in some of the richest countries, there are great concerns regarding low fertility rates and too few people entering the job market. The unemployed people of many nations who wish to migrate from developing countries to developed countries are finding more national borders closed to them. Gaps between rich and poor are widening in almost every location worldwide (UNFPA, 2011).

In 2050, the world population is projected to total 9.15 billion. It is expected that in developing countries, most families will have two or fewer children per family. The largest increases in population growth rates will occur in Africa. Many countries are facing a shrinking pool of working-age individuals (ages 15–64 years), who are needed to support the older adult population. This imbalance may jeopardize pension guarantees and long-term healthcare programs for the elderly. Within the United States, the largest population growth is expected to come from immigration and from growth of the older adult population (Bremner et al., 2010).

The United Nations Family Planning Association (UNFPA) has validated, across nations, the inadequate resources, gender bias, and gaps in serving the world's poor (UNFPA, 2011). Many developing countries have initiated population projects to reduce poverty and have developed laws and policies to protect the rights of women and girls. They have introduced reproductive health services as part of primary health care, increased the skills of birth attendants, and provided more prevention and treatment of HIV/AIDS. Many couples today continue to lack access to birth control. Birth complications remain the leading cause of death of women worldwide, with five million new fatalities per year. Every minute, a woman dies in pregnancy or in childbirth and another 20 to 30 women suffer serious injury or disability; most of these women die in developing countries of preventable or treatable complications. A wide disparity in global survival rates among the rich and poor women within countries is evident (UNFPA, 2011).

World Population Statistics and Related Health Issues

Estimates for the year 2050 range from between 3.2 and 24.8 billion people (The World Bank, 2013).

Life Expectancy

According to IndexMundi (2014a; 2014b), statistics indicated the following for the world:

1. *World life expectancy*—males: 68.09 years and females: 70.24 years.
2. *World birth rate*—18.9 births per 1,000 population. The total fertility rate (2014) ranges from 7.35 births per woman in Niger, 6.57 in Uganda, to 2.22 in Peru.
3. *World death rate*—7.9 deaths per 1,000. The world range leads in South Africa with 17.23 deaths per 1,000 and Russia with 16.03 deaths per 1,000, to the United Arab Emirates with 2.04 per 1,000 and Qatar with 1.55 per 1,000.

WHO's annual statistics report shows that low-income countries have made the greatest progress, with an average increase in life expectancy by 9 years from 1990 to 2012. The top six countries where life expectancy increased the most were Liberia with a 20-year increase (from 42 years in 1990 to 62 years in 2012), followed by Ethiopia (from 45 to 64 years), Maldives (58 to 77 years), Cambodia (54 to 72 years), Timor-Leste (50 to 66 years), and Rwanda (48 to 65 years) (IndexMundi, 2014a; 2014b).

Global Family Planning Needs in Developing Countries

Many emerging economies have experienced very rapid increases in their contraceptive coverage, enabling steady fertility declines. By contrast, the least developed countries, mostly located in Sub-Saharan Africa, are just beginning to use modern contraceptives (Rwanda and Ethiopia are among the few exceptions). An unmet need for family planning remains high in Sub-Saharan Africa. About 25% of couples who would like to postpone their next birth by 2 years do not currently use a contraceptive method. This need could be met by improving knowledge of contraception and increasing the supply of reproductive health services so that couples can better plan their families (Guengant & May, 2013).

Global Health Research

The World Health Organization (2013), in its population data sheet, calls for the following improvements:

1. Increased international and national investment and support for research addressing improved healthcare coverage for all countries.
2. Closer collaboration between researchers and policymakers.
3. Building research capacity by developing a local workforce of well-trained researchers.
4. All countries having comprehensive codes of good research practice.
5. Global and national research networks to coordinate research and increase collaboration and information exchange.

Gaps Between Rich and Poor Countries

A boy born in 2012 in a high-income country can expect to live to the age of around 76, which is 16 years longer than a boy born in a low-income country (age 60). For girls, the difference is even wider; a gap of 19 years separates life expectancy in high-income (82 years) and low-income countries (63 years). Wherever they live in the world, women live longer than men. The gap between male and female life expectancy is greater in high-income countries where women live approximately 6 years longer than men. In low-income countries, the difference is around three years. Women in Japan have the longest life expectancy in the world at 87 years, followed by Spain, Switzerland, and Singapore. Female life expectancy in all the top 10 countries was 84 years or longer. Life expectancy among men is 80 years or more in nine countries, especially as the declining use of tobacco helps people live longer in several countries. At the other end of the scale, life expectancy for both men and women is still less than 55 years in nine Sub-Saharan African countries: Angola, Central African Republic, Chad, Côte d'Ivoire, Democratic Republic of the Congo, Lesotho, Mozambique, Nigeria, and Sierra Leone (CDC, 2014).

WORLD HEALTH STATISTICS

The following facts, from WHO's World Health Statistics report, characterize the current state of world health (WHO, 2014c):

- The top three causes of years of life lost due to premature death are coronary heart disease, lower respiratory infections (such as pneumonia), and stroke.
- Worldwide, a major shift is occurring in the causes and ages of death. In 22 countries (all in Africa), 70% or more of years of life lost (due to premature deaths) are still caused by infectious diseases and related conditions. Meanwhile, in 47 countries (mostly high income), noncommunicable diseases and injuries cause more than 90% of years of life lost. More than 100 countries are transitioning rapidly toward a greater proportion of deaths from noncommunicable diseases and injuries.
- Around 44 million (6.7%) of the world's children, aged less than 5 years, were overweight or obese in 2012. Ten million of these children were in the WHO African Region where levels of child obesity have increased rapidly.
- Most deaths among those under five occur among children born prematurely (17.3%); pneumonia is responsible for the second-highest number of deaths (15.2%).
- Between 1995 and 2012, 56 million people were successfully treated for tuberculosis and 22 million lives were saved. In 2012, an estimated 450,000 people worldwide developed multidrug-resistant tuberculosis.
- Only one-third of all deaths worldwide are recorded in civil registries along with cause-of-death information.

THE CDC GLOBAL HEALTH STRATEGY/HEALTH CHALLENGES

The Centers for Disease Control and Prevention (CDC) created major goals, stated in its Health Challenges report as the following (CDC, 2014a):

1. Health impact—prevent new infections
   a. Reduce TB
   b. Reduce malaria

    c. Reduce child mortality and morbidity

    d. Control or eradicate vaccine-preventable diseases

    e. Reduce noncommunicable diseases

2. Health security—improve capacities to prepare and respond to infectious diseases

    a. Strengthen capacity to prepare for and detect infectious diseases and other emerging health threats

    b. Respond to international public health emergencies and improve country response capabilities

3. Health capacity—build country public health capacity

    a. Strengthen public health institutions and infrastructure

    b. Improve surveillance and use of strategic information

    c. Build workforce capacity

    d. Strengthen laboratory systems and networks

    e. Improve research capacity

4. Organizational capacity—maximize potential of CDC's global programs to achieve impact

    a. Strengthen organizational and technical capacity to better support the CDC's global health activities

    b. Enhance communication to expand the impact of the CDC's global health expertise

MILLENNIUM DEVELOPMENT GOALS

The Millennium Development Goals (MDGs) are the most broadly supported, comprehensive, and specific development goals worldwide. Collectively, they provide benchmarks for resolving extreme poverty and include goals and targets related to income, poverty, hunger, maternal and child mortality, disease, inadequate shelter, gender inequality, environmental degradation, and the Global Partnership for Development. Adopted by world leaders in 2000 and set to be achieved by 2015, the MDGs are both global and local, adapted by each country to address its specific development needs. They provide a framework for the entire international community to work together toward a common end for everyone.

Progress Toward Meeting the Millennium Developmental Goals

In 2014, the United Nations issued *The Millennium Developmental Goals Report 2014*, which contained the following:

    1. *Eradicate extreme poverty and hunger.* Reduce by half the proportion of people living on less than a dollar a day; achieve full and productive employment and decent work for all, including women and young people; and reduce by half the proportion of people who suffer from hunger. The goal of cutting in half the proportion of people in the developing world living on less than $1 per day by 2015 remains within reach. This achievement will be due mainly to the extraordinary economic success in most of Asia. In contrast, previous estimates suggested that little progress was made in reducing extreme poverty in Sub-Saharan Africa. There are half a billion fewer people living below an international poverty line of $1.25 a day. In western Asia, poverty rates are relatively low but increasing.

Progress

The MDG target has been met, and poverty rates have been halved between 1990 and 2010, but 1.2 billion people are still living in poverty (UN, 2014). According to *The Millennium Development Goals Report 2014*, the world reached the poverty reduction target 5 years ahead of schedule as 700 million fewer people in 2010 lived in extreme poverty compared to 1990. Further, the report also highlights that the goal of halving the number of chronically hungry people, while not yet achieved, is within reach. Since 1990 the number has fallen from over 1 billion people to 842 million in 2013.

2. *Achieve universal primary education.*

Progress

In most regions, primary school enrollment rates in 2006 exceeded 90%, and universal enrollment was achieved in many countries. The number of children of primary school age who were not in school dropped from 103 million in 1999 to 73 million in 2006 despite an overall increase in children of that age group. In Sub-Saharan Africa, net enrollment only reached 71%, with 38 million children in that region still out of school. In southern Asia, enrollment reached 90%, with 18 million children still not enrolled. Too many children are still denied a right to a primary education. If current trends continue, the world will not meet the goal of universal primary education by 2015.

3. *Promote gender equality and empower women.* Eliminate gender disparity in primary and secondary education by 2005 and at all levels by 2015.

Progress

For girls in some regions, education remains elusive. Poverty is a major barrier to education, especially among older girls. Women are slowly rising to political power, but usually when boosted by quotas and other special measures. Women are assuming more power in the world's parliaments, boosted by quota systems.

4. *Reduce child mortality.* Child death rates have fallen by more than 30%, with about three million children's lives saved each year, compared to 2000. In 2006, the annual number of deaths among children younger than age five dropped below 10 million. A child born in a developing country is 13 times more likely to die within the first 5 years of life than a child born in a developed country. Sub-Saharan Africa accounts for half of all under-five deaths in the developing world. In eastern Asia, Latin America, and the Caribbean, child mortality rates are approximately four times higher than in developed regions. Mortality rates are higher for children from rural areas and poor families whose mothers lack basic education.

Progress

Large gains have been made in child survival, but efforts must be redoubled to meet the global target. The target is to reduce by two-thirds, between 1990 and 2015, the under-5-year-olds' mortality rate, from 93 children of every 1,000 dying to 31 of every 1,000. Between 1990 and 2012 mortality in children declined by 47% from an estimated 90 deaths per 1,000 live births to 48 deaths per 1,000 live births. The under-five mortality rate is still highest in Africa with a rate of 95 per 1,000 live births. The risk of a child dying before his or her fifth birthday is eight times greater in the WHO African region than in the WHO European region. Inequities among low-income countries were greater than 13 times the average rate for high-income countries. Undernutrition is the major cause of death in children, causing 45% of all deaths. The number of underweight children declined from 160 million in 1999 to 99 million in 2012, a decline from 25% to 15%.

5. *Improve maternal health.* Reduce by three-fourths the maternal mortality ratio; achieve by 2015 universal access to reproductive health.

Progress

Maternal mortality remains high across most of the developing world. In 2005, more than 500,000 women died during pregnancy, childbirth, or within 6 weeks after delivery. Ninety-nine percent of these deaths occurred in developing regions, with Sub-Saharan Africa and southern Asia accounting for 86% of them. In Sub-Saharan Africa, a woman's chance of dying from pregnancy or childbirth complications is 1 in 22, compared to 1 in 7,300 in developed regions.

Maternal mortality has declined by nearly half since 1990, but falls far short of the MDG target. The targets for improving maternal health include reducing by three fourths the maternal mortality ratio and achieving universal access to reproductive health. Poverty and lack of education perpetuate high adolescent birth rates. Inadequate funding for family planning is a major failure in fulfilling commitments to improving women's reproductive health. The number of women dying from pregnancy and childbirth decreased 50% from 1900 to 2013, yet in many developing countries the percentage of deaths still remains high. The key problem remaining for many women is lack of access to quality care. Seven in every 10 births are attended by skilled birth attendants; yet, coverage varies greatly across country by income levels from 99% in high-income countries to 46% in low-income countries.

6. *Combat HIV/AIDS, malaria, and other diseases.* Halt and reverse the spread of HIV/AIDS; achieve by 2010 universal access to treatment; halt and reverse the incidence of malaria and other diseases.

Progress

An estimated 2.3 million people were newly diagnosed with HIV in 2012, which represented a 33% decline in new infections. People living in Sub-Saharan Africa accounted for 70% of all new infections.

Greater than 6.2 million malaria deaths have been prevented between 2000 and 2015, primarily of children under 5 years in Sub-Saharan Africa. The global malaria incidence rate has decreased by 37% and mortality by 58%. Greater than 900 million mosquito nets were delivered to malaria-endemic countries in Sub-Saharan Africa between 2000 and 2014.

In 2012 an estimated 8.6 million people developed tuberculosis (TB) and 1.3 million died from it (including those who also were HIV positive). Globally TB mortality has declined by 45% since 1990 and is expected to be reduced to zero by 2015. The number of cases still remains unacceptably high. Between 2000 and 2013 tuberculosis prevention, diagnosis, and treatment interventions saved approximately 37 million lives. The TB mortality rate decreased by 45% and the prevalence rate by 41% between 1990 and 2013.

7. *Ensure environmental sustainability.* By 2015 cut by half the proportion of people without access to sustainable drinking water and sanitation. Global greenhouse gas emissions resume their upward path, confirming the need for bold action. Forests are a safety net for the poor, but they continue to disappear at an alarming rate (UN, 2013). The global goal of halving the proportion of people without access to safe drinking water was met in 2010 with reduced child mortality and improved nutrition. Still, 747 million people in the world do not have clean water.

Progress

Despite the significant progress, wide disparities exist between urban and rural areas and between different socioeconomic groups. Global emissions of carbon dioxide (CO_2) have increased by almost 50% since 1990. Protected ecosystems covered 14% of terrestrial and coastal marine areas worldwide by 2012. Over 2.3 billion more people have gained access to an improved source of drinking water since 1990, but 748 million people still draw their water from an unimproved source. Between 1990 and 2012, almost 2 billion people obtained access to improved sanitation. However, 1 billion people continue to resort to open defecation. One-third of urban residents in developing regions still live in slums.

8. *Develop a global partnership for development.* Continue to develop an open, rule-based, predictable, nondiscriminating trading and financial system; address the special needs of the least developed countries; deal with landlocked developing countries and small island countries; deal comprehensively with the debt problems of developing countries (UN, 2009, 2010). There is less aid money overall, with the poorest countries most adversely affected (UN, 2014).

Progress

Official development assistance from developed countries increased by 66% in real terms between 2000 and 2014, reaching $135.2 billion. In 2014, Denmark, Luxembourg, Norway, Sweden, and the United Kingdom continued to exceed the UN official development assistance target of 0.7% of gross national income. In 2014, 79% of imports from developing to developed countries were admitted duty free, up from 65% in 2000. The proportion of external debt service to export revenue in developing countries fell from 12% in 2000 to 3% in 2013. As of 2015, 95% of the world's population is covered by a mobile-cellular signal. The number of mobile-cellular subscriptions has grown almost tenfold in the last 15 years, from 738 million in 2000 to over 7 billion in 2015. Internet penetration has grown from just over 6% of the world's population in 2000 to 43% in 2015.

FUTURE GLOBAL HEALTH PATTERNS

The World Health Organization, in its Global Statistics Report, anticipates the following patterns to emerge in global health (WHO, 2014c):

1. Tobacco will cause chronic obstructive pulmonary diseases (e.g., emphysema and lung cancer) and will kill more people than the HIV epidemic.
2. Males living in the former USSR and socialist economies in Europe will have poor and deteriorating health status, including a 28% risk of death in the 15 to 60 age groups.
3. Mental health diseases (depression, alcoholism, and schizophrenia), which have long been underestimated in significance, will be responsible for 1% of deaths and 11% of the total world disease burden.
4. Communicable diseases, maternal and perinatal problems, and nutritional diseases will continue to be major problems in developing countries, while noncommunicable diseases such as depression and heart diseases will also cause premature death and disability.
5. Deaths from noncommunicable diseases will increase by 77% due to the aging of the world population and the decrease in birth rate.
6. Accidents and violence mortality (death) rates may compete with mortality rates of infectious diseases.

Disability Adjusted Life Years and Years Lived with a Disability

"Years of Life Lost" (YLL) is a calculation that subtracts the average life expectancy from the actual age of death. If, for example, a life expectancy is 65 years but that person dies at 45, the calculation would be −20. This calculation is used to put more weight on the death of a child than an older person or someone who lives longer than the average life expectancy). "Disability Adjusted Life Year" (DALY) is calculated by adding the YLL + YLD (Years Lived with a Disability). This measurement is helpful in determining the general health of a person while he or she was alive.

In rank order, the following issues are leading causes of YLL (WHO, 2014c):

1. Ischemic heart disease
2. Lower respiratory infections
3. Stroke
4. Preterm birth complications
5. Diarrheal diseases
6. HIV/AIDS
7. Birth asphyxia and birth trauma
8. Road injuries
9. Chronic obstructive pulmonary disease
10. Malaria
11. Congenital anomalies
12. Neonatal sepsis and infections
13. Self-harm

14. Trachea, bronchus, lung cancers
15. Diabetes mellitus
16. Tuberculosis
17. Cirrhosis of the liver
18. Interpersonal violence
19. Meningitis
20. Protein-energy malnutrition

World Population Challenges

Greater investments in scientific research and technology will be needed in developing countries to meet the increasing demand for the challenges of treatment of illness and disease prevention. UNFPA (2011) indicates that world population challenges will include the following issues:

1. *Migration from rural areas to urban cities.* Half the world's population lived in urban areas as of 2007—a pattern that created a greater need for social services, including reproductive health, especially in poor urban areas.
2. *Stress on the global environment.* Global warming, population growth, resource consumption, deforestation, and decreases in water and cropland further negatively impact health outcomes.
3. *Increased demand for family planning.* More than 350 million couples continued to lack family planning services; by 2025, the demand for such services will increase by 40%.
4. *Pregnancy and childbirth complications.* These issues continue to cause illness and death in women in developing countries, resulting in 8 million women having life-threatening complications and 529,000 deaths from this cause.
5. *Lack of prenatal care.* Thirty-three percent of all pregnant women in the world receive no prenatal care and 60% of all deliveries occur outside a hospital by an unskilled birth attendant.
6. *Skilled birth attendants.* Only 50% of all pregnant women will be delivered by a skilled birth attendant.
7. *HIV/AIDS.* Thirty-eight million people have HIV/AIDS.

Injuries and Violence

Injuries and violence are a major public health issue worldwide and account for nearly 1 out of every 10 deaths every year. The CDC (2014b) notes the following:

- Globally, more than nine people die every minute from injuries or violence (5.8 million people of all ages and economic groups die each year from both unintentional and violence related injuries).
- The three leading causes of injury and violence-related deaths are road traffic incidents (1.3 million), suicides (844,000), and homicides (600,000).
- In addition, millions of people seek medical treatment due to injuries and violence.

- Violence can result in serious injuries and even death, but may also lead to other significant mental and physical health consequences such as depression and anxiety, pregnancy complications, and even chronic diseases such as diabetes and heart disease.
- Violence also erodes the sense of safety and security, essential to the well-being of families and communities.

In addition to deaths, road traffic crashes result in 20 to 50 million injuries every year—nearly half are among pedestrians or people riding motorcycles or bicycles in countries where motorbikes are a principal mode of transportation. These injuries cost $518 billion annually. The Global Helmet Vaccine Initiative in Vietnam is an innovative program that includes helmet distribution, public education, and legislative changes. It has resulted in an increase in helmet usage among motorcycle riders from 30% to over 90%, a 16% decrease in road traffic head injuries, and an 18% decrease in risk of death. Increasing helmet use is a simple, inexpensive, and very cost-effective means of preventing serious head injuries on the road (CDC, 2014b).

Prevention of Child Abuse

Together for Girls is the first global partnership to promote coordinated, effective strategies to prevent sexual violence against girls, one of the most vulnerable groups in society. Societies worldwide want to ensure that children can grow and thrive in safe, nurturing conditions. To support that goal, the Injury Center, a part of the Together for Girls Program, is collaborating with national governments and nongovernmental organizations to protect the health and safety of young girls. Together for Girls was launched in September, 2009 at the annual meeting of the Clinton Global Initiative. This partnership brings together international public, private, and nonprofit organizations, including four UN agencies.

Three core activities have been identified to address the systemic and societal foundations of sexual violence:

1. Collect pertinent data through national surveys.
2. Implement the best prevention and protection strategies.
3. Mobilize an in-depth communications campaign to bring about desired changes in social and behavioral norms.

This initiative builds on a successful partnership formed in Swaziland in 2007, where CDC, UNICEF, and other partners conducted a national survey estimating the magnitude and health consequences of sexual violence against girls. Survey data provided the foundation for the development of critical strategies to address sexual violence, including draft legislation, child-friendly courts, and a national educational campaign aimed at raising awareness about sexual violence and how to prevent it (CDC, 2014b).

GLOBAL HEALTH DISPARITIES

A **health disparity** is a statistically significant difference in health indicators that persists over time. Health disparities are comparative measurements of the burden of disease as well as morbidity and mortality rates, in specific populations. **Healthcare disparities**, by comparison, are differences in access to appropriate healthcare services by various groups because of a multitude of factors; they are mainly associated with social inequalities. Health disparities are differentiated from healthcare disparities, although both concepts are intimately linked. Disparities in access to quality and timely healthcare services contribute to the disparities in health status. Poorer health status compromises the ability of some groups to obtain timely and appropriate health services. Health and healthcare disparities exist worldwide, affecting both developed and developing countries. Population groups both in one nation and across different countries are affected by health disparities. In contrast to developed countries, developing nations have a lower level of material well-being based on per capita income, life expectancy, and rate of literacy. These nations are also referred to as less economically developed, Third World, lower-income nations, or resource-poor countries. In contrast, developed nations are also called industrialized societies, advanced economies, and higher-income nations (King, Harper, & Young, 2012). These terms should be used with caution because they may imply inferiority–superiority relationships among nations.

INDICES OF HEALTH DISPARITIES

1. *Burden of disease.* The impact of a health problem in an area measured by financial cost, mortality, morbidity, or other indicators. It is often quantified in terms of quality-adjusted life-years (QALYs), which allow for comparison of disease burden due to various risk factors or diseases. It also makes it possible to predict the possible impact of health interventions. WHO provides a detailed explanation of how disease burden is measured at local and national levels for various environmental contexts. The global burden of disease is shifting from infectious diseases to noncommunicable diseases, including chronic conditions such as heart disease and stroke, which are now the chief causes of death globally.

2. *Mortality rate.* The number of deaths in a population, scaled to the size of that population, per unit of time. This rate is expressed in units of deaths per 1,000 people per year; thus a mortality rate of 9.5 in a population of 100,000 would mean 950 deaths per year in that entire population.

3. *Infant mortality rate (IMR).* The number of deaths of infants (1 year of age or younger) per 1,000 live births. The IMR is a useful indicator of a country's level of health or development.

4. *Morbidity rate.* The number of individuals in poor health during a given time or number who currently have that disease (prevalence rate), scaled to the size of the population. This rate takes into account the state of poor health, the degree or severity of a health condition, and the total number of cases in a particular population during a particular point in time irrespective of cause.

5. *Life expectancy.* The average number of years of life remaining at a given age or average life span or average length of survival in a specified population; the expected age to be reached before death for a given population in a country, based on the year of birth or other demographic variables.

6. *Birth rate.* The number of childbirths per 100,000 people per year.

7. *Total fertility rate.* The average number of children born to each woman over the course of her life. Fertility rates tend to be higher in developing countries and lower in more economically developed countries.

8. *Disability.* The lack of ability relative to a personal or group standard or spectrum. It may involve physical, sensory, cognitive, or intellectual impairment, or a mental disorder; it may occur during a person's lifetime or be present from birth.

9. *Nutritional status.* A factor influenced by diet, levels of nutrients in the body, and ability to maintain normal metabolic integrity. Body fat may be estimated by measuring skin fold thickness and muscle diameter; levels of vitamins and minerals are measured based on their serum levels, through urine concentration of nutrients and their metabolites, or by testing for specific metabolic responses (CDC, 2003; UNFPA, 2011).

Health Disparities in the United States

Health disparities may be defined more narrowly as persistent gaps between the health status of minorities and nonminorities that continue despite advances in health care and technology. In the United States, ethnic minorities have higher rates of disease, disability, and premature deaths than nonminorities. African Americans, Hispanics/Latinos, American Indians and Alaska Natives, Asian Americans, Native Hawaiians, and Pacific Islanders all have higher rates of infant mortality, cardiovascular diseases, diabetes, HIV/AIDS, and cancer, as well as lower rates of immunizations and cancer screenings, than nonminority groups. Such disparities arise for a number of reasons:

- *Inadequate access to health care.* Caused by economic, geographic, and/or linguistic factors; lack of or decrease in health insurance and education; and poorer quality of health care.
- *Substandard quality of care/lower quality of care.* Caused by patient–provider miscommunication, provider discrimination, and stereotyping or prejudice (Agency of Healthcare Research and Quality, 2006; National Healthcare Disparities Report 2009, 2010).

Challenges of World Population Growth

As of October 2011, the global population of 7 billion continued to grow rapidly at a rate of approximately 76 million per year. The average family size declined from six children per woman in 1960 to three children per woman, mainly due to family planning. Countries that have significant decreases in fertility will have increases in the aging population. Ninety-six percent of the world population growth is attributable to growth in developing countries. As of 2011, Europe and Japan had declining populations, whereas the North American population increased by 1% due to immigration. Actual population sizes and growth patterns today are somewhat lower than those predicted 10 years ago, mainly due to the impact of the HIV/AIDS epidemic. The 38 African countries most affected by HIV/AIDS are projected to have 823 million people by 2015—a population that includes 91 million fewer people than if no AIDS deaths had occurred (UNFPA, 2011).

Global Healthcare Equity

Disparities in health care are now a major challenge for healthcare agencies around the world. As former South African President Nelson Mandela (1998) stated, "The greatest single challenge facing our globalized world is to combat and eradicate its disparities." The burden of disease is growing disproportionately within certain regions of the world, especially in areas commonly affected by "brain drain." Some doctors and nurses from Africa, Asia, and Latin America are leaving the rural areas for cities, while many others are leaving their countries altogether and relocating in developed nations. The irony is that more healthcare providers in developed countries are now working, at least for part of their working lives, in developing countries, even as the "brain drain" pulls some of the most competent healthcare providers out of their home countries, where they are most needed. Regardless of the causes, many developing countries with the least amount of human and economic resources are confronted with the largest burden in public health. In the developed world, the most affluent 15% of the world's population consumes more than 60% of the world's total energy—much more than the developing world (Farmer, Furin, & Katz, 2004).

There is still major evidence that socioeconomic as well as health inequalities exist within and among nations. Although the health of the world population has improved considerably, some countries of the world still have inadequate and inequitable health care within their borders and among their citizens. For example, in 2010, there was an estimated 22.9 million people living with HIV in Sub-Saharan Africa. This has increased since 2009, when an estimated 22.5 million people were living with HIV, including 2.3 million children. The increase in people living with HIV could be partly due to a decrease in AIDS-related deaths in the region. There were 1.2 million deaths due to AIDS in 2010 compared to 1.3 million in 2009. Almost 90% of the 16.6 million children orphaned by AIDS live in Sub-Saharan Africa (Avert.org, 2011). The disappearance of an entire generation of productive men and women (ages 18–45) is evidence that healthcare services have been inadequate in this region, resulting in children and grandparents left behind (Ruger, 2005).

Adequate health care promotes social stability and economic growth. Countries that do not have adequate health care often have inadequate funding, poor government organization, and inadequate access for healthcare services for all of their populations (Go & Given, 2005). Go and Given (2005) report that although developing countries such as India, Mexico, and China would like to expand their healthcare systems and have more high technology, they first must restructure their systems to devote more expenditures to, and place greater emphasis on, education and preventive medicine, rather than trying to first invest in high-technology health care. The three main criteria for an adequate healthcare system include (1) equitable access to quality care in the form of both prevention and treatment services for rural and urban populations; (2) affordability, which means that even if people have no income or health insurance they may receive services; and (3) sustainability, which means that the system has long-term political and financial support.

For example, Mexico, China, and India are emerging economies that are rapidly industrializing and embracing global markets; each has its own unique culture, geography, and history as well. All three countries are working to improve access to their healthcare systems for all of their citizens and are emphasizing preventive health care as a major priority. Ninety percent of Mexicans now have access to preventive care and basic public health services, although some indigenous Indians in isolated rural areas still have no coverage. Sixty-seven percent of India's population is now immunized, although many rural areas have less basic health care than urban areas. In the past, the Indian government paid the entire cost of health care for individuals, but now a shift in healthcare costs has placed greater burden on individuals to cover their own healthcare needs. The Indian government is now spending less and expects that individuals will pay for part of the services that were once completely funded by the government. At present, new medical treatments and medications are becoming more expensive and many people must also pay out-of-pocket for health care because they lack health insurance (Go & Given, 2005). The World Health Report (WHO, 2003) states that a key responsibility of any government's healthcare system is to decrease the health disparities. Lack of political power and basic education represent barriers to accessing the healthcare system for all. The majority of the populations in Mexico, China, and India have equal access, yet only a small elite group has access to state-of-the-art health care.

UNIVERSAL RIGHT TO HEALTH CARE

The right to health care under international law is found in 1948 under the 1948 Universal Declaration of Human Rights ("the Declaration"), which was unanimously accepted by the UN General Assembly as a common standard for the entire world's population. This declaration sets forth each person's right to "a standard of living adequate for the health and well-being of himself and his family . . . including medical care and . . . the right to security in the event of . . . sickness, disability . . . or other lack of livelihood in circumstances beyond his control." The Declaration does not define the components of a right to health, but they are included in the statement regarding medical care. Health is considered to extend beyond health care to include basic preconditions for health, such as potable water and adequate sanitation and nutrition. In addition, the right to health includes freedoms from nonconsensual medical treatment and experimentation (Gable & Meier, 2013).

Within the WHO Constitution and the Declaration of Alma-Ata, health-related human rights have been encouraged. The human right to health has been addressed in international law and implemented through domestic law within numerous nations. The Framework Convention on Global Health (FCGH) states that the right to the highest attainable standard of physical and mental health can be a force to enable even the poorest people to benefit from immense health improvements that we know possible—interventions that are proven and affordable (Gable & Meier, 2013).

Historically, the United States has not wanted to accept international human rights standards or pass the laws necessary to meet them. The United States is currently the only developed country in the world that does not have a plan for universal healthcare coverage and some type of legal right to health care for all its residents (The Atlantic, 2012).

EMERGING GLOBAL HEALTH THREATS

The WHO Report of 2010 indicates that public health issues evolve over time. As a result of planned and unplanned activities or changing environments, humans may come in contact with many different organisms that have the capacity to cause disease. Thanks to the development of antibiotics, people are now able to survive many bacterial infections, which previously would have been the cause of certain death. Even so, infectious diseases continue to cause both new epidemics, such as those linked to HIV/AIDS or the Ebola virus, or reoccurring epidemics, such as those involving tuberculosis or cholera. Many of the emerging health threats around the world today are caused by resistance to antibiotics, new strains of drug-resistant bacteria, or poor adherence to medical regimens (WHO, 2011).

Preventable diseases and injuries are seen more often as humans migrate from rural to urban areas. Also seen more often are unintentional injuries such as traffic accidents, poisonings, and intentional injuries, such as war and street violence. More than 40% of the total disease burden due to urban air pollution occurs in developing countries, and children are most vulnerable to these environmental hazards, because they do not have the ability to detoxify pollutants related to their bodies' immaturity. More than 90% of all deaths due to injuries occurred in low- and middle-income countries. Although tobacco use is declining in developed countries, it is increasing in developing countries (WHO, 2011).

Mental health, neurological disorders, and substance abuse are causing a great amount of disability and human suffering. Many people do not receive any health care for these problems because of inadequate infrastructures, and widely prevalent stigma and discrimination may prevent them from seeking care even when it is available. Many countries lack mental healthcare policies, facilities, or budgets within their healthcare systems. Cost-effective services are available, and research clearly demonstrates that depression, schizophrenia, and alcohol- and drug-related problems can be treated at primary care centers with inexpensive medications and basic training of healthcare personnel. Intentional (suicide, violence, and war) and unintentional (traffic accidents) injuries, which primarily affect young adults, accounted for more than 14% of the adult disease burden of the world, yet in parts of Europe and the Eastern Middle East region, these causes were responsible for more than 30% of the disease burden. In males, violence, traffic injuries, and self-inflicted injuries are within the top 10 disease burdens in the 15- to 44-year-old groups (WHO, 2011).

Measures of Population Health

In order to evaluate the health of a population, one needs to examine four aspects of that population:

1. *Life expectancy.* A measure of mortality rates across the developmental life span, which is expressed in years of life.
2. *Healthy life expectancy (HLE).* Years of active life, reflecting a person's ability to perform tasks that reflect self-care, called the activities of daily living. HLE is a way of measuring not just years of life, but expected years of life divided into healthy and unhealthy life. It is a way to more accurately measure the current health of a population, measuring the extent of morbidity and mortality of a population.
3. *Mortality.* The number of deaths within a specific population, which has often been used as a basic indicator of health.
4. *Disability.* A situation in which a person's abilities or limitations are determined by physical, mental, or cognitive status within society, which is determined by how well the personal environment accommodates the loss of functioning.

Global Health Indicators

Global monitoring of health changes across world populations requires global health indicators. The indicators provide estimates of a country's state of health and may reflect either direct measurements of health phenomena, such as diseases and deaths, or indirect measurements, such as education and poverty. With population statistics available regarding education, access to safe water and sanitation, and rates of diseases, it is possible to fairly accurately measure a population's burden of disease and designate it as low, medium, or high. Unfortunately, few developing countries are able to measure their health statistics accurately; therefore, numbers of births, deaths, persons with specific diseases, and so on may be only estimates—and may not be truly representative of the population. Criteria for good health indicators include the following:

1. *Definition.* The indicator must be well defined and be able to be used internationally.
2. *Validity.* The indicator must accurately measure what it is supposed to measure and must be reliable so that it can be replicable and consistent in different settings, and be easy to interpret.
3. *Feasibility.* Obtaining the information must be easily affordable and not overburden the system.
4. *Utility.* The indicator must provide useful information for various levels of health decision makers (Larson & Mercer, 2004).

MORAL ISSUES IN GLOBAL HEALTH

The creation of global initiatives requires a review of ethical and moral values. In 2003, Lee Jong-Wook, the director-general of the WHO, stated that global health must be guided by an ethical vision. According to Lee, technical excellence and political commitment have no value unless they have an ethically sound purpose. The following are different schools of thought used to justify global initiatives:

1. *Humanitarianism.* Acting virtuously toward those in need. It is often the response to social problems. Humanitarianism is incorporated within all religions, based on compassion, empathy, or altruism. It is the ethical basis of philanthropy by NGOs; it is also the basic philosophy behind U.S. governmental foreign aid policy.
2. *Utilitarianism.* Maximizing happiness for many people. Improving the health of individuals living within a society will be in the best interest for all the people of a society.
3. *Equity by achieving a fair distribution of health capabilities.* Ensuring that all people in a society have a fair and equal chance to achieve good health.
4. *Rights.* Fulfilling obligations so others are dignified; ensures that health care respects human rights and dignity for all people living in a society.
5. *Knowledge and institutions.* Supports the basis for research and development of new health technologies and medications. For example, the development of HIV/AIDS antiretroviral drugs created a new moral dilemma by emphasizing the differences in the drugs' affordability among nations. Corporations have realized what are perceived as "huge" profits by producing and selling the drugs; however, the cost of development and use of resources must be recouped.
6. *Consensus and advocacy groups.* People who are usually in powerful political positions who wish to have health policies established for others in the society.

Global Health Workforce Migrations (Brain Drain)

Presently there is a crisis in human resources, which is a major global health issue at present that threatens the quality and sustainability of healthcare systems throughout the world. Healthcare workers currently find many opportunities for employment abroad, and this has led to major migration for workers moving from low-income countries to higher-income countries. Healthcare worker migration has major effects on the countries from which workers migrate and the receiving countries greatly benefit. The countries from which workers migrate (sending countries) have negative results such as shortages in health service capacity, financial loss in the investment of training and educating the worker, financial loss of income taxes paid to the governments, decline in morale and commitment among remaining workers, loss of expert knowledge in academic centers, and loss of role models for young students. Donor countries ultimately suffer the most from "brain drain."

The gains for recipient countries include relief of shortages of healthcare workers, improved quality of health care, and increased income taxes paid to the governments. Some dispute this argument by saying that many healthcare workers eventually return to their native countries and bring back their gains in medical expertise and experiences. The World Health Organization (WHO) estimates that there is an undersupply of almost 4.3 million doctors, midwives, nurses, and other healthcare professionals. High-income countries have an average of almost 90 nurses and midwives per 10,000 people, as compared to some low-income countries having fewer than 2 per 10,000 people (Aluttis, Bishaw, & Frank, 2014). This imbalance results in North America and Europe gaining 65% of healthcare workers, yet bearing only 20% of global disease. Africa, in contrast, bears 24% of the health burden with only 3% of the global health workforce (Mackey & Liang, 2013).

SUMMARY

This introduction, which serves as a gateway to the rest of this text, has provided an overall perspective on various global health issues. We defined key terms and offered a brief discussion of global health history, the state of the world population, predictions of global health patterns, population growth issues, equity in accessing health care, emerging health threats, global health indicators, migration of healthcare workers, and global health and its relationship to moral values. Within the following chapters, we further address these and many more issues pertaining to global health.

Study Questions

1. What are some of the major health issues regarding the world population growth?
2. What are some causes of the numerous global health disparities?
3. Why is it necessary for wealthier developed countries to share needed funds and technology to assist with developing countries' major health and healthcare problems?
4. What are the Millennium Health Goals and why is important to note their progress worldwide?

Case Study: Unforeseen Costs of Cutting Mosquito Surveillance Budgets

A recent budget proposal to stop the funding for the U.S. Centers for Disease Control and Prevention (CDC) surveillance and research for a mosquito-borne diseases program was found to have the potential to leave a country poorly prepared to handle mosquito-transmitted diseases. Their study showed that decreasing this type of program can significantly increase the management costs of epidemics and total costs of preparedness. The authors' findings demonstrated a justification for the reassessment of a current proposal to slash the budget of the CDC vector-borne diseases program, and emphasized the need for improved and sustainable systems for vector-borne disease surveillance.

Case Study Questions

1. What do you think about the U.S. CDC making budget cuts for surveillance and research for countries with mosquito-borne diseases?
2. Is money really saved in the long term for prevention and control of diseases, such as dengue and West Nile virus, by cutting the surveillance budget? What else could be done to save money?

Data from Vazquez-Prokopec, G., Chaves, L., Ritchie, S., Davis, J., & Kitron, U. (2010). *Neglected Tropical Diseases, 4*(10), 1–4.

References

Agency of Healthcare Research and Quality. (2006). *National healthcare disparities report 2009.* Retrieved from http://www.ahrq.gov/qual/nhdr09/nhdr09.pdf

Aluttis, C., Bishaw, T., & Frank, M. (2014). The workforce for health in a globalized context—global shortages and international migration. *Global Health Action, 7,* 1–7. Retrieved from http://dx.doi.org/10.3402/gha .v7.23611

Avert.org. (2011). *HIV/AIDS statistics for Sub-Saharan Africa.* Retrieved from http://www.avert.org/africa-hiv-aids-statistics.htm

Beaglehole, R., & Bonita, R. (2010). What is global health? *Global Health Action, 3,* 5142.

Beaglehole, R., & Yach, D. (2003). Globalisation and the prevention and control of non-communicable disease: The neglected chronic disease of adults. *Lancet, 362,* 903–908.

Bremner, J., Frost, A., Haub, C., Mather, M., Ringheim, K., & Zuehlke, E. (2010). World population highlights: Key findings from PRB's 2010 world population data sheet. *Population Reference Bureau, 65*(2). Retrieved from www.prb.org

Centers for Disease Control and Prevention. (2003). *Summary measures of population health: Report of findings on methodologic and data issues.* Retrieved from http://www.cdc.gov/nchs/data/misc/pophealth.pdf

Centers for Disease Control and Prevention. (2013). *Health challenges.* Retrieved from http://www.cdc .gov/media/dpk/2013/dpk-2013-review.html

Centers for Disease Control and Prevention. (2014). *Worldwide injuries and violence.* Retrieved from http:// www.cdc.gov/injury/global/

De Cock, K., Simone, P., Davison, V., & Slutsker, L. (2013). The new global health. *Emerging Infectious Diseases, 19*(8), 1192–1197.

Farmer, P., Furin, J. J., & Katz, J. T. (2004). Global health equity. *Lancet, 363,* 1832.

Gable, L. & Meier, B. (2013). Global health rights: Employing human rights to develop and implement the framework convention on global health. *Health and Human Rights, 15*(1), 17–31.

Global Health Initiative consultation document. (2009). Retrieved from http://www.usaid.gov/bd/files/GHI_Consultation_Document.pdf

Go, R., & Given, R. (2005). *Sustainable health care.* Deloitte Research. Tuck Executive Education of Dartmouth. Retrieved from http://www.publicservice.co.uk/pdf/em/issue_3/EM3Robert%20Go%20Ruth%20Given%20ATL.pdf

Guengant, J., & May, J. (2013). *Africa 2050: African Demography* Washington, DC: Centennial Group for Emerging Market Forum.

Healthy People 2020. (2014). *Access to health services.* Retrieved from http://healthypeople.gov20/20/topicsobjectives2020/overview.aspx?topicid=1

Hixon, A., & Maskarinec, G. (2008). The declaration of Alma Ata on its 30th anniversary: Relevance for family medicine today. *Family Medicine, 40*(8), 585–589.

IndexMundi. (2014a). *Birth rate.* Retrieved from http://www.indexmundi.com/world/birth_rate.html

IndexMundi. (2014b). *Death rate.* Retrieved from http://www.indexmundi.com/world/death_rate.html

IOM Report: For the Public Health: Revitalizing Law and Policy to Meet New Challenges (2011). Retrieved from http://www.iom.edu/Reports/2011/For-the-Publics-Health-Revitalizing-Law-and-Policy-to-Meet-New-Challenges.aspx

King, N., Harper, S., & Young, M. (2013). Who cares about health inequalities? Cross-country evidence from the World Health Survey. *Health Policy and Planning, 28*, 558–571.

Koplan, J. P., Bond, T. C., Merson, M. H., Reddy, K. S., Rodriguez, M. H., Sewankambo, N. K., & Wasserheit, J. N. (2009). Consortium of Universities for Global Health Executive Board. Towards a common definition of global health. *Lancet, 373*(9679), 1993–1995.

Larson, C., & Mercer, A. (2004). Global health indicators: An overview. *Canadian Medical Association, 171*(10), 1.

Macfarlane, S. B., Jacobs, M., & Kaaya E. E. (2008). In the name of global health: Trends in academic institutions. *Journal of Public Health Policy, 29*(4), 383–401.

Mackey, T., & Liang, B. (2013). Restructuring brain drain: Strengthening governance and financing for health worker migration. *Global Health Action, 6*, 1–7.

Mandela, N. (1998). *Transcript of the speech at the special convocation of an honorary doctoral degree, Harvard University, Cambridge, Massachusetts, September 18, 1998.* Retrieved from http://www.cambridgeforum.org/cfmandela/13_nelson_mandela.html

National Healthcare Disparities Report 2009. (2010). Retrieved from https://www.google.com/search?sourceid=navclient&ie=UTF-8&rlz=1T4SKPT_enUS419US420&q=National+Healthcare+Disparities+Report+2009.+http://www.healthpolicy.ucla.edu/pubs/Publication.aspx?pubID=40

Office of Disease Prevention and Health Promotion. (2014). *Access to health services: Healthy people.* Retrieved from https://www.healthypeople.gov/2020/topics-objectives/topic/Access-to-Health-Services

Ruger, J. P. (2005). The changing role of the World Bank in global health. *American Journal of Public Health, 95*, 60–90.

Tarantola, D. (2005). Global health and national governance. *American Journal of Public Health Association, 95*(1), 8.

The Atlantic. (June 28, 2012). Retrieved from http://www.theatlantic.com/international/archive/2012/06/heres-a-map-of-the-countries-that-provide-universal-health-care-americas-still-not-on-it/259153/

The World Bank. (2014). *The World Bank Development Report.* Retrieved from http://siteresources.worldbank.org/EXTNWDR2013/Resources/8258024-1352909193861/8936935-1356011448215/8986901-1380046989056/WDR-2014_Complete_Report.pdf

Thirty-fifth Anniversary of the Alma-Ata Primary Health Care Declaration Conference. Retrieved from http://www.goinginternational.eu/wp/de/35th-anniversary-of-the-alma-ata-primary-health-care-declaration-conference/

United Nations. (2009). *The Millennium Developmental Goals Report, 2009.* Retrieved from http://www.un.org/millenniumgoals/reports.shtml

United Nations. (2010). *The Millennium Developmental Goals Report, 2010*. Retrieved from http://www.un.org/
  millenniumgoals/pdf/MDG%20Report%202010%20En%20r15%20-low%20res%2020100615%20-.pdf

United Nations. (2013). *The Millennium Developmental Goals Report, 2013*. Retrieved from http://www
  .un.org/millenniumgoals/pdf/report-2013/mdg-report-2013-english.pdf

United Nations. (2014). *The Millennium Developmental Goals Report, 2014*. Retrieved from http://www
  .un.org/millenniumgoals/2014%20MDG%20report/MDG%202014%20English%20web.pdf

United Nations Family Planning Association. (2011). *State of the world population 2011*. Retrieved from
  www.unfpa.org

United States Implementation of Global Health Initiative. (2009). Retrieved from http://www.pepfar.gov/
  documents/organization/129504.pdf

Universal Declaration of Human Rights. United Nations General Assembly Resolution 217 A (III). (1947).
  New York: United Nations.

Vazquez-Prokopec, G., Chaves, L., Ritchie, S., Davis, J., & Kitron, U. (2010). *Neglected Tropical Diseases, 4*(10), 1–4.

World Health Organization. (2003). *World health report 2003: Shaping the future*. Retrieved from http://
  www.who.int/whr/2003/en

World Health Organization. (2005). *Integrated chronic disease prevention and control*. Retrieved from http://
  www.who.int/chp/about/integrated_cd/en

World Health Organization. (2011). *World health statistics*. Retrieved from: http://www.who.int/whosis/
  whostat/2011/en/

World Health Organization. (2014a). *Globalization*. Retrieved from http://www.who.int/trade/glossary/
  story043/en/

World Health Organization. (2014b). *Trade, foreign policy, diplomacy and health*. Retrieved from http://www
  .who.int/trade/glossary/story043/en/

World Health Organization. (2014c). *World health statistics 2014*. Retrieved from http://www.who.int/
  mediacentre/news/releases/2014/world-health-statistics-2014/en/

World population data sheet. (2013). Retrieved from http://www.prb.org/pdf13/2013-population-data-sheet_
  eng.pdf

Yamin, A. (2005). The right to health under international law and its relevance to the United States. *American
  Journal of Public Health, 95*(7), 1156–1161.

Global Health in Developed Societies: Examples in the United States, Sweden, Japan, and the United Kingdom

Carol Holtz

Objectives

After completing this chapter, the reader will be able to:

1. Compare and contrast population health statistics for the United States, Sweden, Japan, and the United Kingdom.
2. Compare and contrast the major health issues and healthcare systems of the United States, Sweden, Japan, and the United Kingdom.
3. Relate healthcare disparities within and among the countries of the United States, Sweden, Japan, and the United Kingdom.
4. Discuss the high rates of longevity for residents of Japan and Sweden.

INTRODUCTION

This chapter gives examples of developed countries and their major health issues and trends. These countries were chosen because they vary in terms of their healthcare systems, population health statistics, and geographic areas. We will review many of the health issues in greater detail in other chapters of this text.

Many of the developed countries are currently working on controversial legal, religious, and ethical issues that directly relate to health care and healthcare systems of delivery. Specifically, we will address the following topics:

- Access to health care for all residents.
- Issues of funding for nonlegal residents (illegal aliens) and healthcare services provided by government and nongovernment organizations.
- Options for termination of an unwanted pregnancy.
- Women's rights in determining what happens to their bodies (birth control, abortion, contraception, genital mutilation, sexual assault and/or abuse, sterilization, child molestation, prostitution).
- Sex education in schools, clinics, and public health facilities.

UNITED STATES

Location

The United States is located in North America, bordering both the Atlantic and Pacific oceans, between Canada in the north and Mexico in the south. It includes 50 states, the District of Columbia, and several territories and possessions.

Population Statistics

As of March 2015, the U.S. population was 320.5 million, making it the third most populated country in the world, after China's 1.35 billion and India's 1.23 billion population, and a world population of approximately 7.1 billion. According to the 2013 statistics from the U.S. Census Bureau, the majority of the population (81%) lives in cities and suburban areas as compared to the worldwide urban rate of 54%. California and Texas are the most populous states and New York City is the most populous city in the country. Non-Hispanic whites constitute the majority of the population with 77.7%. Immigrants and their U.S.-born descendants are expected to represent most of the future U.S. population increases. Hispanic or Latino Americans represent the largest minority group with 17.1%; black or African Americans represent 13.2%; Asian Americans represent 5.3%; Native Americans/Alaskan natives represent 1.2%; and Native Hawaiian and other Pacific Islanders represent 0.2% (U.S. Census Bureau, 2015).

Economy

The United States has the largest and most technologically powerful economy in the world, with a gross domestic product (GDP) of $16.8 trillion USD, and a per capita annual income of $53,900 annually (World Bank, 2014). In this market-oriented economy, 12% of the population continues to live below the poverty line, which is $24,250 USD for a family of four (U.S. Department of Health and Human Services, 2015). The unemployment rates vary among ethnic groups, gender, socioeconomic groups, and geographic locations. As of March 2015, the overall (over age 20) unemployment rate was 5.5%, although many minority groups and younger residents have much higher rates, such as African Americans with a rate of 12% (Central Intelligence Agency [CIA], 2014b; U.S. Department of Labor, 2015).

The United States is the leading industrial power of the world, highly diversified, and technologically advanced. Its products include steel, petroleum, motor vehicles, aerospace, telecommunications, chemicals, electronics, food processing, consumer goods, lumber, and mining. Food products include wheat, corn, other grains, fruits, vegetables, cotton, beef, pork, poultry, dairy products, forest products, and fish (CIA, 2015).

Trends and Issues

The overall health of the United States is improving because of funding devoted to health education, public health programs, health research, and health care. The average life expectancy for men is 78 years and for women 81 according to Centers for Disease Control and Prevention (CDC) statistics (CDC, 2014c). Longer life expectancies are considered desirable with healthy aging, but aging often is accompanied with an increase in chronic diseases such as hypertension, diabetes, renal disease, cancer, Alzheimer's disease, and other dementias. The probability of children (under 5 years) dying is 7 per 100,000 live births, and the overall U.S. infant mortality rate is 6.4 infant deaths per 1,000 live births (CDC, 2014a, 2015). Yet there remains a significant disparity in infant mortality based on race and ethnicity. African Americans have 2.3 times the infant mortality as compared to non-Hispanic whites. The infant mortality is highest among non-Hispanic blacks, with a rate of 12.4 deaths per 1,000 live births as compared to 5.3 deaths per 1,000 live births in non-Hispanic whites (CDC, 2014a, 2015; Infoplease, 2014).

Heart disease deaths have declined because of public health education emphasizing healthy lifestyles, such as decreasing cigarette smoking, lowering cholesterol through medications and diet, and the increasing new technology in heart procedures and surgery. Despite the fact that the 1964 U.S. Surgeon General's report was published more than 50 years ago, 25% of men and 20% of women in the United States continue to smoke. With respect to infectious diseases, HIV/AIDS rates have declined because of the introduction of antiretroviral medications. Home, workplace, and motor vehicle safety have also helped to extend lives by lowering unintentional injuries for adults and children. Rates of acute infectious diseases of children such as measles, mumps, and rubella have decreased due to immunizations (CDC, 2014d; World Health Organization [WHO], 2014b).

The total national health expenditure as a percent of the U.S. gross domestic product is 17.9%. The United States spends more on health care than any other developed country in the world ($1.7 trillion annually), which is approximately $8,895 per person per year (WHO, 2013a).

Yet in spite of these large expenditures on health care, a growing number of Americans—often referred to as the "working poor"—are caught in the middle, earning too much money to be eligible for Medicaid, not being old enough for Medicare, and not earning enough to pay for a private healthcare policy. In addition to these cost issues, accessing health care for many still presents a problem in the United States. The life expectancy of 78 years in the United States is lower than in many other developed countries. For example, the life expectancy in Japan is 82.1 years; the life expectancy in Germany is 79 years; the life expectancy in Switzerland is

81.3 years; and the life expectancy in the United Kingdom is 79 years (Infoplease, 2014). Considering the fact that the U.S. infant mortality in 2013 was 6.4 deaths per 1,000 live births, this rate was not an especially good rate, when compared to other developed countries such as Sweden, Japan, France, Italy, Spain, Finland, Norway, and many others that have much lower rates (CIA, 2014a; WHO, 2014b).

Admissions and length of hospitalization stays in the United States have decreased. Many procedures that were traditionally done within the hospital are now performed in clinics, physicians' offices, outpatient surgery centers, and rehabilitation centers, leaving more complex procedures and illnesses to be treated within the hospital. Inpatients now have higher acuity levels, whereas inpatient mental health treatment has significantly declined (American Hospital Association, 2014).

Population Characteristics

The racial and ethnic composition of the United States has changed in recent decades. Notably, the Hispanic (Latino) population and Asian and Pacific Islander ethnic groups have grown rapidly. In 2012, the Hispanic/Latino population became the largest ethnic minority, representing 16.3% of the total population, and the Asian minority population accounted for 5.6% of the total U.S. population. During the past 50 years, the U.S. population of adults age 75 and older grew from 3% to 6%, and by 2050, the older adult population is projected to make up 12% of the total population (CDC, 2014c).

Major U.S. Health Issues

The CDC (2014a) has tracked the most common causes of death today in the United States. These are listed in Table 2-1.

Overweight and obesity are directly tied to numerous major health problems in the United States, which include cardiovascular disease, stroke, hypertension, diabetes, some forms of cancer, and skeletal system disorders. Regular exercise can reduce the risk for many diseases and enhance mental health functioning. The rates of overweight and obesity have more than doubled among U.S. school-aged children, 6 to 11 years, and more than tripled among adolescents. Also, among adults 20 to 74 years of age, the obesity rates have more than doubled for similar-year differences. At the same time, inpatient healthcare utilization has been declining.

Overweight and obesity have become nationwide problems among children and adults in all age groups. More than one-third of U.S. adults (34.9%) are obese. Obesity-related conditions include heart disease, stroke, type 2 diabetes, and certain types of cancer, some of the leading causes of preventable death. The estimated annual medical cost of obesity in the United States was $147 billion in 2008 U.S. dollars; the medical costs for people who are obese were $1,429 higher than those of normal weight. Non-Hispanic blacks have the highest age-adjusted rates of obesity (47.8%) followed by Hispanics (42.5%), non-Hispanic whites (32.6%), and non-Hispanic Asians (10.8%). Obesity is higher among middle-age adults, 40 to 59 years old (39.5%) than among younger adults, age 20 to 39 (30.3%) or adults over 60 or above (35.4%) adults (CDC, 2014b).

TABLE 2-1 Leading Causes of Death

Causes	Percent of Total Deaths
1. Heart disease	28.5
2. Malignant tumors	22.8
3. Cerebrovascular diseases	6.7
4. Chronic lower respiratory diseases	5.1
5. Accidents (unintentional injuries)	4.4
6. Diabetes mellitus	3.0
7. Influenza and pneumonia	2.7
8. Alzheimer's disease	2.4
9. Nephritis, nephrotic syndrome, and nephrosis	1.7
10. Septicemia (blood poisoning)	1.4
11. Suicide	1.3
12. Chronic liver disease and cirrhosis	1.1
13. Primary hypertension and hypertensive renal disease	0.8
14. Parkinson's disease (tied)	0.7
15. Homicide (tied)	0.7

Note: *U.S. health behaviors.*
Data from Centers for Disease Control and Prevention (CDC). (2014a). *Causing of death in the U.S.* Retrieved from http://www.cdc.gov/nchs/fastats/health-expenditures.htm

Smoking

Tobacco use is the largest preventable cause of death and disease in the United States. Cigarette smoking kills more than 480,000 Americans each year, with more than 41,000 of these deaths from exposure to secondhand smoke. In addition, smoking-related illness in the United States costs more than $289 billion a year, including at least $133 billion in direct medical care for adults and $156 billion in lost productivity. An estimated 42.1 million people, or 18.1% of all adults (aged 18 years or older), in the United States smoke cigarettes. About 20.5% of men and 15.8% of women in the population smoke. By race/ethnicity about 21.8% of American Indian/ Alaskan Natives, 19.7% of non-Hispanic whites, 18.1% of non-Hispanic blacks, and 12% of Hispanics smoke (CDC, 2014d).

Alcohol

An estimated 17 million Americans use alcohol, and each year, nearly 85,000 people die from alcohol-related causes, making it the third leading preventable cause of death in the United States. The prevalence of fetal alcohol syndrome (FAS) in the United States is estimated to be between two to seven cases per 1,000; the prevalence of fetal alcohol spectrum disorders (FASD) in populations of younger school children may be as high as 2 to 5% in the United States and in some Western European countries (National Institute on Alcohol Abuse and Alcoholism, 2014).

Healthy People 2020

The U.S. Department of Health and Human Services created the *Healthy People 2020* document, the country's new 10-year goals and objectives for health promotion and disease. For the past 30 years *Healthy People* has been committed to improving the quality of U.S. residents' health by producing a framework for public health prevention priorities and actions. The *Healthy People* initiative set national objectives and monitors the progress made toward those goals. Preliminary analyses indicate that the United States has either progressed toward or met 71% of its *Healthy People* targets. *Healthy People* integrates input from public health and prevention experts, a wide range of federal, state, and local government officials, a consortium of more than 2,000 organizations, and also opinions from the general public (CDC, 2014e).

Leading Health Indicators for Healthy People 2020

The leading health indicators are composed of 26 topics which include the statistical evaluations (tracking of incidence, measuring, and reporting) of the following (CDC, 2014e):

1. Access to health care (people with medical insurance and available healthcare providers).
2. Clinical preventive services (adults who receive colorectal cancer screenings, adults whose blood pressure is under control, adult diabetics with A1c values greater than 9%, children aged 19 to 35 months who received DPT, hepatitis B, and A1C vaccinations).
3. Environmental quality (air quality index exceeding 100 and children 3 to 11 years exposed to secondhand smoke).
4. Injury and violence (fatal injuries and homicides).
5. Maternal, infant, and child health (infant deaths and preterm deaths).
6. Mental health (suicides and adolescents with major depression disorders).
7. Nutrition, physical activity, and obesity (adults who meet the federal activity guidelines for aerobic physical activity and muscle strengthening activity, obese children, and total vegetable intake for those 2 years and older).
8. Oral health (those 2 years and older who accessed oral health care in the past 12 months).
9. Reproductive and sexual health (sexually active females who received reproductive health services in the last 12 months, and people who know their HIV serostatus).
10. Social determinants of health (high school education levels).
11. Substance abuse (adolescents using alcohol or other illicit drugs in the past 30 days and adults engaging in binge drinking in the past 30 days).
12. Tobacco (adults who are current cigarette smokers and adolescents who smoked cigarettes in the past 30 days).

U.S. Health and Healthcare Disparities

The best health care in the world is meaningless to those who do not have access to health insurance coverage or who cannot afford it. The increases in healthcare costs combined with economic changes continue to cause some U.S. residents to go without any health insurance or adequate health insurance, giving them less access to health care. Because of the differences in health coverage and access to health care, great health disparities remain in the United States.

The term *health disparities* refers to population-specific differences in the presence of disease, health outcomes, quality of health care and access to health care services that exist across racial and ethnic groups. Disparities represent a lack of efficiency within the healthcare system and therefore account for unnecessary costs. A health disparity is a statistically significant difference in health indicator that persists over time and among groups, for example, maternal and infant mortality. A health disparity also comprises an unequal burden of disease morbidity and mortality often found in racial, ethnic, or socioeconomic groups as compared to the dominant group (CDC, 2014f).

Examples of U.S. health disparities include the following:

- *Infant mortality.* Mortality rates for African American babies remain nearly 2.5 times higher than the corresponding rates for white babies.
- *Life expectancy.* Black men and women have nearly 10 fewer years of life than their white counterparts.
- *Death rates attributable to heart disease, stroke, prostate, and breast cancer.* Rates are significantly higher for the African American population, and diabetes rates are more than 30% higher among Native Americans and Hispanics than among whites (CDC, 2014f).

Health and healthcare disparities exist across racial, ethnic, and socioeconomic groups. Racial and ethnic minorities and low socioeconomic groups tend to receive lower-quality health care than whites, even when insurance status, income, age, and illness severity are comparable. To decrease these healthcare disparities, the United States needs to increase the awareness of the problems among providers, insurers, and policymakers; promote consistency and equity of care; strengthen the culturally competent healthcare approach; and improve diversity of the healthcare workforce to increase patients' choices for healthcare providers. Measurement of health and healthcare quality includes the following considerations: (1) clinical performance measures of how well healthcare providers deliver specific services; (2) assessment by patients of how well providers meet their healthcare needs; and (3) outcome measures that may be affected by the quality of health care received, such as death rates from cancers preventable by screening (CDC, 2014f).

Causes of healthcare disparities in the United States include unequal and inadequate access to insurance coverage. Health insurance directly affects access to health care regardless of race, ethnicity, or socioeconomic status. When they lack or have inadequate health insurance, many people will go without medical care because they cannot afford to pay out of pocket for care. Minority groups and persons without a regular source of health care are less likely to access care. Low-income and uninsured individuals, including those who are not eligible to apply for the Affordable Care Act (Obamacare) health insurance, are particularly unlikely to access health care. Physical barriers to accessing health care include inadequate or no transportation to healthcare services and long waiting times for seeing a healthcare provider. Scarcity of healthcare providers and pharmacy services in the inner cities and in isolated rural areas where there are higher concentrations of minority populations are major issues as well. Language barriers create additional barriers. Persons with limited or no English-speaking and understanding abilities are less likely to be able to set up an appointment for medical care and, therefore, tend to rely on emergency rooms for care when vitally needed. Lack of English skills also inhibits comprehension of healthcare advice and contributes to lack of health literacy. Health literacy is the ability to obtain, process, and understand basic health information to make appropriate health decisions; it is needed to access healthcare systems. A larger number of minority patients have challenges in health literacy (CDC, 2014f).

Lack of diversity in healthcare providers can also be a potential problem. Minority patients, when given a choice, tend to be more comfortable with healthcare providers who are more like themselves and know their culture and language, as well as their health beliefs and practices. Collectively, minority groups in the United States represent 25% of the population, yet members of minorities account for less than 9% of nurses, 6% of physicians, and only 5% of dentists (CDC, 2014f).

In its 2004 report, the *Sullivan Commission* noted that racial and ethnic disparities in healthcare delivery are related to differences in treatment by healthcare providers. Minority groups are less likely than whites to be given appropriate cardiac medicines or to undergo cardiac bypass surgery when necessary. Compared to whites, they are less likely to receive renal dialysis or transplants, the best diagnostic tests, treatment for a stroke or cancer, or the best treatment for HIV/AIDS. Moreover, they often distrust healthcare providers (the majority of whom are white), receive care from less adequate health facilities, and are treated by lower-quality (in terms of education and experience) healthcare providers than whites. African Americans are more likely than whites to seek care from hospitals that have fewer resources and up-to-date technology, have higher surgical mortality rates, and have higher neonatal mortality rates. African Americans are also more likely to receive care from physicians with less training, have less access to specialist physicians, have higher rates of breast and prostate cancer due to less screening, and receive later care and have less access to care. The cancer incidence for black Americans is 10% higher than for whites (Stevens, 2004).

As the United States has been growing more racially and ethnically diverse, its residents are living longer. However, the National Center for Health Statistics has addressed major areas where disparities exist between race and ethnicity and socioeconomic status. Those residents who live in poverty are more likely to be in poor health and less likely to receive adequate health care. Poor people are four times more likely to have psychological stress. There are large disparities in infant mortality rates and life expectancy rates between those persons living in poverty and the remainder of the population. In addition, Latino or Native American adults younger than 64 are more likely to be uninsured than members of other racial or ethnic groups. Diseases and medical conditions such as diabetes or obesity increase with age and are more likely to occur in non-Hispanic blacks and Latinos than in non-Hispanic whites. Some of these disparities may be the result of differences in socioeconomic status, culture, and health practices, stress, environmental exposures, discrimination, and access to health care (CDC, 2014e, 2014f).

Dr. David Satcher (a former U.S. Surgeon General) and colleagues (2005) reported that from 1960 to 2000, the United States made progress in decreasing the black–white gap in civil rights, housing, education, and income, but notes that inequality still exists in health care and general health status. Young adults, 19 to 24 years old, are the most likely to be uninsured in the United States—even though they are at the highest risk of all age cohorts for unintended pregnancy, sexually transmitted diseases, substance abuse, injuries, and other chronic medical diseases. Lack of or inadequate health insurance (particularly with high copayments) is related to less frequent healthcare screenings, delayed diagnosis of illnesses such as cancer, poor care for chronic diseases, and higher rates of mortality when hospitalized. Latino young adults are more likely to be uninsured than any other ethnic group. Clearly, there remain significant disparities in accessing health care in the United States based on race, ethnicity, and socioeconomic status (Stevens, 2004; CDC, 2014f, 2014h).

Because of the lower population density and smaller number of physicians available, patients in rural areas often have to travel longer distances for care, wait longer for appointments, and wait longer in doctors' offices—yet there were no perceived differences in unmet medical needs within the two groups. Nevertheless, physicians in rural areas reported greater difficulty in helping patients (by referral) receive specialty medical care when needed because of a lack of qualified medical specialists in rural areas. Rural residents were also poorer and more likely to lack adequate insurance or be able to pay out-of-pocket expenses for health care (CDC, 2014e).

Overall Quality and Future Needs of U.S. Health Care

There is a substantial gap between the best of health care that can be provided to some individuals and that which is routinely delivered to many people. For example, 95% of hospice patients receive the right amount of pain medications, yet only 8% of alcoholic patients needing treatment receive care in a special facility. The median level of receipt of needed services is 58%. In spite of efforts to focus on effective prevention and chronic illness care, the U.S. healthcare system performs better in making patient diagnoses and treating acute illnesses, such as myocardial infarctions (heart attacks), than in providing outpatient treatments for chronic diseases such as cancer and diabetes. For those without health insurance, the healthcare situation is even worse. The median level of receipt of health care for the uninsured is 50% compared to 65% among people with health insurance (persons 65 years and older are excluded from these statistics because most have Medicare). Patient safety remains a major healthcare problem and clearly needs improvement. Approximately one of every seven hospitalized Medicare patients experienced one or more adverse events. Nosocomial infections (infections acquired during hospital care) are, by far, the most serious problem (CDC, 2014c, 2014f).

Health care varies not only with types of health insurance, but also with geographic location. There are wide variations in the quality of care provided throughout the country. The upper Midwest and New England regions have the highest quality of health care, while the Southwest and South Central regions of the country tend to have the lowest quality of health care. Quality of health care appears to be improving, but at a very slow rate. Outcome measures related to quality health care are also improving (CDC, 2014c, 2014f).

Infectious diseases remain a great cause of morbidity and mortality. The numbers of measles and rubella cases have decreased because of an increase in vaccinations, but some communicable diseases such as chlamydia have increased. In addition, the incidence of new infectious diseases such as H1N1, SARS, H5N1, avian influenza, and some drug-resistant bacteria strains, such as methicillin-resistant *Staphylococcus aureus* (MRSA), has increased. Influenza and pneumonia remain major causes of death, and HIV/AIDS continues to spread (CDC, 2014c, 2014f).

The removal of barriers to receiving health care is greatly needed in the United States. Lack of health insurance continues to represent the major barrier to quality health care. The Office of Healthcare Reform is leading the government effort to improve healthcare access and quality for all residents of the country. Health information technology is needed to support these quality improvements (CDC, 2014c, 2014f).

Payment for Health Care

Health care in the United States is provided by many different resources. The majority of healthcare facilities are owned and operated by private businesses. Sixty-two percent of the hospitals are nonprofit, 20% are government owned, and 18% are for-profit. Health care program payments come from a variety of resources; 60 to 65% of healthcare spending comes from programs such as Medicare, Medicaid, TRICARE, the Children's Health Insurance Program (CHIP), and the Veteran's Administration. Most of the population under 67 is insured by their or a family member's employer; some buy health insurance on their own, and the remainder are uninsured. The health insurance for public-sector employees is primarily provided by the government (Health Care Financing, 2014).

The Affordable Care Act (Obamacare)

The U.S. government passed an act that attempts to correct many of the healthcare access problems particularly for those without health insurance or for those who cannot afford to keep paying for their insurance premiums, which is the Patient Protection and Affordable Care Act (PPACA), and is also commonly referred to as Obamacare, healthcare reform, or the Affordable Care Act (ACA). The Affordable Care Act was signed into law to reform the healthcare industry by President Barack Obama on March 23, 2010, and upheld by the Supreme Court on June 28, 2012. Its goal is to give more Americans access to affordable, quality health insurance, and to reduce the growth in healthcare spending in the United States. The ACA expands the affordability, quality, and availability of private and public health insurance through consumer protections, regulations, subsidies, taxes, insurance exchanges, and other reforms, yet it does not replace private insurance, Medicare, or Medicaid. Provisions stop insurance companies from dropping people when they are sick or if a person makes an honest mistake on the application. It prevents against gender discrimination, stops insurance companies from making unjustified rate hikes, eliminates lifetime and annual limits, gives a person the right to a rapid appeal of insurance company decisions, and expands coverage to millions. Preventive health services include yearly checkups, immunizations, and counseling (Obamacare Facts, 2014).

Of the 17 high-income countries studied by the national Institutes of Health in 2013, the United States had the highest or near-highest prevalence of infant mortality, heart and lung disease, sexually transmitted infections, adolescent pregnancies, injuries, homicides, and disability. Together, such issues place the United States at the bottom of the list (among developed countries) for life expectancy. The Commonwealth Fund ranked the United States last in the quality of health care among similar countries, and notes U.S. care costs the most. In a 2013 Bloomberg ranking of nations with the most efficient healthcare systems, the United States ranked 46th among the 48 countries included in the study (Kaiser Family Foundation, 2011).

Although Americans benefit from many of the investments in health care, the recent rapid cost growth and overall economic slowdown and rising federal deficit, places great strains on the systems used to finance health care, including private employer-sponsored health insurance coverage and public insurance programs such as Medicare and Medicaid. Since 1999, family premiums for employer-sponsored health coverage have increased by 131%, placing increasing cost burdens on employers and workers. Workers' wages growing at a much slower pace than healthcare costs are causing many people to face difficulty in affording out-of-pocket spending (Kaiser Family Foundation, 2011).

Factors driving the growth in U.S. healthcare spending are as follows:

- *Technology and prescription drugs.* New medical technology and prescription drugs are leading contributors to the increase in overall health spending. Some analysts state that the availability of more expensive, state-of-the-art technological services and new drugs fuel healthcare spending not only because the development costs of these products must be recouped by industry, but also because they generate consumer demand for more intense, costly services even if they are not necessarily cost-effective.
- *Chronic disease.* Health care in the United States has changed dramatically over the past century with longer life spans and greater chronic illnesses causing increased demands on the healthcare system, particularly treatment of ongoing illnesses and long-term care services such as nursing homes; it is estimated that healthcare costs for chronic disease treatment account for over 75% of national health expenditures.
- *Aging of the population.* Health expenses have increased as the baby boomers (adults born between 1946 and 1964) began qualifying for Medicare in 2011 and many of the costs shifted to the public sector. Yet the aging of the population contributes minimally to the high growth rate of healthcare spending.
- *Administrative costs.* It is estimated that at least 7% of healthcare expenditures are for administrative costs (e.g., marketing, billing), and this portion is much lower in the Medicare program (<2%), which is operated by the federal government. The mixed public–private system creates overhead costs and large profits that are causing increases in healthcare spending (Kaiser Family Foundation, 2011).

Medication Usage

Utilization of medications differs according to third-party coverage (insurance) and availability. Nearly half of the U.S. population takes at least one prescription medication, and almost one in six takes three or more medications. These medications are predominately prescribed for lowering cholesterol to reduce the risk of heart disease, controlling depression, and/or controlling diabetes. The number of people taking medications and the number of medications taken both increase with age, with five out of six people who are 65 years or older taking at least one medication and nearly half taking three or more (CDC, 2014g).

U.S. Births

The 2013 number for Asian or Pacific Islander women declined 2% in 2013. The general fertility rate was 62.9 births per 1,000 women aged 15 to 44 years, down slightly from 2012 and a record low. Birth rates for teens aged 15 to 19 declined 10% (2013) to 26.6 births per 1,000 women, with rates declining for both younger and older teenagers. The birth rate for women in their early 20s also declined in 2013, to a record low of 81.2 births per 1,000 women, yet birth rates for women in their 30s and 40s rose in 2013 (CDC, 2014c).

The nonmarital birth rate was down 1% in 2013 to 44.8 births per 1,000 unmarried women aged 15 to 44. Preterm birth rates fell to 11.38% in 2013. Preterm birth rates declined 1 to 2% among each of the largest race and Hispanic origin groups in 2013; non-Hispanic white (10.17% in 2013), non-Hispanic black (16.26%), and Hispanic (11.30%). Since 2006, preterm rates have fallen 13% for non-Hispanic white, 12% for non-Hispanic black, and 8% for Hispanic infants; the 2013 rate for non-Hispanic black births is the lowest in more than three decades (CDC, 2014c).

Health of U.S. Ethnic Groups

Significant disparities remain in health among U.S. minority groups as compared to the non-Hispanic white population majority. Among non-Hispanic African American and Mexican American men, those with higher incomes are more likely to be obese than those with low incomes. Higher income women of these ethnic groups are less likely to be obese than low-income women. There is no significant relationship between obesity and education among men. Among women, those with college degrees are less likely to be obese compared with less educated women. By state, obesity prevalence ranged from 20.5% in Colorado to 34.7% in Louisiana in 2012. No state had a prevalence of obesity less than 20%. Nine states and the District of Columbia had prevalence between 20 and 25%. Thirteen states (Alabama, Arkansas, Indiana, Iowa, Kentucky, Louisiana, Michigan, Mississippi, Ohio, Oklahoma, South Carolina, Tennessee, and West Virginia) had a prevalence rate equal to or greater than 30%. Obesity causes approximately 300,000 deaths per year in the United States and is perhaps second only to smoking as a preventable cause of death. Estimates of deaths from obesity are based on body mass index (BMI), which is defined as weight in kilograms divided by height in meters squared. BMI is correlated with body fat and is the measure recommended by the National Heart, Lung, and Blood Institute for use in clinical practice. Much of the overweight/obesity problem relates to trends toward inactivity and overeating, especially of the high-fat "junk" foods (CDC, 2014e). Despite the fact that Americans smoke less, they have lowered their cholesterol levels, and deaths from heart disease and stroke are declining in the general population, deaths are not declining within specific racial and ethnic groups in the United States. Those groups who have not experienced any positive changes in their health statistics include African Americans, Hispanics (Latinos), persons who are poor, and persons with less than a high school education. African American men and women have the highest rates of hypertension, diabetes, and hospitalizations for stroke. Black women also have higher rates of obesity. Hispanics (Latinos) are most likely to lack health insurance, are less likely to receive influenza or pneumonia vaccines, and have the poorest rates of good health. Native Americans have the highest rates of cigarette smoking and alcohol use. Reasons for these disparities include inadequate access to health care, distrust of the healthcare providers, cultural and language barriers, and genetic predisposition to heart diseases and stroke (CDC, 2014e).

Morbidity and Mortality Rates

Mortality rate is a measure of the number of deaths (in general, or due to a specific cause) in a population, scaled to the size of that population, per unit of time, expressed in units of deaths per 1,000 individuals per year. It differs from *morbidity rate*, which refers to the number of people in poor health during a given time period (the prevalence rate) or the number of new cases of the disease per unit of time (incidence rate). The U.S. percent of low birthweight babies (less than 5.5 pounds) is 8.0%; the percent of preterm births (less than 37 weeks gestation) is 11.5% (CDC, 2014e).

Morbidity (disease rate) includes the limitation of activities due to chronic illness. Mortality (death rate) reflects the statistics of life expectancy and infant mortality—the key measures to evaluate the overall health standard of a population. In the United States, there is an upward trend in life expectancy. State variations in infant mortality (for all population groups) range from 9.62 deaths per 100,000 live births in Mississippi to 3.57 deaths per 100,000 live births in Alaska. Infant mortality rates (IMRs) also differ greatly by race, with highs of 20.9 deaths per 100,000 in non-Hispanic blacks, as compared to 2.7 deaths per 100,000 in non-Hispanic whites (CDC, 2014e).

According to the CDC (2014e) the leading causes of infant deaths in the United States are as follows:

1. Congenital malformations, deformations, and chromosomal abnormalities.
2. Disorders related to short gestation and low birthweight.
3. Sudden infant death syndrome.

Health of American Indians/Alaskan Natives

American Indians/Alaskan Natives represent 1.5% of the total U.S. population. More than 538,000 of American Indian/Alaskan Natives (representing one third of the total American Indian/Alaskan Native population) live on reservations or other trust lands where the climate is challenging, the roads are often impassable, transportation is scarce, and healthcare facilities are difficult to access. In some areas, health services and facilities have not kept up with services and facilities in areas with white populations. In the Navajo area, the number of hospital beds has declined steadily and the proportion of doctors and nurses to patients has not kept up with that of the general U.S. population. About 60% of American Indians depend on the Indian Health Service to provide access to health care (CDC, 2014e).

The Indian Health Service (IHS) is part of the U.S. Department of Health and Human Services (HHS). IHS is responsible for providing medical and public health services to members of federally recognized Tribes and Alaska Natives. It is the principal federal healthcare provider and health advocate for the estimated 4.5 million people who are classified as American Indian and Alaska Natives. The IHS provides health care to its clientele at 33 hospitals, 59 health centers, and 50 health stations. The agency employs approximately 2,700 nurses, 900 physicians, 400 engineers, 500 pharmacists, and 300 dentists, as well as other health professionals totaling more than 15,000 in all. It is one of two federal agencies mandated to use Indian preference in hiring. This law requires the agency to give preference hiring to qualified Indian applicants before considering non-Indian candidates for positions. IHS-run hospitals and clinics serve any registered Indian/Alaska Native, regardless of tribe or income. Tribal-contract healthcare facilities serve only their tribal members, with other qualified Indians/Alaska Natives offered care on a space-available basis. This policy makes it difficult for an Indian who leaves the tribal home for education or employment to receive the healthcare services to which they are legally entitled. Thirty-four urban Indian health projects supplement these facilities with a variety of health and referral services. A large part of the overall IHS goal is addressing barriers of access to health care, and giving comprehensive, culturally acceptable, public health services to American Indian and Alaskan Native persons (CDC, 2014e).

There is great diversity among the various tribal communities of American Indians and Alaska Natives in terms of accessing health care, health risk behaviors, and health outcomes. As compared to other U.S. minority groups American Indians/Alaskan Natives have higher rates of tobacco use, infant mortality, delayed prenatal care, violence, attempted suicide, and deaths due to diabetes, accidents, and chronic liver disease. They continue to be among the poorest in the United States, with one in four living below the U.S. federal poverty level. Diabetes and liver diseases within this population are greater than twice that of all other adults in the United States. The greatest mortality rates among American Indians are due to type 2 diabetes despite special federal expenditure programs. Compared with non-Hispanic whites, Indians of all cultural groups have higher levels of obesity and diabetes, and spend less time in physical activities. A special Diabetes Program for American Indians has provided funds for prevention and treatment of diabetes, yet rates are still higher than those of whites. Compared with whites, Indians of all cultural groups have higher levels of smoking and heart disease than whites; have higher death rates of fetuses, infants, children, adolescents and young adults than other groups; have higher preterm deaths and fetal alcohol syndrome (FAS) than other groups; and have lower rates of prenatal care. Infant mortality is 1.7 times higher, and they have twice the rate of sudden infant death syndrome compared to all other U.S. population groups. Their rates of sexually transmitted diseases are 5.5 times higher than that of non-Hispanic whites. Unintentional injuries are the third leading cause of death for those 1 to 44. Death rates for unintentional injuries and motor vehicle accidents are 1.7 to 2 times higher than rates for all other groups in the United States, and suicide rates are 3 times greater than for whites of similar ages (CDC, 2014e; Kunitz, 2008).

Health of African Americans

In 2012, the population of African Americans, including those of more than one race, was estimated at 44.5 million, making up 14.2% of the total U.S. population. Those who identified only as African American made up 13.1% of the U.S. population, which was greater than 39 million people. The U.S. Census Bureau projects that by the year 2060 there will be 77.4 million African Americans, including those of more than one race, in the United States, making up 18.4% of the total U.S. population (CDC, 2014h).

African Americans have twice the uninsured healthcare rates as non-Hispanic whites. Non-Hispanic blacks have a disproportionate burden of diseases, injuries, deaths, and disabilities. The risk factors, incidence, and morbidity rates for diseases and injuries are greater than for non-Hispanic whites. Three of the 10 leading causes of deaths for non-Hispanic African Americans are not among those listed as the 10 leading causes of deaths for non-Hispanic whites. They are homicide (sixth), HIV virus (seventh), and septicemia (ninth). Today, an African American baby is 2.5 times more likely to die before reaching 1 year of age than a non-Hispanic white American baby. Preterm birth is the leading cause of death for African American infants. Higher pregnancy-related mortalities are found among black women compared to white women of similar socioeconomic status including rates of preeclampsia, eclampsia, abruptio placenta, placenta previa, and postpartal hemorrhage, leading to death. Non-Hispanic African American women are at a higher risk for having low and very-low-birth-weight babies. There are lower numbers of females receiving prenatal care during the first trimester of pregnancy. Compared to white American women, middle-class black women have access to fewer financial resources, are more likely to reside in racially segregated areas, and are more affected by lifelong legacies of childhood poverty and psychological stress due to discrimination (CDC, 2014h).

Health of U.S. Hispanic/Latinos

According to U.S. Census Bureau population estimates (2015), there are roughly 52 million Hispanics living in the United States, representing approximately 16.7% of the U.S. total population, making people of Hispanic origin the nation's largest ethnic or race minority. The U.S. Hispanic population for 2050 is estimated to reach 132.8 million, constituting approximately 30% of the U.S. population by that date. Among Hispanic subgroups, in 2010, Mexicans ranked as the largest at 63%. Following Mexicans were Puerto Ricans (9.2%), Cubans (3.5%), Salvadorans (3.3%), Dominicans (2.8%), and the remaining 18.2% were people of other Hispanic or Latino origins (Pew Hispanic Center, 2011).

According to the CDC (2014i) the major causes of mortality in this population are as follows:

1. Cancer
2. Heart disease
3. Unintentional injuries
4. Stroke
5. Diabetes

6. Chronic liver disease and cirrhosis
7. Chronic lower respiratory diseases
8. Influenza and pneumonia
9. Homicide
10. Nephritis, nephrotic syndrome, and nephrosis

The number of Hispanic/Latinos of all ages in the United States in 2012 was 53 million. The number of births per 1,000 women 15 to 44 years was 74.4 and the percent of low-birth-weight babies was 7.0%. The percent of Hispanic/Latinos of all ages in fair or poor health is 10.3%. The percent of Hispanic men 18 years and over who currently smoke cigarettes is 16.7, and the percent of women 18 years and over who currently smoke cigarettes is 8.4%. The percent of persons under 65 years without health insurance coverage is 30.4%. The leading causes of death are cancer, health disease, and accidents (unintentional injuries) (CDC, 2014i).

The Latino/Hispanic Paradox

Despite having lower access to health care, lower education levels, and greater poverty than the majority non-Hispanic white groups, the *Hispanic paradox*, *Latino paradox*, or *epidemiologic paradox* exists. This paradox refers to the research findings that indicate that Hispanic/Latino Americans tend to have health outcomes that are comparable to, or in some cases better than, those of their U.S. non-Hispanic white counterparts. The paradox usually refers in particular to the low infant mortality rates of U.S. Hispanics/Latinos as compared to non-Hispanic whites. This paradox is particularly evident among Mexican-born women. The specific cause of the phenomenon is poorly understood, although the decisive factor could be the possibility that differing birthing or neonatal practices may be involved. Another possibility is the "healthy migrant effect," which hypothesizes that the self-selection of *healthy* Hispanic immigrants into the United States is the reason for the paradox. International immigration statistics demonstrate that the mortality rate of immigrants is lower than in their country of origin. In the United States, foreign-born individuals have better self-reported health than American-born respondents. Furthermore, recent Hispanic/Latino immigrants have better health than those who have lived in the United States for a longer amount of time (McGlade, Saha, & Dahlstrom, 2012).

Health of Asian Americans/Pacific Islanders

In 2011, the population of Asians, including those of more than one race, was estimated at 18.2 million of the U.S. population. In 2010, those who identified themselves only as Asian constituted approximately 4.8% of the American population, which was 14.7 million individuals. The three largest Asian groups in the United States in 2011 were Chinese (4 million) (except Taiwanese descent), Filipinos (3.4 million), and Asian Indians (3.2 million). These were followed by Vietnamese (1.9 million), Koreans (1.7 million), and Japanese (1.3 million) (CDC, 2014e).

The Census Bureau projects that by the year 2050, there will be more than 40.6 million Asians living in the United States, comprising 9.2% of the total U.S. population. The Asian population lives throughout the United States, though the states with the largest Asian populations are California, New York, and Hawaii. Hawaii has the largest concentration or percentage of the total population of Asians (CIA, 2014c, 2014e).

The Office of Management and Budget (OMB) defines Asians as people having origins in any of the original peoples of the Far East, Southeast Asia, or the Indian subcontinent including, for example, Cambodia, China, India, Japan, Korea, Malaysia, Pakistan, the Philippine Islands, Thailand, and Vietnam. According to the 2010 Census, the Asian population category includes people who indicated their race(s) as "Asian" or reported entries such as "Asian Indian," "Chinese," "Filipino," "Korean," "Japanese," and "Vietnamese" or provided other detailed responses. Asian Americans represent the extremes of both health outcomes and socioeconomic status. Asian Americans are less likely to live in poverty (12.8%), more likely to be college graduates or hold graduate degrees (50%), and more likely to be employed in management, business, science, and arts occupations (48.5%) as compared with the total U.S. population (15.9%, 28.5%, 36.0%, respectively). Numerous factors may threaten their health, including infrequent medical visits, language and cultural barriers, and the lack of health insurance (CIA, 2014c, 2014f).

Asian American women experienced the longest life expectancy (85.8 years) of any ethnic group in the United States. The leading causes of death of Asian Americans in 2010 were cancer, heart disease, stroke, unintentional injuries (accidents), and diabetes. Death rates for these conditions are less than other racial/ethnic populations. They are at higher risk for chronic obstructive pulmonary disease, hepatitis B, HIV/AIDS, smoking, and tuberculosis. Liver disease rates are lower than those of other racial and ethnic populations. Asian Americans have a prevalence rate for diabetes of 8.2% compared with the white population's rate of 7.0%. Asian American women (ages 18+) are least likely to have had a Pap test (68.0%) compared with other women: non-Hispanic white (72.8%), non-Hispanic black (77.4%), Hispanic/Latino (73.6%), American Indian/Alaska Native (73.4) (CDC, 2014c, 2014f).

U.S. Child Health

In 2012, the majority of children in the United States enjoyed excellent health (42 million or 57%), and another 19 million children had very good health (26%), yet 7% of children had no health insurance coverage, and 4% of children had no usual place of health care. Six percent of children had unmet dental needs because their families could not afford dental care. Twelve percent of children had one ER visit and 6% had two or more visits. Among children with a usual place of health care, 74% used a doctor's office as their usual place of care; 24%, a clinic; and 1%, a hospital outpatient clinic. Less than 1% used an ER as their usual place of health care (CDC, 2014j).

The U.S. mortality rates for children have fallen sharply during the past few decades. The greatest reduction is attributable to prevention and treatment of acute infectious diseases. Unintentional injury remains the leading cause of childhood death at present in the United States, but children having complex chronic conditions have the second highest death rates. Hospitalization costs for children ages 1 to 18 are typically related to the following causes (ranked from highest to lowest in cost): asthma, mental disorders, trauma, respiratory infections, ear infections, other infections, epilepsy, diabetes, and congenital anomalies. Mortality rates for African American male adolescents (15–19) have risen dramatically in recent years, mainly because of homicide and suicide. In addition, black children experience significant death rates from sickle cell disease. Obesity is now considered a chronic problem for children, which also causes other problems, such as type 2 diabetes (CDC, 2014j; CIA, 2014a).

Health and Health Care of U.S. Older Adults

Older adults are among the fastest growing age groups, as the first baby boomers began turning 65 in 2011. More than 37 million people in this group (60%) will be managing more than one chronic condition by 2030. Older adults are at high risk for developing chronic illnesses and related disabilities. These chronic conditions include diabetes mellitus, arthritis, congestive heart failure, and dementia (CDC, 2014k).

Many experience hospitalizations, nursing home admissions, and low-quality care. They also may lose the ability to live independently at home. Chronic conditions are the leading cause of death among older adults. Preventive health services are valuable for maintaining the quality of life and wellness of older adults. The Patient Protection and Affordable Care Act of 2011 includes provisions related to relevant Medicare services. However, preventive services are underused, especially among certain racial and ethnic groups. Many older adults use many healthcare services, have complex conditions, and require professional expertise that meets their needs. Most providers receive some type of training on aging, but the percentage of those who actually specialize in this area is small. More certified specialists are needed to meet the needs of this group.

The CDC (2014k) recommends the following immunizations for older adults:

- Diphtheria and pertussis for adults up to 64 years (one lifetime dose).
- Tetanus–diphtheria vaccine: all adults, every 10 years.
- Shingles (adults 60 or older).
- Influenza vaccine: adults 50 and older, annually.
- Hepatitis A vaccine: adults at risk.
- Hepatitis B vaccine: adults at risk.
- Measles, mumps, and rubella vaccine: susceptible adults.
- Varicella (chickenpox) vaccine: susceptible adults.
- Meningococcal polysaccharide vaccine: susceptible adults.

For older adults, oral health care is not covered by Medicare, and many have difficulty in accessing this care. The well elderly as well as the chronically ill elderly will need good oral care for routine cleaning, problems with tooth loss, dental caries, and periodontal diseases. At present, there are not enough dentists trained to meet the needs of the elderly in the United States, and many residents do not have sufficient funds to pay for these services on an out-of-pocket basis. In addition to providing medical care benefits, the federal government operates a federal food and nutrition program for older adults who qualify (CDC, 2014k).

The U.S. government appropriates approximately $1 billion annually for all food and nutrition assistance programs for older adults, funded through the Older Americans Act (OAA).

OAA nutrition programs, which are run by the U.S. Department of Health and Human Services and the U.S. Department of Agriculture, reach only 6 to 7% of the people who need them, however. By comparison, the federal government's special Supplemental Nutrition Program for Women, Infants and Children (WIC) is funded at $5 billion and reaches approximately 50% of eligible women, infants, and children (CDC, 2014k).

Occupational Health

The U.S. Occupational Safety and Health Administration (OSHA) is an agency of the U.S. Department of Labor under the Occupational Safety and Health Act, founded in December 1970. OSHA's mission is to "assure safe and healthful working conditions for working men and women by setting and enforcing standards and by providing training, outreach, education and assistance." The agency is also charged with enforcing a variety of whistleblower statutes and regulations (OSHA, 2014).

The total recordable cases of nonfatal occupational injury and illness incidence rate among private industry employers declined in 2010 to 3.5 cases per 100 workers—its lowest level since 2003. The preliminary count of fatal work injuries in the United States in 2010 was 4,547. Overall, fatal work injuries are down 22% since 2006. Fatal work injuries due to fires and explosions increased by 65% in 2010 (OSHA, 2014).

Muscular and skeletal disorders remain the biggest sources of problems reported; these disorders typically come from repetitive motion injuries, which create medical problems such as carpel tunnel syndrome and back injuries. Occupations with the most repetitive motion injuries are as follows:

- Truck drivers
- Nursing aids, orderlies, and attendants
- Laborers, nonconstruction
- Assemblers
- Janitors
- Registered nurses
- Stock handlers and baggers
- Construction workers
- Supervisors, sales jobs
- Carpenters
- Cashiers
- Housecleaners
- Sales workers
- Clerks
- Welders
- Cooks

Occupational safety and health administration issues among farm workers are much higher than the rates among the general U.S. population. Most migrant farm workers have only six years of education, and the majority have access to health care only when absolutely necessary—for example, by visiting hospital emergency rooms or clinics. Fewer than half of the workers have ever been to a dentist. The infectious diseases most often reported among these individuals typically come from parasites from poor drinking water in work camps, and the rate of tuberculosis in this group is six times greater than the rate in the general U.S. population. In addition, HIV/AIDS and sexually transmitted diseases rates among farm workers are much higher than the rates among the general U.S. population (OSHA, 2014).

Complementary and Alternative Medicine

Nearly 40% of Americans use healthcare approaches developed outside of mainstream Western, or conventional, medicine for specific conditions or overall well-being. When describing health approaches with non-mainstream roots, people often use the words *alternative* and *complementary* interchangeably, but the two terms refer to different concepts.

Complementary refers to using a non-mainstream approach together with conventional medicine.
Alternative refers to using a non-mainstream approach in place of conventional medicine.

Most people use non-mainstream approaches along with conventional treatments overlapping with complementary or alternative medicine. Interest in the use of natural products has grown considerably over the past few decades. According to the 2007 National Health Interview Survey (NHIS), which included a comprehensive survey on the use of complementary health approaches by Americans, 17.7% of American adults had used a non-vitamin/non-mineral natural product in the past year. These products were the most popular complementary health approaches among both adults and children. The most commonly used natural product among adults in the past 30 days was fish oil/omega 3s (reported by 37.4% of all adults who said they used natural products); popular products for children (taken in the past 30 days) included echinacea (37.2%) and fish oil/omega 3s (30.5%). Some of these products have been studied in large, placebo-controlled trials, many of which failed to show anticipated effects. Research on others to determine whether they are effective and safe is ongoing.

Examples of mind and body practices include a large and diverse group of procedures or techniques administered or taught by a trained practitioner or teacher. These include the following:

- *Acupuncture* is a technique in which practitioners stimulate specific points on the body—most often by inserting thin needles through the skin.
- *Massage therapy* includes many different techniques in which practitioners manually manipulate the soft tissues of the body.
- Most *meditation* techniques, such as *mindfulness meditation* or *transcendental meditation*, involve ways in which a person learns to focus attention.
- *Relaxation techniques*, such as *breathing exercises*, *guided imagery*, and *progressive muscle relaxation*, are designed to produce the body's natural relaxation response.
- *Spinal manipulation* is practiced by chiropractors, osteopathic physicians, naturopathic physicians, physical therapists, and some medical doctors. Practitioners perform spinal

manipulation by using their hands or a device to apply a controlled force to a joint of the spine. The amount of force applied depends on the form of manipulation used.

- *Tai chi* and *qi gong* are practices from traditional Chinese medicine that combine specific movements or postures, coordinated breathing, and mental focus.

Other examples of mind and body practices include *healing touch* and *hypnotherapy*. (Greater in-depth explanations can be found in the alternative and complementary medicine and treatments chapter of this textbook.)

SWEDEN

The Kingdom of Sweden, a constitutional monarchy, is one of five nations making up the area of northern Europe known as Scandinavia. It has a subarctic climate (part of the country lies within the Arctic Circle), has light all summer, but very little light during the winter. Its area size is slightly larger than the U.S. state of California. It has a population of over 9 million people (2013 estimate). The country is divided into 21 different counties, each with a county administration board and a county council. Each council, in turn, is divided into many municipalities. Sweden has a very high standard of living because of its high-tech capitalism and an extensive social welfare system. It has a gross national income of $43,980 (USD) (Government of Sweden, 2014; WHO, 2013b).

Sweden has one of the highest levels of health care in the world, a very low infant mortality rate, and a high average life expectancy. It has an infant mortality rate of 2.74 per 1,000 live births, one of the lowest in the world. Life expectancy at birth is 82 years: males 78.78 years and females 83.51 years. The maternal mortality rate is 4 per 100,000 and the children under 5 years' mortality rate is 3 per 100,000. Those in the population who have chronic illnesses have a good quality of life due to the country's excellent health care. It also has a literacy rate of 99%. Death rates from diseases such as diabetes and heart disease are declining. The older adult population is growing, and more people are able to live a higher quality of life than in previous years (Government of Sweden, 2014; WHO, 2013b).

Healthcare System

The goal of the Swedish healthcare system is for the entire population to have equal access to good health care, which is funded by the Swedish government and provided to all citizens based on need. The government health welfare system includes health and medical care, care of the elderly, pharmaceutical care, psychiatric care, and dental care (Government of Sweden, 2014).

Sweden's healthcare system is organized by national, regional, and local levels. At the national level, the Ministry of Health and Social Affairs establishes principles and guidelines for care and sets the political agenda for health and medical care. The ministry, along with other government agencies, supervises activities at the lower levels, allocates grants, and periodically evaluates services to ensure correspondence to national goals. At the regional level, responsibility for financing and providing health care is decentralized to the county councils. The county council is a political body whose representatives are elected by the public every 4 years on the same day as the national general election. The executive board or hospital board of a county council exercises authority over hospital structure and management, and ensures efficient healthcare delivery. County councils also regulate prices and level of service offered by private providers. Private providers are required to enter into a contract with the county councils. Patients are not reimbursed for services from private providers who do not have an agreement with the county councils. At the local level, municipalities are responsible for maintaining the immediate environment of citizens such as water supply and social welfare services. Recently, post-discharge care for the disabled and elderly, and long-term care for psychiatric patients was decentralized to the local municipalities (Government Offices of Sweden Ministry of Health, 2014).

Costs for health and medical care amount to approximately 9% of Sweden's GDP. Seventy-one percent of health care is funded through local taxation, and county councils collect income tax. The state finances the bulk of healthcare costs, with the patient paying a small nominal fee for examination. The state pays for approximately 97% of medical costs. When a person in Sweden is sick (declared sick by the doctor) he or she is paid a percentage of his or her normal daily wage from the second day. For the first 14 days, the employer is required to pay this wage, and after that, the state pays the wage until the patient is declared fit. Prescription medicine costs per year are not free, but costs are limited for the patient. When a minimal amount has been paid to the pharmacy, the remainder of medication costs is paid by the government for the rest of the year. All pharmacies are network-connected so medicines can be obtained from any pharmacy in the country. A limit on health care fees per year exists. When visiting a hospital, the entrance fee covers all specialist visits that are requested by the physician. After a minimal amount has been paid, health care for the rest of the year is provided free of charge. Dental care is not included in the general healthcare system but is partly subsidized by the government and is free for children up to 19 years of age (Government Offices of Sweden Ministry of Health, 2014).

There are different categories of charges for health care within the Swedish healthcare system, as follows (Government Offices of Sweden Ministry of Health, 2014):

- *Outpatient healthcare charges.* Charges are applied for visits to a district nurse, doctor, or specialist. Costs vary among the different councils and depend on the type of healthcare provider used. The maximum that any one person pays for health visits per year is 900 SEK ($115 USD); this maximum cost also includes children younger than 18 within the same family.
- *Pharmaceutical charges.* The maximum cost per year for medications is 1,800 SEK ($230 USD). After this cost is reached, a free pass is given, which covers the cost of medications for 12 months from the date of the first purchase.
- *Charges for a portion of dental treatments.* These charges vary depending on the type of treatment and materials used. This category also includes orthodontia work.
- *Costs for inpatient care.* When a patient is admitted to a hospital, the local council can charge the patient a maximum of 80 SEK ($10.24 USD) per day.

Sweden has an extensive social welfare system in which the government pays for child care, maternity and paternity leave, healthcare costs above a ceiling amount, retirement pensions, and sick leave. Parents get 480 days paid leave of absence from their jobs from the time of the birth of a child to his or her eighth year. Child care is free and is guaranteed for all children

1 to 5 years old. For the aging adult, the Swedish Social Security Insurance Agency provides an old-age pension. It also provides for loss of income if a person is unable to work because of illness or because of caring for a child (Government Offices of Sweden Ministry of Health, 2014). During the 1990s, Sweden's welfare state was in crisis due to economic challenges and lack of political support. Some spending cuts and reforms were made, but the healthcare system was left mostly intact. For the first time, however, the private healthcare sector competed with public healthcare providers. The new private healthcare services (which represent 5 to 15% of all health care) began somewhat to undermine the egalitarian system of equal quality health care for all Swedish citizens. At present there are choices of health services, and wealthier citizens often use private healthcare services while lower-income individuals use the public health services (Government Offices of Sweden Ministry of Health, 2014).

Although the country has one of the best healthcare systems and overall health worldwide, several major health issues exist.

Dental Care

The dental health of Sweden has improved considerably for all age groups over the last few decades. The number of children who need tooth fillings has declined, as has the number of older adults who need total tooth extractions. Many differences persist in the level of dental care among county councils (Government Offices of Sweden Ministry of Health, 2014).

Mental Health

The Swedish government takes responsibility for providing mental health care as a part of basic health and medical care. Patients with slight or moderate mental health needs can get care from primary care healthcare providers. Compulsory mental health care is regulated by the Compulsory Mental Care Act. Under this act, patients with serious mental health problems are treated in a special psychiatric care setting, even if they refuse care. This is especially true if the individual threatens the personal safety, physical safety, or mental health of others. Forensic mental health care includes care for people who have committed serious crimes and for those who suffer from mental illness (Government Offices of Sweden Ministry of Health, 2014).The number of psychiatrists in Sweden has increased by nearly 30%; about 5 to 10% still need psychiatric care though only 3 to 4% actually seek psychiatric care. Suicides are a major health problem, and the government is working to decrease this number (Government Offices of Sweden Ministry of Health, 2014).

Sex Education

Sweden is a pioneer country in terms of family planning. Swedish attitudes toward teenage sex education are considered liberal. Sex education is a high priority and has been taught in schools since the 1950s. Since 1975, abortion has been free and is given on demand. Contraceptive counseling is free, and Planned Parenthood services are available in youth clinics. Screening for sexually transmitted diseases is included in these services as well. Contraception and emergency contraception are low in cost and are sold over-the-counter. Teenage pregnancy is rare (Government Offices of Sweden Ministry of Health, 2014). Makenzius and Larsson (2012) researched the habits of those 15 years old and younger who engaged in sexual intercourse and found that these behaviors were also linked to other high-risk behaviors, leading to greater hazardous lifestyles.

Care of Older Adults

The Swedish healthcare system provides care for older and disabled people. Under the Social Services Act, most care for older adults and disabled people, including nursing homes and home services, are provided. These services are not free, but fees are only a fraction (4–5%) of the cost. Home care includes cleaning, shopping, laundry, and cooking as well as personal care such as bathing and dressing. Basic medical services are very comprehensive and include medication administration (such as insulin injections), and emotional and social support. The current growing trend is less care given by social services and more out-of-pocket spending (Szebehely & Trydegard, 2012).

JAPAN

Japan (also known as "Nippon") is an island nation made up of four main islands and 4,000 smaller islands located in the Pacific Ocean, east of the Sea of Japan, China, North Korea, South Korea, and Russia, and north of Taiwan. The four largest islands—Honshu, Hokkaido, Kyushu, and Shikoku—account for 97% of Japan's area. Most of the islands are mountainous, and many are volcanic. Approximately 70 to 80% of the country is covered with forests and mountains and is therefore unsuitable for agriculture, industry, or residential use; as a consequence, the habitable areas, which are mainly located on the coasts, have very high population density. The population of Japan exceeds 127 million, making it the world's 10th largest population. Tokyo, the capital city, in combination with its surrounding smaller cities, has a population of more than 30 million, one of the largest metropolitan areas in the world (CIA, 2014d).

Japan is organized into 47 prefectures, each of which is overseen by an elected governor, legislature, and administrative bureaucracy. Each prefecture is divided into cities, towns, and villages. Japan has a constitutional monarchy with very little power, and an elected parliament called the Diet. The prime minister of Japan is the head of state (CIA, 2014d).

Until recently, Japan had the world's second largest economy, but China has now taken its place in the number two spot, making Japan the third largest economy. It is the world's fourth largest exporter and fifth largest importer and is the only Asian country in the G8 (Group of Eight) and currently serves as a nonpermanent member of the UN Security Council. Japan officially renounced its right to declare war but still maintains a large military for peacekeeping and self-defense purposes. It is a developed country with a very high standard of living (CIA, 2014d).

Japan has one of the world's highest life expectancy rates and has the world's third lowest infant mortality rate. Some of the largest businesses in Japan include Toyota, Nintendo, Canon, Honda, Sony Panasonic, Sharp, and Japan Oil. In addition, Japan is one of the world's leaders in scientific research, including technology, machinery, and biomedical research. Within Japan's population of 127.3 million, the largest group comprises the Yamoto people.

The main ethnic groups are the Ainu and Ryukyuan peoples, and the main social ethnic group is the Burakumin. Today many young Japanese choose not to marry and have children, and the population is expected to drop to 100 million by 2050. As of 2012, Japan's per capita GDP was $36,300. Approximately 84 to 96% of the population practice both Buddhism and Shintoism; a small minority practice Christianity, Taoism, Confucianism, or Buddhism. Most people speak Japanese, and most children today learn both Japanese and English in school. Approximately 75.9% of Japanese children finish high school and attend a university or trade school. The educational system is very competitive, particularly for entrance into universities, and 99% of the population is literate (CI), 2014d; WHO, 2014a).

Health and Health Care

Japan has one of the world's highest life expectancy rates with 84.46 years in the general population: 80 years for males, and 87 years for females. The leading cause of death in people younger than 30 is suicide. The infant mortality rate is 2.13 deaths per 1,000 live births, also one of the lowest rates in the world, and the death rate of children under 5 years is 3 per 1,000. The number of physicians is 2.14 per 1,000 people. The total fertility rate is 1.4 children born per woman and the contraception utilization rate is 54.3% for women ages 20 to 49 years. Government health expenditures represent 10.1% of total government expenditures. In 2014, the total per capita expenditures for health amounted to $3,578, compared to a gross national income per capita of $36,300 (USD). HIV prevalence rate is 0.1% of the population. The unemployment rate is 7.9% of the population (CIA, 2014d; WHO, 2014a).

Mandatory universal healthcare coverage is provided to all residents by a national, employer-based insurance system. Medical care is based on cost sharing, but is free for those on welfare support and living below the poverty line. Long-term care for everyone older than age 65 covers home care, respite care, or institutional care, which is financed by public and private buyers, with premiums based on income and ability to pay. Japan provides universal coverage to all residents through three broad categories of insurance: employer-based insurance, national insurance, and insurance for the elderly. These programs are financed primarily by the national government, private employers, and individual coinsurance payments, but the services are delivered through a mostly privately operated hospital and clinic system. All programs cover a broad range of services, including inpatient and outpatient care, dental care, and some pharmaceuticals. The programs cover little preventive care, however. All programs place a cap on the amount of out-of-pocket spending health consumers may incur in a year (CIA, 2014d; WHO, 2014a).

Healthcare System

Japan's healthcare system is characterized by universal coverage; free choice of healthcare providers for patients; a multipayer, employment-based system of financing; and a predominant role for private hospitals and fee-for-service practices. Virtually all Japanese residents are covered without regard to any medical problems; that is, predisposing conditions or risks for illnesses do not affect coverage. Premiums are based on income and ability to pay. Control of the delivery of care is left largely to medical professionals, and there appears to be no public concern about healthcare rationing. Payment for personal medical services is offered through a universal healthcare insurance system that provides relative equality of access, with fees set by a government committee. People who do not have insurance through their employers can participate in a national health insurance program administered by local governments. Patients are free to select physicians or facilities of their choice and cannot be denied coverage. Hospitals, by law, must be run as nonprofit entities and be managed by physicians (CIA, 2014d; WHO, 2014a).

All patients can select their own healthcare providers, and facilities and cannot be denied coverage. All hospitals must be run as a nonprofit organization and be managed by physicians, and all clinics must be owned and run by physicians. All medical fees are regulated by the government and must be set at an affordable cost (Shibuya, 2011).

The future of Japan's system of good health at low cost with equity is set at beyond universal coverage. All residents of Japan are required to be enrolled in one of the Japanese insurance programs. In contrast, foreigners living in Japan are recommended to join the national health scheme but are not forced to do so. There are a total of eight health insurance systems divided into two categories, Employee Health Insurance and National Health Insurance. National Health Insurance is generally reserved for self-employed people and students, whereas social insurance is normally for corporate employees. National Health Insurance can be broken down into two groups: National Health Insurance for each city, town, or village, and the National Health Insurance Union (CIA, 2014d).

Services are provided either through regional/national public hospitals or through private hospitals/clinics, and patients have universal access to any facility, although hospitals tend to charge higher fees to those patients who arrive without a referral. Compared to the United States, Japan has about three times as many hospitals per capita. Japanese patients visit the hospital 14 times per year, on average, more than four times as often as Americans do. Due to large numbers of people visiting hospitals and doctors for relativity minor problems, space can be an issue in some regions (CIA, 2014d).

Japan's Nuclear Concerns

According to Infoplease (2011), radiation-related health consequences remain a serious concern for the Japanese people. These health risks are dependent upon exposure, which takes into account factors such as amount and type of radiation, weather conditions, proximity to nuclear power plants, and amount of time spent in irradiated areas. The Fukushima Daiichi nuclear power plant experienced serious leakage from the tsunami and earthquake of March 11, 2011. Those persons living between 20 and 30 kilometers from the plant were asked to evacuate the area, and risks of exposure included food contamination.

UNITED KINGDOM

The United Kingdom of Great Britain and Northern Ireland is a country located in Western Europe. A member of the European Union, the nation is usually known as the United Kingdom, or inaccurately known as Great Britain, Britain, or England. The United Kingdom has four parts consisting of England, Wales, and Scotland (all located on the Island of Great

Britain) and Northern Ireland (located on the island of Ireland). The capital and largest city is London. As of January 2012, England's government was headed by Prime Minister David Cameron (the leader of the Conservative Party) and Queen Elizabeth II. The queen's role is mainly ceremonial; the U.K. government is a constitutional monarchy with executive power given to the prime minister (CIA, 2014e).

Population

In 2014, the population of the United Kingdom totaled approximately 63.7 million people. Life expectancy is 80.42 years with 78.26 years for men and 82.69 years for women. Total expenditures on health as a percentage of the GDP amounted to 9.3% in 2011. On a per capita basis, $3,399 is spent on health care annually. The United Kingdom is a leading world financial power and trading center, with a capitalist economy. It has the third largest economy in Europe after Germany and France, ranking fourth largest in the world, with a per capita income of $37,300 (2013 estimate). Over the past 20 years, the government has decreased private ownership and has continued the growth in the direction of a welfare state. The United Kingdom produces 60% of its food and other needs through the efforts of only 1% of its labor force. Coal, natural gas, and oil supplies are available from domestic sources. Insurance, banking, and other business services provide for the high per capita incomes in the country. The United Kingdom is Europe's largest manufacturer of cars, armaments, computers, petroleum products, televisions, and mobile phones. It is ranked sixth in the world for tourism. Language spoken is mainly English, but other indigenous languages include Welsh, Scottish Gaelic, Irish Gaelic, Cornish, Lowland Scots, Romany, and British Sign Language (CIA, 2014e).

Health and Healthcare System

The National Health System (NHS) was established in 1948 to provide free health care for all residents of the United Kingdom. It was designed to be free at the point of need, meaning that every time a resident needs a doctor or receives inpatient hospital treatment, it is provided free of charge. This system is funded by federal taxation and run by the Department of Health. In addition, private healthcare providers are available; people pay for such services either through their insurance or as out-of-pocket expenses at the time of use (BBC, 2005).

There are 2.77 physicians per 1,000 people and hospital beds are 3 per 1,000 people. The net migration rate is 2.56 persons per 1,000 people. The maternal mortality rate is 12 per 100,000 live births; infant mortality rate is 4.44 deaths per 1,000 live births (CIA, 2014e).

Funding for health care comes from direct taxation. England, Northern Ireland, Scotland, and Wales each have their own systems of publicly funded health care that is free at the point of service. The United Kingdom's expenditure was 7.8% of the UK's GDP, about 1.45 above the average country in the European Union. Each NHS system also provides dental care through private dental practices.

The basic concepts underlying the U.K. healthcare system are

- Health care should be "free at the point of service." No copayments are needed for services.
- Health care is funded through income taxes.

- A strong primary healthcare base should be established for the NHS. Every U.K. resident should be able to choose a physician or healthcare service. The system also provides general practitioners (physicians) with incentives to practice in underserved areas.
- Reductions in the inequalities of health care have been made. Areas that have greater health problems and are poorer now receive more funding.
- Bonuses are given to general practitioners who reach population-based targets for health prevention.
- All subspecialists are paid on the same salary scale.
- Basic prescription drugs are price controlled, while research that produces new drugs is rewarded. The government works out an agreement with the private pharmaceutical companies to create price controls for drugs. In Northern Ireland, Scotland, and Wales there is no longer any prescription charges; however, in England, a prescription charge of 8.25 English pounds per item (2015) is charged for patients under 16 years of age (18 years if going to school full time) or over 60 years, and those with certain medical conditions (CIA, 2014e).

During the last few years, the private sector has funded some of the buildings and structures within the NHS, and some local communities are currently making some of their own healthcare decisions. Although there are differences in the healthcare system within each country in the United Kingdom, there is a single secretary of state for health, who answers to the U.K. parliament. The Department of Health is responsible for local planning, regulation, inspection, and policy development. Healthcare services are classified as either primary or secondary, and are managed by the local NHS organizations called trusts. The primary trusts are often outsourced to private companies. Primary care is delivered by local general practitioners, surgeons, dentists, and opticians (i.e., primary care trusts, or PCTs). The PCTs, who decide the amount and quality of services provided by hospitals, receive approximately 75% of the overall budget. In addition, the PCTs control hospital funding. Hospitals and specialized services, such as mental health, are managed by organizations called acute trusts. Usually, outpatient services such as surgery and ophthalmology have long waiting lists (CIA, 2014e).

Private health care offers similar services, and patients who use this system of care generally pay through private health insurance. Insurance premiums are paid by either employers or individuals who pay out of pocket by themselves. There are more than 300 private hospitals in the United Kingdom. The current situation of the NHS is that the current system is no longer sustainable and no longer affordable. If services were limited to only emergency and welfare service, however, the NHS approach would be economically feasible. In the future, specialty care services are likely to be united with primary care services. The system is failing to meet expectations because of underfunding and the fact that it is centrally controlled (National Health Service [NHS], 2015).

The NHS provides

- Comprehensive service to all people of all ages, genders, disabilities, race, sexual orientation, religion or belief, and respecting human rights.
- Access to the NHS is based on clinical need, not ability to pay.
- Care that aspires to the highest standards of excellence and professionalism to provide high-quality and safe care.

- A provision for the needs of patients, families, and caregivers.
- Work across organizational boundaries and in partnership with other organizations which are of interest to patients, the community, and the general population.

Rights to care include service that

- Is free of charge.
- Is nondiscriminatory.
- Never refuses on reasonable grounds.
- Is obtainable from any NHS provider or with preapproval from any EEA.
- Provides assessment by the local NHS to meet locally assessed needs.
- Provides patients with the right to drugs and treatments that have been recommended by their doctors if clinically appropriate for them.
- Provides the approved vaccinations under the NHS national immunization program.
- Offers respect, consent, and confidentiality (NHS, 2015).

Within the United Kingdom, there is a persistent disparity in health care and health issues. Scotland has the lowest life expectancy among the U.K. countries, at 74.6 years for men and 77.2 years for women, compared with 77.2 years for men and 81.5 years for women in England. The rate of hospital inpatient admissions varies from 205 per 1,000 population in Northern Ireland, to 135 per 1,000 population in Scotland. The death rate from heart disease is highest in Scotland and lowest in England. From 1996 to 2006, smoking rates among teens and young adults dropped 18% in England, 15% in Scotland, and 12% in Wales. An increased number of women are breastfeeding, with the highest rates (77%) seen in England and Wales; in contrast, only 64% of women breastfeed their children in Northern Ireland. The infant mortality rate in the United Kingdom is 1.8 deaths per 1,000 live births, higher than the IMR in many countries in the European Union, yet lower than the rate in the United States. The HIV rate within the general population is two cases per 1,000 adults (13–49 years) (CIA, 2014e).

Cardiovascular disease (CVD) and stroke are two of the major causes of death or disability on an annual basis (NHS, 2013). Heart attack deaths have decreased by 50% in less than a decade, according to a major study of more than 800,000 patients in England (NHS, 2012).

Deaths from heart and circulatory disease are falling, but it remains the UK's biggest killer. In 2009, over 180,000 people died from CVD in the United Kingdom—one in three of all deaths. Twenty-eight percent of premature deaths in men and almost 20% of premature deaths in women were from CVD in 2009. Stroke is the single largest cause of severe disability and the third most common cause of death in the United Kingdom. Each year 11,000 people die of stroke in England and Wales. Most people diagnosed with CVD or stroke take aspirin and lipid-reducing medications (British Heart Foundation, 2010).

Uncontrolled hypertension is the greatest cause of stroke. In the United Kingdom approximately 5.7 million adults, or 12% of the population older than 16 years, have a blood pressure exceeding 160/95 mm Hg. In addition, 10.3 million (21%) have a blood pressure of 140/90 mm Hg. An estimated 58,000 cardiovascular problems occur in these patients because of hypertension, which would not exist if the patients' blood pressure were within normal limits. Failure to control blood pressure contributes to huge monetary costs to the NHS for treating cardiovascular problems (NHS, 2015).

Cancer causes problems for one in four people, with the most common form (one-third) lung cancer. Eighty to 90% of all lung cancers are attributable to smoking. In women, 20% of all cancer cases involve breast cancer: England has one of the highest rates of breast cancer in all of Western Europe. Cancer in the United Kingdom is one of the three leading causes of death for people of all ages, except for preschool children. Cancer causes approximately 62,000 deaths per year (NHS, 2015).

Smoking has been identified as the single greatest preventable cause of illness and premature death in the United Kingdom. In this country, the overall smoking rates for all ages are 27% of men and 24% women, though these rates are higher among younger adults and lower among persons 75 years or older. Cigarette smoking in the United Kingdom has been found to increase as household income decreases (NHS, 2015).

Alcohol consumption has been reported by 42% of men and 26% of women in the United Kingdom, who stated that they consumed alcohol at least three days per week. Statistics on alcohol reveal that in 2002, 47% of men drank more than four units of alcohol at least one day in the previous week, and 22% of women drank at least three units of alcohol one day in the past week. Total expenditures on alcohol amounted to 5.7% of family income (NHS, 2012).

Overweight and obesity have been diagnosed in 65.4% of men and 55.5% of women in the United Kingdom. Overweight is defined as 25 kg/mm^2 and obesity as more than 30 kg/mm^2. Obesity rates are higher in lower-income households (Office of National Statistics UK, 2011).

Accidents account for 10,000 deaths per year in England. England has lower death rates from car accidents than anywhere else in Europe, but rates of death of children from pedestrian accidents are among the highest in Europe. Road accident rates are higher in rural areas than in larger cities. Older adults are at risk for death and disability from falls. Osteoporosis affects more women and contributes to the number of broken bones, especially wrists and hips, incurred by this population (NHS, 2015).

Infant and Child Health
In 2010 the infant mortality rate was 4.2 deaths per 1,000 live births, the lowest ever recorded for England and Wales. Infant mortality rates were high among babies of mothers aged under 20 years and over 40 years at 5.6 and 5.8 deaths per 1,000 live births respectively. Perinatal mortality rates were also higher for mothers in the under 20 and 40 and over age groups, at 8.3 and 10.2 deaths per 1,000 live births respectively. Very-low-birthweight babies (under 1,500 grams) had the highest infant and perinatal mortality rates, at 164.7 and 250.9 deaths per 1,000 live births, respectively. Infant mortality rates were highest for babies registered jointly by parents living at different addresses and those registered solely by their mother, at 5.5 and 5.4 deaths per 1,000 live births, respectively (NHS, 2015).

SUMMARY
Table 2-2 compares population and health statistics for Japan, Sweden, the United Kingdom, and the United States (Kaiser Family Foundation, 2011).

TABLE 2-2 Healthcare Statistics for Japan, Sweden, the United Kingdom, and the United States

Indicator	Date/Date Range	Data Type	Data			
			Japan	Sweden	United Kingdom	United States
Demography and Population						
Population	2011	Number	126,475,664	9,088,728	62,698,362	313,232,044
Adult sex ratio	2011	Number	1.02	1.02	1.03	1.00
Median age	2011	Number	44.8	42.0	40.0	36.9
Population younger than age 15	2010	%	13%	17%	18%	20%
Urban population	2010	%	86%	84%	80%	79%
Birth rate	2011	Rate per 1000	7.31	10.18	12.29	13.83
Total fertility rate	2011	Number	1.21	1.67	1.91	2.06
Contraceptive prevalence rate	2000–2010	%	54.3%	NA	84.0%	78.6%
Death rate	2011	Rate per 1000	10.09	10.20	9.33	8.38
Infant mortality rate	2011	Rate per 1000 2.78 2.74 4.62 6.06				
Female infant mortality rate	2011	Rate per 1000	2.58	2.57	4.15	5.37
Male infant mortality rate	2011	Rate per 1000	2.98 2	.90	5.07	6.72
Under-five mortality rate	2009	Rate per 1000	3	3	6	8
Maternal mortality ratio	2008	Rate per 100,000	6	5	12	24
Life expectancy: female	2009	Number	86	83	82	81
Life expectancy: male	2009	Number	80	79	78	76
Population growth rate	2011	%	–0.28%	0.16%	0.56%	0.96%

(continues)

TABLE 2-2 **Healthcare Statistics for Japan, Sweden, the United Kingdom, and the United States (*Continued*)**

Income and the Economy

GDP per capita	2009	U.S. dollars	$32,418	$37,377	$35,155	$45,989
GNI per capita	2009	U.S. dollars	$33,440	$38,050	$35,860	$45,640
Country income classification	As of July 2011	Text	High income	High income	High income	High Income

HIV/AIDS

People living with HIV/AIDS	Data from most recent year available	Number	8100	8100	85,000	1,200,000
Adults living with HIV/AIDS	2009	Number	8100	8100	85,000	1,200,000
Adult HIV/AIDS prevalence rate	2009	%	< 0.1%	0.1%	0.2%	0.6%
Women living with HIV/AIDS	Number of women living with HIV/AIDS and women as a percentage of adults living with HIV/ AIDS, 2009	%	33%	31%	31%	26%
Men living with HIV/AIDS	Number of men living with HIV/AIDS and men as a percentage of adults living with HIV/ AIDS, 2009	%	65%	69%	69%	77%
Children living with HIV/AIDS	2009	Number	NA	NA	NA	NA
AIDS deaths	2009	Number	<100	<100	<1000	17,000
AIDS orphans	2009	Number	NA	NA	NA	NA

Tuberculosis

Indicator	Year	Unit				
New TB cases	2009	Number	26,000	580	7400	13,000
People living with TB	2009	Number	33,000	750	9100	14,000
TB prevalence rate	2009	Rate per 100,000	26	8	15	5
TB death rate	2009	Rate per 100,000	1	0	1	0
TB incidence in HIV+ people	2009 Number	110	14	260	1300	
TB incidence in HIV+ people per 100,000 population	2009 Rate per	100,000	0	0	0	
HIV prevalence in incident TB cases	2009	%	0.4%	2.4%	3.5%	10.0%
Other Diseases, Conditions, and Risk Indicators						
DTP3 immunization coverage rate	2009	%	98%	98%	93%	95%
Percent with water	2008	%	100%	100%	100%	99%
Access to sanitation	2008	%	100%	100%	100%	100%
Population undernourished	2005–2007	%	NA	NA	NA	NA
Low-birth-weight babies	2000–2009	%	8%	NA	8%	8%
Child malnutrition	2000–2009	%	NA	NA	NA	1.3%
Female prevalence of obesity	2005	%	2%	11%	24%	42%
Male prevalence of obesity	2005	%	2%	12%	22%	37%
Female prevalence of smoking	2006	%	13%	23%	24%	19%
Male prevalence of smoking	2006	%	42.4%	17.3%	26.1%	25.4%

(continues)

TABLE 2-2 Healthcare Statistics for Japan, Sweden, the United Kingdom, and the United States (*Continued*)

Programs, Funding, and Financing			Japan	Sweden	United Kingdom	United States
Health expenditures per capita	2008	$	$2817	$3622	$3222	$7164
Total expenditures on health	2008	%	8.3%	9.4%	8.7%	15.2%
Government health expenditures as a percentage of total government expenditures	2008	%	17.9%	13.8%	15.1%	18.7%
Government health expenditures as a percentage of total health expenditures	2008	%	80.5%	78.1%	82.6%	47.8%
Social security expenditures on health	2008	%	81.5%	0.0%	0.0%	27.8%
Out-of-pocket expenditures on health	2008	%	80.6%	92.8%	63.7%	24.4%
Health Workforce and Capacity						
Physicians	2000–2010	Rate per 10,000	21	36	27 2	7
Nurses and midwives	2000–2010	Rate per 10,000	41	116	103	98
Community health workers	2000–2010	Rate per 10,000	NA	NA	NA	NA
Births attended by skilled health personnel	2000–2010	%	100%	NA	NA	99%
Hospital beds	2000–2009	Rate per 10,000	139	NA	39	31

This chapter has examined the health and health care of the countries of the United States, Sweden, Japan, and the United Kingdom. Included in this comparison were population statistics, types of government healthcare programs, economics and healthcare spending, and healthcare personnel.

Study Questions

1. Why do you think the United States has the world's highest rate of obesity? How does this problem relate to chronic health diseases such as cardiovascular disease, hypertension, and diabetes?
2. In spite of the country having the highest level of per capita expenditures, why does the United States still have a relatively high rate of infant mortality as compared to other developed countries?
3. What are some reasons that contribute to Japan and Sweden having the world's best longevity rates? Even though it spends the most dollars per capita on health care, why is the United States so far behind in terms of longevity?
4. What are some health disparities within the United Kingdom, and how might they be solved?

Case Study: Addressing U.S. American Indians (Native Americans)/Alaskan Natives and Diabetes

The mortality rate for American Indians, which includes Alaskan Natives (Native Americans), has increased primarily due to the effects of type 2 diabetes. The U.S. Department of Indian Health Service has provided a Special Diabetes Program for Indians resulting in increased spending for health care; however, the rate for age-adjusted deaths has increased as compared to white Americans.

Infectious diseases are decreasing while chronic diseases, such as type 2 diabetes, are increasing in this population. Data collected were mainly from Navaho Indians living in the western part of the United States. Other major health issues include obesity, cardiovascular diseases, smoking, and hypertension. Also discussed was the high rate of sedentary lifestyles as compared to historically much greater daily physical activities.

Case Study Questions

1. Create a culturally congruent plan for reduction of exceptionally high levels of type 2 diabetes among American Indians/Alaskan Natives.
2. Why do American Indians have higher levels of increased smoking, obesity, and sedentary life styles, which contribute to the type 2 diabetes rates than whites?
3. Why is the Indian Health Service an important part of health care that is historically "owed" to American Indians/Alaskan Natives?

Data from Kunitz, S. (2008). Changing patterns of mortality among American Indians. *American Journal of Public Health, 98*(3), 404–411.

References

American Hospital Association. (2014). *Trends affecting hospitals and health systems*. Retrieved from http://www.aha.org/research/reports/tw/chartbook/ch3.shtml

British Heart Foundation. (2010). *CVD in the UK*. Retrieved from http://www.bhf.org.uk/heart-health/statistics/mortality.aspx

Centers for Disease Control and Prevention. (2014a). *Causing of death in the U.S.* Retrieved from http://www.cdc.gov/nchs/fastats/health-expenditures.htm

Centers for Disease Control and Prevention. (2014b). *U.S. overweight and obesity*. Retrieved from http://www.cdc.gov/obesity/data/

Centers for Disease Control and Prevention. (2014c). *National vital statistics system*. Retrieved from http://www.cdc.gov/nchs/nvss.htm

Centers for Disease Control and Prevention. (2014d). *Adult cigarette smoking in the U.S.* Retrieved from http://www.cdc.gov/tobacco/campaign/tips/resources/data/cigarette-smoking-in-united-states.html

Centers for Disease Control and Prevention. (2014e). *Healthy People 2020*. Retrieved from http://www.cdc.gov/nchs/healthy_people/hp2020.htm

Centers for Disease Control and Prevention. (2014f). *Health disparities*. Retrieved from http://www.healthypeople.gov/2020/about/foundation-health-measures/Disparities

Centers for Disease Control and Prevention. (2014g). *Prescription drug use*. Retrieved from http://www.cdc.gov/nchs/data/hus/hus13.pdf

Centers for Disease Control and Prevention. (2014h). *Minority health*. Black. Retrieved from http://www.cdc.gov/minorityhealth/populations/REMP/black.html

Centers for Disease Control and Prevention. (2014i). *Hispanic health*. Retrieved from http://www.cdc.gov/minorityhealth/populations/REMP/hispanic.html

Centers for Disease Control and Prevention. (2014j). *Child health*. Retrieved from http://www.cdc.gov/nchs/fastats/child-health.htm

Centers for Disease Control and Prevention. (2014k). *Aging*. Retrieved from http://www.cdc.gov/aging/data/

Centers for Disease Control and Prevention. (2015). *National Center for Health Statistics*. Retrieved from http://www.cdc.gov/nchs/

Central Intelligence Agency. (2014a). *Infant mortality rates*. Retrieved from https://www.cia.gov/library/publications/the-world-factbook/rankorder/2091rank.html

Central Intelligence Agency. (2014b). *U.S. unemployment rates*. Retrieved from https://www.cia.gov/library/publications/the-world-factbook/rankorder/2129rank.html

Central Intelligence Agency. (2014c). *Ethnic groups*. Retrieved from https://www.cia.gov/library/publications/the-world-factbook/fields/2075.html

Central Intelligence Agency. (2014d). *Japan*. Retrieved from https://www.**cia**.gov/library/.../ja.htm

Central Intelligence Agency. (2014e). *United Kingdom*. Retrieved from https://www.cia.gov/library/publications/the-world-factbook/geos/uk.html

Central Intelligence Agency. (2015). *World Factbook*. United States. Retrieved from https://www.cia.gov/library/publications/the-world-factbook/geos/us.html

Government Offices of Sweden Ministry of Health, 2014. (2014). *Ministry of Health*. Retrieved from http://www.government.se/sb/d/2061

Health Care Financing. (2014). Retrieved from http://www.merckmanuals.com/home/fundamentals/financial_issues_in_health_care/overview_of_health_care_financing.html

Infoplease. (2011). *The 2011 nuclear crisis in Japan*. Retrieved from http://www.infoplease.com/world/disasters/japan-nuclear-2011.html

Infoplease. (2014). *Life expectancy at birth for countries*. Retrieved from http://www.infoplease.com/world/statistics/life-expectancy-country.html

Kaiser Family Foundation. (2011). *State health facts*. Retrieved from http://statehealthfacts.org/

Kunitz, S. (2008). Changing patterns of mortality among American Indians. *American Journal of Public Health, 98*(3), 404–411.

Makenzius, M. & Larsson, M. (2012). Early onset of sexual intercourse is an indicator for hazardous lifestyle and problematic life situation. *Scandinavian Journal of Caring Sciences, 27*(1), 20–26. doi: 10.1111/scs.2013.27-1/issuetoc

McGlade, M., Saha, S., & Dahlstrom, M. (2012). The "Latina epidemiologic paradox": Contrasting patterns of adverse birth outcomes in U.S.-born and foreign-born Latinas. *Women's Health Issues, 22*(5), 501–507. doi: 10.1016/j.whi.2012.07.005

National Health Service. (2012). *Massive decline in deadly heart attacks*. Retrieved from http://www.nhs.uk/news/2012/01January/Pages/heart-attack-death-rate-reduction.aspx

National Health Service. (2015). *About the NHS: Overview*. Retrieved from http://www.bing.com/search?q=National+Health+Service+UK&FORM=R5FD

National Institute on Alcohol Abuse and Alcoholism. (2014). Retrieved from http://www.niaaa.nih.gov/

NationMaster.com. (2010). Retrieved from http://www.nationalmaster.com/country/ja-japan/hea-health

Obamacare Facts. (2014). Retrieved from http://obamacarefacts.com/obamacare-facts/

Occupational Safety and Health Administration. (2014). Retrieved from https://www.osha.gov/

Office of National Statistics UK. (2011). *Infant and perinatal mortality in England and Wales by social and biological factors, 2010*. Retrieved from http://www.ons.gov.uk/ons/rel/child-health/infant-and-perinatal-mortality-in-england-and-wales-by-social-and-biological-factors/2010/index.html

Pew Hispanic Center. (2011). *Hispanics account for more than half of the nation's growth in a decade*. Retrieved from http://www.pewhispanic.org/2011/03/24/hispanics-account-for-more-than-half-of-nations-growth-in-past-decade/

Satcher, D., Fryer, G., McCann, I., Troutman, A., Woolf, S., & Rust, G. (2005). What if we were equal? A comparison of the black-white mortality gap in 1960 and 2000. *Health Affairs, 24*(2), 459–463.

Shibuya, K. (2011, October 1). The future of Japan's system of good health at low cost with equity: Beyond universal coverage. *The Lancet, 378*(9798), 1265–1273. doi:101016/SO140-6736(11)61098-2

Stevens, S. (2004). Reform strategies for the English NHS. *Health Affairs, 23*(3), 37–44.

Sullivan Commission. (2004). Missing persons: Minorities in health professions. In *The Sullivan report*, pp. 1–208.

Szebehely, M. & Trydegard, G. (2012). Homecare for older people in Sweden: A universal model in transition. *Health and Social Care in the Community, 20*(3), 300–309. doi: 10.1111/j.1365-2524.2011.0146xEpub2011Dec5

U.S. Census Bureau. (2015). *Population profile*. Retrieved from http://www.census.gov/

U.S. Department of Health and Human Services. (2015). *Poverty guidelines*. Retrieved from http://aspe.hhs.gov/poverty/15poeverty.efm

U.S. Department of Labor. (2015). *Bureau of Labor Statistics unemployment rates*. Retrieved from http://data.bls.gov/timeseries/LNS14000000

The World Bank. (2014). *World Development Report*. Retrieved from http://data.worldbank.org/data-catalog/world-development-report-2014

World Health Organization. (2013a). *US health expenditures*. Retrieved from http://www.cdc.gov/nchs/fastats/health-expenditures.htm

World Health Organization. (2013b). *Sweden*. Retrieved from http://www.who.int/countries/swe/en/

World Health Organization. (2014a). *Japan. Health profile*. Retrieved from http://www.who.int/countries/jpn/en/

World Health Organization. (2014b). *United States of America. Health profile*. Retrieved from http://www.who.int/countries/usa/en/

Developing Countries: Egypt, China, India, and South Africa

Carol Holtz and Ibrahim Elsawy

Objectives

After completing this chapter, the reader will be able to:

1. Discuss family planning, infertility, abortion, and sterilization practices in Egypt, China, India, and South Africa.
2. Explain how communism affects health and health care in China.
3. Discuss women's rights issues in South Africa.
4. Compare the health and healthcare systems of Egypt, China, India, and South Africa.

INTRODUCTION

This chapter addresses the health conditions of four developing countries: Egypt, China, India, and South Africa. These countries were selected for examination because they differ in culture, economics, politics, geographic regions, and types of health care and health issues.

EGYPT

Background

Egypt (the Arab Republic of Egypt) is located in the far northeastern part of the African continent, bordered on the north by the Mediterranean Sea, on the east by the Red Sea, on the west by Libya, on the south by Sudan, and on the northeast by the Gaza Strip and Israel. Egypt is traversed by the Suez Canal, which is located between its Asian and African territories.

The country's total land area is 1,002,450 square kilometers. Most of Egypt is located in Africa, but part of its land, the Sinai Peninsula, is located in Asia. The majority of its population of approximately 83 million people live on the banks of the Nile River or on the coasts of the Mediterranean Sea, the Red Sea, and the Suez Canal. The Nile River flows northward from Egypt from Sudan and into the Mediterranean Sea. The largest defined landmass within Egypt is the Sahara Desert, which is very sparsely populated. The largest cities include Cairo (the capital), Alexandria, and other cities in the Nile Delta. Ninety-eight percent of the Egyptian population live on just 4% of the country's land (Arab Republic of Egypt, 2010).

Most of Egypt's rainfall occurs during the winter months, with only 0.1 to 0.2 inches of precipitation falling each year. Before the construction of the Aswan Dam, the Nile River flooded annually, producing good soil and good harvests in its floodplains. Arabic is the official language; English and French are the most commonly used foreign languages. The majority ethnic groups are Egyptian, Bedouin Arab, and Nubian. Education is compulsory for children aged 6 to 15 years, and the literacy rate is 58% (About Egypt, 2010).

Egypt has a distinguished cultural heritage, accumulated over the thousands of years of its history. Most of Egypt's famous landmarks were built during the Pharaonic period, which includes more than 50 pyramids and many temples located along the Nile. Each of the Egyptian successive civilizations (Pharaonic, Greco-Roman, Coptic, and Islamic) contributed to the areas of philosophy, literature, and the arts. Because of its long-held ties with Europe, Egypt has been a cultural pioneer in the modern Arab world. In 2002, with the support of the United Nations Educational, Scientific and Cultural Organization (UNESCO), the new Bibliotheca Alexandria was inaugurated. This world-recognized special historical site is located in Alexandria. The goal of the reconstruction of the ancient Library of Alexandria is to revive the legacy of this universal center for science and knowledge (About Egypt, 2010).

Egypt has a legislative body comprised of the House of Representatives and the Shura Council, or Majilis al-Shura. The Shura Council is composed of at least 150 members, one-tenth of whom were appointed by the president (Saleh, 2013).

The Egyptian population consists of 94% Muslims and 6% Christians. The two main Islamic institutions in Egypt are the oldest and the most important Islamic institutions in the country:

- Al-Azhar, built by the Fatimids to spread the Shiite sect in North Africa. Later Salah El-Din converted it to Sunni University, which became one of the main pillars of Sunni Islam in the world.
- Dar el Eftaa, founded in 1895 and headed by the Grand Mufti of Egypt.

The Coptic Orthodox Church, one of the oldest Christian churches in the world, and the Roman Orthodox Church of the Arab Republic of Egypt are located in Alexandria (Arab Republic of Egypt, 2010).

Economy

Table 3-1 presents statistics on Egypt's current economy.

TABLE 3-1 Egypt's Economy

GDP	$218.91 billion
GDP growth	5.2% per year
Inflation, GDP deflator	10.1% per year
Agriculture, value added	10% of GDP
Industry, value added	29% of GDP
Services and other revenue sources, value added	61% of GDP
Exports of goods and services	21% of GDP
Imports of goods and services	28% of GDP
Gross capital formation	19% of GDP

Data from The World Bank. (2010). Arab Republic of Egypt.

Health

Table 3-2 presents population health statistics for Egypt.

Healthcare Systems

The majority of Egyptians have access to health care for basic health services, managed by the Ministry of Health and Population (MOHP), the Health Insurance Organization (HIO), private health practitioners, and nongovernmental organizations (NGOs). The HIO covers 45% of the population, and there is a growing and unregulated private healthcare sector. Pharmaceuticals account for nearly one-third of all healthcare costs (WHO, 2011a).

Communicable Diseases

Within the last decade there has been a huge decline in deaths from communicable diseases in Egypt, largely due to the high rate of vaccinations for preventable diseases. Schistosomiasis (a parasitic disease caused by flatworms), TB, malaria, and HIV, as well as Hepatitis A, B, and C remain the most serious infectious diseases today (WHO, 2011a). In addition, there is an increasing burden of antibiotic resistance. The incidence of TB in Egypt is 25 per 100,000 (2010 statistics). Of those in Egypt with TB, 16 to 40% are antibiotic resistant (Mohamoud, Mumtaz, Riome, Miller, & Abu-Raddad, 2013).

HIV in Egypt, as is the case with other Arab countries, carries tremendous stigma. The prevalence rate is <.1% but may be higher. One problem is a lack of knowledge of the disease due to the culturally conservative background of the people of the area. Malaria has been identified from Egyptian mummies from their DNA, which suggests that this disease has existed since antiquity. The Al-Fayoum Governorate in the northwestern part of Egypt today has a high rate of malaria risk. Up to 69% of the population of this area is infected, particularly the children (Boutros & Skordis, 2010).

TABLE 3-2 Egypt's Population Health Statistics, 2011

Birth rate	28.9 per 1,000
Underweight children	7.5%
Population younger than age 15 years	31.7%
Population 65 years or older	3.7%
Total births per woman	3
Adult literacy rate (among persons 15 years or older)	71%
Population with sustainable access to improved water sources	94%
Population with sustainable access to improved sanitation	94%
Smoking rate of adults	19%
Total government expenditure per capita on health	$124
Total government expenditure on health as a percentage of GDP	6.4%
Out-of-pocket expenditure on health per capita	58.7%
Human Resources (per 10,000)	
Physicians	28.3
Dentists	4.2
Pharmacists	16.7
Nurses and midwives	35.2
Hospital beds	17.3
Primary healthcare units and centers	0.7
Primary Health Care (per 100)	
Population with access to healthcare services	88
Contraception prevalence	57.6
Prenatal care	52
Births attended by skilled personnel	84
Health Status	
Life expectancy	72.3 years
Infant mortality rate (per 1,000 live births)	17
Under-five mortality rate	21.8 per 1,000
Maternal mortality rate	55 per 100,000
Probability of not reaching 40 years of age	10.3%
Smoking prevalence (among males 15 years or older)	40%

Data from World Health Organization. (2011a). *Egypt: Country health profile.* Retrieved from http://www.who.int/gho/countries/egy/country_profiles/en/.

The hepatitis C (HCV) rate in Egypt is the highest in the world, with a rate of 14.9% of the population. It is estimated that 100,000 to 500,000 new cases are reported annually. The incident rate reported by the Minister of Health is 6.9 per 1,000 people. Historically, the high rate of this disease is linked to the widespread use of parenteral tartar emetic and the use of unsterilized needles and reuse of glass syringes. Currently in Egypt there is a public education prevention program to curb future infection transmissions of hepatitis C (Mohamoud, Mumtaz, Riome, Miller, & Abu-Raddad, 2013; Waked et al., 2014).

A study conducted in Egypt and supported by USAID to prevent typhoid fever in rural communities used the intervention of handwashing with soap. Studies indicate that 9,000 to 42,000 cases of typhoid are reported each year. Typhoid fever is transmitted by the fecal–oral route, so it is appropriate to build prevention strategies against this infection—yet only 40% of all households in Egypt had soap and water available for handwashing at the time the intervention was undertaken. The scarcity of water and problems with waste disposal are related issues for handwashing. As part of the intervention, proper handwashing techniques were taught, and general education of disease transmission was performed. Results indicated improvement in handwashing rates in the rural Fayoum region of Egypt (Lohinivak, El-Sayeed, & Talaat, 2008).

Maternal and Infant Health

Despite health clinics that are accessible to the general public, maternal and infant mortality rates in Egypt are high, with an infant mortality rate of 17 deaths per 1,000 live births and a maternal mortality rate of 55 deaths per 1,000 live births. In addition, the 21.8 per 1,000 death rate for children younger than five is considered high. These rates reflect exceptionally high mortality rates among women and children in rural Upper Egypt. Child survival initiatives, such as cord care, delivery instrument antisepsis, and infant warming have reduced the rate of mortality of children younger than five (Darmstadt et al., 2009).

As is true in most developing countries, most births in Egypt take place in the home. A major contributing factor to maternal and infant morbidity and mortality is unhygienic conditions, which increase the likelihood of infections within both the mother and the newborn. Tetanus typhoid immunization is one method of reducing deaths due to tetanus, but many other infections can occur at the time of birth. Infection ranks third among the causes of maternal mortalities in Egypt. A cohort study explored the use of a clean delivery kit as a means of reducing infant and maternal infections. Kits were distributed from primary health facilities, and birth attendants received training on how to use the kits. Results from the study of 334 women indicated that neonates of mothers who had the use of the kits were less likely to develop sepsis from cord infection and mothers had fewer postpartum infections (Darmstadt et al., 2009).

Pregnancy outcomes in Egypt are poorer as compared to those in other developing nations with similar per capita gross national products (GDPs). The national rate of low birth weight in Egypt is 12% of all live births, but for 30% of low-birth-weight infants in Egypt, the mortality rate is 2.5 times that of full-term infants. These increased risks of mortality for low-birth-weight children persist throughout the first year of life and beyond, with this risk factor also associated with increased cognitive disabilities. A special antenatal nutrition project in Al-Minia, in Upper Egypt, demonstrated an ability to improve birth weight in newborns. Women in this project received food supplements and nutrition education as well as prenatal care and home visits. Results indicated that infant birth weights increased, which ultimately resulted in healthier babies who were less likely to contribute to the infant mortality rate (Ahrani et al., 2006).

Noncommunicable Diseases

Neuropsychiatric (19.8%), digestive diseases (11.5%), chronic respiratory diseases (6.9%), cardiovascular diseases (6.7%), and diabetes are major noncommunicable diseases whose incidence continues to increase in Egypt. Smoking, substance abuse, failure to use car seats and seat belts, lack of exercise, and consumption of fatty and salty foods are major contributors to the disease burden. Diabetes mellitus affects nearly 3.9 million people in Egypt, and its prevalence is expected to increase to 9 million by 2025. A study conducted in 2011 in Cairo indicated that type 1 diabetes mellitus care needs to be carefully monitored, as complication rates were nearly 50% among patients in the study. Regular exercise for patients in this study demonstrated a significant positive effect for children and adolescents (Ismail, 2011).

The rate of diabetes in Egypt has significantly increased and Egypt is now ranked eighth highest in the world in diabetes incidence. According to a research study conducted in 2010 by the Zagazig University School of Medicine, the number of people with diabetes rose to 16.5 million people: half of this group did not know they had the disease, and the other half was receiving treatment. The disease has risen 83% over the past 15 years—a very large increase compared to international rates. The Middle East and the Arab world are the countries suffering from diabetes the most, specifically Egypt and the Gulf countries. The increase of the disease is due to unhealthy lifestyles and poor nutritional habits, in addition to genetic factors (Abdo & Mohamed, 2010).

Table 3-3 lists the top five most frequently occurring cancers in Egypt. Breast cancer accounts for 38% of all new cancer cases among women living in this country. The age-standardized rate (ASR) for breast cancer incidence in Egypt is 37.3 per 100,000, and the mortality rate is 20.1 per 100,000. Incidence of breast cancer is lower in Egyptian women than in U.S. women, possibly due to a lower rate of cancer screening, and mortality rates for Egyptian women are higher than those for U.S. women (WHO, 2010).

TABLE 3-3 Top Five Cancers in Egypt		
Males	**Females**	**Both Sexes**
1. Bladder	1. Breast	1. Breast
2. Liver	2. Non-Hodgkin's lymphoma	2. Bladder
3. Non-Hodgkin's lymphoma	3. Ovary	3. Non-Hodgkin's lymphoma
4. Lung	4. Colorectal	4. Liver
5. Leukemia	5. Leukemia	5. Leukemia
Data from World Health Organization. (2011a). *Egypt: Country health profile.* Retrieved from http://www.who.int/gho/countries/egy/country_profiles/en/		

Mortality and Burden of Disease

Table 3-4 provides child mortality data for Egypt in 2009 and 2010. Table 3-5 lists adult mortality rates, defined as the probability of dying between 15 and 60 years of age per 100,000 population; a breakout is provided for the maternal mortality rate. Table 3-6 identifies age-standardized mortality rates by cause. Table 3-7 lists causes of death for Egyptian children younger

TABLE 3-4 Child Mortality in Egypt, 2009 and 2010

	Year	Rates
Under-five mortality rate (probability of dying by age 5 per 1,000 live births)	2010	22
Number of under-five deaths (thousands)	2010	41
Infant mortality rate (probability of dying between birth and age 1 per 1,000 live births)	2010	19
Number of infant deaths (thousands)	2010	35
Neonatal mortality rate (per 1,000 live births)	2010	9
Number of neonatal deaths (thousands)	2010	18
Stillbirth rate (per 1,000 total births)	2009	13

Data from World Health Organization. (2011a). *Egypt: Country health profile.* Retrieved from http://www.who.int/gho/countries/egy/country_profiles/en/

TABLE 3-5 Adult Mortality in Egypt, 2008 and 2009

	Year	Number of Deaths Among Persons Aged 15–60 Years per 1,000 Population
Male	2009	215
Female	2009	130
Both sexes	2009	174
Maternal mortality ratio (per 100,000 live births; interagency estimates)	2008	82 (range: 51–130)

Data from World Health Organization. (2011a). *Egypt: Country health profile.* Retrieved from http://www.who.int/gho/countries/egy/country_profiles/en/

TABLE 3-6 Age-Standardized Mortality Rates by Cause, 2008 (per 100,000 population)

Mortality rate from communicable disease	76
Mortality rate from noncommunicable disease	749
Mortality rate from injuries	34

Data from World Health Organization. (2011a). *Egypt: Country health profile.* Retrieved from http://www.who.int/gho/countries/egy/country_profiles/en/

TABLE 3-7   Causes of Death Among Children Younger Than Age Five Years, 2008 (percentage of all deaths)

Prematurity	30
Pneumonia	11
Diarrhea	6
Birth asphyxia	5
Injuries	5
Neonatal sepsis	1
HIV/AIDS	0
Measles	0
Malaria	0
Other	23

Data from World Health Organization. (2011a). *Egypt: Country health profile.* Retrieved from http://www.who.int/gho/countries/egy/country_profiles/en/

TABLE 3-8   HIV/AIDS, Malaria, and Tuberculosis in Egypt, 2008 and 2009

	Year	Data (Range)
Deaths due to HIV/AIDS (per 100,000 population per year)	2009	0.6 (0.5–0.9)
Deaths due to malaria (per 100,000 population per year)	2008	0.2 (0.1–0.2)
Deaths due to tuberculosis among HIV-negative people (per 100,000 population per year)	2009	1.10 (0.74–1.50)
Prevalence of HIV among adults aged 15 to 49 (%)	2009	<0.1
Incidence of tuberculosis (per 100,000 population per year)	2009	19.0 (16.0–22.0)
Prevalence of tuberculosis (per 100,000 population)	2009	30.0 (13.0–49.0)

Data from World Health Organization. (2011a). *Egypt: Country health profile.* Retrieved from http://www.who.int/gho/countries/egy/country_profiles/en/

than age five. Table 3-8 provides mortality data related to HIV/AIDS, tuberculosis, and malaria.

Road Traffic Injuries

Road traffic injuries are a major cause of mortality and morbidity worldwide. Estimates in Egypt indicate 42 deaths per 100,000 of the population, which is one of the highest of the Eastern Mediterranean region. The high burden of road traffic injuries and deaths include pedestrians, children, and those on bicycles and motorcycles (WHO, 2012a).

Female Circumcision

Female circumcision has been a tradition in Egypt since the Pharaonic period. The prevalence of female circumcision is widespread in Egypt; 91% of all women age 15 to 49 have been circumcised and 94 to 96% of women older than 49 have been circumcised. Urban women are less likely to be circumcised than rural women. The likelihood that a woman is circumcised also declines with the woman's education level and is markedly lower among women in the highest wealth quintile than in other quintiles (78% versus 92% or higher). The majority of circumcised women (63%) report that (midwives) were responsible for performing the procedure. Trained medical personnel (primarily doctors) performed most of the remaining circumcisions (Egypt Demographic and Health Survey, 2008). Girls in Egypt usually undergo the procedure prior to or around puberty. According to the Department of Health, doctors in Egypt carry out a large majority (72%) of circumcisions in girls under 17 years and dayas (traditional birth attendants) perform 21%. The issue of marriageability is often cited as the strongest motivation for circumcision. The expectation is that if a woman is not circumcised in a community where this is the norm, the girl's chances of getting married will be severely reduced and high social status and livelihood will be endangered (Fahmy, El-Mouelhy, & Ragab, 2010).

Spousal Violence in Egypt

Nearly three-fourths of women visiting family health centers in Alexandria, Egypt, have experienced spousal violence in their lifetimes. Approximately half of the women experienced physical violence (Spousal Violence in Egypt, 2010). Violence against women and exposure to physical abuse is common in Egypt as in other parts of the Arab world. A study of 5,249 married women within a 12-month period of time revealed women's experiences with physical violence by their husbands. The study indicated a 29.4% exposure rate, 60% of those who experienced marital violence were exposed within the last 12 months, with the majority of women not having any medical insurance for treatments (El-Rashidi, 2013; Monazea & Khalek, 2010).

Mental Health

A national household survey of prevalence of disorders in five governorates, using the Mini International Neuropsychiatric Interview–Plus (MINI-Plus) instrument, indicated that almost 17% (range: 11 to 25.4% in different governorates) of adults in Egypt had mental disorders, with the common being mood disorders (6.4%), anxiety disorders (4.9%), and somatoform disorders (0.6%). Psychoses were seen in 0.3% of the population (WHO, 2005).

Environmental Problems

Air pollution, especially in Cairo and Alexandria, is a major source of chronic respiratory diseases. According to the Country Cooperation Study, Egypt receives 98% of its fresh water from the Nile River; unfortunately, there is excessive water pollution in the Nile due to large discharges of pesticides, nutrients, and heavy metals from industry in Cairo, making obtaining clean water a major health challenge for the country's population. Tap water assessments indicate that lead levels are at a high risk level as well. A recommendation by the WHO suggested that lead and other heavy metal residuals should be lowered for health safety of the population (Lasheen, El-Kholy, Sharaby, Elsherif, & El-Wakeel, 2008).

Egypt's Response to the Millennium Development Goals

Tables 3-9 to 3-15, presented in this subsection, profile Egypt's responses to WHO's Millennium Development Goals (WHO, 2011a):

- Millennium Development Goal MDG 1: Poverty and hunger (see Table 3-9).
- Millennium Development Goal MDG 4: Child mortality (see Table 3-10).
- Millennium Development Goal MDG 5: Maternal health.
  - Maternal mortality (see Table 3-11).
  - Births attended by skilled health personnel, 2008: 79%.
  - Reproductive health (see Table 3-12).
- Millennium Development Goal MDG 6: HIV/AIDS, malaria, and other diseases (see Table 3-13).

TABLE 3-9   Egypt: Hunger Indicators, 2008

	Male	Female	Both Sexes
Percentage of children younger than 5 years who are underweight	8.1	5.4	6.8
Percentage of children younger than 5 years who are stunted	33	28.4	30.7

Data from World Health Organization. (2011a). *Egypt: Country health profile.* Retrieved from http://www.who.int/gho/countries/egy/country_profiles/en/

TABLE 3-10   Egypt: Child Mortality Indicators, 2009 and 2010

	Year	Data
Under-five mortality rate (probability of dying by age 5 per 1,000 live births)	2010	22
Number of under-five deaths (thousands)	2010	41
Infant mortality rate (probability of dying between birth and age 1 per 1,000 live births)	2010	19
Number of infant deaths (thousands)	2010	35
Measles (MCV) immunization coverage among 1-year-olds (%)	2009	95

Data from World Health Organization. (2011a). Egypt: Country health profile. Retrieved from http://www.who.int/gho/countries/egy/country_profiles/en/

TABLE 3-11 Egypt: Maternal Mortality Indicators, 2008

Maternal mortality ratio (per 100,000 live births; interagency estimates)	82 (range: 51–130)
Births attended by skilled health personnel	79%

Data from World Health Organization. (2011a). *Egypt: Country health profile.* Retrieved from http://www.who.int/gho/countries/egy/country_profiles/en/

TABLE 3-12 Egypt: Reproductive Health Indicators, 2006 and 2008

	Year	Data
Contraceptive prevalence	2008	60.3%
Contraceptive prevalence, among women aged 15–19	2008	23.4%
Adolescent fertility rate (per 1,000 girls aged 15–19 years)	2006	50
Antenatal care coverage: at least one visit	2008	74%
Antenatal care coverage: at least one visit, among women aged 15–19	2008	76.5%
Antenatal care coverage: at least four visits	2008	66%
Unmet need for family planning	2008	9.2%
Unmet need for family planning: women aged 15–19	2008	7.9%
Births attended by skilled health personnel, among women aged 15–19	2008	78.8%

Data from World Health Organization. (2011a). *Egypt: Country health profile.* Retrieved from http://www.who.int/gho/countries/egy/country_profiles/en/

TABLE 3-13 Egypt: HIV/AIDS, Malaria, and Tuberculosis Indicators, 2008 and 2009

	Year	Data
Prevalence of HIV among adults aged 15–49 (%)	2009	<0.1
Deaths due to malaria (per 100,000 population per year)	2008	0.2 (0.1–0.2)
Incidence of tuberculosis (per 100,000 population per year)	2009	19.0 (16.0–22.0)
Prevalence of tuberculosis (per 100,000 population)	2009	30.0 (13.0–49.0)
Deaths due to tuberculosis among HIV-negative people (per 100,000 population per year)	2009	1.10 (0.74–1.50)
Case detection rate for all forms of tuberculosis	2009	63 (54–75)
Smear-positive tuberculosis treatment: success rate (%)	2008	89

Data from World Health Organization. (2011b). *Global health observatory data repository.* Retrieved from http://apps.who.int/ghodata/?vid=710

- Millennium Development Goal MDG 7: Environment sustainability (see Table 3-14).
- Not a Millennium Development Goal MDG. The following is a table relating summarizes nutrition in Egypt (Table 3-15).

TABLE 3-14 Egypt: Water and Sanitation Indicators, 2008

	Urban	Rural	Total
Population using improved drinking-water sources	100%	98%	99%
Population using improved sanitation facilities	97%	92%	94%

Data from World Health Organization. (2011b). *Global health observatory data repository.* Retrieved from http://apps.who.int/ghodata/?vid=710

TABLE 3-15 Egypt: Nutrition Indicators, 2008

	Male	Female	Both Sexes
Children younger than 5 years: overweight	19.8%	21.2%	20.5%
Children younger than 5 years: stunted	33%	28.4%	30.7%
Children younger than 5 years: underweight	8.1%	5.4%	6.8%
Children younger than 5 years: wasted for age	8.8%	7.1%	7.9%

Data from World Health Organization. (2011a). *Egypt: Country health profile.* Retrieved from http://www.who.int/gho/countries/egy/country_profiles/en/

Traditional Health

In the Arab Republic of Egypt, a national policy on traditional medicine/complementary alternative medicine (TM/CAM) is part of the national drug policy that was issued in 2001. Herbal medicine regulation in Egypt began in 1955, and is achieved through the same laws as are applied to conventional pharmaceuticals. Herbal medicines are regulated in the forms of prescription medicines, over-the-counter medicines, self-medication, and dietary supplements. Control mechanisms exist for both manufacturing and safety assessment requirements. There are 600 registered herbal medicines, though no herbal medicines are included on the national essential drugs list. In Egypt, herbal medicines are sold in pharmacies by licensed practitioners as over-the-counter products and as prescription medicines (WHO, 2011a).

Care of the Aging in Egypt

As life expectancy in Egypt is increasing with great morbidity, aging is becoming a greater social and health issue in Egypt, especially for lower- and middle-class people due to economic restrictions and lifestyle changes. Women are working during the day, and there is no one home to care for the older adults in many households. There is currently a shortage of institutions providing in- and out-patient care. Geriatric homes (nursing homes) are needed to reduce caregiver strain in families (Boggatz & Dassen, 2005).

CHINA

Description

China is the world's fourth-largest country in area (after the countries of Russia, Canada, and the United States), and is located in east Asia, bordering numerous countries, including the Russian

Federal Republic, India, Pakistan, Vietnam, and Mongolia. China, which is slightly smaller than the United States, has climates varying from tropical in the south to subarctic in the north. At present it has a great amount of air pollution—mostly greenhouse gases and sulfur dioxide particles from use of coal and other carbon-based fuels. It also has water pollution, hazardous waste, deforestation, and soil erosion problems (Central Intelligence Agency [CIA], 2011a).

Population

As of 2012, China has a population of 1.39 billion people (WHO, 2014a). Health and vital statistics of the Chinese population, as compiled by the World Health Organization (2014a), include the following:

Sex ratio: 1.333 males to 1 female
Infant mortality rate: 16 per 1,000 live births
Life expectancy: males—74 years and females—77 years
Total fertility rate: 1.54 children
HIV rate: 0.1% (2012 statistics)
Per capita government health expenditure: $480 USD
Total expenditure on health as a % of GDP (2012): 5.4%
    Major infectious diseases:
    1. Food or waterborne diseases: bacterial diarrhea, hepatitis A, and typhoid fever
    2. Vector-borne diseases: Japanese encephalitis and dengue fever
    3. Soil contact diseases: hantaviral hemorrhagic fever
    4. Animal contact diseases: rabies
    5. Viral: H1N1

Ethnic Groups in China

The Han ethnic group makes up 91.9% of the population; the remainder comprise Zhaung, Uygur, Hui, Yi, Tibetan, Miao, Manchu, Mongol, Buyi, Korean, and other nationalities. The official religion of China is atheist, but 1 to 2% is Daoist, Buddhist, or Muslim, and 3 to 4% is Christian. The standard language is Mandarin; other dialects spoken in the country include Cantonese, Shanghaiese, Fuzhou, Hokkien-Taiwanese, Xiang, Gan, and Hakka. China has a 91.6% literacy rate (CIA, 2011a).

Government

The government of China (also called the People's Republic of China [PRC]) is communist, and the capital is in Beijing. China has 23 provinces and 5 autonomous regions (CIA, 2011a).

Economy

Since 1978, the Chinese economy has moved from a centrally run and planned Soviet style of government to a market economy. Business and agriculture are now more locally run, rather than being controlled by the central communist government. The overall economic system continues to function within strict communist political control, however. The change in management style of business has increased the GDP four times and boosted per capita income to $8,288 in 2011 (CIA, 2011a).

China has now moved beyond Japan to become the world's second-largest economy, and it may overtake the United States in terms of national income within the next 10 years, though it remains far behind in per capita income. The country now has hundreds of millions of people who have moved out of poverty and has a large group of students and tourists who visit the West. In spite of China now having many billionaires, as well as numerous millionaires, the average income for most of its residents is still among the world's lowest (China Surges Past Japan, 2010).

History of the Healthcare System

China has one of the longest historical records of medicine of any existing civilization in the world. Both traditional medicine and new technology are components of the Chinese healthcare system. In 1949, Chairman Mao Zedong established a rural preventive healthcare program, emphasizing disease prevention. At that time, the ministry of public health was made responsible for all health care. Large numbers of more sophisticated urban physicians were sent to the countryside to practice. In addition, less trained "barefoot doctors" were sent to small rural communities to help supply the needs for local rural health care. They worked out of village medical centers, providing preventive and primary medical care. In addition, township health centers containing 10 to 30 bed hospitals were established as part of the so-called rural collective health system. Only seriously ill patients went to county hospitals, which served a much larger population base. In large urban areas, health care was provided by paramedical personnel, who were assigned to factories and neighborhood health stations. Patients with serious illnesses went to the district or municipal hospitals.

In the 1950s, China was isolated by the Western powers, and the Soviet Union was its only ally. During this era, medical schools and hospitals in China were built with the help of Russians. There was an emphasis on public health and prevention of illness. The government mobilized the people to begin massive patriot health campaigns aimed at environmental sanitation and preventing disease. An example was the assault on the "four pests" (rats, sparrows, flies, and mosquitoes), as well as the efforts directed toward eradicating snails that carried schistosomiasis disease. Other health campaigns were devoted to water quality and waste management (CIA, 2011a). Unfortunately, much of the country's agricultural sector was ignored or handled poorly by overplanting and not harvesting all the crops, leaving them to rot. Thus, many of the agricultural programs failed. As many as 20 to 30 million people starved to death, and infant mortality rose to 300 per 1,000 (CIA, 2011a).

In the 1960s, campaigns to prevent sexually transmitted diseases, such as syphilis, were successful. By the 1970s, China was able to set up affordable primary health care in the rural areas. During the 1980s, its health policy was restructured based on market-driven reforms. The barefoot doctors were needed less, as a more sophisticated system of health care was established. With a 1% growth rate and a population of 1.3 billion people, China became very concerned about population growth and began restricting family size by implementing the "one child per family" policy. Diseases such as tuberculosis, hepatitis, hookworm, and schistosomiasis still remained problems. Later, other more chronic diseases such as HIV/AIDS, cancer, cardiovascular disease, and heart diseases became frequent causes of mortality, similar to other developed societies (CIA, 2011a).

According to Freedom House (an organization that judges how much freedom citizens of various countries have), China is near the bottom of the list of countries for limiting freedom. It is possible that these restrictions actually helped the healthcare system in China, however. From the 1950s to the 1970s, health care in China improved greatly under a very strict authoritarian rule. Brothels and opium dens were officially closed, the four pests (flies, mosquitoes, rats, and sparrows) were greatly reduced, and the training of a million barefoot (lay) doctors by urban doctors was accomplished. Health care through prevention was promoted. The communist government claimed that the incidence of sexually transmitted diseases, schistosomiasis, and leprosy decreased, access to health care for all was promoted, and infant mortality decreased. It is almost impossible to verify all of these claims, however, because China was a closed system that allowed few outsiders to document facts. The irony today is that as China becomes freer and turns toward a more market-driven economy, some advances in health care have actually been reversed. For example, universal access to health care for all is gone, and poor rural Chinese have great difficulty today getting prevention and treatment under the current partial out-of-pocket payment system (CIA, 2011a).

China, through its market reforms, has experienced tremendous economic growth. One of the results of the economic upturn has been the establishment of a fee-for-service private medical practice with few governmental restrictions. Private medical practice was not allowed during the Cultural Revolution, but it reemerged in the 1980s after the dissolving of the Cooperative Medical System (CMS) during the Maoist times, when many people lived in communes. At present, rural families must pay out-of-pocket fees for medical services; these often prohibitive costs render health care inaccessible for many (CIA, 2011a).

The Chinese barefoot doctors today in the small remote villages of the far west are often supported by a very small government salary each month and typically work out of their homes rather than a clinic, which enables them to maintain their farms when there are no patients. The doctors charge a small fee to the patients for their services, and the remainder of their salaries comes from drug sales. Often doctors overprescribe medicines simply to increase their incomes. Village doctors have inadequate training and often do not take patient histories or keep medical records as part of China's economic reforms. The Chinese government has increasingly cut the funds made available for health care, so by 2000, 60% of all healthcare costs were paid for by the individual. The typical city doctor earns $600 to $1,200 per month and sees 60 to 80 patients per day. The government has recently budgeted $350 million dollars to establish disease control and prevention centers in poor areas. Many poor areas had difficulty treating severe acute respiratory syndrome (SARS) cases when this disease emerged in China because of the inadequate resources (Life as a Village Doctor in Southwest China, 1997).

Access to Health Care and Costs

Since the 1980s, the Chinese government has had a laissez-faire policy for health care in rural areas. As part of that policy, it reverted to a self-pay system for clinic visits and hospitalization, which are now both very expensive relative to income. One average hospitalization stay costs

50% more than the average annual income. Access to health care in many areas is now priced on a sliding scale based on the ability to pay, yet many people are still unable to afford health care. In urban areas, medical care includes the use of high technology. The government health insurance program has given more equal access to health care, but cost inflation is now a major governmental concern. Copayments were first started to make the users more aware of health costs when accessing medical care. Medications and high-tech tests are now charged to patients and not covered by the government insurance. The majority of China's population lives in rural areas. Those who live in urban areas are in many ways advantaged. The distinction between rural and urban subpopulations is reinforced by a system of population registration that limits migration from rural to urban areas (Liu & Darimont, 2013).

Chinese health care has changed greatly in recent years. The most recent is the attempt to establish a healthcare provision that is a middle path between public health care and commercial private insurance. Before the economic reform in 1978 all people in China were guaranteed basic health care, yet more recently in the last 10 years there has been a decline in quality of public health care. The budgets of local governments have been decreased, and many private healthcare services began especially with the shift into the market economy. The Chinese healthcare system is separated into two parallel systems, one for providing health care to urban populations and the other for providing health care for rural areas. The decision about which system a citizen belongs to depends on the household registration (hukou). Once the household members are registered as rural residents, it is difficult for any members to transfer to an urban registration, though sometimes it is allowed at great financial cost. Hence many migrant workers live in urban areas without any entitlement to receive the social benefits of the urban residents (Hu, Cook, & Salazar, 2008; Liu & Darimont, 2013).

All employers must participate in Urban Employee Basic Health Insurance (UEBNI) to insure their employees. This plan currently covers 20% of the population (about 237 million people). Six percent is paid by the employers and 2% is paid by the employees. The remainder is paid by the government. Additionally, each person saves a percentage of their wages into an individual medical savings account maintained by the Office of Human Resources and Social Security. Children, students with severe disabilities, poor elderly greater than 60 years, and residents living in deprived areas receive extra government subsidies (Liu & Darimont, 2013).

The old cooperative medical system has been financed primarily through the rural collective economy and administered by the village municipalities. All funds are managed at the district level. The medical financial assistance healthcare program is voluntary and does not provide care to all groups of people. Regulations for payments are set up by local governments. In recent years, China has made great efforts to improve its public health system. Funds have been expended to modify and enlarge the disease prevention and control centers and to establish emergency centers and hospitals throughout the country. The major infrastructure has been improved. The ministry of health set up 10 national medical teams for disaster relief and disease prevention in some of the major cities. The SARS epidemic was controlled rapidly through this new infrastructure (Liu & Darimont, 2013).

In 1949, when the Communists came to power, there were only 2,600 hospitals in China. About 4.5% of the gross domestic product (GDP) is allocated to health care, half of which comes from the private sector. By comparison the average healthcare expenditure of countries in the European Union is 9% of GDP, while in the United States, it is closer to 16% (Hays, 2011).

The makeup of the current healthcare workforce in China differs from that in many other nations. China has more doctors than nurses. In 2005, there were 1.9 million licensed doctors and 1.4 million licensed nurses. The density of healthcare providers is much greater in urban as compared to rural areas—specifically, a three-to-one ratio. Most doctors and nurses have only a junior college or high school level of education. Approximately one third of physicians and nurses have been educated at the college level or higher. The majority of the higher-educated healthcare workers can be found in the urban areas, which creates a great disparity in the quantity and quality of healthcare providers in urban versus rural areas (Anand, Fan, & Zhang, 2008).

Ouyang and Pinstrup-Andersen (2012) addressed the health inequalities of the ethnic majority Han population and the minorities. The Han are the dominant ethnic group of China, comprising 91.6% of the population, and the other ethnic groups together comprise 8.4%, representing 114 million people. The general health and nutritional status of the minority groups were significantly lower than the majority Han population.

Health Priorities

China's Five-Year Plan (2011–2015) consists of goals including:

1. Rebalancing the economy (which includes environmental protection and social services to increase economic growth).
2. Reduction of social inequality by increasing social safety nets, increasing minimum wages, and increased investment in the infrastructure and healthcare insurance.
3. Environmental reforms from corporations and individuals.

Economic growth and urbanization have created sedentary lifestyles with greater Western diets, smoking, alcohol and air pollution, which have all led to increases in obesity, cardiovascular diseases, and cancer. About 80% of all deaths in China are now due to noncommunicable diseases and injuries with cardiovascular disease being the most common, and cancer, the second most common (Gross, Strasser-Weippl, & Lee-Bychkovsky et al., 2014).

China has experienced such rapid growth in social and economic development it has created a demand for high-quality health care within the country. The life expectancy of the average person has increased, and this trend is expected to create an aging population with chronic health problems. Currently the leading cause of death in those 1 to 44 years is injury. Approximately 750,000 deaths and 3.5 million hospitalizations occur each year. More people are now using motorcycles and cars, resulting in fewer people who are walking or using bicycles. As a result of such changes in diet and activity, cardiovascular disease is increasing rapidly. Nearly 2.6 million deaths occur annually from this problem, but by 2020 it is projected that 13 million people will die each year from cardiovascular disease (Yang et al., 2013).

The leading causes of deaths in China are as follows:

1. Stroke (1.7 million deaths)
2. Ischemic heart disease (948,700 deaths)
3. Chronic obstructive pulmonary disease (934,000 deaths)
4. Cancers
5. Mental disorders, substance abuse
6. Infections
7. Injuries

Noncommunicable diseases have risen because of the urbanization of the population, rising incomes, and longer life spans. Poor diets, an increase in hypertension, tobacco use, high cholesterol and elevated fasting glucose levels, and control of air pollution are highest health issues in China (Yang et al., 2013).

Environmental Health Issues

Air pollution is a major public concern. It is associated with higher risks for ischemic heart disease, strokes, lung cancer, and chronic obstructive pulmonary disease. Air pollution has been estimated to cause nearly one to two million premature deaths in China in 2010, which is responsible for nearly 20% of the global air pollution deaths (Alcorn, 2013).

China's movement toward a market economy has increased incomes and improved health for its population, but created some difficult environmental problems. Biomass fuel and coal are burned in most of China for cooking and heating especially in most rural areas, and a significant number of urban areas, which contributes to a major problem with indoor air pollution. In addition, the country has intense pollution from coal combustion for industry, which is damaging the air, water, and ultimately the agriculture, which in turn affects the residents' health. Of the 10 most polluted cities of the world, China is home to 7 of them. China is also the world's second-highest emitter (after the United States) of carbon dioxide pollution, mainly from industry. With the help of the United Nations and the United States, China hopes to develop a multimillion-dollar energy strategy to combat pollution (Zhang, Mo, & Weschler, 2013).

Respiratory diseases are now a widespread and serious issue. Driven by China's tremendous industrial growth, the pollution that causes these diseases is taking a heavy toll on both the environment and public health. High rates of smog from industrial and traffic pollution are associated with very high rates of respiratory infections and chronic illnesses. China relies heavily on coal that contains high levels of sulfur; this fuel is used to satisfy 70% of the country's domestic energy needs. Outdoor air tends to be more polluted in large cities than in rural areas, a result of industrial plants and vehicle emissions. Most residents in China spend the majority of their days indoors, and are exposed to coal and oil combustion from power plants, industry, pesticides, building materials, furniture, wall coverings and heating (Zhang, Mo, & Weschler, 2013).

Tobacco smoking, especially among adult males, is another growing environmental problem in China that has caused many respiratory diseases and deaths. China makes and sells more cigarettes than any other country in the world and has more than 350 million smokers, which represents about one-third of the population. Rates are highest among adult men who have a 67% smoking rate; in contrast, only 4% of all females smoke. Cigarette smoking is now the leading cause of preventable deaths in China (and the rest of the world). It seems inevitable that China will see a tremendous increase in mortality from smoking-related diseases such as chronic obstructive pulmonary disease (COPD), lung cancer, and pulmonary tuberculosis. The China National Tobacco Corporation is the largest tobacco manufacturer in the world. As part of an effort to stem the tide of smoking, the Minister of Health publishes an annual tobacco control report and campaigns have been launched to increase tobacco taxes and put health warnings on tobacco products beginning in January 2009 (Gonghuan, 2010).

Water pollution is another major problem in China. Half of all Chinese water sources are considered too polluted for human consumption. Air and water pollution in China cause 2.4 million premature deaths per year from cardiopulmonary and gastrointestinal diseases. Increases in the use of fossil fuels in industrial and residential use increases the country's production of greenhouse gases, which also cause significant health risks to the population. Significant health disparities exist between poor and wealthy populations, related to the exposure to polluted air and water especially in poorer households (Zhang, Mauzerall, Zhu, Liang, Ezzati, & Remais, 2010).

Lead poisoning is a concern among many residents. In 2009, approximately 2,000 children living near zinc and manganese smelting plants in two provinces were found with unsafe levels of lead in their blood—a revelation that provoked riots (Watts, 2009). A rapidly growing economy and population has increased the deterioration of the water supply in rivers and lakes due to large discharges of industrial and domestic waste water, poorly planned disposal of solid waste, and extensive use of fertilizers and pesticides. In addition to the contamination of water, the supply of clean water is inadequate for the population (Gross, Strasser-Weippl, & Lee-Bychkovsky et al., 2014).

Food contamination is another major health hazard in China. A major food safety incident in China was made public in 2008. An estimated 300,000 infants and young children were made ill, and six died after melamine was deliberately added to diluted raw milk as well as other food and feed products. This additive led to formation of kidney stones and renal failure. Twenty-two manufacturers of infant formula sold this contaminated product, in what is considered one of the largest ever food contamination incidents—which also had implication for international food safety (Gossner et al., 2009). Findings from a 2011 study demonstrated that about 10% of the Chinese rice is contaminated with harmful chemicals (Gross, Strasser-Weippl, & Lee-Bychkovsky et al., 2014).

Mental Health

Mental health is a major issue in China today because of the rapid social and economic changes. Changes that some members of the population face today include financial losses from bad business deals and gambling; higher rates of extramarital affairs, family violence, and divorce; rising rates of substance use and abuse; weakening of traditional family values and relationships; large numbers of rural migrants seeking employment in larger urban environments; a widening gap between the rich and poor; work-related stress; and a faster pace of life. Eighty percent of the country's healthcare budget goes to the urban residents, even though they represent only 30% of the total population. Funds for mental health are very limited for the rural population, most of whom cannot afford the out-of-pocket costs for mental health care. Shanghai, the largest population in China, boasts having the most comprehensive mental healthcare system in the country (Chang & Kleinman, 2002).

Thirteen percent of the Chinese population has psychological problems, and 16 million people in China suffer from serious mental illness. Every year in China, some 280,000 people commit suicide, accounting for 25% of the entire world's suicide statistics. Another 20 to 50 million people attempt suicide each year. Suicide is the fifth-leading cause of death for Chinese people 15 to 35 years of age. The suicide rate in China is three times higher in rural areas as compared to urban areas. This rate is 25% higher among women than men, a trend that is the opposite of that found in many other nations of the world. The higher rates of female suicides in rural areas are primarily due to poverty, the low status of rural women, forced marriages, family violence and conflict, chronic stress, and no hope for the future. Men in rural areas are often absent from the homes for long periods of time, leaving the women to work in the fields, take care of children, cook, and care for the house (Pochagina, 2005).

Nutrition

Throughout China, there has been a change in diet and physical activity and overall body composition patterns. During the past 10 years, the number of people living in China in absolute poverty has significantly declined. The proportion of those considered extremely poor decreased from 20 to 6% of the total population during the same period. As a result of this change in economic status, the prevalence of obesity and diet-related noncommunicable diseases has increased more rapidly in China than in other developed societies. Diets have shifted from high-carbohydrate to high-fat and high-density energy foods, leading to overweight and obesity—and their associated diseases, such as diabetes, stroke, cancer, and cardiovascular diseases (CIA, 2011a).

Cardiovascular Disease

Cardiovascular disease is the leading cause of mortality in the world, including in China and other developing countries. China and other developing nations have been experiencing an epidemic in cardiovascular disease during the last few decades mainly because of lifestyle and diet changes. Currently, there is a growing prevalence of metabolic syndrome and overweight individuals among adults in China. Metabolic syndrome is characterized by a cluster of problems that consists of abdominal obesity, increased blood pressure and glucose concentration, and elevated cholesterol levels. Obesity is a risk factor not only for cardiovascular disease but also type 2 diabetes, hypertension, and cancer. Excess weight is also a cause for osteoarthritis and gallbladder disease (CIA, 2011a).

Infectious Diseases

Major infectious diseases in China include the following (CIA, 2011a):

- Food- and water-borne diseases (bacterial diarrhea, hepatitis A, and typhoid fever)
- Vector-borne diseases (Japanese encephalitis and dengue fever)
- Soil-contact diseases (hantaviral hemorrhagic fever and renal syndrome)
- Animal contact diseases (rabies)

HIV/AIDS

The general population of China knows little about the sexual practices that increase the risk of contracting HIV infection. HIV/AIDS prevention in the general population has been rare. Those now living in China with HIV/AIDS face severe discrimination and have limited access to healthcare services, especially in the rural areas. The government has promised to provide free HIV tests to anyone who wants one and to fully cover treatment costs for poorer patients. The CIA (2011a) has estimated that 0.1% of the total Chinese population is infected with HIV, which ranks China 115th worldwide in number of cases. It translates into 700,000 adults living with HIV/AIDS, which ranks as the 17th largest population with this disease in the world. The estimated number of deaths from this cause—39,000 per year—places China at 15th worldwide in AIDS deaths.

Tuberculosis

China reported the worldwide second-highest number of new tuberculosis (TB) cases (1.31 million) and the second-highest number of TB deaths (201,000 TB cases) in 2007, behind only India. China has 4.5 million TB cases currently, and each year 1.4 million people develop the disease. TB killed 160,000 people in China in 2008, according to WHO. TB also represents a drain on China's health budget because of the high incidence of people with a drug-resistant strain of the disease, which is much more difficult and expensive to treat; these patients need to take drugs for up to two years and one out of every two patients dies. Regular TB costs 1,000 yuan ($158.60) to treat in China, whereas drug-resistant TB costs range from 100,000 to 300,000 yuan ($15,900 to $47,600) per person. China spent $225 million fighting TB in 2008, up from $98 million in 2002, according to WHO. (These figures do not take into account the amounts that patients pay out of their pockets, which typically amounts to between 47 and 62% of their hospital bills.) The World Bank funded the first TB survey in China, which was followed by a new program that aimed to treat the existing cases and prevent new ones (Lyn, 2010).

Population Control

China has only 7% of the world's arable land, yet 22% of the world's population. To feed, house, and promote good health care for this country's citizens despite the relatively scarce resources, the "one child per family" policy was established by Chinese leader Deng Xiaoping in 1979 to limit China's population growth. The advantages of such a policy are that each child will have a healthier life, family costs will be lower, and the child will get a better education. Women will be able to focus on their careers as well as on care for their families. The government claims that this policy has prevented mass starvation (Rosenberg, 2011).

Fines, pressures to abort a pregnancy, and even forced sterilization occur with subsequent pregnancies after the first. The policy includes ethnic Han Chinese living in urban areas. Citizens living in rural areas and minorities living in China are not subject to the law. The "one child" policy has estimated to have reduced the population of the country by as much as 300 million people in the past 20 years. A new law in addition to the "one child" regulation states that if both parents have no siblings, they may have two children, thus preventing too dramatic a population decrease (Rosenberg, 2011).

One problem with this population control policy is that Chinese parents usually rely on their children, especially their sons, for support in their old age. The result is that most couples want a male child as their only child. In turn, sex selection during pregnancy (e.g., through ultrasound and subsequent abortion of female fetuses) has resulted in a ratio of 114 males to 100 females among children from birth to four years old. Over time, the population control policies have caused serious problems for female infants, including abortion, neglect, abandonment, and even infanticide (Rosenberg, 2011).

China is a lineage-based society and *bare branches*, a term used for unmarried men who represent the end of the line for their families, are poorly regarded in China. They often suffer discrimination, which frequently extends to their parents, ultimately causing an increase in shame, leading to greater alcoholism and mental health disorders (Rosenberg, 2011).

Traditional Medicine

The practice of traditional Chinese medicine was strongly promoted by Chinese leaders, and it has remained a major part of health care although Western medicine gained acceptance in the 1970s and 1980s. The goal of China's medical personnel is to synthesize the use of both Western and traditional Chinese medicine, yet this practice has not always worked seamlessly. Physicians trained in traditional medicine and those trained in Western medicine are very separate groups with different basic ideas. Traditional Chinese medicine uses herbal treatments, acupuncture, acupressure, moxibustion, and cupping of skin with heated bamboo. These approaches are very effective in treating minor ailments and chronic diseases, and they produce far fewer side effects. Some more serious and acute problems are also treated with traditional medicine. For more information regarding this topic see Chapter 11 entitled, "Global Use of Complementary and Integrated Health Approaches."

Road Traffic Accidents

Road traffic accidents in China kill more than 250,000 people (21.3/100,000 people) annually, which is more than in any other country in the world. Accidents are the fourth leading cause of premature deaths. Interventions to decrease speeding and drunk driving began in the cities of Suzhou and Dalian in 2010. Underreporting of accidents impedes the gathering of statistics for the various regions. Social marketing campaigns are attempting to reduce the incidence of drunk driving and speeding, but no great outcomes so far have been reported (Bhalla, Li, Duan, Wang, Bishai, & Hyder, 2013).

INDIA

History

The Indus Valley civilization, one of the world's oldest, was a vibrant presence during the second and third millennia BCE. Aryan tribes from the northwest came to the Indian subcontinent in 1500 BCE, merging with the earlier Dravidian people and creating the classical Indian culture. Many years later in the nineteenth century, India came under British rule. Nonviolent resistance to British rule, led by Ghandi and Nehru, brought India to independence in 1947. Violence in the new state eventually led to a partition of the nation, creating two countries, India and Pakistan. Later, a war in 1971 resulted in East Pakistan becoming the country of Bangladesh (CIA, 2011b).

Geography

India is located in southern Asia, bordering the Arabian Sea and the Bay of Bengal, between Burma and Pakistan. It has a large land area, ranking seventh in the world. The climate includes monsoons in the south and a more temperate climate in the north. The country's natural resources include coal (India has the fourth-largest reserves in the world), iron ore, manganese, mica, titanium ore, natural gas, diamonds, and petroleum, among others. Within this country there is an abundance of deforestation, soil erosion, overgrazing, air pollution from industry and vehicle emission, and water pollution from raw sewage and agricultural pesticides, making water nonpotable throughout the country (CIA, 2011b).

Population

India has a population of 1.24 billion people, ranking the country second in the world in population size. The population is growing at a rate of 2% annually, which will create the world's largest population, surpassing China by 2030. By 2050, India's population is expected to reach 1.6 billion people. The population increase is due to increases in life expectancy, decreases in infant mortality, and emphasis on eradication of diseases such as hepatitis, tetanus, and polio among infants. The gross national income is $3,910 USD. Life expectancy is 64 years for men and 68 years for females. The total expenditure on health per capita is $157 USD. The annual percentage on health as a percentage of the GDP is 4.1%. The maternal mortality ratio is 190 per 100,000 live births. The HIV rate is 169 per 100,000 population (WHO, 2014b).

The majority of India's people (70%) live in a rural agrarian economy and have incomes of less than $1 per day (CIA, 2011b). Only 29% of the total population lives in urban areas. Twenty-two percent of the population is malnourished and 48% of the children have stunted growth. This country's poor health conditions contribute to two thirds of the global morbidity. Those people living in rural areas have many more healthcare access challenges. The ratio of hospital beds for the rural population is 15 times lower than for urban areas. The ratio of doctors to people in rural areas is six times lower than in the urban population. The infant mortality rate in the poorest 20% of the population is two and a half times greater than the wealthiest 20% of the population. India also ranks third in Southeast Asia in greatest out-of-pocket expenses for health. Only 17% of healthcare expenses are paid by the government and the remainder is paid by out-of-pocket payments (WHO, 2014b).

Infectious Diseases

India has about 2.40 million people living with HIV, with an adult HIV/AIDS prevalence of 0.31% (2009). Children up to 15 years old account for 3.5% of all infections, while 83% are in the age group 15 to 49. Of all HIV infections, 39% (930,000) are among women. India's epidemic is largely concentrated in a few states in the industrialized south and west, and in the northeast. The four states of South India (Andhra Pradesh—500,000, Maharashtra—420,000, Karnataka—250,000, Tamil Nadu—150,000) account for 55% of all HIV infections in the country. West Bengal, Gujarat, Bihar, and Uttar Pradesh are estimated to have more than 100,000 people with HIV/AIDS, accounting for another 22% of HIV infections in the country (Sabharwal & Lamba, 2014; The World Bank, 2012).

Food- and water-borne diseases cause a high rate of bacterial diarrhea, hepatitis A and E, and typhoid fever. Vector-borne diseases include chikugunya, dengue fever, Japanese encephalitis, and malaria. Rabies comes from contact with an infected animal, and leptospirosis is traced to contact with infected water. India's malaria and TB rates are ranked third in the world (Sabharwal & Lamba, 2014).

Chronic Diseases

India is now faced with a double burden of long-term chronic illnesses and serious acute illnesses. Cardiovascular diseases, cancer, degenerative diseases, and diabetes have become major health issues in addition to the acute communicable diseases mentioned previously.

Culture

Indians practice a number of different religions: Hindu (80.5%), Muslim (13.4%), Christian (2.3%), Sikh (1.9%), other (1.8%), and unspecified (0.1%). English is the official language, though Indians use many other languages as well. Hindi is the most widely spoken of these languages (used by 41% of the population), but 14 other languages are also spoken. Approximately 61% of the population is literate, being able to read and write, and the average education level is 10 years. Inequality of opportunity has caused the lower-caste Hindus, Muslims, tribal people, and other minority populations to be disproportionately represented within the poor, the uneducated, and those with most health problems (CIA, 2011b).

Government and Economy

India is a federal republic with New Delhi as its capital city. The country contains 28 states and seven union territories. The economy is developing into an open-market economy, which encompasses traditional village farming, modern agriculture, handicrafts, and a wide range of services, including information technology and software workers. India's annual per capita income is $3,400 (2010 estimate). The country has a significant labor force of 467 million people (second largest in the world) and has 81 million people using the Internet (the fourth-largest group of users in the world). The unemployment rate is 10.7%. The Indian pharmaceutical market has grown rapidly in the past few years and the federal government uses price controls to ensure that vital drugs are available to the general population (CIA, 2011b).

Health Care

India has the world's largest democracy and the second most populous country in the world. Twenty-two percent of the residents are malnourished and 48% of the children have stunted growth, conditions that are responsible for two thirds of the burden of morbidity. There remains a significant disparity in access to and equity of health care for different ethnic and socioeconomic groups within the population. In addition, the ratio of people to hospital beds for rural residents is 15 times lower than for urban residents, and the ratio of doctors to rural residents is six times lower than for urban residents. The infant mortality rate for the poorest 20% of the population is two and a half times higher than that of the richest 20% of the population. India ranks third in the Southeast Asia region with the highest out-of-pocket expenditures for health care. The private health sector of the population has a monopoly of the ambulatory urban and rural healthcare services. The government has a general obligation to provide free and universal access to healthcare services to all and ensure that no one is denied health services. The healthcare system continues to suffer from inadequate funding and poor health management, and numerous health problems related to malnutrition, starvation, and disease, especially in the rural areas (Sabharwal & Lamba, 2014).

Health care is the responsibility of each state or territory of India. Each state is expected to pay for 80% of healthcare facilities, and the federal government pays 15%, mainly through national healthcare programs. Health care in India can be traced back 3,500 years to the inception of Ayurvedic traditional medicine, which is still used today. India has historically suffered from great famines, which have been eradicated, yet continues to experience significant problems with undernutrition. Undernutrition rates in children in India are higher than Sub-Saharan Africa. Approximately 46% of children from birth to three years are undernourished (Rao, 2009). A preference for male babies has led to an imbalanced ratio of 93.5 girls per 100 boys, in contrast to the natural gender ratio at birth of 105 males to 100 females. Maternal and infant death rates remain high. The vast majority of the Indian population suffers from waterborne and airborne infections. Most of the country lacks a basic infrastructure, as its development has not kept up with the growing economy. Almost one million people die each year due to inadequate health care, and 700 million people lack access to specialist care, which mainly exists in large urban areas. Forty percent of the healthcare facilities in India are understaffed (Rao, 2009).

The number of hospital beds is low with only 0.7 per 1,000 population, compared to the world average of 3.96 hospital beds per 1,000 population. In addition, India lacks an adequate number of trained healthcare personnel for its growing healthcare industry. Rural healthcare services are mainly provided by smaller primary healthcare centers, which rely on trained paramedics for most of the care. Serious cases are sent to urban areas, where specialists and acute care facilities are available. Skilled birth attendants are needed, yet are still not provided in adequate numbers to decrease the high rates of maternal and infant mortality (Rao, 2009).

Indigenous traditional medicine is practiced throughout the country. The main forms are Ayurvedic medicine, which addresses mental and spiritual well-being as well as physical well-being. In addition, Unani herbal medicine is practiced. Today only 25% of the Indian population has access to Western medicine (Rao, 2009).

The government has made a major commitment to telemedicine to reach the majority of the poor, rural, underserved population. Health insurance is inaccessible to the majority of Indians, and 75% of healthcare expenses are paid on an out-of-pocket basis, which is very difficult for the many people who live in poverty. Emergency and specialty care is well beyond the reach of most of the poor lower-class residents. Among those in the urban middle and upper classes, approximately 50% have private health insurance (Rao, 2009).

The National Rural Health Mission was begun in 2005 to provide major improvements in health care for the rural population. Primary healthcare clinics, which have social activist leanings, help support public health priorities such as childhood immunizations and compliance with TB treatments. The National Rural Health Mission program was established to address issues of poverty and provide 100 days of work at minimal wage to one family member per household. In addition, an increase in primary school enrollment, particularly among girls, was established as a goal (Rao, 2009).

SOUTH AFRICA

Geography

South Africa is located at the southern tip of the continent of Africa. It is bordered by Botswana, Lesotho, Mozambique, Namibia, Swaziland, and Zimbabwe, as well as the Atlantic and Indian oceans. Its climate is mostly arid, with a subtropical region found along the country's east coast. Natural resources include gold, chromium, antimony, coal, iron ore, manganese, nickel, phosphates, tin, uranium, gem diamonds, platinum, copper, vanadium, salt, and natural gas (CIA, 2012).

Population

South Africa's population as of 2013 was approximately 53 million people of diverse origins, cultures, languages, and religions. The growth rate is 1.34%, birth rate is 19.1 per 1,000 population, and the death rate is 16.99 per 1,000. Life expectancy is 49.2 years overall, with 50.08 years for men and 48.29 years for women. The infant mortality rate is 43.78 deaths per 1,000 live births. The probability of dying under age five is 45 per 1,000 live births. The total expenditure on health per capita (2012) was $982 with a percent of the GDP as 8.8%. The literacy rate is 93% of the population, and there is a 51.9% unemployment rate (CIA, 2012; WHO, 2012b).

There are 11 official languages consisting of Afrikaans, English, Ndebele, Northern Sotho, Sotho, Swazi, Tswana, Tsonga, Venda, Xhosa, and Zulu. Despite the fact that English is the recognized language for commerce and science, it is ranked fourth and spoken by only 9.6% of South Africans as their primary language.

Religions include Zion Christian (11.1%), Pentecostal (8.2%), Roman Catholic (7.1%), Methodist (6.8%), Dutch Reformed (6.7%), Anglican (3.8%), and other Christians (36%), Muslims (1.5%), Hindus (1.3%), and Jews (0.2–15.1%) (CIA, 2012b).

South Africa spends 8.5% of its GDP on health care, ranking 54th in the world. The ratio of physicians in the population is 9.76 per 1,000, and there are 2.6 hospital beds per 1,000 people.

South Africa is considered a middle-income nation with a progressive constitution that guarantees the right to health care. The National Health Insurance (NHI) delivers universal health coverage.

Ethnic groups in South Africa include the following (CIA, 2012):

- Black African (79.6%)
- White (9.1%)
- Colored (8.9%)
- Indian/Asian (2.5%)

Languages spoken in South Africa include the following:

- IsiZulu (23.8%)
- IsiXhosa (17.6%)
- Afrikaans (13.3%)
- Sepedi (9.4%)
- English (8.2%)
- Setswana (8.2%)
- Sesotho (7.9%)
- Xitsonga (4.4%)
- Other (7.2%)

South Africa has the largest population of people of European descent in Africa, the largest Indian population in Africa, and the largest colored (mixed European and African) group in Africa. It is one of the most ethnically diverse countries in Africa. The country has had a long history of racial problems between the black majority and the white minority. The country's Apartheid policy, a system of racial segregation in South Africa enforced through legislation, was introduced in 1948 and ended in 1990. Crime remains a major problem in South Africa, which ranks first in the world in number of murders by firearms, manslaughter, rape, and assault cases. It also ranks fourth in the world in robbery incidence, according to a survey conducted by the United Nations from 1998 to 2000. Problems also persist with illegal drug transportation and sales (CIA, 2012b).

The South African population is relatively young, with approximately one-third younger than age 15. Fertility is declining, and there is an increase in persons older than 60 years. The country's healthcare services include not only services for obstetrics, pediatrics, and adolescents, but also those for the aging population. A large proportion of the population (18% in some areas) is illiterate. Half of all households use electricity for cooking. Since 1994, life expectancy in South Africa has declined by 20 years, mainly because of the increase in HIV/AIDS incidence. The global burden of disease is quite high, and morbidity and mortality rates are very high due to HIV/AIDS, violence and injury, chronic diseases, mental health disorders, and maternal, neonatal, and child mortality (Chopra, Lawn, Sanders, Barron, Abdool Karim, & Jewkes, 2009).

Government

The government is a republic, formally named the Republic of South Africa (RSA), with a legal system based on Roman-Dutch law and English common law. The system of government is also called a parliamentary democracy. South Africa has three capital cities: Cape Town, the largest, is the legislative capital; Pretoria is the administrative capital; and Bloemfontein is the judicial capital. The country comprises nine provinces (CIA, 2012).

Economy

South Africa has a two-tiered economy. One segment is similar to other economically strong developed countries, and the other is more like developing countries with only the basic infrastructure. South Africa has well-developed financial, legal, communication, energy, and transportation systems. It has the world's 10th-largest stock exchange and a modern infrastructure. It has the best telecommunications system in Africa. At the same time, South Africa has a very high unemployment rate (25%) and most of the country's citizens live on less than $1.25 per day. The country's wealth is unevenly distributed, with the minority whites having a much larger portion of the wealth and the majority blacks having a very challenging existence with difficulty finding well-paying jobs (Index Mundi, 2013).

The country has an overall per capita GDP of $11,500 (2013 estimate) (Index Mundi, 2013). Its industries include mining (South Africa is the world's largest producer of platinum, gold, and chromium), auto assembly, metalworking, machinery, textile, iron and steel, chemicals, fertilizers, ship repair, and foods The main agricultural products are corn, wheat, sugarcane, fruits, vegetables, beef, poultry, mutton, wool, and dairy products (OECD, 2013).

Healthcare System

South Africa's healthcare system consists of a large public sector and a smaller, yet fast-growing private sector. Basic primary health care is offered free to all residents of the country, but is highly specialized; high-tech care is limited to only those who can afford private care. The dilemma is that the government contributes approximately 40% of healthcare costs for the public health, yet 80% of the population uses the services. The number of public hospitals continues to grow, and companies in the mining industry operate their own 60 hospitals and clinics in different locations within the country (Coovadia, Jewkes, Barron, Sanders, & McIntyre, 2009).

The South African healthcare system faces many challenges. The country's history of very high rates of communicable and noncommunicable diseases, combined with the legacy of colonialism, Apartheid, and post-Apartheid turmoil, have led to major racial and gender discrimination, a migrant labor system, destruction of family life, great disparities in family incomes, and extreme violence, which have all affected the health and healthcare system of the nation. For many decades, black people were forced to work for the white minority for very low wages. Before 1994, politics restricted health and health care for blacks. The public healthcare system has now been transformed into an integrated national service, but is plagued by a lack of management and leadership. Some of the main problems related to health include poverty-related illnesses such as infectious diseases (HIV/AIDS, TB, and malaria), maternal mortality, malnutrition, and high rates of noncommunicable diseases. HIV/AIDS accounts for 31% of the disability-adjusted life-years, and violence and injury continue to cause premature deaths (Coovadia, Jewkes, Barron, Sanders, & McIntyre, 2009).

South Africa is considered a middle-income country because of its economy, yet its disease rates are higher than those of many low-income countries. It is one of only 12 countries in the world where child mortality has increased, rather than decreased, since the 1990 Millennium Developmental Goals were established (Coovadia, Jewkes, Barron, Sanders, & McIntyre, 2009). There are great disparities between the country's public and private healthcare systems. Less than 15% of the population uses private health care, yet 46% of all healthcare expenditures are devoted to private healthcare services. There is also a disparity in funding among the provinces within South Africa's healthcare system (Coovadia, Jewkes, Barron, Sanders, & McIntyre, 2009).

Major Health Issues

As noted previously, South Africa is challenged by very high rates of injury, the problem of under-development of the country as a whole, and numerous residents with chronic diseases. The largest rise in death rates for adults has occurred among the young adult group, who are dying in increasing numbers from HIV/AIDS. Deaths from tuberculosis, pneumonia, and diarrhea are also increasing rapidly. The leading cause of death in South Africa is HIV/AIDS (infants and young adults), followed by homicide (young adult men), tuberculosis, road traffic accidents, and diarrhea. Large numbers of deaths from noncommunicable diseases occur in the 60 and older group of the population. Causes of death for children younger than five years are ranked as follows:

1. HIV/AIDS
2. Low birth weight
3. Diarrhea
4. Lower respiratory infections
5. Protein-energy malnutrition
6. Neonatal infections
7. Birth asphyxia and birth trauma
8. Congenital heart disease
9. Road traffic accidents
10. Bacterial meningitis

Health care in South Africa varies from the most basic primary health care, offered free by the state, to highly specialized, hi-tech health services available in the both the public and private sector. The private sector, on the other hand, is run largely on commercial lines and caters to middle- and high-income earners who tend to be members of medical schemes. It also attracts most of the country's health professionals. This two-tiered system is not only inequitable and inaccessible to a large portion of South Africans, but institutions in the public sector have suffered poor management, underfunding, and deteriorating infrastructure. While access has improved, the quality of health care has fallen (South Africa.info, 2014).

National, Provincial and Local Health Care

Prior to South Africa's first democratic elections, hospitals were assigned to particular racial groups, and most were concentrated in white areas. With 14 different health departments, the system was characterized by fragmentation and duplication. But in 1994 the dismantling began, and transformation is now fully underway; nonetheless, high levels of poverty and unemployment cause health care to remain primarily a burden of the state. The Department of Health holds overall responsibility for health care, with a specific responsibility for the public sector.

Provincial health departments provide and manage comprehensive health services, via a district-based, public health care model. Local hospital management has delegated authority over operational issues, such as the budget and human resources, to facilitate quicker responses to local needs. Public health consumes around 11% of the government's total budget, which is allocated and mostly spent by the nine provinces. Hundreds of NGOs make an essential contribution to HIV/AIDS and TB, mental health, cancer, disability, and the development of public health systems. The part played by NGOs from a national level, through provincial and local, to their role in individual communities—is vitally important to the functioning of the overall system (SouthAfrica.info, 2014).

National Health Insurance

The Department of Health is focused on implementing an improved health system, which involves an emphasis focused on public health, as well as improving the functionality and management of the system through stringent budget and expenditure monitoring.

Known as the "10-point plan," the strategic program is improving hospital infrastructure and human resources management, as well as procurement of the necessary equipment and skills.

Under this plan, health facilities—such as nursing colleges and tertiary hospitals—are being upgraded and rebuilt to lay the way for the implementation of the National Health Insurance (NHI) scheme. The NHI is intended to bring about reform that will improve service provision and healthcare delivery (SouthAfrica.info, 2014).

Facilities

There are 4,200 public health facilities in South Africa. Since 1994, more than 1,600 clinics have been built or upgraded. Free health care for children under six and for pregnant or breastfeeding mothers was introduced in the mid-1990s. The National Health Laboratory Service is the largest pathology service in South Africa. It has 265 laboratories, serving 80% of South Africans. The labs provide diagnostic services as well as health-related research (SouthAfrica.info, 2014).

Doctor Shortages

In March 2012, 165,371 qualified health practitioners in both public and private sectors were registered with the Health Professions Council of South Africa, including 38,236 doctors and 5,560 dentists. The physician-to-population ratio is estimated to be 0.77 per 1,000 people in the population, but because the majority (73%) of GPs works in the private sector, there is just one practicing doctor for every 4,219 persons (SouthAfrica.info, 2014).

In response, the Department of Health has introduced clinical health associates, mid-level health care providers, to work in underserved rural areas. In an attempt to boost the number of doctors in the country, South Africa signed a cooperation agreement with Cuba in 1995. South Africa has since recruited hundreds of Cuban doctors, and South Africa is able to send medical students to Cuba to study (SouthAfrica.info, 2014).

Infectious Diseases

Life expectancy has increased because of expansion of HIV/AIDS and TB treatment and care. South Africa has one of the highest TB rates in the world and has 17% of the global burden of multiresistant tuberculosis. Diagnosis and treatment is costly using a substantial portion of the medical budget with a treatment success rate of about 40% (SouthAfrica.info, 2014).

HIV/AIDS

Currently 6.4 million people, a 17.9% prevalence rate, in South Africa are living with HIV/AIDS (2012), an increase from 4.6 million in 2008, which is attributed to antiretroviral therapy (ART). The country continues to have the world's highest rate of people with HIV/AIDS, as well as the world's highest mortality rate from this disease. In 2013 there were 235,000 deaths from AIDS. Domestic investment in HIV is $735 million USD (2012). More than 2 million people in 2013 were accessing ART (antiretroviral therapy), representing 54% of those in need. Although the government plans to increase ART accessibility to 4.6 million people in a few years, HIV/AIDS continues at an extremely high rate with 900 people infected and 500 dying each day. In May 2012, the government said it had cut the mother-to-child transmission rate from 3.5% in 2010 to less than 2%. It also said the rate of new infections had dropped from 1.4% to 0.8% in the 18 to 24 age groups (WHO, 2012b).

South Africa has the largest antiretroviral treatment programs in the world. Life expectancy has increased by five years since the height of the epidemic. These efforts have been largely financed from its own domestic resources. The country now invests more than $1 billion annually to run its HIV and AIDS programs. HIV prevalence is almost 40% in Kwazulu Natal compared with 18% in Northern Cape and Western Cape. HIV prevention initiatives are having a significant impact on mother-to-child transmission rates in particular, which are falling dramatically. New HIV infections overall have fallen by half in the last decade. Moreover, while South Africa is yet to make significant inroads into the reduction to TB deaths, the country has made great progress in the scaling up of ARV access for co-infected people. In South Africa there were still 370,000 new HIV infections in 2012, the world's highest (UNAIDS, 2013).

The HIV epidemic in South Africa fuels the TB epidemic. People with HIV are at a far greater risk of developing active tuberculosis as a weakened immune system facilitates the development of the disease. Similarly, TB can accelerate the course of HIV: about 1% of the South African population develops TB every year and the number of TB cases continues to rise. Seventy percent of people living with HIV in South Africa are co-infected with TB (AVERT, 2014).

Another HIV/AIDS risk factor is the very high rate of violence against women in South Africa. The incidence of rape in South Africa is considered to be among the highest in the world, yet these crimes are seldom reported. Rates of rapes of female children are exceptionally high. A myth that having sex with a virgin will cure AIDS remains to blame for part of the increase in child rape. In addition, a very high incidence of violence at the hands of husbands or boyfriends occurs. Women can be beaten if they refuse to have sex with their partners. Women often remain in abusive relationships for financial dependency reasons. No matter why it occurs, violence against women increases the risk of HIV and STI infections (UNAIDS, 2013).

In South Africa, 30% of women are heads of households. These women are often poor, have no financial aid from men, and consequently have a very unfavorable economic position and little power. Selling sex can often be a survival strategy for these women, albeit one that makes them even more vulnerable to HIV. Young girls may trade sex for money, clothes, or food.

Another problem in South Africa is the increasing number of orphans who are left behind when both of their parents die of AIDS. Some grandparents are trying to provide care for as many as 10 to 20 grandchildren after they have lost their children. Other AIDS orphans are left alone to care for themselves. There is a lost generation of street children who have no education and have few economic resources. Some sell themselves for sex to keep themselves and siblings fed. Some are HIV infected and some are not, but many will die regardless of their situation (Sowell, 2000).

Tuberculosis

South Africa is one of the countries with the highest burden of TB. WHO estimates the incidence of 500,000 cases of active TB in 2011. About 1% of the population (about 50 million people) develops active TB disease each year. This is the third-highest incidence of any country worldwide, after India and China, and the incidence has increased by 400% over the past 15 years. Out of the 500,000 incident cases in South Africa it is estimated by WHO that about 330,000 (66%) people with HIV/AIDS also have a TB infection (TBFacts.org, 2014). The high rate also reflects South Africa's poor standard of living, which is characterized by poverty and overcrowding. Other factors include the increase and extent of drug resistance, particularly multidrug resistance (MDR).

Cholera

South Africa last experienced an upsurge in the incidence of cholera where more than 6,000 reported cases of cholera were reported in February 2009. More than 50 people died from this disease. Most of the victims were from Mpumalanga and Limpopo. Cholera is an intestinal illness caused by the *Vibrio cholerae* organism. Cholera results in the loss of large volumes of watery stool (excrement), leading to rapid dehydration and shock, and often resulting in death without treatment. The fatality rate for untreated cholera is 50%. Persons with cholera develop rapid breathing, vomiting, and painless diarrhea, and they go into metabolic acidosis. Appropriate oral or intravenous rehydration therapy is needed to replace lost fluids and electrolytes. In South Africa, cholera represents a significant burden. Approximately 200,000 cases are reported to the World Health Organization every year. However, WHO believes the true number of cases annually is between 3 to 5 million, with 100,000 to 120,000 deaths. Cholera is contracted by consuming food or water contaminated with the fecal bacteria Vibrio cholerae.

The symptoms are usually mild, but about 20% of cases include symptoms of watery diarrhea. Cholera deaths result from poor sanitation and poor-quality water supplies and an estimated 18 million South Africans have no basic sanitation. Across the continent of Africa, more than 38% of all people have no access to safe water—a percentage higher than that found in any other place in the world. In South Africa, some 12 million people lack safe water and 20 million lack sanitation facilities. By 2020, South Africa's population demands will exceed its water supply by 6%. Health maintenance is dependent on an adequate water supply and adequate sanitation facilities (toilets). It is vital in hospitals and healthcare clinics to have adequate clean water and sanitation for prevention and treatment of diseases and illnesses. A clean and adequate supply is necessary for simple handwashing in patient care. In short supply areas, it is necessary for healthcare workers to disinfect water if unclean and teach similar techniques to patients. Techniques of disinfection include boiling, use of chlorine tablets, filtration, and clean storage (WHO, 2012b).

Malaria
Malaria is a serious disease transmitted to humans by the bite of the *Anopheles* mosquito. Symptoms include fever and a flulike illness characterized by chills, headache, muscle aches, and fatigue. Malaria can also cause anemia and jaundice. If not treated promptly, this infection can lead to kidney failure, coma, and death. Malaria can be prevented by antimalarial drugs, such as atovaquone/proguanil, doxycycline, and mefloquine. Chloroquine is not effective for malaria prevention in South Africa. Protection from mosquito bites is also very important (WHO, 2013).

Malaria is a major health problem in Sub-Saharan Africa and affects great numbers of young children and pregnant women. It is the main cause of 20% of all deaths of young children in Africa. Approximately 95% of the infections in South Africa are due to *Plasmodium falciparum,* a microbe that lives in the gut of the *Anopheles* mosquito. Transmission is seasonal, with the largest number of cases occurring October to February. Use of drugs for treatment and vector control by spraying has proved effective in deterring infection. South Africa, along with five other countries, was given permission by the United Nations Environmental Programme to use DDT for public health use only. The application of DDT in 2000 led to significant improvements in the mortality and morbidity associated with this disease. It should be noted, however, that DDT is a banned pesticide in the United States and in most developed and developing countries (SouthAfrica.info, 2014; WHO, 2012b).

Violence and Injury
South Africa has many disturbing social issues that have proved challenging to manage. It is estimated that 500,000 women are raped each year in the country. Approximately 28% of men state that they have committed rape. Gender-based violence is especially high, with South African female homicide rates six times the global average; 50% of the female victims are killed by their spouses or partners. In addition, this country is ranked by the United Nations as second in the world for murder and first for assaults and rape. Violence and injury are the second leading

cause of death, and the injury rate is almost twice the global average. Approximately 16,000 road-related (motor vehicle collision) deaths occur yearly. Children also are subject to very high rates of sexual, physical, and emotional abuse and neglect (Coovadia, Jewkes, Barron, Sanders, & McIntyre, 2009).

Maternal and Infant Health

South Africa has a major problem with maternal and infant health. The infant mortality rate is 42.5 per 1,000 live births. Each year approximately 75,000 children die, and 23 die within their first month of life. In addition, 23,000 babies are stillborn, a factor closely associated with the 1,660 maternal deaths that occur annually. The major causes of maternal deaths are HIV/AIDS infections. Strengthening HIV/AIDS health care will require at least a 2.4% increase in funding for HIV prevention and treatment programs (Coovadia, Jewkes, Barron, Sanders, & McIntyre, 2009).

Since 1978, the country has had a decentralized basic primary healthcare system, instead focusing on a district healthcare system run by local governments. Disparities exist between municipalities, depending on the funding from the local area. Poor municipalities with little funding have little allocated for their healthcare budgets. Rural areas are poorly funded as compared to urban areas. Poor women, especially in rural areas, are often seen by a nurse or nurse-midwife for prenatal care and delivery, whereas urban women more often receive prenatal care and delivery from a physician. The poorest women had antepartal healthcare coverage yet in 2013 only 39.6% received care before 20 weeks' gestation. In addition there are considerable differences in the quality of maternal health care in rural as compared to urban sites (Wabiri, Chersich, Khangelani, Blaauw, & Ntabozuko, 2013).

South Africa is one of the most inequitable countries worldwide. The wealthiest 10% of the population account for greater than 50% of the county's income. Child mortality is double in the rural Eastern Cape, and four times higher for black than for white residents. Maternal mortality rates are as high as 84.9 deaths per 100,000 live births in the Western Cape to 289.1 maternal deaths per 100,000 live births in the Free State Province. These deaths are mainly due to HIV and other nonpregnancy-related infections (41%), obstetrical hemorrhage (14%), and hypertension (14%). There are huge deficiencies in the knowledge and skills of healthcare providers in these impoverished areas.

Adverse nutrition and health conditions continue to be deficient in the Kwa Zulu-Natal, and those in the Eastern Cape provinces of South Africa households reported to have tap water are 50%, and toilets, 82%; wood is the main energy source for cooking. Diarrhea rates are high at 35% for Umkanyakude and Zululand, and 55% for Tambo. The prevalence of stunting for children older than 12 months was 22 to 26%. Interestingly, the prevalence of overweight and obesity in adults in these same districts was 42 to 60% (Shoeman et al., 2010).

Smoking and Diet

There is a significant increase in the use of tobacco in South Africa, which in turn is causing more lung diseases, especially lung cancer. Campaigns to deter youth from smoking and encourage smokers to stop are being led by healthcare organizations in increasing numbers.

South Africans are undergoing a major change in diet in types and quantity of foods consumed, moving away from traditional plant foods to high-fat and high-sugar foods with low fiber. As a result of this change, overweight and obesity are now chronic problems among South African people. Urban people are more likely to be obese than rural people, and those older than 65 years are less likely to be obese. South Africans are now more sedentary than they previously were as well (WHO, 2012b).

Racial/Ethnic Inequalities

Racial inequalities continue to exist in the wake of the policy of Apartheid. Significant disparities in standards of living persist, with most blacks continuing to lack adequate public health services, such as clean water, a proper sewage system, and access to health care, making them much more vulnerable to disease. Unemployment is much higher within the black or African populations compared to other ethnic groups. Whites are the most employed group. Half of all Africans live in formal housing (solid structures with indoor plumbing and electricity), compared with 95% of whites. Poverty-related health problems such as infectious diseases, maternal and infant deaths, and malnutrition remain widespread (Coovadia, Jewkes, Barron, Sanders, & McIntyre, 2009; Kon, 2008).

Healthcare Personnel

There is a shortage of nursing and other healthcare personnel in South Africa, as well as a problem of maldistribution of resources. The majority of trained nursing and allied health professionals work in the private sector, which serves much less of the general population than does the public sector. In addition, more trained health personnel work in urban areas than in rural areas. Doctors, especially those with more subspecialty training, are more likely to work in the private sector and in urban areas (79%) as well. Moreover, there has been a trend of skilled health personnel leaving South Africa for other countries, such as the United States, Canada, New Zealand, the United Kingdom, and Australia. South Africa is actively trying to recruit nurses and doctors, especially to work in the underserved areas. In addition to healthcare personnel trained in Western medicine, there are 200,000 traditional healers who practice in South Africa (Coovadia, Jewkes, Barron, Sanders, & McIntyre, 2009).

Chronic Diseases

South Africa, a developing country, currently is experiencing a vast increase in the prevalence of chronic diseases, which historically were more associated with developed countries. Health problems such as hypertension, elevated cholesterol, alcohol and tobacco use, and obesity are now being observed in South Africa in greater frequencies. Risks for chronic diseases reflect individuals' age, gender, tobacco and alcohol use, diet, and physical activity. Other risk factors include family history and genetic background. Most chronic diseases are preventable with modification of lifestyle behaviors, and changes in activity and diet can greatly influence the risk for numerous chronic diseases. The leading causes of deaths in South Africa include the following:

- HIV/AIDS
- Heart disease

- Homicide and violence
- Stroke
- Tuberculosis
- Lower respiratory infections
- Road traffic accidents
- Diarrhea diseases
- Hypertension
- Diabetes

All of these conditions are chronic diseases, with the exceptions of homicide, violence, and traffic accidents (Coovadia, Jewkes, Barron, Sanders, & McIntyre, 2009).

SUMMARY

This chapter has addressed the health and health care of four developing countries. Although Egypt, China, India, and South Africa are located in different regions of the world, and they have a variety of languages, customs, values, health practices, types of government, and health care per capita allocations; they also share some commonalities and similar health challenges. Although the data presented here can be used for cross-country comparisons, the definitions of health problems and data collection methodology may greatly differ, so that these comparisons, at best, may be only a good estimate for a certain time and geographical location.

Study Questions

1. How are the health issues of infant mortality and nutrition similar for the countries of Egypt, China, India, and South Africa?
2. Compare and contrast the health beliefs and practices of traditional medicine in China with those in India. How do cultural influences affect health and health care differently? What are some basic commonalities?
3. What are some contributory factors leading to the exceptionally high rate of HIV/AIDS in South Africa?

Case Study: Smoking and Health Concerns Versus Tobacco Production in China

"As the health impact of smoking, including rising heart disease and lung cancer, gradually emerges, unless there is effective government intervention, it will affect China's overall economic growth due to lost productivity," said Yang Gonghuan, deputy director of the Chinese Center for Disease Control and Prevention. Lost productivity from smoking-related health problems will hamper China's economic growth, and related costs incurred by smoking far exceed the tobacco industry's contribution in terms of profits and jobs it generates. China's addiction to huge revenues from the state-owned tobacco monopoly is hindering antismoking measures, potentially costing millions of lives in the country with the world's largest number

TABLE 3-16 Healthcare Statistics for Egypt, China, India, and South Africa

Indicator	Date/Date Range	Data Type	Data China	Egypt	India	South Africa
HIV/AIDS						
People living with HIV/AIDS	Data from most recent year available	Number	740,000	11,000	2,400,000	5,600,000
Adults living with HIV/AIDS	2009	Number	730,000	10,000	2,300,000	5,300,000
Adult HIV/AIDS prevalence rate	2009	%	0.1%	<0.1%	0.3%	17.8%
Women living with HIV/AIDS	Number of women living with HIV/AIDS and women as a percentage of adults living with HIV/AIDS, 2009	%	32%	24%	38%	62%
Men living with HIV/AIDS	Number of men living with HIV/AIDS and men as a percentage of adults living with HIV/AIDS, 2009	%	NA	81%	61%	38%
Children living with HIV/AIDS	2009	Number	NA	NA	NA	330,000
AIDS deaths	2009	Number	26,000	<500	170,000	310,000
AIDS orphans	2009	Number	NA	NA	NA	1,900,000
ARV need	2009	Number	NA	3,300	NA	2,600,000
ARV treatment	2009	Number	65,481	359	320,074	971,556
ARV coverage Rate	2009	%	NA	11%	NA	37%
Tuberculosis						
Tuberculosis HBCs	2010	Text	Yes	No	Yes	Yes
New TB cases	2009	Number	1,300,000	15,000	2,000,000	490,000
New TB smear-positive cases	2008	Number	640,000	6,500	890,000	200,000
New TB case rate	2009	Rate per 100,000	96	19	168	971

(continues)

TABLE 3-16 Healthcare Statistics for Egypt, China, India, and South Africa (*Continued*)

People living with TB	2009	Number	1,900,000	25,000	3,000,000	400,000
TB prevalence rate	2009	Rate per 100,000	138	30	249	808
TB death rate	2009	Rate per 100,000	12	1	23	52
TB prevalence in HIV-positive people per 100,000 population	2007	Rate per 100,000	1	0	4	345
Malaria						
Malaria cases	2009	Number	14,491	94	1,563,344	6,072
Malaria deaths	2009	Number	12	2	1,133	45
Other Diseases, Conditions, and Risk Indicators						
Yellow fever cases	2009	Number	NA	NA	NA	0
Yellow fever deaths	2004	Number	0	0	0	0
Diphtheria cases	2009	Number	0	0	NA	1
Measles cases	2009	Number	52,461	608	NA	5,857
Polio cases	2009	Number	0	0	752	0
DTP3 immunization coverage rate	2009	%	97%	97%	66%	69%
Vitamin A supplementation coverage rate	2009	%	NA	NA	66%	NA
Percentage with water	2008	%	89%	99%	88%	91%
Access to sanitation	2008	%	55%	94%	31%	77%
Population undernourished	2005–2007	%	10%	NA	21%	NA
Low-birth-weight babies	2000–2009	%	3%	13%	28%	NA

Child malnutrition	2000–2009	%	6.8%	6.8%	43.5%	NA
Female prevalence of obesity	2005	%	2%	46%	1%	35%
Male prevalence of obesity	2005	%	2%	22%	1%	7%
Female prevalence of smoking	2006	%	4%	1%	4%	9%
Male prevalence of smoking	2006	%	59.5%	27.6%	33.2%	29.5%
Programs, Funding, and Financing						
Financial development assistance for health per capita	2007	U.S. dollars	$0.18	$1.23	$0.50	$6.60
USAID NTD program countries	Fiscal year 2010	Text	No	No	Yes	No
USAID maternal assistance	Fiscal year 2010	Text	No	Yes	Yes	No
U.S. food assistance program countries	Fiscal year 2008	Text	No	No	Non-emergency	No
USAID Nutrition program countries	Fiscal year 2010	Text	No	Yes	Yes	No
Health expenditure per capita	2008	U.S. dollars	$265	$261	$122	$843
Total expenditure on health	2008	%	4.3%	4.8%	4.2%	8.2%
Government health expenditures as a percentage of total government expenditures	2008	%	10.3%	5.9%	4.4%	10.4%
Government health expenditures as a percentage of total health expenditures	2008	%	47.3%	42.2%	32.4%	39.7%

(continues)

TABLE 3-16 Healthcare Statistics for Egypt, China, India, and South Africa (*Continued*)

Social Security expenditures on health	2008	%	66.3%	21.6%	17.2%	3.0%
Out-of-pocket expenditures on health	2008	%	82.6%	97.7%	74.4%	29.7%
Health Workforce and Capacity						
Physicians	2000–2010	Rate per 10,000	14	28	6	8
Nurses and midwives	2000–2010	Rate per 10,000	14	35	13	41
Community health workers	2000–2010	Rate per 10,000	8	NA	1	NA
Births attended by skilled health personnel	2000–2010	%	96%	79%	47%	91%
Hospital beds	2000–2009	Rate per 10,000	30	21	9	28
Demography and Population						
Population	2011	Number	1,336,718,015	82,079,636	1,189,172,906	49,004,031
Adult sex ratio	2011	Number	1.17	1.03	1.07	1.02
Median age	2011	Number	35.5	24.3	26.2	25.0
Population younger than age 15	2010	%	18%	33%	32%	31%
Urban population	2010	%	47%	43%	29%	52%
Land area	2009	Number	9,560,981	1,001,449	3,287,263	1,221,037
Population density	2010	Number	140	80	362	41
Birth rate	2011	Rate per 1000	12.29	24.63	20.97	19.48
Total fertility rate	2011	Number	1.54	2.97	2.62	2.30
Adolescent fertility rate	2000–2008	Rate per 1000	5	50	45	54

	Year	Unit				
Contraceptive prevalence rate	2000–2010	%	59.9%	56.3%	60.3%	84.6%
Death rate	2011	Rate per 1000	17.09	7.48	4.82	7.03
Infant mortality rate	2011	Rate per 1000	43.20	47.57	25.20	16.06
Female infant mortality rate	2011	Rate per 1000	39.14	49.14	23.52	16.57
Male infant mortality rate	2011	Rate per 1000	47.19	46.18	26.80	15.61
Under-five mortality rate	2009	Rate per 1000	62	66	21	19
Maternal mortality ratio	2008	Rate per 100,000	410	230	82	38
Life expectancy: female	2009	Number	55	66	73	76
Life expectancy: male	2009	Number	54	63	69	72
Population growth rate	2011	%	−0.38%	1.34%	1.96%	0.49%
Income and the Economy						
GDP per capita	2009	$	$10,278	$3296	$5673	$6828
GNI per capita	2009	$	$10,050	$3280	$5680	$6890
Population living on less than $1.25 per day	Data from most recent year available	%	3.3% (2006)	10.5% (2005)	0.4% (2005)	4.0% (2005)
Unemployment rate	Data from most recent year available	%	23.3% (2010)	10.8% (2010)	9.7% (2010)	4.3% (2005)
Country income classification	As of July 2011	Text	Upper middle income	Lower middle income	Lower middle income	Upper middle income
External country debt	2009	U.S. dollars	$42,101	$237,692	$33,257	$428,442

ARV: antiretroviral therapy.
Data from Kaiser Family Foundation. (n.d.). *Customized data sheet.* Retrieved from http://www.globalhealthfacts.org/data/factsheet.aspx?loc=59, 76,105, 1958&ind=1,2

of smokers. The warnings, issued in a report prepared by a group of prominent public health experts and economists, came amidst growing calls for the government to give stronger support to tobacco-control measures. China is the world's largest tobacco producing and consuming country, with more than 300 million smokers on the mainland. Each year, about 1.2 million people die from smoking-related diseases on the mainland and the figure will increase to 3.5 million by 2030, according to estimates from the World Health Organization (WHO). The report underscores increasing concern that the country's economic potential will be jeopardized due to escalating medical costs and lost productivity if the government fails to take serious action to combat smoking.

Case Study Questions

1. What are some major health risks related to smoking and what is the impact on health for the Chinese people?
2. Why do you think that government owned tobacco production in China continues in spite of knowledge about health risks?
3. How would you suggest that smoking in China be decreased?

Condensed from Shan, J. (2012). Report: Smoking industry harming economic health. *China Daily*. Retrieved from http://www.chinadaily.com.cn/china/2011-01/07/content_11805846.htm

References

Abdo, N. M., & Mohamed, M. E. (2010). Effectiveness of health education Program for type 2 diabetes mellitus patients attending Zagazig University Diabetes Clinic, Egypt. *Journal of Egypt Public Health 2010, 85*(2–4), 113–130.

About Egypt: General information (2010). Retrieved from http://cabinet.egy/AboutEgypt/GeneralInfo.aspx

Ahrani, M., Houser, R., Yassin, S., Mogheez, M., Hussaini, Y., Crump, P. . . . Levinson, F. J. (2006). A positive deviance-based antenatal nutrition project improves birth-weight in Upper Egypt. *Journal of Health, Population, and Nutrition, 24*(4), 498–509.

Alcorn, T. (2013). China's skies: A complex recipe for pollution with no quick fix. *Lancet, 8;381*(9882), 1973–1974.

Anand, S., Fan, V., & Zhang, J. (2008). Health care reform in China 5. China's human resources for health: Quantity, quality, and distribution. *Lancet, 372*(9651), 1774–1782.

Arab Republic of Egypt, Ministry of Foreign Affairs. (2010). Retrieved from http://www.mfa.gov.eg/English/insideegypt/history/Pages/default.aspx

AVERT. HIV/AIDS in South Africa. (2014). Retrieved from http://www.avert.org/hiv-aids-south-africa.htm

Bhalla, K., Li, Q., Duan, L., Wang, Y., Bishai, D., & Hyder, A. (2013). The prevalence of speeding and drunk driving in two cities in China: A mid project evaluation of ongoing road safety interventions. *Injury, 44*(4), 49–56. doi: 10.1016/S0020-1383(13)70213-4

Boggatz, T., and Dassen, T. (2005). Ageing, care dependency, and care for older people in Egypt: A review of the literature. *International Journal of Clinical Nursing, 14*(8b), 56–63.

Boutros, J., & Skordis, J. (2010). HIV/AIDS Surveillance in Egypt: Current status and future challenges. *Eastern Mediterranean Health Journal, 16*(3), 251–258.

Central Intelligence Agency. (2011a). *The world factbook: China.* Retrieved from http://www.cia.gov/cia/publications/factbook/goes/ch.html

Central Intelligence Agency. (2011b). *The world factbook: India.* Retrieved from http://www.cia.gov/cia/publications/factbook/goes/ind.html

Central Intelligence Agency. (2012). *The world factbook: South Africa.* Retrieved from https://www.cia.gov/library/publications/the-world-factbook/geos/sf.html

Chang, D., & Kleinman, A. (2002). Growing pains: Mental health care in a developing China. In A. Cohen, A. Kleinman, & B. Saraceno (Eds.), *The World Mental Health Casebook* (pp. 85–97). New York: Kluwer.

China surges past Japan as number 2 economy. (2010, August 17). Retrieved from http://www.boston.com/business/articles/2010/08/16/china_surges_past_japan_as_no_2_economy_us_next/

Chopra, M., Lawn, J., Sanders, D., Barron, P., Abdool Karim, S. & Jewkes, R. (2009). Health in South Africa. *Lancet.* doi: 10.1016/S0140-6736(9)

Coovadia, H., Jewkes, R., Barron, P., Sanders, D., & McIntyre, D. (2009). Health in South Africa. *Lancet.* Retrieved from http://www.thelancet.com/series/health-in-south-africa

Dang, S., Yan, H., Yamamoto, S., Wang, X., & Zeng, L. (2004). Poor nutritional status of younger Tibetan children living at high altitudes. *European Journal of Clinical Nutrition, 58*, 938–946.

Darmstadt, G., Hasaan, M., Balsaran, Z., Winch, P., Darmstadt, G., Gipson, M., & Santosham, M. (2009). Impact of clean delivery-kit use on newborn umbilical cord and maternal puerperal infections in Egypt. *Journal of Health, Population and Nutrition, 27*(6), 746–755.

Department of State, Bureau of African Affairs. (2005). *South Africa.* Retrieved from http://www.state.gov.r/pa/ei/bgn/2898.htm

Egypt Demographic and Health Survey. (2008). Retrieved from: http://www.measuredhs.com/pubs/pdf/FR220/FR220.pdf

El-Rashidi, S. (2013). *Egyptian women demand cultural revolution against domestic violence.* Retrieved from http://english.ahram.org.eg/NewsContent/1/64/85640/Egypt/Politics-/Egyptian-women-demand-cultural-revolution-against-.aspx

Fahmy, A., El-Mouelhy, M, & Ragab, A. (2010). Female genital mutilation/cutting and issues of sexuality in Egypt. *Reproductive Health Matters, 18*(36), 181–190. doi: 10.1016/S0968-8080(10)36535-9

Gonghuan, Y. (2010). China wrestles with tobacco control. *Bulletin of the World Health Organization, 88*, 251–252.

Gossner, C., Schlundt, J., Embarek, P., Hird, S., Lo-F Wong, D., Beltran, J., . . . Tritscher, A. (2009). The melamine incident: Implications for international food and feed safety. *Environmental Health Perspectives, 117*(12), 1803–1808.

Gross, P., Strasser-Weippl, K., & Lee-Bychkovsky, L. et al. (2014). Challenges to effective cancer control in China, India, and Russia. *The Lancet Oncology Commission, 15*(489–538). Retrieved from http://news.medlive.cn/uploadfile/20140418/13978078983689.pdf

Hays, J. (2011). *Health Care in China: Doctors, insurance and costs.* Retrieved from http://factsanddetails.com/china.php?itemid=335&catid=13&subcatid=83

Hu, X., Cook, S., & Salazar, M. (2008). Internal migration in China. *Lancet, 372*, 117–120.

Index Mundi. (2013). *South Africa.* Retrieved from http://www.indexmundi.com/south_africa/

International Agency for Research on Cancer. (2010). *Cancer in Egypt.* Retrieved from http://www.iarc.fr/en/publications/scientific-papers/2010/index.php

Ismail, H. (2011). Self-related health and factors influencing responses among young Egyptian type 1 diabetes patients. *BioMedCentral, 11*, 216–223.

Kon, Z., & Lackan, N. (2008). Ethnic disparities in access to care in post-Apartheid South Africa. *American Journal of Public Health, 98*(12), 2272–2277.

Lasheen, M., El-Kholy, G., Sharaby, C., Elsherif, I., & El-Wakeel, S. (2008). Assessment of selected heavy metals in some water treatment plants and household tap water in greater Cairo, Egypt. *Management of Environmental Quality, 19*(3), 367.

Life as a village doctor in southwest China. (1997). *Newsweek/Healthweek.* Retrieved from http://www.nurseweek.com/features/dispatches/China/971023.html

Lohinivak, A., El-Sayeed, N., & Talaat, M. (2008). Clean hands: Prevention of typhoid fever in rural communities in Egypt. *International Quarterly of Community Health Education, 28*(3), 215–227.

Lyn, T. (2010). *China fights growing problem of tuberculosis.* Retrieved from http://www.reuters.com/article/2010/01/06/us-tuberculosis-china-idUSTRE60501Z20100106

Mohamoud, Y., Mumtaz, G., Riome, S., Miller, D., & Abu-Raddad, L. (2013). The epidemiology of hepatitis C virus in Egypt: A systematic review and data synthesis. *BMC. Infectious Diseases, 13,* 288. doi: 10.1186/ 1471-2334-13-288

Monazea, E., & Khalek, E. (2010). *Domestic violence high in Egypt, affecting women's reproductive health.* Retrieved from http://www.prb.org/Publications/Articles/2010/domesticviolence-egypt.aspx

Organisation for Economic Co-operation and Development. OECD South Africa. (2013). Retrieved from http:// www.oecd.org/eco/surveys/South%20Africa%202013%20Overview%20FINAL.pdf

Ouyang, Y., & Pinstrup-Andersen, P. (2012). Health inequality between ethnic minority and Han populations in China. *World Development, 40*(7), 1452–1468.

Pochagina, O. (2005). Suicide in present day China. *Far Eastern Affairs, 33*(2), 60–73.

Population—China. Putting on the brakes on reproduction. *Canada and the World,* 18–21.

Rao, M. (2009). Tackling health inequalities in India. *Perspectives in Public Health, 129*(5).

Rosenberg, M. (2011). *China's one child policy.* Retrieved from http://geography.about.com

Sabharwal, A., & Lamba, P. (2014). Public health in India: Challenges ahead. *OIDA International Journal of Sustainable Development, 7*(2), 17–24.

Saleh, N. (2013). *The 2012 Constitution of Egypt.* Retrieved from http://en.wikipedia.org/wiki/Egyptian_Shura_ Council_election,_2013

Shan, J. (2012). Report: Smoking industry harming economic health. *China Daily.* Retrieved from http://www .chinadaily.com.cn/china/2011-01/07/content_11805846.htm

Shoeman, S., Faber, M., Adams, V., Smuts, C., Ford-Ngomane, N., Laubscher, J. & Dhansay, M. (2010). Adverse social, nutrition and health conditions in rural districts of the KwaZulu-Natal and Eastern Cape provinces, South Africa, *23*(3), 140–147.

SouthAfrica.info (2014). Retrieved from http://www.southafrica.info/about/health/health.htm

Sowell, R. (2000). AIDS orphans: The cost of doing nothing. *Journal of the Association of Nurses in AIDS Care, 11*(6), 15–16.

Spousal violence in Egypt. (2010). Retrieved from: http://www.prb.org/Publications/Reports/2010/ spousalviolence-egypt.aspx

TBFacts.org. (2014). Retrieved from http://www.tbfacts.org/tb-statistics-south-africa.html

UNAIDS, South Africa (2013). Retrieved from http://www.unaids.org/en/regionscountries/countries/ southafrica

Waked, I., Doss, W., El-Sayed, M., Estes, C., Razavi, H., Shiha, G., Yosry, A., & Esmat, G. (2014). The current and future disease burden of chronic hepatitis C virus infection in Egypt. *Arab Journal of Gastroenterology, 15*(2), 45–52. doi: 10.1016/j.ajg.2014.04.003

Wabiri, N., Chersich, M., Khangelani, Z., Blaauw, D., & Ntabozuko, D. (2013). *Equity in Maternal Health in South Africa: Analysis of Health Service Access and Health Status in a National Household Survey.* doi: 10.1371/journal.pone.0073864. Retrieved from http://www.jourlib.org/paper/3017344

Watts, J. (2009). Lead poisoning cases spark riots in China. *Lancet, 374*(9693), 868.

World Bank. (2010). *Arab Republic of Egypt.* Retrieved from http://worldbank.org/WBSITE/EXTERNAL/ COUNTRIES/MENEXT/EGYPTEXTN/), menuPK:287182~pagePK:141132~piPK:141109~thesit ePK:256307,00.html

World Bank. (2012). *HIV/AIDS in India.* Retrieved from http://www.worldbank.org/en/news/feature/2012/07/ 10/hiv-aids-india

World Health Organization. (2005). *Mental health atlas.* Retrieved from http://www.who.int/mental_health/ evidence/atlas

World Health Organization. (2010). *Cancer in Egypt.* Retrieved from http://www.bing.com/search?q =WHO%2C+International+Agency+for+Research+on+Cancer%2C+2010&src=IE-SearchBox& FORM=IE8SRC

World Health Organization. (2011a). *Egypt: Country health profile.* Retrieved from http://www.who.int/gho/ countries/egy/country_profiles/en/

World Health Organization. (2011b). *Global health observatory data repository.* Retrieved from http://apps .who.int/ghodata/?vid=710

World Health Organization. (2012a). *Road safety in Egypt.* Retrieved from http://www.who.int/violence_injury_ prevention/road_traffic/countrywork/egy/en/

World Health Organization. (2012b). *South Africa statistics.* Retrieved from http://www.who.int/countries/zaf/en/

World Health Organization. (2013). *World malaria report.* Retrieved from http://www.who.int/malaria/ publications/country-profiles/profile_zaf_en.pdf

World Health Organization. (2014a). *China: Statistics.* Retrieved from http://www.who.int/countries/chn/en/

World Health Organization. (2014b). *India: Health profile.* Retrieved from http://www.who.int/countries/ind/en/

Yang, G., Wang, Y., Zeng, Y., Gao, G., Liang, X., Zhou, M., Wan, X., Yu, S., Jiang, Y., Naghavi, M., Vos, T., Wang, H., Lopez, A., & Murray, C. (2013). Rapid health transition in China, 1190–2010: Findings from Global Burden of Disease study 2010. *Lancet, 8*(381). doi: 10.1016/S0140-6736(13)61097-1

Zhang, J., Mauzerall, D., Zhu, T., Liang, S., Ezzati, M., & Remais, J. (2010). Environmental health in China: Progress towards clean air and safe water. *Lancet, 375,* 1110–1119.

Zhang, Y., Mo, J., & Weschler, C. (2013). Reducing health risks from indoor exposures in rapidly developing urban China. *Environmental Health Perspectives, 121*(7), 751. doi: 10.1289/ehp.1205983

4

Global Perspectives on Economics and Health Care

Govind Hariharan and T. Mark Haney[1]

INTRODUCTION

The world has seen dramatic transformations in the delivery, cost, and effectiveness of health care over the last century. A century ago, living to 50 years was considered an anomaly, whereas the present generations worry about whether they have saved enough to live to 100 years and beyond. At the same time that very expensive and effective robotic surgical equipment is used to enhance health in some parts of the world, in other parts the struggle to feed their children enough to avoid a cruel and debilitating fate from malnourishment continues. Such variations in availability, access, and prevalence of medical care highlight the emphasis placed by organizations such as the Bill and Melinda Gates foundation to find cost-effective ways of providing health care and preventing disease.

Across the world there is tremendous variation in the way health care is provided and funded and most importantly in healthcare outcomes. Yet concern about the financing of health care has become a matter of great concern in every economy. In developed countries, rapid growth in medical innovations and technology and the cost of caring for an aging population have combined to make soaring healthcare costs a primary concern. On the other hand developing countries plagued with a struggling economy find themselves hard-pressed to find sources of funding for providing even basic medical care for a growing population.

Economics is the study of how to allocate scarce resources across unlimited wants and needs. It is no wonder then that in a world faced with the problem of ever-growing demands on its healthcare resources amid tightening budgets, the field of health economics has grown exponentially more important in academic and policy settings. Health economists are often interested in analyzing whether healthcare resources are used efficiently and whether the proper incentives and healthcare systems exist or can be created to ensure efficiency. The current system for the provision of health care in countries such as the United States is rather complex, often with the patient receiving care from providers who are paid by a third party such as a private or public health insurance organization. Since the early 1970s, the emergence of managed care organizations in the United States (often centered around health insurance companies) with its emphasis on cost effectiveness, return on investments, and aligning incentives properly, highlighted the importance of using economic principles in health care. However, in 2013, there were close to 45 million people in the United States without any health insurance coverage. Providing unpaid medical care for these uninsured segments of the population results in cost shifting that makes health insurance more expensive. This was a primary argument in the enactment of the Affordable Care Act popularly known as Obamacare in 2013 with a principal focus to bring more Americans under an insurance umbrella.

In this chapter, we compare and contrast five countries: Canada, India, Japan, Ukraine, and the United States. The choice of these particular countries for analysis was driven by the stark differences in their systems for providing health care and in their economic strength. Of these five countries, Canada, Japan, and the United States are highly industrialized countries with high per capita gross domestic product (GDP) and high levels of expenditure on health care, as shown in Table 4-1. Yet there are significant differences between them in their levels of public and private expenditures on health care, the type of health systems they use, and, by some measures, the levels of the health of their population. India has a rapidly growing economy with the second largest population in the world faced with problems of inequality. Ukraine is a newly independent former Soviet republic recovering from an economic recession and with an archaic healthcare system.

In section 1, we briefly describe the history and structure of the healthcare systems in each country, pointing out some of the critical problems in each. In section 2, we conduct a comparative analysis. In section 3, we develop the economic concept of productivity, explain the various techniques for applying it in healthcare settings, and analyze the productivity of healthcare resources in each country. In section 4, we discuss some of the key issues in the development of an ideal healthcare system.

TABLE 4-1   Basic Economic and Demographic Characteristics (2013 or latest available)

Indicator	Canada	India	Japan	Ukraine	United States
Population (in thousands)	35,182	1,252,140	127,144	45,239	320,051
Gross national income per capita (international $)	41,170	5,080	36,440	8,670	52,620
Total health expenditure per capita (international $)	4,759	215	3,741	687	9,146

Data from World Health Organization. (2015). Global Health Observatory Data Repository. Retrieved from http://www.who.int/gho/en/

PROFILES OF FIVE HEALTHCARE SYSTEMS

The five countries under analysis here show a wide range of structures from predominantly private systems in Japan to the central universal program in Canada, from a health insurance–based system in the United States to a Ukrainian system with no health insurance. In this section, we begin with a profile of each country's healthcare system and then briefly conduct a comparative study. The data for the profiles are derived from various sources at the Organization for Economic Cooperation and Development (OECD) and the Global Health Observatory Data Repository (GHODR) at the World Health Organization (WHO).

Profile of the Canadian Healthcare System

Canada is the second-largest country in land area in the world and has a relatively small population of slightly over 33.5 million. Canadians have enjoyed significant improvements in life expectancy over the last four decades. Canadian life expectancy is higher than the average for OECD countries (OECD, 2015a). In 2013, life expectancy for women was 83.58 while it was 79.326 for men (World Bank, 2015). The interesting aspect of recent Canadian life expectancy patterns has been the narrowing of the gap between men and women. According to Or (2000) per capita GDP and tobacco, alcohol, and fat consumption are all strongly correlated with premature mortality. Over the last three decades, there has been a dramatic reduction in smoking rates (especially among men); overall smoking rates have dropped from 22% in 2000 to 15% in 2013 (OECD, 2015a). Similarly, alcohol consumption has declined by 23% over the last 30 years although it has increased recently in Canada. Between 2000 and 2013, alcohol consumption increased from around 7.8 liters per capita to 8 liters per capita. It should be noted that as with other OECD countries, alcohol consumption is heavily concentrated, with 20% of the population accounting for 70% of total alcohol consumption. However, obesity, especially among women, remains a problem with 52.10% of population over 15 years reporting to be obese in 2013 as compared to 48.20% in 2001 (OECD, 2015b). Diabetes is also quite prevalent, with 9.41% of adults reportedly diabetic (World Bank, 2015). The reduction in male smoking and the higher rates of female obesity may be responsible for the narrowing gap in life expectancy across gender.

Canadian infant mortality is low at 4.3 per 1,000 live births with neonatal mortality rate at 3.2 and under-five mortality rates at 4.9 in 2014 (World Bank, 2015). The under-five mortality rate differential between male and female children is not as low as Japan's but is lower than the United States at 5.3 and 4.5 respectively. The low infant mortality rates are perhaps a result of the very high rate (100%) of births that are attended by skilled medical personnel. Obesity among children is very high in Canada at 7.6%, with girls having much lower rates of obesity (5.2%) compared to boys (9.6%).

Prior to 1971, the Canadian healthcare system was very similar to that of the United States. It was predominantly based on employer-provided health insurance with a smaller role played by various government programs. Both hospitals and physicians operated privately with physicians' fees determined by the market and hospitals paid on a negotiated fee-for-service basis. During this period, a little over 7% of the GDP was spent on health care.

In 1971, Canada adopted a system of universal health insurance, called the Canadian Medicare System, that was provided by the government and funded by value-added taxes and income tax. All basic services were covered and patient copayments were nominal. Physicians were paid on the basis of a fee schedule determined by the government, and hospitals were allocated a budget by the provincial government with the overall budget set nationally. Although health insurance was provided to all by the government, the provision of health care remained largely in private hands. However, the private health providers in Canada are heavily regulated with price controls on most activities, services, and products. Hospitals also are restricted from raising funds on their own for capital investments and instead have to obtain funds from the provincial government. Although there are significant differences in overall spending on health care between Canada and the United States, Canadian health expenditures have not grown as rapidly as those in the United States, mostly as a result of the government regulation of prices and the government setting the budget allocation for health care.

In the early 1990s, Canada went through an economic recession that resulted in significant cost-cutting measures. This significantly affected healthcare expenditures, which were the largest single item in the provincial government budgets. As a result, between 1992 and 1997, total health expenditure (THE) as a percentage of GDP declined significantly. Since then it has continued to increase and according to the OECD was 11% in 2013. Public expenditure on health accounted for 70% of THE while private expenditure as a percentage of THE was 30%, with 15% of it comprising out-of-pocket expenditure in 2013. Hospitals occupy an important role in the Canadian health system, and inpatient costs represented 22% of total health expenditure in 2013 while outpatient services accounted for 34%. Payment to physicians (mostly fee for service) at $946 per capita was the fastest-growing health expenditure between 2007 and 2013, growing at a rate of 2.2%. The average per capita expenditure on drugs was $959 in 2013 with close to 90% of it being prescribed medication. In 2014, there were 28 physicians and 16 nurses per capita. The number of hospital beds per capita decreased marginally during the 2000s and was 29 per capita in 2014. Canada has the longest waiting times for medical care among OECD countries, with 60% waiting for four weeks or more for a specialty appointment.

Canada has often been cited by some as an example of the type of system the United States should adopt to provide universal coverage, though it has at least as many opponents.

Profile of the Indian Healthcare System

With a population of more than a billion, India is the second-largest country in the world (second only to China). It is a country of haves and have-nots with significant proportions of the population living in poverty while some segments are extremely well off. The economy grew very rapidly during the 1990s and early 2000s. Growth rates during some years were in the double digits, and though the economy has continued on the fast track in this century there has been a recent slowdown. Like China, India has benefited greatly from participating in the global economy and is fast becoming an economic superpower.

India obtained its independence from Great Britain in 1947 and has for much of its independent life adopted a socialist approach to the provision of most services. However, the provision of healthcare services has to a large extent been provided and funded by private entities. Over 50% of all inpatient services and 60% of outpatient services are provided by the private sector. Many of the newer private hospitals are staffed by Western-educated medical personnel with the latest medical technologies available to them. Health care for the poorer and disadvantaged segments of the population, on the other hand, are primarily provided for by government-owned and ill-equipped health facilities. Public ownership is divided between central (national), state, municipal, and *panchayat* (village) governments. Public facilities own and operate many teaching hospitals, secondary hospitals, rural referral hospitals, primary health centers, and clinics or dispensaries.

In 1951 life expectancy at birth was only 36.7 years. It increased steadily to 64.1 years by 2009. In 2013, life expectancy at birth for women was 69.09 and 66.3 for men (World Bank, 2015). Only 2.1% of adults reported being obese in 2009 (self-reported data with attendant errors). Alcohol consumption was 0.7 liters per capita, and 14.3% of the population over 15 smoked daily, all of which are among the lowest compared to OECD countries. On the negative side, although significant progress has been made since India's independence, communicable diseases such as tuberculosis continue to affect large segments of the population. In addition, HIV/AIDS has assumed virulent proportions, and problems with access to clean drinking water and access to infant and maternal health care remain major barriers to advancement in health care.

While Indians have enjoyed significant improvements in life expectancy over the last four decades there is much room for improvement. Overall smoking rates have been slowly falling, but smoking prevalence rates among men remains high at 22.8% compared to women at 2.4%. As is the case in countries such as Japan, smoking rates among women has been increasing during this time frame. Obesity, especially among women, remains a problem with 24.7% of population over 15 years reporting to be obese in 2013 compared to 19.5% of men.

Similarly, infant mortality was 146 per 1,000 live births in 1950 and declined to 50.3 by 2009. Infant mortality remains extremely high in India at 37.9 per 1,000 live births with neonatal mortality rate at 27.7 and under-five mortality rates at 47.7 in 2014 (World Bank, 2015). The under-five mortality rate differential between female and male children is also high at 49.2 and 46.3 respectively. The high infant mortality rates are perhaps a result of the very low rate of live births that are attended by skilled medical personnel, and the very low rate of pregnant women receiving prenatal care of at least four visits. As with adults, obesity among children is very low in India at 1.9% of girls and 2.4% of boys.

According to data from WHO, total health expenditure (THE) in India was 4% of GDP in 2013 with government expenditure accounting for 32% of the private expenditure on health. Health care is financed mostly with out-of-pocket payments. Private health insurance is still a very nascent industry in India, and out-of-pocket expenditures (which includes employers who are mostly self-insured) was 86% of private health expenditures on health and 58% of THE. The high out-of-pocket payments often pose a problem since, according to a World Bank report by Peters and colleagues in 2002, almost one-quarter of all hospitalizations push people into poverty because of the loss of jobs and the high cost of private medical facilities. Within public expenditure the central government allocation for health out of its total budget remained stagnant in the 1990s and 2000s, whereas state allocations actually declined.

Health insurance covers about 10% of the population, with government employees covered under government plans and some private-sector employees covered under employer-provided plans. Since 2000 various plans have been rolled out by the government to provide affordable health insurance for the needy, but coverage for those insured in such plans is often restricted to ill-equipped public health facilities.

In 2013, India had about 0.7 physicians per 1,000 population and about 0.9 nurses per 1,000 population. Primary care physicians working in the public sector are paid a low and fixed salary set at the national level. As a result, most physicians work in their own clinics where fees are determined in competitive factors. Available hospital capacity is still very low in India with only 0.7 hospital beds per 1,000 population (World Bank, 2015). During the 1990s with liberalization of controls many private hospitals and hospital chains with large capital investments in advanced technology and with highly trained staff began to grow rapidly. These new facilities provide care for the many beneficiaries of the booming economy. In addition, these new facilities have made significant inroads into providing services for the "health tourists" from Western economies attracted by the lower cost of advanced care in these facilities.

The stark disparity in healthcare use between different socioeconomic classes and rural–urban regions in India has been a matter of great concern to the government of India for many decades now. The best indicator of this is the disparity in infant mortality rates. The under-five mortality rates for the lowest wealth quintile is triple that of the highest quintile. It is also twice as high in rural regions as compared to urban regions and for mothers with no education compared to mothers with higher education. Similar disparities also exist with immunizations (see Table 4-2). Such

TABLE 4-2   Inequities in Health in India in 2010 or Latest Available

Indicator	Value
Under-five mortality rate (per 1,000 live births)—rural	82
Under-five mortality rate (per 1,000 live births)—urban	51.7
Under-five mortality rate (per 1,000 live births)—lowest wealth quintile	64.3
Under-five mortality rate (per 1,000 live births)—highest wealth quintile	30.6
Under-five mortality rate (per 1,000 live births)—mother with no education	124.4
Under-five mortality rate (per 1,000 live births)—mother with higher education	50.5
Measles immunization coverage among one-year-olds (%)—rural	45.3
Measles immunization coverage among one-year-olds (%)—urban	69.2
Measles immunization coverage among one-year-olds (%)—lowest wealth quintile	28.4
Measles immunization coverage among one-year-olds (%)—highest wealth quintile	81.2
Measles immunization coverage among one-year-olds (%)—mother with no education	34
Measles immunization coverage among one-year-olds (%)—mother with higher education	75.8

Data from WHO. (2015). *Global Health Observatory Data Repository*. Retrieved from http://www.who.int/gho/en/; WHOSIS. (2006). Statistical Information System. World Health Organization.

TABLE 4-3 Health Disparity Across States in India

State	Per Capita Net State Domestic Product (Rupees)	Life Expectancy at Birth	Infant Mortality Rate per 1,000 Live Births	% Below Poverty
Andhra Pradesh	9,982	63.1	55	15.77
Bihar	4,123	60.2	62	42.6
Gujarat	12,975	62.8	62	14.07
Kerala	10,627	73.5	14	12.72
Punjab	15,310	68.1	52	6.16

Data from Government of India. (2005). Financing and delivery of health care services in India (Background Papers, table 1, p. 7). New Delhi, India: National Commission on Macroeconomics and Health.

disparities in health care at young ages are undoubtedly likely to result in widening disparities at older ages.

In addition to the inequalities between rural and urban regions, there are also significant variations across states in India in every aspect of income and health, as shown in Table 4-3. The state of Punjab has the highest per capita income and the lowest percent of population below poverty. The best-performing state in terms of its health is the state of Kerala; it also has the highest literacy rates (especially for women) and density of physicians and healthcare facilities per capita. Excluding Kerala, India appears to have a positive relationship between high incomes and better health.

As one of the fastest-growing economies in the world India has to take urgent steps to address the huge disparities in healthcare provision. Sustained growth in the economy requires a source of healthy worker power.

Profile of the Japanese Healthcare System

Since the end of World War II, Japan has evolved from being an economy devastated by war to the second-largest economy in the world with a GDP of $32,018 per capita in 2003. It has a population of around 125 million of which 20% are 65 years or older. By 2020 this segment is expected to be over one-quarter of the population. The rapid aging of the population is a matter of great concern especially for healthcare provision and funding. Japan has some of the best health outcomes in the world, and it continues to improve in the health status of the population. There is also very little disparity within the country in healthcare access.

Life expectancy in Japan was 50 years for men and 54 years for women at the end of World War II. It has since grown to the highest among industrialized countries at 86.6 and 80.21 years at birth for women and men respectively in 2013 (World Bank, 2015). Infant mortality is very low at 2 per 1,000 live births with neonatal mortality rate at 1 and under-five mortality rates at 2.9. The under-five mortality rate differential between male and female children is also very low at 2.9 and 2.5 respectively. The very low infant mortality rates are perhaps a result of the very high 99.8% of births that are attended by skilled medical personnel. The leading cause of death in Japan is malignant neoplasm followed by cardiovascular disease. High stress levels have been blamed for the very high levels of suicides (19.7 deaths per 100,000 population), especially among working men. Although the prevalence of smoking is decreasing, the rates among men are among the highest at 36.3% in 2014 compared to other industrialized countries. While recent approaches to reduce smoking have paid dividends it is becoming increasingly more prevalent among women at 11.3% in 2014 (World Bank, 2015). Obesity among women is not as prevalent as in most other industrialized nations, with 19.7% of women being obese but the rate is much higher for men, with 29% reportedly obese. Japan also has the lowest obesity rates among children under five years at only 1.5% being obese with girls having lower rates of obesity prevalence (1.1%) compared to boys (1.9).

The Japanese enjoy universal coverage and free access to all health facilities. Enrollment in an insurance plan was made mandatory for all Japanese in 1961. Most people (around 75 million) obtain their insurance through employer-related groups. The rest are covered under a national health insurance plan. Employers contribute around 4.5%, and employees contribute 3.5% of their pay toward the insurance premium. Both the employer groups and the national plans have copayments and catastrophic caps on out-of-pocket payments. Balance billing, which is the practice of charging full fees and billing the patient for the amount unpaid by insurer is prohibited, and prices to providers are set by the government. The fees for physicians are lower than in the Medicare Relative Value Scale used in the United States and is an important reason for the lower health cost in Japan (Phelps, 2003). Hospitals are mostly private, but the large hospitals and teaching hospitals are public. Most doctors work in private clinics and earn much more than the specialists working in the hospitals. The Japanese public visit their physicians regularly at an average rate of 15 times per year (Phelps, 2003). However, the number of minutes spent with the doctor is lower than in the United States. The prevalence of a fee-for-service system makes usage levels high for physician visits as the patient does not bear much additional cost from frequent visits. Due to the same reason, pharmaceutical spending is very high in Japan at 20% of total spending on health.

Total health expenditure went up considerably since the 1990s, accounting for 10.2% of GDP in 2013 according to WHO data (WHO, 2013). Health spending per capita was $3,966. The rapid aging of the population has been a primary cause of high health expenditures in Japan as in many other countries. Among industrialized nations, Japan has the worst old age support ratio (number of working-age people per retirement-age person) of 2.4 and is expected to decline even further to 1.3 by 2050 (OECD, 2013). A sizable portion of total health expenditure (around one third) was for the aged and is growing. Likewise, per capita expenditure for the aged was over three times the average. In 2000, in response to the large increase in long-term nursing care, the government introduced long-term care insurance. However, private insurance remains small accounting for only 14% of total health expenditure. Although hospital admissions are lower than in the United States, the average length of stay in Japan is among the highest in the world at 17.2 days. This explains why 39% of total health spending in 2013 was for inpatient care with hospitals providing over 90% of it. Outpatient care expenditure accounted for 34% of THE. Public funds were used for 82% of total health expenditure with the majority coming from the Social Security Fund. Private expenditure accounted for 18% in 2013, with 80%

of it being household out-of-pocket payment. The low levels of private payment often result in patients going directly to specialists even for minor ailments. The fee-for-service system also results in overtreatment and has been blamed for the high average length of stay. In 2014, there were 2.29 physicians per 1,000 population and 11.48 nurses and midwives per 1,000 population.

Profile of the Ukrainian Healthcare System

Ukraine is the second-largest country in Europe. It is a newly independent state formed as a result of the breakup of the Soviet Union in 1991. In the 2001 census it had a population of 48.4 million, with 67% living in urban areas. During the era of the Soviet republic, Ukraine was severely affected by major disasters including civil wars, famines, German invasion, and World War II. The Chernobyl nuclear accident in 1986 was a major catastrophe with significant consequences to life. The civil war over the last three years has further devastated the country. The Ukrainian economy suffered through a major economic recession in the last decade that it had begun to recover from when the war pushed its economy further back. Since obtaining its independence, Ukraine has developed the foundations for a more democratic system, but its healthcare system continues to be shackled by Soviet-style incentive systems.

Since its independence the population of Ukraine has fallen by 3.6 million or around 7.5%. In 2009 it had a population of 45.7 million. The country finds itself faced with the unfortunate situation of poor economic health, a civil war, and a shrinking and aging population. Its fertility rate is the lowest in Europe, and its birth rate fell by 40% during the 1990s. This has been attributed by some to the increased rates of abortion. For example, in 2002, there were 82.8 abortions for every 1,000 live births. As a result of the low birth rates the proportion of the population under age 15 has declined over the last 10 years.

Between 1990 and 1999 GDP in Ukraine fell by 62%. This was not only a period of declining incomes, but it was accompanied by hyperinflation. Economic recovery since that time has been very slow. In 2000, only around 66% of the adult population was actively employed, and more than one-quarter of the population lived in poverty. Thus, the ability of the government to finance the growing demand for health care is very limited.

In the postwar Soviet state, healthcare services with universal access to care was provided in a multitier structure with much of the responsibility for care being at the district (*rayon*) level and regional (*oblasts*) level. The republic provided more of the guidelines and norms governing the lower tiers. Healthcare services were provided at hospitals, sanitary and epidemiological stations, polyclinics, and specialized healthcare facilities. Size and staffing of these facilities was determined by population size. Much of the provision of care was initiated at the clinics and by primary physicians. During the 1970s and 1980s, there was considerable growth in the network of specialized facilities and units. This shifted priority away from primary care and physicians to specialists (WHO, 1999). The goal of the planning authorities was to increase capacity as measured by beds and personnel, and as a result Ukraine had the highest number of beds and physicians per capita in the world. The incentive structure was such that 80% of healthcare expenditure went toward inpatient care, and long hospital stays were common even for minor disorders. During the waning years of the Soviet Republic a new economic

TABLE 4-4 Source of Finance (% of Total Health Expenditure)				
Source of Finance	1996	2000	2009*	2013*
Public (tax, nontax revenue)	81.4	66.4	55.03	54.0
Private (out-of-pocket insurance)	18.3	32.1	44.97	46.0
Private health insurance	0.3	0.7	2.0	3.0

Data from Lekhan, V., Rudiy, V., & Nolte, E. (2004). Health care systems in transition: Ukraine. WHO Regional Office for Europe, European Observatory on Health Systems and Policies; *WHO. (2015). Global Health Observatory Data Repository. Retrieved from http://www.who.int/gho/en/

mechanism was introduced to transform the system to a performance-based system rather than a capacity-based system.

After independence in 1991, the economy experienced a painful restructuring stage with very little ability to fund the increasing need for health care. This phase of transition to a free-market economy, as with many other former Soviet economies, saw dramatic increases in prices of pharmaceuticals as well as basic necessities such as energy. The Ukrainian Constitution in 1996 stated that the function of the state was to "create conditions for effective medical services accessible to all citizens." Although Ukraine has universal access to health care for its citizens, most medical expenses are not covered except for children and other socially vulnerable groups. Thus, out-of-pocket payments are quite high as shown in Table 4-4.

Even by 2013, private insurance only accounted for slightly over 3% of private health care spending. The structure of the present-day system continues to be similar to the Soviet system. Most of the primary health clinics (PHCs) (6,456 of them in 2000) are funded and operated at the district (*rayon*) levels. The regions fund and operate both the multispecialty and specialized hospitals. They also establish the number of beds and staffing levels. The area serviced by a PHC is broken up into catchment areas (*uchastok*) each with a certain number of residents and a primary care physician. Although patients have free choice of physicians on paper, there are many obstacles to it. They can also go to a specialist directly, and more 60% do so. The incentive system is such that this is even lucrative for primary care physicians who get paid for referrals. Over 80% of public healthcare expenditure is funded locally. This results in significant inequalities across regions in the level of healthcare provision, and in 2001 a system of interbudget transfers was set up to remove regional imbalances. The budget allocation is based on the number of beds for hospitals and visits for clinics. There is very little incentive to be efficient, and the system encourages use of consultants and admissions.

Since 1991, healthcare expenditure in Ukraine has declined by 60%. The vast majority of healthcare facilities are publicly owned (24,166 such facilities in 2000) (WHO, 2000). Since 2000, there has been an attempt to increase the role played by privately owned facilities, but such a development is still nascent. The share of inpatient expenditure has dropped since independence but continues to be high at over 60% of total healthcare expenditure, mostly as a result of reductions in the number of beds. By 2006, there were around 8.7 hospital beds per 1,000 population and had increased to 9 by 2013. Capital investments in health care, while it has increased during the 1990s, remains low at only 7% of total health expenditures. Replacement of outdated medical technology and equipment has been very low at about 2%.

Private health insurance remains very limited with only 2% of the population covered by such policies in 2000. This is primarily a result of the high cost of such insurance and the inability of much of the population to afford it. In 1998, Ukraine developed a plan to provide mandatory state social insurance. This was to cover the entire population with insurance premiums paid by employers and employees equally with employee premium levels set at a fixed proportion of income. However, the high rates of unemployment and a poor state revenue base made this impractical, and the plan was rejected by Parliament in 2003.

Ukraine faced a severe health crisis in the early 1990s when life expectancy actually fell by 4.4 years for men and 2.4 years for women. Life expectancy of Ukrainians has since improved to 71.16 by 2013 (World Bank, 2015). The differential between men and women, however, remains among the highest in the world at 66 and 75 years, respectively. Recent years of civil war in Ukraine continues to make the situation dire. Infant mortality is lower than in India but higher than industrialized countries at 8.6 per 1,000 live births with neonatal mortality rate at 5.5 and under-five mortality rates at 9. Under-five mortality rate differential between female and male children is low at 8.1 and 9.9 respectively. The low infant mortality rates compared to India are perhaps a result of the much higher 7.67 nurses and midwives per 1,000 live births and the 99% of births that are attended by skilled medical personnel. Cardiovascular disease is the primary cause of death in Ukraine. The prevalence of smoking is extremely high, with the rates among men among the highest in the world at 51.4% in 2013. Smoking has also become increasingly more prevalent among women at 14.4% (World Bank, 2015). Obesity is very high with 52.4% of women being overweight, but the rate is slightly lower than it is for men with 56.3% reportedly overweight. Ukraine also has very high overweight rates among children under five years at only 26.5% being obese, with girls having lower rates of overweight prevalence (25.5%) compared to boys (27.3).

Ukraine has a very large number of physicians per capita. In 2013, there were 3.5 physicians per 1,000 people (World Bank, 2015). Of this only about one-quarter are primary care physicians with the remaining being specialists. The staffing model and low remuneration has resulted in about 1,300 vacant positions for physicians in 2000. In 1991, it was the highest among our comparison countries at 11.9 nurses per 1,000 and had fallen to 7.8 by 2002. Recent data suggest that that trend has continued with 7.7 total nurses and midwives per 1,000 population. This is primarily because of low pay and low social prestige. Healthcare professionals are paid fixed salaries based on a national pay scale. Since 2000, the government has been making efforts to provide performance-based salary increments, but the economic and civil crisis has stymied much of those efforts. Given the high rates of obesity, smoking, and alcohol consumption, the importance of maintaining the high levels of healthcare professionals in Ukraine cannot be overemphasized.

Profile of the United States Healthcare System

The United States is the richest country in the world and is a leader in technological innovation. It is no wonder then that it has evolved into a leader in the provision of sophisticated health care. According to OECD data in 2013, total health spending as a share of GDP was 17%, and health expenditures per capita were $9,146. This was higher than any other country including others in the OECD. The United States also has one of the fastest growth rates in real health expenditures per capita (over 5% for most of the last two decades) and spends the most on pharmaceuticals among OECD member countries at $947 per capita in 2004. Yet over the past four decades the increase in life expectancy at birth of 7.6 years is less than the 14 years gained in Japan and 8.6 years in Canada over the same time period. This has resulted in the claim by many that the United States has reached a level of production of health care at which further improvements in health care will require very large increases in expenditure, an issue that we will explore further in the next section.

The U.S. healthcare system relies extensively on private insurance to provide financial coverage for its people. More than 70% of the population under age 65 are enrolled in private health insurance plans, mostly through their employers. The American health system is distinguished by the unique role of managed care organizations. Managed care organizations evolved in the early 1970s primarily as a response to the rapidly growing cost of care in the United States. In the previously common practice known as "fee for service" providers charged a fee per unit of service rendered. Such a fee for service method resulted in significant overprovision of services because the provider would be paid more for each additional service they provided. In managed care organizations, payment for services rendered by providers of care is usually a negotiated capitation or per enrollee rate. In the early days of managed care, HMOs, in which the same organization that provided insurance itself provided care, were the norm. Since then numerous other variants with different degrees of contractual arrangements between the insurance company and healthcare providers have evolved.

Government provision of health insurance in the United States is undertaken through Medicare and Medicaid, which were initiated in 1966. Health insurance for the population aged 65 and older is provided through Medicare. Part A of Medicare covers hospitalization and some skilled nursing facility charges, and the supplemental Part B covers physician and laboratory charges and medical supplies. Most prescription drugs are not covered under Medicare, but the passage of the Prescription Drug Act in 2005 provides some relief from the soaring costs of pharmaceutical products. The working population pays a Medicare tax to pay for the benefits received by the elderly. The rapid growth in the elderly population caused by the aging of the baby boom generation and their longer life spans, coupled with low birth rates and working populations, has made the financial viability of such a program a matter of immediate and great concern. The Medicare system has been unable to meet its current obligations with current revenue since around 1995, and it is expected that it will deplete all of its accumulated funds within the next decade. Numerous attempts have been made to rein in the growth of Medicare expenditures, including contracting with managed care organizations and stricter controls on charges by hospitals and physicians.

Medicaid is a safety net program for people with low income, mostly women, children, and the elderly and disabled, who receive federal or state financial assistance. The program typically covers charges for physician visits, inpatient and outpatient hospital stays, and nursing home stays. However, each state has tremendous discretion in determining benefits covered. As a result, there are significant variations across states in the level of benefits provided by Medicaid. Although initially it was a federal–state program with matching federal funds, this program has increasingly become reliant on state tax revenue. As a result of escalating healthcare costs, Medicaid programs have become the largest single item in many states budgets. As with Medicare, attempts to control growing Medicaid expenditures have included contracting with managed care organizations.

A potentially significant recent development has been the passage of the Affordable Care Act in 2010 (Obamacare Facts, 2010). This act attempts to potentially overhaul healthcare provision in the United States by, among other things, prohibiting insurance coverage denial due to preexisting conditions, and bans (restricts) use of lifetime (annual) limits on expenditure. The more significant and controversial aspects of the act began to take effect in 2014 with the creation of state-run medical insurance exchanges and mandatory insurance coverage. Many aspects of this act are still under litigation, and hence it is too early to include a detailed analysis of this act here.

In 2002, there were 5,794 hospitals in the United States, and 3,025 of them were nongovernment owned. Most of these hospitals are not for profit with only about 766 of them being investor owned. Hospital charges account for over one-third of healthcare costs in the United States with a total bill of $650 billion. Medicare paid 43.5% of this bill, private insurance paid 31.2%, Medicaid paid 18.3%, and the uninsured accounted for 3.8%. Those aged 65 years and older make up about 13% of the total population but accounted for about 35% of all hospital stays. The top three principal diagnoses for this age group were hardening of the heart arteries, pneumonia, and congestive heart failure The mean charge per stay was $17,300, with infant respiratory distress syndrome having the highest average charge at $91,400 (see Table 4-5).

TABLE 4-5 Mean Hospital Charges

Principal Diagnoses with the Highest Mean Charges	Mean Charges ($)	Mean Length of Stay (in days)
1. Infant respiratory distress syndrome	91,400	24.2
2. Premature birth and low birth weight	79,300	24.2
3. Spinal cord injury	76,800	12.8
4. Leukemia (cancer of blood)	74,500	14.1
5. Intrauterine hypoxia and birth asphyxia (lack of oxygen to baby in uterus or during birth)	72,800	15.6
6. Cardiac and circulatory birth defects	71,400	8.9
7. Heart valve disorders	70,900	8.8
8. Polio and other brain or spinal infections	63,200	13.0
9. Aneurysm (ballooning or rupture of an artery)	55,300	7.7
10. Adult respiratory failure or arrest	48,500	10.0

Reproduced from Agency for Healthcare Research and Quality. (2003). Hospitalization in the United States. *HCUP Fact Book, 6*. Retrieved from http://archive.ahrq.gov/data/hcup/factbk6/factbk6c.htm

In the United States as opposed to most other OECD countries, private expenditure on health is larger than public expenditure, mostly financed through private insurance. The share of private insurance is therefore higher than in any other country in the OECD. However, around 15% of the population does not have any form of insurance and relies on emergency rooms for medical care. Emergency rooms are required by law to provide essential care regardless of insurance status. The cost of providing uncompensated care to them is recovered by hospitals when feasible by charging more for their insured patients. Faced with the strong forces of competition from other providers, healthcare facilities in locations where such uncompensated care is large often are faced with an inability to pass on much of the costs and hospital bankruptcies are quite prevalent. The high cost of inefficiency to the hospitals under the new reimbursement mechanisms has also resulted in significant reductions in the number of hospital beds. The United States now has among the fewest number of hospital beds per capita among OECD countries at 2.9 per 1,000 population in 2013.

The United States has fewer physicians and nurses per capita than the OECD average (OECD, 2006). In 2013, there were 2.45 physicians and around 10.8 nurses per 1,000 population. Because of the increasing prevalence of managed care organizations and the adoption of the relative value fee schedule for physician reimbursement rates, the number of general practitioners has been growing while the number of some specialists (anesthesiologists, for example) has been declining.

Life expectancy differential of Americans between men and women remains high at 76.5 and 81.3 years respectively, and both are lower than life expectancy in comparison countries such as Canada and Japan (World Bank, 2015). Infant mortality similarly is higher than the comparison countries at 5.6 per 1,000 live births with neonatal mortality rate at 3.6 and under-five mortality rates at 6.5. The under-five mortality rate differential between female and male children is high at 5.9 and 7.1 respectively. The fact that the infant mortality rates are higher compared to other industrialized countries is in spite of the much higher number of nurses and midwives (9.815) per 1,000 live births and the higher level and share of health spending out of GDP (17%). The prevalence of smoking has drastically declined through regulator policies and peer pressure and has now dropped to 21 and 16.3% of men and women, respectively. Obesity and overweight remain among the highest for both men and women at 72.1 and 62.6% respectively. The United States also has high overweight rates among children under five years with 6.9% of girls and 5.2% of boys being overweight.

The United States spends the most in absolute amounts as well as a share of its GDP, and both have continued to increase rapidly. Between 2003 and 2013, the ratio of health spending to GDP grew from 9.5 to 10.7% in Canada, from 8 to 10.2% in Japan, and from 15.1 to 17.1% in the United States (OECD, 2015b). In 2013, the United States spent $9,086 (purchasing power parity) per person on health compared to $4,629 in Canada and $5,713 in Japan. Total spending on health grew at 5.3% in 2014 compared to 2.9% in 2013 (CMS, 2015). Spending on hospitals accounted for $2,964 of this compared to $1,338 for Canada and $1,673 for Japan. On pharmaceutical products the United States spent $1,034 compared to $761 by Canada and $756 by Japan. On services provided by physician offices the United States spent $1,856 compared to $720 by Canada and $668 by Japan. For the United States alone, spending for hospital care grew at 4.1% in 2014 compared to 3.5% in 2013, spending for physician services grew at 4.6%

compared to 2.5%, and spending for prescription drugs grew at 12.2% compared to 2.4%. The question of why the United States with the prevalence of managed care and other cost-control mechanisms finds its healthcare costs soaring has been a question that has puzzled many. Three reasons are often cited for the rapid increase in healthcare costs: pharmaceutical price increases, utilization of new technology, and healthcare costs associated with aging.

Retail prescription drugs, which accounted for about 11% of national health expenditures in 2003 according to Smith et al. (2003), were responsible for close to 10% in 2014 (CMS, 2015). According to a study done by the American Association of Retired Persons (AARP, 2006), during the 2000 to 2005 period manufacturers' prices for the most widely used brand-name prescription drugs grew at an average annual rate of around 6%. Without exception prescription drug prices grew faster than the overall inflation rate during the last three decades. The growth in utilization of expensive new technology has been another key driver of the rising cost of health care in the United States according to many studies (Commonwealth Fund, 2012; Hay, 2003). According to Rothenberg (2003), "Changes in medical technology accounted for 20 to 40% of the yearly rise in healthcare spending in the late 1990s."

As pointed out in the discussion of hospital costs earlier, the elderly (65 and older) make up 13% of the population but consume 36% of health care. According to Stanton and Rutherford (2005), the elderly had an average healthcare expenditure of $11,089 compared to $3,352 for working age people in 2002. Figure 4-1 shows that 43% of the highest spenders are in the 65 and older age group. This age group is the fastest-growing group among the U.S. population. The United States in 2010 had by far the largest number of centenarians at 70,490 compared to Japan at 44,449 according to the Population Division of the United Nations. The number of

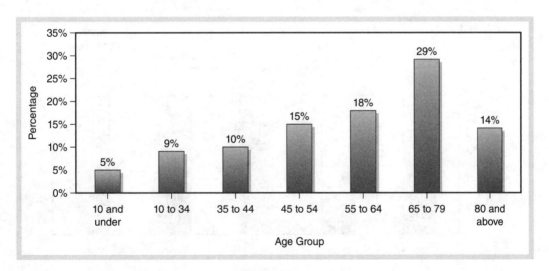

FIGURE 4-1 Distribution of Top 5% of Healthcare Spenders
Modified from Conwell, L., & Cohen, J. (2005). Characteristics of persons with high medical expenditures in the U.S. civilian noninstitutional population, 2002. *MEPS Statistical Brief No. 73.* Retrieved from http://meps.ahrq.gov/mepsweb/data_files/publications/st73/stat73.pdf

centenarians in the United States grew by over 6% during the 1990s, according to Krach and Velkoff (1999). There were 120 centenarians per 10,000 population aged 85 and older in 1990 while in Japan there were about 29. Manton and Waupal (1995) found that life expectancy at age 85 is significantly higher in the United States than in England, France, Japan, or Sweden. Although this can be seen as a feather in the cap for our healthcare system, it is also a cause for great concern due to the associated high costs. Total health spending per capita by those age 85 and over was the highest of any age group at $34,784 in 2010 compared to the second highest age group of 65 to 84 years, which was $15,857 (CMS, 2015).

COMPARATIVE ANALYSIS OF HEALTHCARE SYSTEMS

The five countries under study here show tremendous variation in the size of expenditures, role of government, and health insurance (see Figure 4-2 and Table 4-6). For consistency we have used the same data source extracted from the World Health Organization Statistical Information System (WHOSIS) for our analysis. WHOSIS is one of the few data sets that collects comparable data for these five countries. While WHOSIS has been subsumed into a new Global Health Observatory Data Repository (GHODR) system, some of the key data that are used here for cost impact studies are not yet readily available to the public and hence we have refrained from updating the data in this section. The OECD has much more detailed data on some variables, but it does not collect data on Ukraine and India and hence is of limited value here.

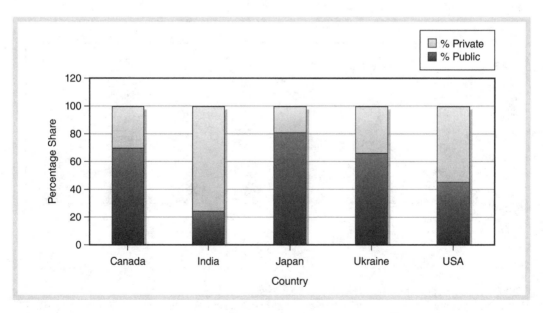

FIGURE 4-2 Per Capita Health Expenditure Shares
Data from WHOSIS. (2006). Statistical information system. World Health Organization.

TABLE 4-6 Expenditure Breakdown 2013

Country	Per Capita Total Health Expenditure ($)	Per Capita Government Health Expenditure ($)	Share of Private in Total Health Spending (%)	Out-of-Pocket Expenditure as Percentage of Private Expenditure on Health (%)	Private Prepaid Plans as Percentage of Private Expenditure on Health (%)
Canada	5,718	3,991	30	50	41
India	61	20	68	86	5
Japan	3,966	3,255	18	80	14
Ukraine	313	170	46	94	2
United States	9,146	4,307	53	22	63

Data from World Health Organization. (2015). Global Health Expenditure Database. Retrieved from http://apps.who.int/nha/database

The United States leads in healthcare spending and spends per capita about $9,146 compared to India's $6. The share of government expense in total health expenditure is similarly different across countries. Whereas the government in India spends only $20 per capita annually on health care, the U.S. government spends over $4,300 (see Table 4-6). Japan's healthcare system is mostly publicly provided, with the government covering close to 80%, while in India the government barely covers 30% of health expenditures. Ukraine, which has universal coverage, still has a high share of private spending as benefits provided are so limited that patients are forced to make sizable out-of-pocket payments. Eighty-six percent of private health spending is out of pocket in Ukraine compared to about 22% in the United States. Private health insurance pays for over 63% of private spending in the United States while it pays for only 2% in Ukraine where health expenditures are mostly financed by out-of-pocket payments. Thus, there are large differences in how health care is paid for across these countries.

The next question we can ask is does the type of system matter for the healthcare outcomes? Measures of health outcomes that are commonly used are life expectancy and infant mortality rates, and their values are shown in Table 4-7. The mostly public health financing system in Japan appears to do the best under either measure followed by Canada, which has the second most public financing of health care. In addition to the health system, lifestyle and other differences often play a big role as well, as we point out later.

As we can see in Table 4-7, in spite of its high levels of spending, the United States does not perform as well as other industrialized nations in these broad health outcomes. India is perhaps the worst performing on the aggregate. Because measures of life expectancy do not always reflect the true health of the person, an alternate measure called Healthy Life Expectancy (HALE) has recently been developed. HALE attempts to measure the number of healthy life years the person can expect to live. In Table 4-8, HALE numbers are shown for the comparison countries at birth for the overall population and for males and females. They follow the same ranking as

TABLE 4-7 Health Outcomes 2013

Country	Life Expectancy in Years		Infant Mortality Rate (per 1,000 Live Births)
	Females at Birth	Males at Birth	
Canada	83.8	79.3	4.3
India	69	66.2	37.9
Japan	86.61	80.21	2
Ukraine	76.22	66.34	7.7
United States	81.3	76.5	5.6

Data from World Bank. (2015). *Health, nutrition, and population statistics.* Retrieved from http://datatopics.worldbank.org/hnp/Home

TABLE 4-8 Healthy Life Expectancy (HALE) in Years

Population	At Birth 2000	At Birth 2013	Males 2013	Females 2013
Canada	69.7	72	71	73
India	51.2	58	56	59
Japan	73.5	75	72	78
Ukraine	57.5	63	59	67
United States	67.4	69	68	71

Data from WHO. (2006). World Health Statistics 2006. World Health Organization, Geneva; WHO. (2015). *Global Health Observatory Data Repository.* Retrieved from http://www.who.int/gho/en/

life expectancy measures. It is also interesting to note that the gains made in HALE since 2000 for the countries starting at a lower level of economic prosperity and health spending—Ukraine and India—are significantly larger. Perhaps this is a sign of diminishing productivity from health spending (as more is spent, the gains become smaller) or is due purely to transfer of knowledge from developed to developing economies. It is, however, difficult to argue that this is a result of the financing system because, as we pointed out earlier, each of these five countries has very different levels of public versus private health spending shares.

The structure of the healthcare system and the reimbursement arrangements (capitation versus fee for service) can influence how much health care is provided per dollar spent. A crude illustration of this notion is displayed in Table 4-9. A more accurate investigation is undertaken in the next section. We compute the number of expected years of life at birth per dollar of per capita health expenditure by dividing life expectancy at birth and infant mortality rates by per capita health expenditure. The larger numbers in the table represent the more productivity in

TABLE 4-9 Health Outcome per Dollar of per Capita Health Expenditure

Country	Life Expectancy per Capita Dollar		HALE per Capita Dollar	
	Females at Birth	Males at Birth	Females at Birth	Males at Birth
Canada	0.146	0.138	0.127	0.124
India	1.131	1.081	0.967	0.918
Japan	0.021	0.020	0.019	0.018
Ukraine	0.243	0.211	0.214	0.188
United States	0.008	0.008	0.007	0.007

Computations by authors.

TABLE 4-10 Selected Risk Factors 2013

Country	Prevalence of Overweight Adult Males (%)	Prevalence of Overweight Adult Females (%)	Prevalence of Adult Male Tobacco Smokers (%)	Prevalence of Adult Female Tobacco Smokers (%)
Canada	69.0	59.8	19.5	14.2
India	24.7	19.5	22.8	2.4
Japan	29.0	19.7	36.3	11.3
Ukraine	56.3	52.4	51.4	14.4
United States	62.6	72.1	21.0	16.3

Data from World Bank (2015). *Health, Nutrition and Population Statistics.* Retrieved from http://datatopics.worldbank.org/hnp/Home

terms of each dollar spent per capita. Life expectancy per dollar spent (and HALE per dollar spent) is lowest in the United States across gender. The huge disparity in healthcare expenditures per capita across countries without an equally large disparity in outcomes is what drives this result, but the point still remains.

There is a good deal of evidence in the literature that shows that lifestyle factors play a major role in determining the level of health. The Japanese diet rich in fish has often been argued to be a principal reason for the healthier Japanese population. Table 4-10 displays prevalence rates for some key lifestyle risk factors. No clear pattern emerges from this. Smoking is highly prevalent among Japanese males and is second only to Ukrainian males. Obesity is most prevalent in the United States, and given the links between obesity, diabetes, and heart disease it is a cause for major concern. India has very low levels of obesity but high levels of smoking prevalence among males.

Thus, it is clear that there are wide variations in healthcare systems, expenditures, and outcomes across this selection of countries. In the following section, we describe and analyze production and productivity of health care in these countries.

HEALTHCARE PRODUCTIVITY AND COSTS

In this section, we describe the concept of productivity and costs in health care and how they are used in making healthcare expenditure decisions. We then use cross-country data to estimate the production and cost of health improvements. We also compare the productivity and cost of health care across the sample of five countries.

Why does the United States have such high levels of medical expenditure per capita compared to the other countries but not much better outcomes? Phelps (2003), using data on perinatal mortality rates for five industrialized nations including Canada, Japan, and the United States, points out that the "United States with higher medical spending than any other country is closer to the "flat of the curve" than other countries in the sense that additional spending on medical care is less likely to produce increases in health outcomes."

In Figure 4-3 we plot per capita healthcare spending on male life expectancy at birth for our sample of five countries. As per capita healthcare spending increases from a low of $82 in India to $2,244 in Japan, life expectancy increases rapidly from 61 years to 79 years. Further increases in spending such as for Canada at $2,989 and United States at $5,711 actually see lower life expectancy of 78 and 75 years, respectively. This could be taken to suggest that healthcare spending in Canada and the United States is beyond the stage of effectiveness in increasing medical outcomes, which is an issue that we explore further in this section. The association depicted here must be considered with great caution because of the very small number of observations and other factors such as lifestyle that play a role.

Economists often describe the production of health care using the concept of a production function. A production function describes the relationship between inputs and outcomes. It specifies for any given technology of production, the maximum amount of output that could be produced by a given combination of amounts of inputs. Outputs or outcomes could be cancer detection, mortality rates, length of hospital stay, or other measures of morbidity, and inputs could be tests, treatment procedures, and expenditures. With better technology, methods, and processes the same amount of inputs, such as physician time, can produce more output. The average product of an input (often referred to as productivity of an input) is the amount of output

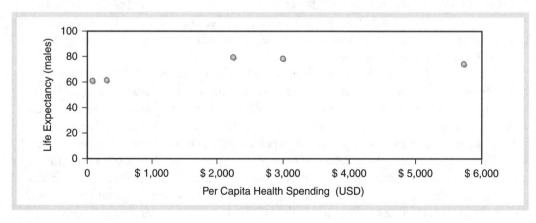

FIGURE 4-3 Health Spending and Life Expectancy

produced per unit of input whereas marginal product of an input refers to the amount of additional output produced using an additional unit of that input. At very low levels of health care, every additional test (unit of treatment) has a large and positive effect in improving health outcome. As the number of tests and procedures performed on the patient increases, each additional test has a smaller and smaller effect on outcomes. Such a tendency is what is referred to as diminishing marginal productivity. Across disease groups, across countries, and across patients this pattern often tends to occur and may explain why the United States does not do much better in some measures of health outcomes even though it spends significantly more than many other industrialized countries.

Neuhauser and Lewicki (1975) were one of the first to use economic analysis to advise medical decision making. They looked at the use of the sixth stool guaiac test for detecting colon cancer cases. The stool guaiac test can be repeated in order to detect more cases because of the existence of false positives or negatives in each round of testing. Table 4-11 shows the number of tests conducted and the resulting number of cases detected. As can be seen, while more cases are detected with more tests, each additional test detects fewer and fewer additional cases of colon cancer. In moving from the fifth to the sixth test, almost no additional cases are detected. Figure 4-4 plots the production function for cancer detection using the sixth stool guaiac test. The curve flattens out from the third test on indicating that very little additional cases are detected through additional testing. Figure 4-5 plots the marginal product of the sixth stool guaiac test showing the number of additional cases detected through additional tests.

Many studies such as Pritchett and Summers (1996) and Bhargava, Jamison Lau, and Murray (2001) find evidence that higher incomes permit individuals to afford better nutrition, health care, and thereby health. Similar studies (McGinnis & Foege, 2004) have shown that education and lifestyle factors play an important role in many dimensions of health. At a cross-country level, the production of health (as measured by HALE) should depend on the country's income (per capita gross national income [GNI]) and education (literacy rate) as well as lifestyle factors (smoking prevalence). We extracted data from the WHO World Health Statistics database for 58 countries (the reduction in sample size is due to the lack of data on smoking prevalence in many countries). Our regression result below suggests that not only does HALE

TABLE 4-11 Cancer Detection

Number of Tests	Number of Cancer Cases Detected	Additional Cases Detected
1	65.9469	65.9469
2	71.4425	5.4956
3	71.9005	0.458
4	71.9387	0.0382
5	71.9419	0.0032
6	71.9422	0.0003

Data from Neuhauser, D., & Lewicki, A. M. (1975). What do we gain from the sixth stool guaiac? *New England Journal of Medicine, 293,* 226–228.

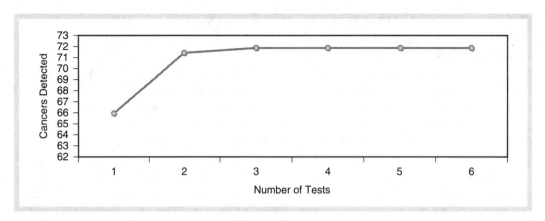

FIGURE 4-4 Production Function for Cancer Detection

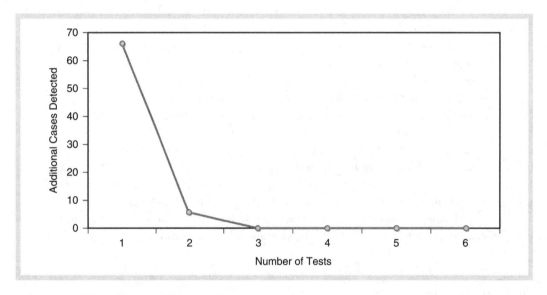

FIGURE 4-5 Additional Cases Detected

increase with literacy rate and GNI, the effect of GNI on HALE gets smaller as GNI increases suggesting that it becomes less and less effective at generating higher HALE. Smoking prevalence was not significant probably because GNI already captures most of its effect.

Figure 4-6 shows the position of each of our sample of countries in this relationship (with literacy rate fixed at mean value of 80%). As can be seen, United States, Japan, and Canada are at the stage where further increases in GNI is not likely to bring about any increase in HALE, while India and Ukraine are likely to see significant improvements in HALE as their economy grows. These results should be regarded with great caution; they are for illustrative purposes only as there are potentially multiple directions of causality between income and health

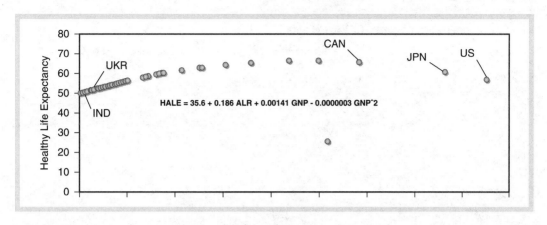

FIGURE 4-6 Health Activity Life Expectancy Versus GNP (Literacy Rate Fixed at Mean Value of 80%)

(Chapman & Hariharan, 1994), which we have not controlled for. Bloom et al. (2004) also provide evidence that improvements in health have a significant positive effect on the rate of growth of GDP per capita. There are also problems associated with using cross-country regressions that we have not addressed.

Although productivity studies can characterize which tests or treatments or which countries are most effective in providing health care, the cost of treatments must play a central role when making decisions on the allocation of scarce resources. In a world faced with growing demands on its scarce healthcare budgets, the most pressing and controversial decisions are often associated with the questions of how much health care to provide. Whether governments, healthcare providers, or private individuals make such decisions, cost considerations invariably become critical in addressing them.

There are many methods developed by economists and others to include cost considerations in making better decisions. The most controversial of these is benefit-cost analysis (BCA). In BCA the monetized value of all the benefits (better or longer life, for example) is compared against the cost of obtaining such a benefit. The controversy in the use of BCA to allocate healthcare resources is often centered on the methods for monetization of health benefits. For example, one commonly used dollar value for increases in life expectancy is the value of a statistical life (VSL) (Viscusi & Aldy, 2002). The VSL is often arrived at by using the amount individuals have been willing to accept as appropriate compensation for a reduction in life expectancy (e.g., accepting a wage premium for jobs with a higher risk of death). Table 4-12 lists some estimates of VSL for a sample of countries. For example, the value of a statistical life in India is $3.3 million compared to $9.7 million in Japan.

Critics of this approach point to the difficulty of inferring from a small increase in risk of death to a large increase, as well as the wide range of these estimates and measurement errors in these studies. In one report, Jamison (2006) calculates the value of investments in health by comparing changes in annual healthcare costs to changes in annual population health outcomes monetized using VSL. They calculate that in the United States, the cost per disability adjusted life year in

TABLE 4-12   International Estimates of Value of a Statistical Life

Country	Estimates of Value of Statistical Life (millions of US$)
United Kingdom	5.7–74.1
Canada	5.1–5.3
India	4.1
Taiwan	0.7
Japan	9.7
Hong Kong	1.7
Australia	11.3–19.1
South Korea	0.8
Austria	3.9–6.5
United States	5–12
Ukraine	3.3

Data from Viscusi, K. W., & Aldy, J. E. (2002). The value of a statistical life: A critical review of market estimates throughout the world. *Journal of Risk and Uncertainty, 27*(1), 5–76.; Wallsten, S., & Kosec, K. (2005). The economic cost of the war in Iraq (Working Paper 05-19). AEA-Brookings Joint Center for Regulatory Studies.

U.S. dollars ranges from as low a cost as $3 for taxing tobacco products to over $25,000 for performing coronary artery bypass surgery. In a study on the effects of technological change on cost and care, Cutler and McClellan (2001) identified two channels through which improved medical technology affects health: substitution of newer technology for older, less-effective technology, and expansion, in which more people are treated with the new technology. Their results suggest that while improved technology comes at a higher cost the benefit from them outweighs the cost.

As a result of some of these criticisms and the difficulties in identifying all of the costs and benefits across generations, other approaches have become popular in healthcare decision making. Perhaps the most popular method for advising decision making in the allocation of scarce medical resources is cost-effectiveness analysis (CEA). CEA measures the cost per additional or incremental unit of health outcome and uses that to guide decisions on which procedure or test should be used and how much of it should be undertaken. The popularity of CEA over benefit-cost analysis (BCA) comes from the lack of a need to monetize health outcomes or benefits. CEA can be used for both the decision on which test or intervention to use as well as for how much of any given test or treatment. In the Neuhauser and Lewicki (1975) study, the cost per additional case detected increases rapidly with each additional test (Table 4-13). The first screening test is highly cost effective: it gains an additional cancer detected for only $1,175. Further tests detect fewer and fewer cases and thus entail progressively higher costs per case detected. The additional cost per cancer detected gained due to the sixth test are over $40 million, making it highly cost ineffective. However, in order to decide on the number of tests that is reasonable to conduct, it becomes necessary to draw a subjective line. One attempt to do this can be found in Chapman and Hariharan (1994, 1996) in which the value of statistical life provides the cutoff.

TABLE 4-13   Stool Guaiac Test Cost Effectiveness

Number of Tests	Total Cost of Diagnosis ($)	Additional Cost of Detection ($)	Cost per Cancer Detected ($)	Marginal Cost per Cancer Detected ($)
1	77511	77511	1175.354717	1175.354717
2	107690	30179	1507.366064	5491.484096
3	130199	22509	1810.8219	49146.28821
4	148116	17917	2058.919608	469031.4136
5	163141	15025	2267.677112	4695312.5
6	176331	13190	2451.009282	43966666.67

International Comparisons of Cost

Because of a lack of comparable data across countries, especially for developing countries, international comparisons of healthcare productivity has until recently been difficult. The World Health Organization in 1998 began an elaborate study to compute the costs of health care for a wide range of countries using a standardized metric. They computed the unit cost of care for primary, secondary, and tertiary care bed days and outpatient visits as well as for health centers at different levels of population coverage. Table 4-14 lists the unit cost of care for hospitalization (bed days), outpatient visits, and health center visits for our sample of five countries. As expected the differences are quite

TABLE 4-14   Unit Cost for Health Care

	Canada	India	Japan	Ukraine	USA
Cost per Bed Day					
Primary	140.09	14.71	138.85	30.11	906.64
Secondary	182.76	19.19	181.14	39.29	1182.81
Tertiary	249.64	26.21	247.42	53.66	1615.58
Cost per Outpatient Visit					
Primary	55.43	3.96	54.85	9.16	366.17
Secondary	78.62	5.62	77.80	12.99	519.38
Tertiary	116.30	8.31	115.09	19.22	768.31
Cost per Health Center Visit					
50%	29.05	6.43	28.95	6.79	30.46
80%	29.05	6.43	28.95	6.79	30.46
95%	31.58	6.99	31.47	7.38	33.11

Data from WHO. (2006). *Choosing interventions that are cost effective (WHO-CHOICE)*. Retrieved from http://www.who.int/choice/publications/discussion_papers/en/index.html

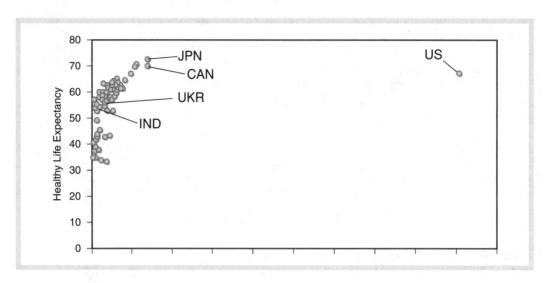

FIGURE 4-7 Healthy Life Expectancy Versus Unit Costs (Health)
Data from World Health Organization. (2006). World Health Statistics 2006, World Health Organization, Geneva.

stark. While Canada and Japan have similar unit costs, the United States has inpatient and outpatient costs that are about seven times as high. India has the lowest unit costs across the board followed by Ukraine. Unlike inpatient and outpatient costs, health center care costs for the three wealthier countries are not significantly different from each other indicating that the major cost difference between the United States and other industrialized countries must be found in hospitals.

To make any reasonable statements, sample sizes much larger than our five countries are required. We therefore extracted a set of 58 countries from the WHO-Choice data with recent information on healthy activity life expectancy and unit cost per primary bed day. If the higher unit costs in developed countries are from better quality of care it should be reflected in higher HALE in those countries. We used unit cost per bed day rather than per outpatient or health center visit because hospitalization is more often required for treating ailments with a high risk of death. As can be seen in Figure 4-7, omitting the United States as an extreme outlier, the data does show that higher unit costs result in higher healthy life expectancy.

Figure 4-7 is a scatterplot of healthy life expectancy and unit costs of primary bed care for the 58 countries. The United States is an extreme outlier here because of its very high unit cost of inpatient care.

We also regressed healthy life expectancy on unit cost and unit cost squared to see if the increase in HALE gets progressively smaller as unit costs increase and find that to be true:

$$HALE = 41.4 + 0.454 \text{ UNIT COSTS} - 0.00194 \text{ UNITCOST2}$$

Figure 4-8 shows the positive relationship between unit costs and health outcomes, as measured by healthy life expectancy. Thus, there is some evidence that higher unit costs do translate into better health outcomes.

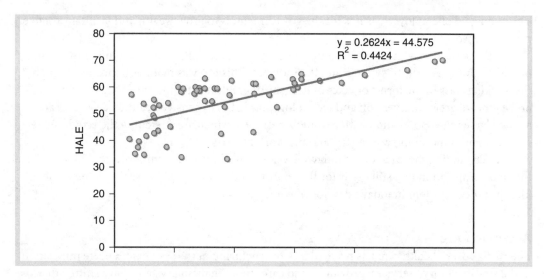

FIGURE 4-8 Unit Costs and Health Outcomes

To summarize, there appears to be some evidence suggesting that perhaps as Phelps and others have pointed out the United States may be at a stage where additional improvements in health are more difficult to achieve while countries such as India and Ukraine may find it easy and less expensive to achieve improvements in health.

KEY COMPONENTS OF AN IDEAL HEALTHCARE SYSTEM
After exploring the healthcare systems of several countries, examining the differences and similarities among them, and comparing certain outcomes and costs, can we now identify the attributes of an effective healthcare system? An effective system would provide the best *value* for the nation and for the health care of each inhabitant of that country. Each system has evolved over time based on its unique circumstances around politics, culture, religion, and economic resources.

In the macro view, the incentive, or *value*, to develop a healthcare system as a country is to build wealth. In defining an ideal healthcare system, we will focus on a country that is committed to growing wealth as a nation, contrasted with a country that is focused on building wealth for a focus minority of the country. The developed healthcare system provides needed stability for the country to build a reliable workforce that optimizes productivity and contributes to a more unified nation. Additionally, health care itself creates an industry that in itself contributes to the wealth of the country.

Traditionally, healthcare systems have focused on intervention and technology. The primary beginnings focused on growing the human resources of trained professionals, primarily physicians and nurses. Trained professionals led to the need for technology. Due to the limited economic resources of the country, private investment into the healthcare system was vital. This private investment came from the individual end user, or from employer-sponsored insurance.

The main goal of employers, as it is for the government, is to grow wealth and facilitate a stable, productive workforce.

As the focus of health care was on the working class, the culture and religion of the country provided for the elderly, the young, and the indigent. This too was mainly supported through the working class in the forms of taxes or cost shifting. But most important is that as this focus on healthcare grew, intervention and technology has led to expensive healthcare systems and a much larger aged population with chronic conditions, which are stretching the economic resources of both the country, industry, and the working class.

Understanding these factors as today's developed healthcare systems grow and in terms of the value proposition that still exists for the country and industry, what are the elements of an ideal healthcare system in today's developed countries?

Access to Care

The rising cost of health care has resulted in a restructuring of the system and more innovation in the stratification of services, providers, and care sites. Financing systems have shifted the cost to be more on the individual. New care sites are being developed to service individual healthcare needs anywhere the population is gathered.

Preventive, Screening, and Monitoring

The wearing of seat belts challenged a value proposition, which was supported only through a penalty system. But the real success of seat belt wearing arrived when a child challenges the parent or grandparent: "Grandpa, why are you not wearing your seatbelt?" The need of the child to understand safety demanded compliance of the adult. Prevention has to start with education of the young. Prevention is the lowest cost of health care with the highest return on health status and cost avoidance. Yet, in focusing on the development of a healthcare industry, the wealth proposition won as the country's professional base and wealth grew. Now faced with a large population of senior citizens with chronic disease, prevention now demands a stronger value proposition toward avoiding unnecessary cost to the healthcare system. Prevention includes education, diet and exercise, early screening, regular primary care visits, and ongoing monitoring of chronic conditions. This was evident in the Japanese healthcare model where the barriers were removed for citizens making regular and frequent visits to their doctor. This probably was the reason for many of their strong outcome measures.

An excellent example to demonstrate the effectiveness of screening can be built around lung cancer. In a population of 200,000 residents, approximately 25% will meet screening criteria for an early screening for lung cancer. That criterion is 40 years of age with a history of smoking, occupational exposure, or significant secondhand smoke. Based on the initial studies findings as published in the *New England Journal of Medicine* (October 26, 2006), 1.3% will show up positive for lung tumors on the baseline screen and 0.03% will show up positive on the annual follow-up screen. These numbers represent 665 individuals with lung tumors that are symptom free. Early intervention conservatively results in a 50% reduction in treatment cost. Assuming a conservative $40,000 savings in avoided healthcare cost (radiation therapy, chemotherapy, major surgery, etc.) per individual, the healthcare system saved $13.3 million in cost avoidance. In addition to the large cost avoidance, early intervention results in a reduction of sick leave (office visits, hospital stay, and rehab time). Assuming three weeks per individual, 1,995 weeks of productivity is regained. Assuming an average of $30,000 annual salary, a little more than $1 million of productive salary is regained.

Palliative Care

At the opposite end of the spectrum is palliative care, or more simply stated, focusing on quality of life versus quantity of life for individuals with chronic or life-limiting diseases. In a population where the demands of the aging population outgrow the economic resources of the country, a culture of palliative care can help balance the economic equation in a more positive manner.

For many individuals, the last few years of healthcare expenditures may represent the majority of their lifetime healthcare cost. This is due to expensive technology and drugs to extend life. The value proposition of the higher cost interventions in the last few years of life diminishes in both quality of life and quantity of life metrics. By including the patient and family in education of the options and the desires of the patient, some of this expensive care can be, and should be, diverted.

Population Management

Following the 80/20 rule of thumb, 80% of a country's, or a company's, healthcare cost may be spent on 20% of their healthcare insurance participants. This is a very valid scenario for all healthcare systems. Management of this top 20% must be focused and deliberate if costs are to be controlled. Management may include the previous preventive and palliative methods, and management may include punitive or incentivized methods such as higher insurance premiums based on lifestyle or behavioral habits. Examples include diet and exercise in weight management and smoking cessation.

Provider and Setting

In today's high-tech environment, new diseased-targeted treatments are being discovered routinely. Many of these discoveries have opened the door to new forms of providers and settings for healthcare delivery. Now there are many therapies that can be administered by providers that are not doctors (e.g., physician assistant and nurse practitioners) and some care visits can be provided by a technician as in a regular A1C blood draw for a diabetic monitoring. By partnering alternative providers with new technology that provides for opportunities for monitoring and screening in alternative settings, many of these healthcare services can be offered in new settings that include employer clinics, school clinics, churches, retail settings, or in the home.

As the cost curve rises for the consumers of care, these lower-cost options must be developed to stabilize a changing value proposition.

Technology and Institutional Care

Due to the growth of the world's population and along with it a higher percentage of individuals with chronic disease, the demands for high-cost technology and institutional care will stay high. More of this type of care will carry a higher burden of the cost on the individual consumer, as government and employers work to balance their need for a strong workforce in an ever-growing cost equation.

Balancing the Value Equation: Financing

Within the value equation, there must exist in the financing a system that balances the incentives in payment for services. The U.S. model for years has made payment to institutions of care based on the diagnosis and procedure for the visit. The U.S. model made payments to providers (doctors, nurse practitioners, etc.) based on activity that is created (fee for service). In this system, the two entities are incentivized in two different directions. The hospital needs to manage their services to optimize the payment by assuring that care is targeted toward the specific disease and no more. The doctor is incentivized to create activity that results in additional payment to the doctor. In the U.S. system, many doctors own the technology for which they control the prescribing authority, therefore incentivizing over utilization. The ideal system would have a system of payment that incentivizes the system to manage utilization at all levels. The design of this payment system should shift more financial responsibility to the consumer to encourage lower cost and lower utilization, without negatively effecting, or creating barriers to, the utilization of preventive care.

Litigation

In cultures where health care is viewed as a right and is unlimited, another incentive to overutilize resources is the need of providers to practice defensive medicine due to the threat of costly lawsuits. As discussed earlier, the value of the first test diminishes substantially as a second, third, or fourth test is performed. Yet, in an environment of defensive medicine, this type of serial testing occurs.

The overall frequency of suits, cost of trials, and higher awards has led to higher insurance premiums and significant legal cost. These practices continue to strain the healthcare system. Judicial systems must be created that can assure that a balance exists that supports a highly reliable healthcare system while eliminating low-value litigation activity.

Public Health/Safety Net

Many healthcare models address providing care for those that cannot afford to pay. In an ideal healthcare system, the care for these individuals should be blended into the base model in a seamless delivery model that is not recognized as different to the base healthcare system. An example of this approach has been used in housing. Traditional housing for underprivileged families was at one time to develop special housing units that served this needy population. This congregated a challenged population and acted as a barrier to success. The families and the support systems for this community would bear a disproportionate share of the burden of this population. Newer methods of housing in some communities blend housing needs by allocating a percentage of new houses in a new neighborhood to be designated for the local housing author-ity. These agency-placed families live as neighbors, the children are blended into the schools, and the burdens are spread evenly across the system.

In the idea healthcare system, the consumers who need the support of a safety net would be placed into existing provider practices as a small percentage of the overall practice. The care should be the same as all other consumers. This plan will require the necessary ratio of providers-to-consumer in each community to avoid overload of any specific practice and a financial plan for testing and treatment.

Global Perspectives

As we have seen, there can be no one ideal healthcare system to suit the needs of every country. The culture of each country must devise a system that balances individual expectations against societal expectations, and decides which members of its society will have access to and cover-age for health care. The value of care will be determined by providing the greatest benefit to the nation paid for by the financial resources that country can or decides to dedicate to health care. The value of care will be characterized by the quality, access, and breadth of services available to the population, rendered in a customer-friendly way. The effective system must have suf-ficient resources to meet the needs of the population, including medical professionals, physical facilities, technology, infrastructure, and an efficient organizational structure to deliver the care. Finally, the government of an evolving or nationalized system must raise money from the tax-payers to fund a functional administrative organization to act as the major consumer of goods and services, in conjunction with private payers in certain settings, and distribute payment to the care providers in an effective and equitable manner.

U.S. Healthcare Evolution

Many measures of health care place the United States among the best places in the world to re-ceive care, as can be attested to by the rich and powerful from other nations who come to the United States for care; but many other measures place the United States low on the list of devel-oped countries. It is this wide dispersion of outcomes superimposed on the highest per capita spending and highest national healthcare costs as a percentage of GDP that is driving the reexam-ination of the U.S. healthcare system during the present healthcare reform debate and legislation. As planners look at innovative ways to improve the value of health care, that is, prioritized benefit minus cost, we must remember that any changes must evolve from the intersection of the unique American culture, resources, and finances. It is clear that Americans as a whole would support changes that improve the system, but even basic questions such as who is eligible for care are still unsettled. Should the U.S. system provide health care only for its citizens and legal residents, or should everyone—including illegal aliens—receive the same benefits? The recognition that two-thirds of all Medicare spending goes for care rendered in the final stages of life opened the vola-tile discussion of controlling costs for end-of-life care and futile care. How to handle those issues is yet to be determined and has raised concerns of healthcare rationing. Nationalized healthcare systems have recognized that there must be some controls over which procedures will be paid for, and countries such as Great Britain have empowered panels to review tests and treatments to select which give the best outcomes at the lowest cost, and only those approved procedures will receive payment. This payment approval methodology is still being debated in the United States. Payment to medical providers is being shifted to incentives for quality, but which metrics should be tracked is still controversial. The medical education component of the healthcare system is under scrutiny and several proposals for overhaul have been presented. Finally, the question of how to pay for health care is far from settled. The original foundation for the Patient Protection and Affordable Care Act (PPACA), the mandate for every individual to purchase healthcare insurance, is so controversial that several states have sued the federal government in a challenge to the constitutionality of the mandate. The ultimate status of the health insurance exchanges outlined by PPACA is uncertain and continues to be under consideration. Payment cuts to medical professionals and hospitals are part of the plan, but it is uncertain what effect this step would have on access to care, and whether operating cost reductions will reduce the workforce, which would have a hugely deleterious effect on consumer spending and thus reduce the GPD.

In addition to governmental efforts, the private sector is also working to make the healthcare system more effective. Insurance companies are becoming more active in chronic care management, and employers are offering employee wellness programs. Professional organizations and medical specialty groups are developing hosts of disease-specific, evidence-based best practice guidelines. The ascendency of integrated healthcare networks promises a coordinated and seamless approach to care with those networks assuming clinical and fiscal responsibility for their patients.

It is clear that the healthcare system in the United States is undergoing a dramatic evolution, but it is equally clear that to attempt change that is too rapid and too sweeping would have drastic and unanticipated consequences. The best approach would be a measured melding of free-market forces and governmental policy to drive toward an effective system that reflects the culture, resources, and finances of the United States.

References

Agency for Healthcare Research and Quality. (2003). Hospitalization in the United States. *HCUP Fact Book*, 6.

American Association of Retired Persons. (2006). Trends in manufacturer prices of brand name prescription drugs used by older Americans—2005 year-end update. *AARP Public Policy Institute Data Digest, 134.*

Bhargava, A. D. T., Jamison Lau, L. J., & Murray, C. J. L. (2001). Modeling the effects of health on economic growth. *Journal of Health Economics, 20*, 423–440.

Bloom, D., Canning, D., & Sevilla, J. (2004). The effect of health on economic growth: A production function approach. *World Development, 32*(1), 1–13, doi:10.10161jworlddev.2003.07.002

Bularajan,Y., Seloaraj, S., & Subramanian, S. U. (2011). Health care and equity in India. *Lancet, 377*(9764), 505–515. doi:10.106/50140-6736(10)61894-6

Canadian Broadcast Corporation. (2002, October). 1,000,000 vehicles per year in Woodstock, Ontario, starting 2008. CBC, Toronto, Ontario.

Carliner, B. (2005). Health care costs cripple U.S. manufacturers. *Economic Strategy Institute*, Retrieved from http://www.econstrat.org/blog/?p=26

Chapman, K. S., & Hariharan, G. (1994). Controlling for causality in the link from income to mortality. *Journal of Risk and Uncertainty, 8*(1), 85–94.

Chapman, K. S., & Hariharan, G. (1996). Do poor people have a stronger relationship between income and mortality than the rich: Implications of panel data for health-health analysis. *Journal of Risk and Uncertainty*, *12*, 51–63.

Centers for Medicare and Medicaid. (2015). *Fact sheets*. Centers for Medicare and Medicaid Services. Retrieved from https://www.cms.gov/Newsroom/MediaReleaseDatabase/Fact-sheets/2015-Fact-sheets.html

Commonwealth Fund. (2012*). Explaining high health care spending in the United States: An international comparison of supply, utilization, prices and quality*. Retrieved from http://www.commonwealthfund.org/Publications/Issue-Briefs/2012/May/High-Health-Care-Spending.aspx

Conwell L., & Cohen, J. (2005). Characteristics of persons with high medical expenditures in the U.S. civilian noninstitutionalized population, 2002, *MEPS Statistical Brief No. 73*. Retrieved from http://www.meps.ahrq.gov/mepsweb/data_files/publications/st73/stat73.pdf

Cutler, D. M., & McClellan, M. (2001). Is technological change in medicine worth it? *Health Affairs*, *20*, 11–29.

Families USA Foundation. (2005). Paying a premium: The added cost of uninsured. Washington, D.C.

Government of India. (2005). Financing and delivery of health care services in India. (Background Papers, Table 1, p. 7). National Commission on Macroeconomics and Health, New Delhi, India.

Hay, J. W. (2003). Hospital cost drivers: An evaluation of 1998–2001 state-level data. *American Journal of Managed Care*, *9*, 13–24.

Hogan, C., Lunney, J., Gabel, J., & Lynn, J. (2001). Medicare beneficiaries' cost of care in the last year of life. *Health Affairs*, *20*(4), 188–194.

Jamison, D. T. (2006). Economics and cost-effectiveness: Disease Control Priorities Project. International Bank for Reconstruction and Development/World Bank.

Krach, C. A., & Velkoff, V. A. (1999). Centenarians in the United States. Current population report, special studies. Washington, DC: U.S. Census Bureau.

Lekhan, V., Rudiy, V., & Nolte, E. (2004). Health care systems in transition: Ukraine. WHO Regional Office for Europe, European Observatory on Health Systems and Policies.

Manton, K. J., & Vaupal, E. W. (1995). Survival after the age of 80 in the United States, England, France, Japan and Sweden. *New England Journal of Medicine*, *333*(18), 1232–1235.

McGinnis, J. M., & Foege, W. H. (2004, March 10). Actual causes of death in the United States, 2000. *JAMA*, *291*(10), 1238–1245.

Neuhauser, D., & Lewicki, A. M. (1975). What do we gain from the sixth stool guaiac? *New England Journal of Medicine*, *293*, 226–228.

Obamacare Facts. (2013). Retrieved from http://obamacarefacts.com/affordablecareact-summary/

Or, Z. (2000). Determinants of health in industrialized countries: A pooled cross-country time series analysis. *OECD Economic Studies*, *30*, 53–77.

Organisation for Economic Co-operation and Development. (2001, October). OECD health at a glance: How Canada compares. *OECD Policy Brief*.

Organisation for Economic Co-operation and Development. (2006). *OECD health data 2006: How does the United States compare?* Retrieved from http://www.oecd.org/dataoecd/29/52/36960035.pdf

Organisation for Economic Co-operation and Development. (2011). *Health at a Glance 2011: OECD Indicators*. OECD Publishing. doi:10.1787/health_glance-2011-en

Organisation for Economic Co-operation and Development. (2013). *Economic survey*. Retrieved from http://www.google.com/url?sa=t&rct=j&q=&esrc=s&source=web&cd=3&ved=0ahUKEwif0ML30p_LAhVMKh4KHYtGDXwQFggpMAI&url=http%3A%2F%2Fwww.oecd.org%2Feco%2Fsurveys%2FOverview%2520Japan%25202013%2520English.pdf&usg=AFQjCNGSuF11lMkdiCF-Ljw2Dg3U0p_o_Q&bvm=bv.115339255,d.dmo

Organisation for Economic Co-operation and Development. (2015a). *Health at a glance 2015*. Retrieved from http://www.oecd-ilibrary.org/social-issues-migration-health/health-at-a-glance_19991312

Organisation for Economic Co-operation and Development. (2015b). *Health data 2015*. Retrieved from https://data.oecd.org/health.htm

Pan American Health Organization. (1999). *United States of America*. Retrieved from http://www.paho.org/
English/DD/AIS/unitedstates_graf_eng.pdf

Peters D. H., Yazbeck, A. S., Sharma, R. P., Ramana, G. N. V., Pritchett, L. H., & Wagstaff, A. (2002). *Better
health systems for India's poor: findings, analysis, and options*. Washington DC: World Bank.

Phelps, C. E. (2003). *Health Economics* (3rd ed.). Boston, MA: Addison-Wesley.

PricewaterhouseCoopers. (2002). The factors fueling rising healthcare costs (prepared for the American
Association of Health Plans). Washington, DC: PricewaterhouseCoopers.

Pritchett, L., & Summers, L. H. (1996). Wealthier is healthier. *Journal of Human Resources, 31*, 841–868.

Rothenberg, B. M. (2003). *Medical technology as a driver of healthcare costs: Diagnostic imaging*. Blue Cross and
Blue Shield Association. Retrieved from http://www.bcbs.com/betterknowledge/cost/diagnostic-imaging
.html

Smith, C., Cowan, C., Sensenig, A., Catlin, A., & Health Accounts Team. (2003). Health spending growth slows
in 2003. *Health Affairs, 24*(1), 185–194.

Stanton, M. W., & Rutherford, M. K. (2005). The high concentration of U.S. healthcare expenditures (Agency
for Healthcare Quality and Research Pub. No. 06-0060). *Research in Action, 19*.

United BioSource. (2002). *Estimating the value of investments in health care: Better care, better lives*. Retrieved
from http://www.unitedbiosource.com/pdfs/HP_FullReport.pdf

Viscusi, K. W., & Aldy, J. E. (2002). The value of a statistical life: A critical review of market estimates throughout the world. *Journal of Risk and Uncertainty, 27*(1), 5–76.

Wallsten, S., & Kosec, K. (2005). The economic cost of the war in Iraq (Working Paper 05-19). AEA-Brookings
Joint Center for Regulatory Studies.

White House. (2011). *Affordable Care Act*. Retrieved from http://www.whitehouse.gov/healthreform/
healthcare-overview#healthcare-menu

World Bank. (1993). Ukraine: The social sectors during transition—A World Bank country study. Washington,
DC: World Bank.

World Bank. (2015). *Health, Nutrition and Population Statistics*. Retrieved from http://datatopics.worldbank
.org/hnp/Home

World Health Organization. (1999). Ukraine country health report. WHO Liaison Office in Kiev, Ukraine.

World Health Organization. (2000). *Highlights on health in Ukraine*. Retrieved from http://www.euro.who.int/
document/e72372.pdf

World Health Organization. (2004). Regional overview of social health insurance in South-East Asia. Regional
Office for South East Asia, India.

World Health Organization. (2005). *Country profile: Japan*. Retrieved from http://www.wpro.who.int/
countries/05jpn/JPN.htm

World Health Organization. (2006). World Health Statistics 2006, World Health Organization, Geneva.

World Health Organization. (2013). *Japan*. Retrieved from http://www.who.int/countries/jpn/en/

World Health Organization. (2015). *Global Health Observatory Data Repository*. Retrieved from http://www
.who.int/gho/en/

World Health Organization Statistical Information System. (2006). Statistical Information System, World Health
Organization.

Footnote

1. This chapter is dedicated to the memory of Dr. Lipson, a health care visionary, leader, and
mentor.

SECTION II

SPECIAL GLOBAL HEALTH AND HEALTHCARE ISSUES

Human Trafficking: The Pandemic of Modern Slavery

5

Mary de Chesnay

Objectives

After completing this chapter, the reader will be able to:

1. Define human trafficking and associated terms.
2. Describe global efforts to address human trafficking.
3. Compare and contrast the health issues and treatment of sex trafficking survivors.
4. Identify resources within global communities to assist survivors.

INTRODUCTION

The purpose of this chapter is to educate readers on the extent of the problem of human trafficking, the effects of slavery on human beings who are victimized, what global efforts are being made to address the problem, and how nurses and other healthcare providers can participate in the abolition of the modern pandemic of human trafficking. Although demographics are difficult to measure, there is no doubt that slavery is alive and thriving in the modern world. Bales (2012) estimated that 35.8 million people worldwide were currently enslaved. He maintained that human trafficking was the fastest-growing criminal enterprise, third behind drugs and arms smuggling. Bales also estimated that about 80% of human trafficking victims are women and children, mostly in the sex trade, although women and children forced into labor are likely to be sexually abused as well. Note that children of both genders are victimized as sex slaves, but most are girls. The younger they are the more vulnerable they are to the manipulations of the Romeo pimps, those that seduce young girls.

At this writing, projections are that human trafficking has risen to the number two spot behind drugs and that 35.8 million people are currently living in slavery with 61% of those enslaved living in five countries: India, China, Pakistan, Uzbekistan, and Russia (Global Slavery Index, 2014). The current number of enslaved people represents at least triple the number of those captured in the trans-Atlantic slave trade to the New World. Segal (1995) estimated that almost 12 million Africans were brought to the New World though it is not known how many died during the difficult sea voyage.

Statistics on human trafficking are notoriously unreliable in that they describe a population largely invisible to the general public because they are labeled as something else. For example, migrant workers may be poorly paid, but they are not all held as slaves. Children who are exploited for sex are called prostitutes or child brides. Babies who are transferred from birth mothers might be given up by women who are overwhelmed, but they are not all sold for profit by traffickers. Perhaps the most useful way to evaluate the published statistics is to acknowledge that many people are trafficked for the profit of another and that one person held as a slave is one too many.

A complicating factor in determining the number of trafficking victims in developed countries is that citizens tend to believe it cannot happen to them—that human trafficking takes place "over there" but not "here." This kind of denial is understandable because the traffickers are adept at hiding their slaves behind the closed doors of respectable businesses or out in the open as in the sex trade, which many observers would assume is voluntary because of the way the girls dress and act in public. What the general public does not see is the abuse, neglect, and deprivation used by the traffickers to keep the girls (or boys) under control.

Kara, a Harvard economist, conducted multicountry studies and estimated that human trafficking generated over $32 billion, representing more than the combined annual revenue of Starbucks, Google, and Nike (Kara, 2009). However, a new report indicates the figures are much higher—up to $150 billion USD per year, representing more than three times higher profits than Kara's estimate in 2009 (International Labor Office, 2014). While drugs and arms are sold once, the labor of human beings can be sold repeatedly, generating enormous profits for traffickers with little risk of discovery. Because enslaved victims are deprived of adequate food and rest and their injuries are often left untreated, their will to fight and escape is eroded. Even when attempts are made to rescue them, they may resist because their fear of the traffickers is much greater than their trust in well-meaning strangers who may not understand the full extent of their abuse. When victims are rescued, they are asked to place themselves at further risk by testifying against their well-financed and powerful traffickers. Without the testimony of victims, traffickers go free and victims are left in an even more vulnerable position.

Nurses and other healthcare providers might encounter human trafficking victims in a variety of contexts but are probably most likely to see victims of sex trafficking in healthcare settings. For this reason, special attention is given in this chapter to the identification and treatment of sex trafficking victims.

DEFINITIONS OF HUMAN TRAFFICKING

One of the paradoxes of working with the population of trafficking victims is whether to define them as victims or survivors. The term *victim* connotes a person who is powerless and has little control over his or her own body, schedule, money, family, and time. This is certainly true for those whose labor or bodies are used for the financial gain of the traffickers. Yet rescued victims will often resist and even become angry at being so labeled. From a psychological standpoint it is easy to understand their reaction as an attempt to maintain some limited control, because naming and labeling connotes power. For this reason, I use the term *victim* in order to convey the vulnerability of these people and the term *survivor* when talking with them to emphasize whatever resilience they have.

UN Protocol Definition

In 2000 the Palermo Protocol (also known as the United Nations Definition) defined human trafficking "as the recruitment, transportation, transfer, harbouring or receipt of persons, by means of the threat or use of force or other forms of coercion, of abduction, of fraud, of deception, of the abuse of power or of a position of vulnerability or of the giving or receiving of payments or benefits to achieve the consent of a person having control over another person, for the purpose of exploitation" (UN Protocol, 2000). The declaration specifically mentions sexual exploitation, forced labor, organ trafficking, and the exploitation of children (defined as younger than 18) even if the above conditions are not met.

Trafficking Victims Protection Act

Also in 2000, the United States passed the Trafficking Victims Protection Act (TVPA), which adopted the UN definition and extended special protection to foreigners trafficked into the United States. It is important to understand that the definition includes a variety of activities for which people can be prosecuted. For example, taxi drivers hired by pimps to transport customers from an airport to a motel for sex with minors can be prosecuted for human trafficking, not just the pimps or handlers themselves. Hotel employees who rent rooms by the hour can be prosecuted if law enforcement can gather sufficient evidence that the employees know the rooms are used by victims of the sex trade.

TYPES OF HUMAN TRAFFICKING

Forced Labor

Forced labor is prevalent in many parts of the world. In the United States, we might think most often of migrant workers who arrive as undocumented workers from Mexico and Central America to work in agriculture, and domestic workers who are brought in as nannies and housekeepers but are treated as slaves. However, any industry can use forced labor. The following sources describe forced labor across a variety of industries:

- Fishing in Thailand (Taylor, 2014)
- Brick making in India and Afghanistan (U.S. Department of State TIP Report, 2014)
- Chocolate production in western Africa, Asia, South America (Mull, 2005)
- Making clothing in Italy (Aronowitz, 2001).

Recruitment into forced labor is often accomplished with the willing participation of victims, who are tricked into applying for jobs in other countries with the understanding that they will earn a certain amount—enough to send home to their families. They are asked for travel money and may be given legitimate travel documents, but once in the new country, their passports are confiscated and they are told they owe much more money, which they must work off. In reality, the amount places them in substantial and ever-increasing debt. *Debt bondage* then becomes a secondary form of slavery and is commonly used in forced labor and the sex trade.

Case Study: Forced Labor

Twelve Pakistani men saw a newspaper ad for construction jobs in Kuwait. The recruiters flew the men to Saudi Arabia where the traffickers confiscated their passports and sent them to Sierra Leone, where they were kept in crowded and unsanitary housing and forced to work 20-hour days. After a month, one man escaped to a local mosque where he was able to find help to contact a nongovernmental organization (NGO) to rescue the men. They were able to return home, but their wages were confiscated by the traffickers who disappeared before they could be arrested.

Sex Trafficking

Sex trafficking is distinguished from prostitution in that sex trafficking victims do not control their own lives and are unwilling participants in their sexual encounters. Some men and women do choose prostitution, but many enter the life as children under circumstances of extreme deprivation, neglect, and abuse within their families. In some cultures parents in poor communities sell their children in order to obtain money for the rest of the family. Children in some cultures may cooperate fully to help their families because the value for family is more important to them than their own needs. Sometimes women in developing countries apply for domestic or nanny jobs in richer countries and are either sold into the sex trade or abused sexually by members of the families they serve. In the United States, the commercial sexual exploitation of children is referred to as domestic minor sex trafficking (DMST).

Case Study: Sex Trafficking

Effia was an 18-year-old, single mother of two small children. Effia left her children with her mother in Nigeria while she responded to a recruiter from France who promised her a job in Paris as governess to his daughter. When she arrived in Paris, she was taken to an apartment with six other young women who were informed they were now prostitutes. She resisted and was gang-raped until she was "broken," at which time she was sold to a brothel run by a criminal organization.

Organ Trafficking

Organ trafficking may be both voluntary and involuntary in that poor people are more likely to be conned into selling their body parts (particularly kidneys) for the thriving black market. Not enough people choose to designate organ donation after their deaths relative to the number of people needing organs. Long waiting periods on the donation lists increase the demand for black-market organs, especially for affluent people who can afford to pay high prices. Unfortunately, sometimes the organs are removed without proper attention to blood typing and sanitary conditions, leading to infection, rejection, and death of the recipient (Anker & Feeley, 2012).

Involuntary organ donation takes place when highly vulnerable people such as infants or young children or vulnerable adults are kidnapped for removal of organs. No attention is given to sanitation and the "surgeons" are untrained or poorly trained in medical techniques. Needless to say, these victims tend not to survive.

Case Study: Organ Trafficking

Jaime, a 28-year-old married father of six was desperate for money to feed his growing family and sought a way to sell his kidney to a group that offered $1,500 per kidney. He traveled to Manila and underwent surgery in unsanitary conditions. Jaime later developed sepsis and died. His kidney was sold by the traffickers to a wealthy American who bypassed the waiting list and paid $35,000 for Jaime's kidney.

Baby Trafficking

There are at least two forms of baby trafficking: black-market adoptions (Varnis, 2001) and the selling of infants for organs as mentioned above. In some parts of the world, prostituted women give birth on baby farms and the infants are then sold by the traffickers while the mothers return to work in the brothels. Pimps might use babies as leverage against the mothers to ensure their continued cooperation.

Case Study: Baby Trafficking

Elena, an 18-year-old woman from Moldova, was conned into traveling to Paris to be a model. She was quickly assigned to a brothel where she was gang-raped until "broken." She became pregnant almost immediately and her blond, blue-eyed baby was taken from her to be sold to a wealthy American couple who were told the mother died in childbirth.

Debt Bondage

Debt bondage refers to the continuous enslavement of victims by increasing the debt they owe the traffickers for arranging their jobs, transportation, living accommodations, and daily expenses. It is common for traffickers to tell victims that their travel expenses were greater than expected or that they must now pay the traffickers for food, clothing, shelter, and special fees.

Case Study: Debt Bondage

Jose traveled from Mexico to the United States as part of a so-called construction crew to build houses in Southern California. He and his compadres were told they would be housed in a special place on the property so they could save money to send home to their families. When he arrived, he and his fellow travelers were locked in a converted boxcar with a few buckets for sanitation and told their travel expenses were greater than anticipated so they would need to pay more to the traffickers. This left them with no extra money.

Child Brides

Though not specifically categorized as victims of human trafficking, child brides enter into involuntary marriages mostly through cultural traditions. Once married, they are treated as sexual slaves, housekeepers, and mothers of heirs for their husbands. Their lives are characterized by hard work and child-rearing, and they are rarely given opportunities to develop as human beings: they are not educated and they are prohibited from activities that they might choose.

Case Study: Child Brides

Zakia was 10 when her Afghani father sold her as a bride to a wealthy man to whom he was in debt. Her new "husband" promised the father he would not consummate the marriage until she was 13, but he forced himself on her during their "wedding night." She endured three years of abuse, degradation, and forced labor until she became pregnant at menarche. She delivered a stillborn son after 22 hours of labor. She then developed obstetric fistula and her husband abandoned her by the side of road because he could not stand the smell. Her family refused to take her back since she had dishonored them by giving birth to a stillborn baby.

Child Soldiers

Similarly, child soldiers are involuntarily conscripted into guerilla armies by being kidnapped from their villages. They are forced by the leaders to commit atrocities upon threat of their own deaths. Even if they manage to escape, they may suffer major psychoses (Amone-P'Olak, Nyeko Otim, Opio, Ovuga, & Meiser-Stedman, 2015). The Child Soldiers Prevention Act of 2008 (CSPA) was signed into law on December 23, 2008 (Title IV of Pub. L. 110-457), and took effect on June 21, 2009. The CSPA requires publication in the annual *Trafficking in Persons* (TIP) *Report* a list of any foreign governments identified during the previous year as having governmental armed forces or government-supported armed groups that recruit and use child soldiers. Child soldiers are defined in the act as any child under the age of 18 who is forced to participate in armed conflicts even in a support role such as messenger or cook. The act also covers children under the age of 15 who voluntarily participate (U.S. Department of State TIP Report, 2015).

Case Study: Child Soldiers

Ishmael was 10 when his village in Sierra Leone was attacked by a guerrilla band. He was forced to shoot his father or the guerrillas would rape and kill his mother. He did so, but the leaders raped and killed or kidnapped the women anyway. He spent the next 7 years fighting as a child soldier until he escaped to a rescue organization, where he was sent to a rehabilitation camp.

THE TRAFFICKERS

In the United States, we have a stereotype of a pimp as a young man who dresses in outlandish costumes and drives an expensive car. He is portrayed as highly desirable to beautiful women. He is usually portrayed as African American and lives in an inner-city neighborhood where he is looked up to by younger boys who want to grow up to be just like him. While some pimps fit this stereotype, it is a highly misleading picture of modern traffickers, who might be of any race, may be members of gangs or organized syndicates, and might be white men or women of any age.

According to the UN's Global Initiative to Fight Human Trafficking (GIFT), traffickers often use women to recruit because they are seen as less threatening to potential victims. For example, one young woman from an affluent community in California explained that she was complimented on her makeup by a woman claiming to be a Hollywood makeup artist and offered her a job in Los Angeles. From Nigeria to Italy, traffickers are primarily women with men in a secondary role and some traffickers are former victims (UNGIFT, 2008). For the most part, traffickers worldwide are male and often associated with criminal syndicates. In the United States, the gangs have found trafficking in women to be even more profitable than dealing drugs, which can only be sold once.

A stereotype of traffickers is that they are kidnappers who pluck unsuspecting victims off the street. While this does happen, it is not the norm. Traffickers, particularly sex traffickers, are excellent profilers who are able to identify the vulnerable and con them or force them into slavery. In developing countries, young girls who seek a better life accept jobs as nannies or domestic workers, are promised high salaries in foreign countries, then tricked into brothels or enslaved into domestic service, where they are likely to be abused by the men of the house. In the United States, runaways escape intolerable homes only to find themselves conned by men who present themselves as saviors, buy them food and provide shelter, and claim to love them. Soon they tell the girl she must help out with the rent by dating his friends. By the time she catches on to his real motivation, she is trapped. Similarly, men in poor countries are conned into taking jobs as laborers in foreign countries, but when they arrive they are housed in crowded conditions without adequate food, hydration, or sanitation.

Vulnerable populations are at particular and substantial risk of being trafficked. For example, some customers prefer deaf children who cannot speak up for themselves. Transgendered children find themselves on the street when they are rejected by their families. The traffickers may specialize in certain types of clients who demand specific people to abuse.

Sex tourism is a growth industry and some countries are known for marketing the sexual services of children to affluent foreigners. The customers or "Johns" are traffickers as well as the travel agents and controllers who profit financially (de Chesnay, 2016).

HEALTH OF SEX TRAFFICKING SURVIVORS

Mental and Physical Issues

Almost any disease or injury can be manifested in sex trafficking victims, who are prone to regular deprivation of food and sleep and beatings by customers and pimps. In a study by de Chesnay et al. (2013a), 300 stories by 178 survivors were content analyzed for first-person accounts of illnesses and injuries, and reports ranged from expected illnesses such as sexually transmitted infections (STIs) to drug abuse, all types of mental illnesses, and minor to severe injuries. One pimp told me that "one of my girls disrespected me so I had to discipline her." His way of doing that was to run over her with his car.

For the traffickers, the goal is to make money, and the health and welfare of their "stable" of girls is irrelevant. One might think they would treat their victims well considering that healthy workers would be able to endure more work, but this is not the case. In contrast, the traffickers usually house the girls together in secure places, feed them minimally with no attention to proper nutrition, and provide medical care only when they have to, such as in the case of multiple complaints from "johns" about sexually transmitted infections.

Identifying Victims

The most common types of trafficking likely to be encountered by nurses are sex trafficking and to a lesser extent forced domestic labor. The most common victims are women and children of both sexes. The intimidation, beatings, and deprivation traffickers use to keep victims under control are so severe that it is difficult first to identify victims and then to convince them to cooperate. For example, one patient from the Far East told me she could not afford to be rescued because she was convinced the Chinese traffickers sent her earnings to her family at home. Another victim tried to escape and the trafficker drove her past her little brother's school and threatened to take him if she did not cooperate. Sex trafficking victims do not seek medical help unless the trafficker allows them to do so and the circumstances are such as would prohibit them from working. For example, hemorrhaging from a botched abortion might cause the trafficker or pimp to let the girl go to the emergency department, but there would be an accompanying person trusted by the trafficker who would speak for the patient with a lie about how she became injured.

The Polaris Project website has a list of red flag indicators that nurses (or anyone) might use to identify potential trafficking victims. Readers are referred to the website for a substantial amount of information about trafficking (www.polarisproject.org/). A few of the indicators are disorientation (not knowing what city she is in because victims are often moved around), not controlling her own money, having her papers confiscated, and not being able to come and go as she wishes.

Treatment

Best Practices

One of the many difficulties in treating patients who are victims of sex trafficking is that the customary evidence-based practices for illnesses and injuries do not work because the patients do not control their own time, bodies, or money. For example, the usual treatment for most STIs is a 10-day course of antibiotics and protection from spreading the disease through abstinence or at least a condom. However, the choice of using a condom is not that of the victim but rather belongs to the customer.

To prevent unwanted pregnancies, abstinence or birth control is best practice. However, Romeo pimps (those men who recruit girls by pretending to fall in love with them) will often impregnate new recruits deliberately to bind her to him with the hope that he will eventually marry her and they will live happily ever after. In some countries, trafficked women who become pregnant are allowed to carry to term and the newborns are sold in the lucrative black market adoption trade.

System of Care

Georgia was the first state in the United States to develop a statewide response to DMST, and the pioneers who spearheaded this effort determined that the best practice for intervention involves a team effort by professionals in many disciples: medical, social services, legal, criminal justice, the business community, and the general public (de Chesnay, 2013b). The basic idea is that the first priority is safety for the victim so safe houses and shelters must be available to house escapees. Returning victims to their homes may not be feasible; for example, in the United States, the children most vulnerable to trafficking often come from highly dysfunctional homes. Foreigners who are trafficked outside their home countries have their passports confiscated until they work off their debt. If they manage to escape their traffickers, it is unlikely that they will be able to make their way through the unfamiliar city to their embassy. Even if they make it home, victims live under the fear that the traffickers who found them once will find them again.

Once a safe haven is provided, the survivor is evaluated for other needed services, such as medical and psychiatric treatment. Social workers have been in the forefront in this country for providing counseling services and, of course, permanent housing and connections with law enforcement and prosecutors. Foreign nationals trafficked into the United States may qualify for t-visas that enable them to remain here. In other countries many NGOs provide similar services. The United States has a national hotline number easy to remember because of the way it is written (888-3737-888). The U.S. State Department publishes an annual Trafficking in Persons (TIP) Report and their website has a list of phone numbers of resources for victims in the countries they evaluate. The TIP Report is a valuable resource that updates the public on the extent to which the countries surveyed are creating and enforcing legislation to combat human trafficking (U.S. Department of State, 2015).

One source from a shelter told me she estimated the cost of basic medical care to treat each sex trafficking survivor was $30,000. This number rises substantially if surgery is needed. One victim who required extensive gynecological surgery to repair genital trauma needed $150,000 to cover her medical and surgical expenses.

Case Study: System of Care

Jenny was a 14-year-old freshman high school student when she was persuaded by a boy she met at a friend's party to go to New York with him to try out for a small part in a Broadway show. Her affluent parents were on vacation in Europe at the time, and she easily convinced her alcoholic aunt (with whom she was staying) that she would be well-chaperoned. Once they arrived they were met by a limousine and taken to an estate outside the city where she quickly learned she had been sold to a trafficker. She endured a hellish life for three years, being moved around the country until she ended up in Atlanta where she was arrested by a police officer knowledgeable of DMST. He investigated her story instead of simply jailing her as a prostitute. Ashamed to return home, she entered a shelter in the state of Georgia which provided immediate medical care for her numerous injuries from repeated beatings and gonorrhea. She also received trauma-focused cognitive behavioral therapy (TFCBT), legal services, and skills training to complete her high school equivalency test. After a year at the shelter and help from multiple sources, she entered college to study nursing and became a peer counselor at the shelter. The lawyer she worked with in Georgia was able to provide important information to the New York authorities that enabled them to prosecute the original traffickers.

Case Study Questions

1. Define the elements of the system of care for Jenny that would include professionals from social services, law enforcement, health care, and the business community.
2. Identify at least three prevention strategies that could reduce the demand for sex trafficking and prevent girls like Jenny from being victimized.
3. Discuss the prognosis for Jenny based upon the resources described.

SUMMARY

This chapter has educated readers about the growing and violent world of human trafficking. Though commonly denied as a problem or thought to be limited to poor countries, human trafficking is a global social issue with consequences for professionals in many disciplines. Traffickers repeatedly ensnare unsuspecting and highly vulnerable marginalized people, although some victims inadvertently participate in their own capture by being conned into applying for legitimate jobs overseas in which they can make more money to send home to their families. Women and children are at particular risk of sexual abuse because even if they are trapped in forced labor and not specifically trafficked for the sex trade, they are likely to be abused by the men with whom they come in contact. There are no evidence-based treatment protocols because the research base to establish them has not been done. However, creating a community-based system of care in which a variety of professionals cooperate to meet the diverse needs of trafficking victims seems to be the best option at present. In addition to social, legal, and medical services, survivors need job training to learn new ways of making a living.

Study Questions

1. Define human trafficking and compare and contrast the types of activities for which people can be prosecuted.
2. Compare and contrast the types of human trafficking.
3. Explain how one can identify a victim of sex trafficking.
4. Discuss the elements of a system of care for victims of sex trafficking.

References

Amone-P'Olak, K., Nyeko Otim, B., Opio, G., Ovuga, E., & Meiser-Stedman, R. (2015). War experiences and psychotic symptoms among former child soldiers in Northern Uganda: The mediating role of post-war hardships—the WAYS Study. *South African Journal of Psychology, 45*(2), 155–167. doi:10.1177/0081246314556567 · 0.46

Anker, A., & Feeley, T. (2012). Estimating the risks of acquiring a kidney abroad: A meta-analysis of complications following participation in transplant tourism, *Clinical Transplantation, 26,* E232–E241. doi: 10.1111/j.1399-0012.2012.01629.x

Aronowitz, A. A. (2001). Smuggling and trafficking in human beings: The phenomenon, the markets that drive it and the organizations that promote it. *European Journal on Criminal Policy and Research 9,* 163–195. doi: 10.1023/A:1011253129328

Bales, K. (2012). *Disposable people: New slavery in the global economy.* Berkeley, CA: University of California Press.

de Chesnay, M. (2013a). Community models and resources. In M. de Chesnay (Ed.), *Sex trafficking: A clinical guide for nurses* (pp. 51–62). New York: Springer.

de Chesnay, M. (2013b). Psychiatric-mental health nurses and the sex trafficking pandemic. *Issues in Mental Health Nursing, 34,* 901–907.

de Chesnay, M. (2016). The Samfie man revisited: Sex tourism and trafficking. In M. de Chesnay and B. Anderson (Eds.), *Caring for the vulnerable* (pp. 549–564). Burlington, MA: Jones and Bartlett.

de Chesnay, M., Chalk-Gaynor, C., Emmons, J., People, E., & Williams, C. (2013). First-person accounts of illnesses and injuries sustained while trafficked. In M. de Chesnay (Ed.), *Sex trafficking: A clinical guide for nurses* (pp. 131–150). New York: Springer.

Global Slavery Index. (2014). *Walk Free Foundation.* Retrieved from http://d3mj66ag90b5fy.cloudfront.net/wp-content/uploads/2014/11/Global_Slavery_Index_2014_final_lowres.pdf

International Labor Office. (2014). *Profits and poverty: The economics of forced labour.* Geneva: International Labor Office.

Kara, S. (2009). *Sex trafficking: Inside the business of modern slavery.* New York: Columbia University Press.

Mull, L., & Kirkhorn, S. (2005). *Child labor in Ghana cocoa production: Focus upon agricultural tasks, ergonomic exposures, and associated injuries and illnesses.* Association of Schools of Public Health. Retrieved from http://www.ncbi.nlm.nih.gov/pmc/articles/PMC1497785/#__ffn_sectitle

Polaris Project. (n.d.). *Homepage.* Retrieved from http://www.polarisproject.org/

Segal, R. (1995). *The black diaspora: Five centuries of the black experience outside Africa.* New York: Farrar, Straus and Giroux.

Taylor, E. (2014). Human trafficking and the fishing industry in Thailand. *Cornell International Law Journal Online.* Retrieved from http://cornellilj.org/wp-content/uploads/2014/12/E.-Taylor-Thai-Fishing-Thai-Trafficking.pdf

UNGIFT. (2008). *The Vienna Forum to Fight Human Trafficking, 13–15 February 2008, Austria Center Vienna Background Paper.* Retrieved from http://www.unodc.org/documents/human-trafficking/2008/BP016 ProfilingtheTraffickers.pdf

United Nations. (2000). *Protocol to Prevent, Suppress and Punish Trafficking in Persons Especially Women and Children, supplementing the United Nations Convention against Transnational Organized Crime.* Retrieved from http://www.ohchr.org/EN/ProfessionalInterest/Pages/ProtocolTraffickingInPersons.aspx

United States Department of State. (2015). *Trafficking in Persons Report for 2015.* Retrieved from http://www.state.gov/j/tip/rls/tiprpt/

Varnis, S. (2001). Regulating the global adoption of children. *Social Science and Public Policy, 1,* 39–46. Retrieved from http://web.b.ebscohost.com.proxy.kennesaw.edu/ehost/pdfviewer/pdfviewer?vid=7&sid=e7224a21-3f3b-47fd-9831-d23f89541997%40sessionmgr112&hid=101

6

Social Determinants of Health

Dula F. Pacquiao

Objectives

After completing this chapter, the reader will be able to:

1. Define social determinants of health.
2. Describe how social determinants create health inequities.
3. Analyze the significance of social justice in addressing health inequity.

INTRODUCTION

Globalization has increased awareness of health inequities across population groups in local, national, and global contexts (Labonté, 2012; Population Reference Bureau, 2010). These inequities are manifested in group differences in health status, outcomes, and access to health services. European countries and the World Health Organization (WHO) have adopted the notion of social inequality and injustice as the explanation for differences in morbidity and mortality in populations. Margaret Whitehead is credited for bringing to the forefront the moral and ethical dimensions of health inequity as differences which are not only unnecessary and avoidable but, also unfair and unjust (Whitehead, 1992).

SOCIAL DETERMINANTS OF HEALTH

According to the WHO (2013), social determinants are the conditions in which people are born, grow, live, work, and age that are shaped by the distribution of money, power, and resources at global, national, and local levels, which are mostly responsible for health inequities. Health inequities are attributed to systemic inequality in the allocation of resources and power. They are linked with social injustices producing health inequity because of unfair distribution of goods, services, and privileges across populations. Equity refers to fairness in the distribution of goods and services based on need. Needs are not necessarily equal (Bambas & Casas, 2001), thus, equal opportunity or equal allocation of resources that ignore differences in needs, generally fail to achieve equity of outcomes. Social justice has become the focal emphasis for addressing health inequities by emphasizing a collective societal moral obligation to create equity or fairness in the allocation of risks and rewards to everyone (Braverman, 2014).

Raphael (2004) defines social determinants of health as the economic and social conditions that influence the health of individuals, communities, and jurisdictions. They determine the extent to which a person or group possesses the physical, social, and personal resources to identify and achieve personal aspirations, satisfy needs, and cope with the environment. Social determinants of health pertain to the quantity and quality of a variety of resources that a society makes available to its members such as income, food, housing, employment, and health and social services. British Prime Minister Gordon Brown stated that health inequalities stemming from social injustice are barriers to the development and prosperity of communities, nations, and continents (Marmot & Bell, 2009). Indeed, people do not get sick randomly but in relation to their living, working, environmental, social, and political contexts, as well as biological and environmental factors that are unevenly distributed in the population (Bambas & Casas, 2001).

Social determinants have been identified at both individual and group level (Diez-Roux, 2004; Kaufman, 2008). At the individual level factors such as race/ethnicity, gender, employment, discrimination, social class, and income are used to demonstrate their causal effects on health. At the group level, social factors that can influence or interact with health status include social capital, social networks, and segregation. These social factors are determinates of the conditions under which people live and work that impact both their daily life and health outcomes (Burris, Kawachi, & Sarat, 2002). Often individual and societal variables are reciprocally linked to produce health vulnerability.

In the United States, the term *health disparity* is used by government agencies such as the U.S. Department of Health and Human Services (USDHHS), the Centers for Disease Control and Prevention (CDC), and the National Institutes of Health (NIH). Health disparity is defined as:

> A type of difference in health that is closely linked with social or economic disadvantage. Health disparities negatively affect groups of people who have systematically experienced greater social or economic obstacles to health. These obstacles stem from characteristics historically linked to discrimination or exclusion such as race or ethnicity, religion, socioeconomic status, gender, mental health, sexual orientation, or geographic location. Other characteristics include cognitive, sensory, or physical disability. (CDC, 2011; USDHHS, 2009).

The USDHHS established the national goal of eliminating health disparities through its *Healthy People* initiative by setting goals and objectives for national health promotion and disease prevention and identifying targeted health indicators to be achieved over a 10-year period. Carter-Pokras and Baquet (2002) traced health disparity to a "chain of events signified by a difference in environment affecting access to, utilization of and quality of care that lead to a particular health status or health outcome" (p. 427). Environment incorporates both physical and social factors that impact health status. Exposure to pollutants, overcrowded and unsafe residential areas, and neighborhoods with absent or marginal resources are associated with poor health.

Conventional explanations such as lack of access to medical care and unhealthy lifestyles only partially explain differences in health status (Marmot & Bell, 2009). The seminal Whitehall I and II studies of British civil servants (Marmot, Rose, Shipley, & Hamilton, 1978; Marmot et al., 1991) found a social gradient in health among Caucasians who were not poor and had equal access to health services. Whitehall I examined cardiovascular disease prevalence and mortality rates of more than 18,000 British white male civil servants between the ages of 20 and 64 for more than 10 years using a prospective cohort design (Marmot, Rose, Shipley, & Hamilton, 1978). These subjects had similar access to universal healthcare coverage. Higher mortality from all causes including coronary artery disease and lower life expectancy were observed among those in the lower grades of employment as compared to those in higher grades. Lower status was associated with higher prevalence of significant risk factors including obesity, smoking, reduced leisure time, lower levels of physical activity, higher prevalence of underlying illness, higher blood pressure, and shorter height. Controlling for these risk factors accounted for no more than 40% of differences between civil service grades in cardiovascular disease mortality. After controlling for these risk factors, the lowest grade continued to have a relative risk of 2.1 for cardiovascular disease mortality compared to the highest grade.

Twenty years later, the Whitehall II study documented a similar gradient in morbidity in 10,308 men and women using a longitudinal, prospective cohort study of employees in the London offices of the British Civil Service (Marmot et al., 1991). The initial data collection included a clinical examination and self-report questionnaire followed by nine waves of data collection. The Whitehall Studies revealed the social gradient for a range of different diseases: heart disease, some cancers, chronic lung disease, gastrointestinal disease, depression, suicide, sickness absence, back pain, and general feelings of ill health. Higher social position was associated with better health. Marmot (2006) labeled this phenomenon as the *status syndrome*. The lower individuals are in the social hierarchy, the less likely they are able to meet their needs for autonomy, social integration, and participation (Marmot, 2006). The Whitehall studies confirmed that access to healthcare services does not guarantee equity of health outcomes suggesting that health status is more significantly shaped by life conditions—social determinants.

Powers and Faden (2008) argued that social injustice does not arise solely from distribution of goods and services but also in the allocation of nondistributive aspects of well-being. Well-being is affected by the nature of a person's social relationships with others that impose systemic constraints on the development of well-being with profound and pervasive adverse effects on all aspects of well-being. People who are victims of social subordination, discrimination, and stigma experience lack of respect, lack of attachment, and determination, which are essential aspects of well-being. Justice needs to integrate the distributive and nondistributive aspects of well-being. Social justice is concerned with human well-being that has multiple, irreducible dimensions, each representing something of independent moral significance.

GLOBAL HEALTH INEQUITIES

United States

In contrast to most developed countries, the United States does not provide universal health access for all its citizens (Schroeder, 2007). Although the United States spends the most for health care in the world, it lags behind other developed countries and some less developed countries in many health outcomes (OECD, 2014). Health coverage for able adults below 65 years of age is generally acquired through employer-sponsored health insurance. This system of access to care is grounded in a basic inequity favoring high-wage earners with good benefits over low-income groups whose employers may not have the ability to provide optimal health coverage or any coverage at all for their employees. While Medicare is available for adults 65 years and older, procurement of supplemental benefits depends on the financial capacity of the individual or his or her family.

The Patient Protection and Affordable Care Act or the Affordable Care Act (ACA) was signed into law by President Obama on March 23, 2010, to provide access to health coverage to more than 40 million Americans. The ACA expands healthcare coverage to most U.S. citizens and permanent residents by requiring most people to have or purchase health insurance (Health care.gov, 2012). The ACA has failed to reach its goal of expanding access to affordable health insurance for a great number of Americans because of lack of political will to reform the healthcare insurance system. While access to health care does not guarantee equity in health outcomes, lack of universal access perpetuates social and health inequity. In the United States, the Agency for Healthcare Research and Quality [AHRQ] (2012) reported continuing evidence of suboptimal quality of care and access to health services among minority and low-income groups. Health disparities and access to care have shown no improvement for disadvantaged groups. The CDC (2011) reported that despite progress over the past 20 years, racial/ethnic, economic, and other social disparities in health persist in the United States. Racial and ethnic minorities experience greater rates of poverty, unemployment, lack of health insurance, shorter life expectancy, and higher morbidity and mortality rates than white Americans, as shown in Table 6-1 (AHRQ, 2012; CDC, 2011).

Racial and ethnic minorities receive lower-quality health care and intensity of care compared with whites across a wide range of preventive, diagnostic, and therapeutic services and disease states (Washington et al., 2008). Both Hispanics and African Americans had significantly higher uninsured rates (CDC, 2011) with non-Hispanic whites comprising approximately half of the uninsured adults (Moonesinghe, Zhu, & Truman, 2011). The adjusted rate of preventable hospitalizations was higher among non-Hispanic blacks and Hispanics compared with the rate for non-Hispanic whites (Moy, Barrett, & Ho, 2011). Among adults aged 65 years or more, racial and ethnic differences in influenza vaccination coverage persisted, with non-Hispanic blacks consistently having the lowest coverage each year (Setse et al., 2011).

European, Latin, and Caribbean Countries

Income, education, and occupation have all been shown to predict morbidity and mortality (Miranda, Messer, & Kroeger, 2012; Seith & Kalof, 2011; Williams, John, Oyserman, Sonnega,

TABLE 6-1   Health Disparities in the United States

Health Disparity	Most Vulnerable/Disadvantaged Groups
Life expectancy from birth	African Americans
Mortality	
Cancer	African Americans
Complications of Diabetes	African Americans
Coronary disease and stroke	African Americans
Homicide	African Americans
Motor vehicular deaths	American Indian and Alaskan Natives
Suicide	American Indian and Alaskan Natives
Morbidity	
Childhood asthma	Puerto Ricans and African Americans
Diabetes	African Americans and AIANs
HIV	African Americans, AIAN males, MSM
HTN and its complications	African Americans
Obesity	African Americans and Mexican Americans
Infant mortality	African Americans
Low birth weight	African Americans
Extremely preterm birth	African Americans
Preterm birth	African Americans
Health Behaviors	
Smoking	AIAN

Data from Centers for Disease Control and Prevention. (2011). *Health Disparities and Inequalities Report*. Atlanta, GA: Author.

Mohammed, & Jackson, 2012). Individual indicators of socioeconomic status (income, education, and occupation) are found to affect self-reported health status worldwide, independently and collectively. People of high income have more than 50% greater odds of reporting good health than those with low income even when education and occupational class remained the same. Those with high education have more than 60% greater odds of reporting good health than people with lower educational achievement (Babones, 2010).

A study comparing all-white British civil servants with whites and blacks in the United States found that socioeconomic status was related to health (Adler, Singh-Manoux, Schwartz, Stewart, Matthews, & Marmot, 2008). Subjective social status (SSS), the perception of one's socioeconomic position, was also associated with health status. Occupation was a more important determinant of SSS among British civil servants compared to education and income among the U.S. subjects. SSS was significantly related to global health and depression in all groups, and to hypertension in all groups except African American males. Socioeconomic factors did not predict SSS scores for black Americans as well as they did for the British subjects and white Americans. Overall, relationships of SSS and health were stronger for the British and white American subjects than for African Americans suggesting race as a potential factor affecting the latter's SSS.

A longitudinal study of inpatient psychiatric admissions of adolescents in London found that young blacks are nearly six times more likely than their white counterparts to be admitted with psychosis, followed by Other (other ethnic groups and those with mixed ethnic background) and Asians. Young people with psychosis in the Black and Other groups were around three times more likely to experience formal detention on admission (Corrigall & Bhugra, 2013). Bask (2011) examined accumulation of problems associated with welfare recipients using two waves of data from annual surveys of living conditions in Sweden in 1994 to 1995 and 2002 to 2003. The analysis focused on such factors as chronic unemployment, economic problems, health problems, experiences of threat or violence, crowded housing, lack of a close friend, and sleeping problems. Being single (with or without children) and immigrant was associated with the most clusters of problems. Interestingly, education and economic factors were not significant, which was attributed by the author to the fact that Sweden is a welfare state with an ambitious universal social policy agenda involving redistributive activities and extensive spending on public welfare.

In Latin and Caribbean countries, the poor tend to use fewer public resources than middle- and upper-income groups. Large, patterned health inequalities between socioeconomic groups as well as between gender and ethnic groups suggest links between health outcomes and material and social living conditions. There is a growing impact of macro-determinants reflected by inequalities in health and overall well-being of populations (Bambas & Casas, 2001).

Canada

Low-income Canadians are less likely to see a specialist when needed, have more difficulty getting care on weekends or evenings, and more likely to wait five days or more for an appointment with a physician. Canadians with below-average incomes are three times less likely to fill a prescription due to cost and 60% less able to get a needed test or treatment due to cost than above-average income earners (Mikkonen & Raphael, 2010). Men living in the wealthiest neighborhoods live on average more than 4 years longer than men in the poorest neighborhoods; the comparative difference for women was found to be almost 2 years; those living in the most deprived neighborhoods had higher suicide and death rates. Adult-onset diabetes and heart attacks are far more common among low-income Canadians. Food insecurity is common in households led by lone mothers and aboriginal households. Food insufficient households were more likely to report having diabetes, high blood pressure, and food allergies than households with sufficient food. Children in food insecure households are more likely to experience a whole range of behavioral, emotional, and academic problems than children living in food secure households (Mikkonen & Raphael, 2010).

Social exclusion is evident among recent immigrants and aboriginal populations in Canada. Recent immigrants have higher unemployment rates and lower labor force participation than Canadian-born workers. Compared to non-Aboriginal Canadians, First Nation Aboriginal people earn much less income, have twice the rate of unemployment, are more likely to live in crowded conditions, and are much less likely to graduate from high school. Aboriginal Canadians live the shortest lives, have higher rates of infant mortality, suicide, major depression, alcohol, and childhood sexual abuse (Mikkonen & Raphael, 2010).

SOCIAL PATHWAYS TO POOR HEALTH

Krieger (2012) has posited that societal patterns of disease are the biologic consequences of life conditions produced by a society's economic and political structure. People incorporate in their bodies the social and economic conditions of their lives from utero to death. Studies of racial residential isolation concentrating poor African Americans in neighborhoods with overcrowded housing, low-quality health services and schools, violent and polluted environments, and limited availability of affordable healthy foods create cumulative health risks and limited opportunities for economic mobility that perpetuate social and environmental injustices resulting in poor health (Kwate, 2008). Class and racial inequality differentially affect the environmental exposures of dominant and subordinated classes, creating class and racial/ethnic health differences (Dennis, Webb, Lorch, Mathew, Bloch, & Culhane, 2012; Reardon & Bischoff, 2011). A society's economic, political, and social relationships affect both how people live and their environment, and shape different distribution of diseases. Patterns of morbidity and mortality are linked with social inequalities.

Studies of chronic stress associated with experiences of discrimination, marginalization, and lack of control over one's life circumstances create a "wear and tear" effect on the body, or allostatic load, which is linked with sustained high levels of cortisol and other stress hormones that increase one's susceptibility to chronic diseases such as hypertension, cardiac disease, diabetes, cancer, and increased incidence of preterm births (Barker, 2007; McEwen, 2009; Sheridan, Sarsour, Jutte, D'Esposito, & Boyce, 2012; Shuey & Wilson, 2008; Williams et al., 2012). Poor intrauterine conditions associated with increased levels of maternal stress hormones and malnutrition have been correlated with coronary disease in adulthood (Burton, Barker, Moffett, & Thornburg, 2011). The effects of chronic stress on the brain are linked with high-risk behaviors and impaired decision making. Williams et al. (2012) stressed the importance of addressing social determinants as more significant in improving health than physical pathologies alone. Understanding the fundamental causes of poor health facilitates accurate assignment of responsibility and identification of measures to rectify the problem (Krieger, 2008).

According to Powers and Faden (2008) inequalities produce other inequalities in the social determinants of well-being and ultimately in the essential dimensions of well-being themselves. It is important to know how inequalities of one kind result in inequalities of another kind to create clusters of disadvantages that emerge as nearly impossible to escape from. The interactive effect of social determinants can compound, sustain, and reproduce a multitude of deprivations in well-being, bringing some persons below the level of sufficiency for more than one dimension, rendering them with the highest risks and greatest number of risks—a state of vulnerability. Children growing up in poverty are exposed to marginal life conditions—living in neighborhoods characterized by high unemployment, crimes, dilapidated housing, low-quality schools, and lack of resources. Consequently, they experience food insufficiency, violence, and higher rates of asthma, emotional illness, school absenteeism, and academic failure. Such life conditions create clusters of disadvantages that perpetuate their vulnerability throughout life as well as succeeding generations that follow them. Thus, social determinants create a life course of disadvantages and continuing experiences with adversities through life.

Longitudinal studies worldwide confirmed the association between low birth weight and mortality from coronary heart disease in adult men and women (Barker, 2007). Significant correlations were found between mortality rates from coronary artery disease and neonatal mortality across geographic regions in England and Wales. Barker hypothesized that under-nutrition in utero permanently changes the body's structure, function, and metabolism in ways that lead to coronary heart disease in later life. Barker's developmental origins hypothesis attributes neonatal and adult mortality to prenatal and early postnatal conditions (poverty, in-adequate housing, overcrowding, and other adverse environmental factors after birth), which create the stage for early death and development of coronary heart disease. Similarly, a 27- year prospective study of northern Swedish cohort starting in the ninth grade found that accumula-tion of adverse social circumstances over the life course plays a greater role for cardiovascular risk factors in adulthood than birth weight (Gustafsson, Janlert, Theorell, Werterlund, & Hammarstrom, 2010).

Cumulative disadvantages create poor health and dependency of certain groups that in turn perpetuate their vulnerability to negative social relations and diminished potential for self-determination and socioeconomic mobility. Social determinants of health are multicausal and multifaceted social structural barriers to achieving a level of sufficiency in well-being. Social de-terminants demand social action in order to stop the cycle of vulnerability. Vulnerable popula-tions have multiple and cumulative risks not limited to health. The embodiment of these social disadvantages is ultimately manifested in poor health. Because of the interaction and interlock-ing nature of these disadvantages, amelioration of the effects should target the root cause and not just the outcomes of poor health. Conditions that produce lifelong adversities throughout childhood, adulthood, and future generations should be addressed early in life. The social and cultural reproduction of vulnerability should be prevented.

Macrosocial approaches go beyond disease-based care or care of the sick and the disabled in healthcare institutions. Policies and programs must be informed by the tenets of health eq-uity which gives priority to vulnerable groups. Priorities should be based on the moral obliga-tion of attaining a level of sufficiency for the vulnerable. Egalitarianism falsely assumes that equal opportunity ensures equitable outcomes because there is no equal opportunity without consideration of need differences across groups. The tenets of individualism and egalitarian-ism predispose blaming the victim because of the belief that one deserves the benefits of one's work within a climate of equal opportunity. Health equity demands fairness in allocation of goods, services, and goodwill in order to ensure that the vulnerable attain a level of sufficiency of well-being.

CONCLUSION

This chapter defined social determinants of health and how they create local, regional, and global health inequities. Legal, moral and ethical issues are also examined. Solutions for correcting health inequities were explored, giving suggested remedies. Some examples of social determinants included: availability of resources to meet daily needs (e.g., safe housing and local food markets); access to educational, economic, and job opportunities: access to health care services; quality of education and job training; availability of community-based resources in support of community living and opportunities for recreational and leisure-time activities; transportation options; public safety; social support; and language/literacy.

Case Study: A Community Cooperation Approach to Combat Social and Health Challenges

In an urban community in the northeastern part of the United States, the majority of the residents are poor African Americans affected by higher prevalence and mortality rates from cancer, cardiovascular disease, HIV, and homicide. There is also a high incidence of childhood asthma and preterm births as well as high rates of infant mortality. The community has one of the highest rates for crime, unemployment, and school dropout. While some large corporations and academic institutions are located in this community, most residents do not have the advanced skills to qualify for these jobs.

The community is situated amongst 10 Superfund sites, many of which have not been cleaned. A number of abandoned homes and buildings, as well as dilapidated infrastructure are evident in the community. The neighborhood is considered a food desert, as residents do not have access to large food chains offering a variety of fresh, healthy produce at affordable prices. Fast-food venues, liquor stores, and bodegas (small, retail stores offering limited healthy and fresh produce) predominate in the neighborhood. Many residents depend on food banks to provide for their families.

Typical of many urban communities in the United States, this area was previously a bustling industrial metropolis that deteriorated after the industrial boom and government programs that pushed for suburban growth. Loss of economic revenues and jobs concentrated in the neighborhood poor minorities who were unable to compete for employment elsewhere. The neighborhood also suffered from public and private disinvestment, resulting in dilapidated and decaying infrastructure, and loss of critical social and healthcare services. Lack of revenues has impacted the number and quality of schools, health, and social services.

In one of the poorest districts of this urban community, a newly elected member of the municipal council, who is African American, has emerged as a champion of the community. Several generations of his family have remained in the neighborhood and maintained a network of influential black American friends who were former residents. The community champion decided to conduct monthly town meetings so he invited local community members, members of his social network, and interested participants from local organizations. He generally holds these meetings in the center of the district on Saturdays and makes refreshments available to attendees.

Residents who have attended express their various concerns, the most important of which are the high crime rate, unresponsive police force, open drug dealing, and loitering in the neighborhood. Residents are hesitant to report crimes and confront offenders because of fear of retaliation. Consequently, they are shut in their homes, unable to go out and walk on their streets and often have difficulty in sleeping. Fear of crimes has prevented family members from using a neighborhood park, shop at bodegas, or walking to bus stops. To address these problems, the community champion did the following:

1. Invited the chief of police to one of these meetings to address the community's concerns.
2. Conducted neighborhood walks with residents to promote their collective ownership of their neighborhood, enhance their feeling of being safe on their own streets, and encourage watching out for each other.
3. Arranged for the city to install cameras to deter crimes in the most vulnerable neighborhoods.
4. Provided residents with names and contact information of municipal officials responsible for specific aspects of their lives such as sanitation, policing, transportation, and the like.
5. Created a community advisory group with members of the community and local businesses to promote job opportunities and access to essential goods and services.
6. Promoted increased accountability of the police to the local community and created relationships between community members and the police.

Other entities in the city began to develop other initiatives to complement the efforts in this district. A private, non-profit organization in partnership with a local university monitors air pollution in the city. Another organization in partnership with the local government promotes local gardens by renting vacant city lots at a low cost to residents and providing technical assistance, such as soil analysis, clean dirt, and seeds; they ask that the produce be shared with other residents. Soil analysis is performed by a local university to determine the fitness of the soil for planting edible foods given the history of soil contamination in the city.

Initial outcomes from the town meetings have demonstrated increased awareness of the community's concerns by professionals and the local government. These meetings have promoted development of social networks comprised of local community members and individuals and groups outside of the district. This network is composed of local politicians, academicians, health professionals, students, and community organizations. Community members are encouraged to bring their concerns, make observations about implemented strategies and outcomes, and connect with existing groups within the city. There has been an increase in the community's vigilance in collecting evidence of the outcome of implemented programs, such as the response of the police to their calls during emergencies. The role of a trusted community champion with a long history of engagement in the community and his social network of influential community advocates is critical to building a cohesive community to foster collective effort for improvement. This champion and his social network epitomize culturally congruent advocates with in-depth knowledge and proven commitment to the community.

Building a healthy community requires the development of mutual trust and reciprocity with the local people. It is grounded on prolonged engagement with the local community, understanding the multifaceted causes of problems, and building partnerships and coalitions across different sectors, levels, and disciplines. Health promotion is beyond disease-based care. It needs to empower communities to create life changes that can eventually translate to better health. Living in poverty and in a denigrated environment with little opportunity for socioeconomic mobility creates lifelong adversities and vulnerability in populations. Indeed, prevention of asthma, cancer, obesity, cardiovascular diseases, diabetes, HIV, and infant mortality is not possible without improving the life conditions and the ability of the local community to advocate for itself.

Case Study Questions

1. What social determinants of the health of the population were addressed in the case study?
2. Identify three key elements to building healthy communities.
3. In what way does the approach by the community champion address the fundamental causes of poor health in the community?
4. What would be the shortcomings of solely initiating programs on disease prevention, such as vaccination, education on disease prevention, and early screening?

References

Adler, N., Singh-Manoux, A., Schwartz, J., Stewart, J., Matthews, K., & Marmot, M.G. (2008). Social status and health: A comparison of British civil servants in Whitehall-II with European- and African-Americans in CARDIA. *Social Science & Medicine, 66,* 1034–1045.

Agency for Healthcare Research and Quality. (2012). *National Healthcare Disparities Report 2011. AHRQ Publication No. 12-0006.* Gaither, MD: DHHS. Retrieved from www.ahrq.gov/qual/qrdr11.htm.

Babones, S. (2010). Income, education, and class gradients in health in global perspective. *Health Sociology Review, 19*(1), 130–143.

Bambas, A., & Casas, J. (2001). Assessing equity in health. Conceptual criteria. In PAHO, *Equity and Health: Views from the Pan American Sanitary Bureau,* Publication 8 (pp. 12–21). Washington DC: Author.

Barker, D. (2007). The origins of the developmental origins theory. *Journal of Internal Medicine, 261,* 412–417.

Bask, M. (2011). Cumulative disadvantage and connections between welfare problems. *Social Indicators Research, 103,* 443–464.

Braverman, P. (2014). What are health disparities and health equity? We need to be clear. *Public Health Reports, 129*(S2), 5–8.

Burris, S., Kawachi, I., & Sarat, A. (2002). Integrating law and social epidemiology. *Journal of Law, Medicine & Ethics, 30*(4), 510–521.

Burton G., Barker, D., Moffett, A., & Thornburg, K. (Eds.) (2011). *The placenta and developmental programming.* UK: Cambridge University Press.

Carter-Pokras, O., & Baquet, C. (2002, September–October). What is a health disparity? *Public Health Reports, 117,* 426–434.

Centers for Disease Control and Prevention. (2011). *Health Disparities and Inequalities Report.* Atlanta, GA: Author.

Corrigall, R., & Bhugra, D. (2013). The role of ethnicity and diagnosis in rates of adolescent psychiatric admission and compulsory detention: A longitudinal case-note study. *Journal of the Royal Society of Medicine, 106,* 190–195.

Dennis, E., Webb, D., Lorch, S., Mathew, L., Bloch, J., & Culhane, J. (2012). Subjective social status and maternal health in a low-income urban population. *Maternal and Child Health Journal, 16,* 834–843.

Diez-Roux, A. (2004). The study of group-level factors in epidemiology: Rethinking variables, study designs and analytical approaches. *Epidemiologic Reviews, 26*(1), 104–111.

Gustafsson, P., Janlert, U., Theorell, T., Werterlund, H., & Hammarstrom, A. (2010). Fetal and life course origins of serum lipids in mid-adulthood: results from a prospective cohort study. *BMC Public Health, 10,* 484. Retrieved from http://www.biomedcentral.com/1471-2458/10/484.

HealthCare.gov. (2012). *Affordable Care Act.* Retrieved from http://www.health care.gov/law/full/

Kaufman, J. (2008). Social epidemiology. In K. J. Rothman, S. Greenland, & T. L. Lash (Eds.), *Modern epidemiology* (pp. 532–548). Philadelphia, PA: Lippincott Williams & Wilkins.

Krieger, N. (2008). Proximal, distal, and the politics of causation: What's level got to do with it? *American Journal of Public Health, 98*(2), 221–230.

Krieger, N. (2012). Methods for the scientific study of discrimination and health: An ecosocial approach. *American Journal of Public Health, 102*(5), 938–944.

Kwate, N. (2008). Fried chicken and fresh apples: Racial segregation as a fundamental cause of fast food density in black neighborhoods. *Health & Place, 14*(1), 32–44.

Labonté, R. (2012). Global action on social determinants of health. *Journal of Public Health Policy,* 1–9. doi:10.1057/jphp.2011.61

Marmot, M. (2006). Status syndrome: A challenge to medicine. *Journal of the American Medical Association, 295*(11), 1304–1307.

Marmot, M., & Bell, R. (2009). Action on health disparities in the U.S.: Commission on Social Determinants of Health. *JAMA, 301*(11), 1169–1171.

Marmot, M., Rose, G., Shipley, M., & Hamilton, P. (1978). Employment grade and coronary heart disease in British civil servants. *Journal of Epidemiology and Community Health, 32,* 244–249.

Marmot, M., Smith, G., Stansfeld, S., Patel, C., North, F., Head, J., White, I., Brunner, E., & Feeney, A. (1991). Health inequalities among British civil servants: The Whitehall II study. *Lancet, 337*(8754): 1387–1393. doi:10.1016/0140-6736(91)93068-K.

McEwen, B. (2009). The brain is the central organ of stress and adaptation. *NeuroImage, 47,* 911.

Mikkonen, J., & Raphael, D. (2010). Social determinants of health: The Canadian facts. Toronto: York University School of Health Policy and Management.

Miranda, M., Messer, L., & Kroeger, G. (2012). Associations between the quality of the residential built environment and pregnancy outcomes among women in North Carolina. *Environmental Health Perspectives, 120*(3), 471–477.

Moonesinghe, R., Zhu, J., & Truman, B. (2011). Health insurance coverage—United States, 2004 and 2008. *MMWR, 60*(Suppl.), 35–37.

Moy, E., Barrett, M., & Ho, K. (2011). Potentially preventable hospitalizations—United States, 2004–2007. *MMWR, 60*(Suppl.), 80–83

NSMC (2010). *Social Determinants of Health: Case Study of smoking cessation in UK Changing behavior, improving lives.* Retrieved from http://www.thensmc.com/content/health-equity-social-determinants/Casestudies#national

Office of Economic Cooperation and Development. (2014). *Health statistics.* Retrieved from http://www.oecd.org/els/health-systems/health-statistics.htm

Population Reference Bureau. (2010). *2010 World population data sheet.* Washington, DC: Author.

Powers, M., & Faden, R. (2008). *Social justice: The moral foundations of public health and health policy.* New York: Oxford University Press.

Raphael, D. (2004). Introduction to the social determinants of health. In D. Raphael (Ed.), *Social determinants of health: Canadian perspectives* (pp. 2–19). Toronto: Scholars Press.

Reardon, S., & Bischoff, K. (2011). *Growth in Residential Segregation of Families by Income,* 1970–2009. US 2010 Project. Russell Sage Foundation.

Schroeder, S. (2007). We can do better—Improving the health of the American people. *New England Journal of Medicine, 357,* 1221–1228.

Seith, D., & Kalof, C. (2011). *Who are America's poor children?* National Center for Children in Poverty. Mailman SPH, Columbia University.

Setse, R., Euler, G., Gonzalez-Feliciano, A., Bryan, L., Furlow, C., Weinbaum, C., & Singleton, J. (2011). Influenza vaccination coverage—United States, 2000–2010. *MMWR, 60*(Suppl.), 38–41.

Sheridan, M., Sarsour, K., Jutte, D., D'Esposito, M., & Boyce, W. (2012). The impact of social disparity on prefrontal function in childhood. *PLoS ONE, 7*(4), e35744. doi:10.1371/journal.pone.0035744

Shuey, K., & Wilson, A. (2008). Cumulative disadvantages and black-white disparities in life-course health trajectories. *Research on Aging, 30*(2), 200–225.

U.S. Department of Health and Human Services. (2009). *Healthy People 2020 Draft. 2009.* Washington, DC: U.S. Government Printing Office.

Washington, D., Bowles, J., Saha, S., Horowitz, C., Moody-Ayers, S., Brown, A., & Cooper, L. (2008). Transforming clinical practice to eliminate racial-ethnic disparities in health care. *Journal of General Internal Medicine, 23*(5), 685–691.

Whitehead, M. (1992). The concepts and principles of equity and health. *International Journal of Health Services, 22*, 429–445.

Williams, D., John, D., Oyserman, D., Sonnega, J., Mohammed, S., & Jackson, J. (2012). Research on discrimination and health. *American Journal of Public Health, 102*(5), 975–978.

World Health Organization. (2013). *Social determinants of health*. Retrieved from http://www.who.int/social_determinants/sdh_definition/en/

7

Global Perspectives on Mental Health

Mary Ann Camann and Astrid H. Wilson[1]

Objectives

After completing this chapter, the reader will be able to:

1. Analyze the implications of mental health for overall health in a population or geopolitical area.
2. Discuss legal and ethical issues related to global mental health.
3. Discuss policies, programs, and research that support mental health treatment among countries and areas.
4. Identify factors that result in client-centered services that are culturally appropriate and build on health and move an individual toward recovery.
5. Describe factors that are barriers to mental health care.
6. Evaluate case examples related to delivery of mental health services and recovery.

OVERVIEW

The importance of mental health and mental illness as components of population health is increasingly being recognized as vital to the overall health of a country. Additionally, lack of mental health care is a known factor in the economic burden placed on individuals and their families facing mental health issues, which adds to the personal burden of suffering and disability associated with such conditions. The 66th World Health Assembly (2013) adopted the World Health Organization's (WHO) Comprehensive Mental Health Action Plan 2012–2020 that sets important new directions for mental health focused on provision of community-based care and human rights.

WHO (2013) defines mental health as "a state of complete physical, mental and social well-being and not merely the absence of disease or infirmity" (p. 3). Also emerging is a concept of recovery from mental illness that goes beyond treatment to include an individual's sense of hope, sense of meaning, and opportunities for satisfying material needs, social relationship, meaningful activities, and ability to use services of the mental healthcare system. Recovery concepts challenge assumptions about chronicity and the need to remove persons with mental illness from the population.

In this chapter, current issues related to the global understanding of mental health and mental illness are presented in a policy-making and policy implementation context. The extent of the effects of mental illness on health worldwide is explored, along with an overview of the prevalence of mental illness and application of the concept of disease burden to community health and recovery status. Issues related to mental health and illness, such as cultural variations in understanding of the course and treatment and related stigma, are discussed. A review of current global mental health issues and the policy, belief structure, and resource allocation that underpin program development in various parts of the world are presented. Finally, the most recent findings on mental illness as compiled in WHO's 2014 *Mental Health Atlas* project are presented as they point toward issues that will need continued attention.

GLOBAL PERSPECTIVE: THE INFLUENCE OF RESEARCH AND TECHNOLOGY

The first annual World Mental Health Day, initiated by the World Federation for Mental Health (WFMH), was held nearly two decades ago to call attention to the lives of persons who experience mental illness. World Mental Health Day was a public acknowledgment of the effects of mental health and illness on overall health and productivity worldwide. Still, in 2015, there are thousands of people with mental health conditions globally who are deprived of their human rights. They are stigmatized and marginalized and even abused in mental health facilities and their communities. Poor quality care coupled with limited qualified health professionals and undesirable facilities leads to further violations. The theme of the 2015 World Mental Health Day was "Dignity in Mental Health":

> WHO will be raising awareness of what can be done to ensure that people with mental health conditions can continue to live with dignity, through human rights oriented policy and law, training of health professionals, respect for informed consent to treatment, inclusion in decision-making processes, and public information campaigns. (WHO, 2015a, p. 1)

The National Alliance on Mental Illness (NAMI) announced the First Annual Global Peer Supporter Celebration. The day recognized the success of using peer support in managing mental health and addiction challenges which is now a major part of global mental health care. The core of peer support can be summarized in a quote from Thomas Jefferson, "Who then can so softly bind up the wound of another as he who has felt the same wound himself?" The specialty of peer support views those who experience mental health and substance abuse as needing to move away from focusing their lives on problems and symptoms to viewing themselves as being able to engage in recovery (Weaver, 2015).

NAMI also used a media campaign of radio messages to encourage Congress to pass comprehensive mental health legislation. The radio tour consisted of about 20 interviews to news programs and talk shows. It was anticipated that these messages were heard on 8,600 networks or stations and heard by 17 million listeners. The focus of the interviews was to speak out about mental health. Some of the interviews related to the Oregon tragedy where nine persons were killed and which elicited discussion of issues of violence and gun control. NAMI suggested that the vast majority of people living with mental illness are not violent and, regardless of individual views on gun control, mental health reform is needed for the sake of those and family members affected by mental health issues (Carolla, 2015).

In addition to the aforementioned work of WFMH, NAMI, and WHO, another influence on mental health was President George Bush's proclamation of the years 1990–1999 to be called the Decade of the Brain, focusing on continued study of the brain so as to expand upon the growing knowledge of brain neuroanatomy and physiology. The Library of Congress and the National Institute of Mental Health of the National Institutes of Health sponsored a unique interagency initiative to advance the goals set forth in the proclamation by President Bush: to enhance public awareness of the benefits to be derived from brain research through "appropriate programs, ceremonies, and activities." The increasing knowledge shed light on the needs of millions of Americans affected each year by disorders of the brain, ranging from neurogenetic diseases to degenerative disorders such as Alzheimer's disease, stroke, schizophrenia, autism, and impairments of speech language and hearing. These efforts drew attention to the mapping of the brain's biochemical circuitry; the study of how the brain's cells and chemicals develop, interact, and communicate with the rest of the body; and breakthroughs in molecular genetics and understanding of the connection between the body's nervous and immune system. The emerging science provided a new foundation upon which to build new understanding of mental illness as well as understanding of the various factors that support mental health. Philosophical and religious leaders as well as the general public had the opportunity to learn a new paradigm for understanding mental illness that was based on the visualization of brain activity through advanced imaging such as positron emission tomography (PET) scans, and begin to reconcile this biological view with long-held beliefs about human identity and understanding of the self (Boyle, 2001).

The acceptance of the developing neuroscience had implications around the world for the subsequent development of mental health policy and programs. The work that was done during the Decade of the Brain also brought together many public and private entities in the United States and abroad for discussion about the science of brain function as well as the economic implications of health and diseases. During this time, WHO, the World Bank, and Harvard University also worked on the development of a single measure of disease burden to capture the effects of various illnesses on daily life—specifically, the disability-adjusted life year (DALY), which expresses years of life lost to premature death and years lived with a disability. The DALY is a measure that can aid in analyzing and prioritizing health challenges globally regionally and nationally and nationally. "The results of the WHO study confirmed what many health workers in mental health promotion and injury prevention had suspected for some time: that neuropsychiatric disorders and injuries were major causes of lost years of healthy life" (Lopez, 2005, p. 1186).

In 1999, the Surgeon General's *Report on Mental Illness in the United States* was issued as the first such report in the nation's history and heralded an "understanding of the importance of mental health in the overall health and well-being and to the strength of a nation and its people" (U.S. Department of Health and Human Services [USDHHS], 1999, p. 1). Donna Shalala, then Secretary of Health and Human Services, noted in the introduction to the report that "We are coming to realize . . . that mental health is absolutely essential to achieving prosperity . . . [and there is] an opportunity to dispel the myths and stigma surrounding mental illness" (USDHHS, 1999, p. 1). The report marked the beginnings of more inclusive, population-based mental health policies. It also focused on the disparities in the availability of, and access to, services in the mental health field, and the stigma and hopelessness that often surrounded the issue. It set the tone for national policy and echoed the themes of WHO's (1999) *World Health Report*.

Closely following the Surgeon General's report, *World Health Report 2001: Mental Health: New Understanding, New Hope* was issued and firmly placed mental health in the arena of global health. This report marked the continuation of a collaborative effort to develop a global campaign focused on depression management, suicide prevention, schizophrenia, and epilepsy (WHO, 2001a). In keeping with the emphasis on disease burden, it was acknowledged that most illnesses—both mental and physical—are influenced by a combination of biological, psychological, and social factors, setting the stage for advocacy for the cause of mental health and treatment of mental illness all over the world. Following that groundbreaking report came WHO's (2002b) Mental Health Global Action Programme (mhGAP), which sought to "provide a clear and coherent strategy for closing the gap between what is urgently needed and what is currently available to reduce the burden of mental disorders, worldwide" (p. 1).

In all regions of the world mental, neurological, and substance use (MNS) disorders have a significant impact on morbidity and premature mortality. Globally, it is estimated that lifetime prevalence rates of mental disorders in adults are 12.2 per 1,000 (48.6%), and 12-month prevalence rates are 8.4 (29.1%). In addition MNS disorders affect the global burden of disease, measured in disability-adjusted life years and 30% of the total burden of noncommunicable diseases. Unfortunately, the countries with low and lower-middle incomes bear the burden of neuropsychiatric disorders. The stigma and violations directed toward people with these disorders, which in turn increases their vulnerability, accelerates them toward poverty and interferes with their treatment and rehabilitation. The focus of the 2008 mhGAP is summed up as, "Restoration of mental health is not only essential for individual well-being, but is also necessary for economic growth and reduction of poverty in societies and countries" (WHO, 2008a, p. 12).

LEGAL AND ETHICAL ISSUES

Global Burden of Disease

The 1996 Global Burden of Disease (GBD) study was created to measure the burden of disease and injury in a manner that could also assess the cost-effectiveness of interventions, in terms of the cost per unit of disease burden prevented. Disease burden represents the gap between a population's actual health status and a reference point—that is, the expected years of healthy life.

The measure of disease burden takes into consideration egalitarian principles of how long a person should live regardless of socioeconomic status, race, or level of education. Disease burden also addresses the time lived with disability as well as lost healthy time due to death. Most people can agree that some disabilities are more serious than others and produce variations in the effects of the illness on the healthy days of individuals (Murray & Lopez, 1996).

An additional study was conducted based on data from 187 countries from 1990 through 2010 that included a complete reassessment of GBD for 1990 and estimates for 2005 and 2010. Of the top causes of disability worldwide in 2010, measured in years lived with a disability, five were psychiatric conditions: major depression disorder, drug use disorders, Alzheimer's disease and other dementia, anxiety disorders, and self-harm. Altogether psychiatric and neurological conditions accounted for 29% of all disability adjusted years. In 1990, there were 2.497 billion global DALYs; and in 2010 the number decreased slightly, to 2.482 billion DALYs. The authors reported that they would have expected the number of DALYs to increase by 37.9% on the basis of population growth alone. They attributed the small decrease of 0.6% to progress in reducing DALY rates according to age, sex, country, and cause (Murray & Lopez, 2013). GBD findings that focused on mental illness in terms of loss of productivity cut across world regions and economic status levels, thereby setting the stage for worldwide health officials to continue to address mental health as an important and economically significant public health issue.

Demographics of Mental Illness

The picture of global mental health and illness is complicated, and mental health is recognized by the public health community as essential for good health. "An estimated 26% of Americans age 18 and older suffer from a diagnosable mental disorder in a given year. The estimated lifetime prevalence of any mental disorder among the U.S. adult population is 46%" (Centers for Disease Control and Prevention, 2011).

Mental health disorders can be found in people of all regions, all countries, and all societies. The estimated lifetime prevalence of having one or more of the disorders considered here varies widely across the world mental health surveys, from 47.4% in the United States to 12.0% in Nigeria. The inter-quartile range (IQR; 25th–75th percentiles across countries) is 18.1 to 36.1%. Symptoms consistent with the existence of one or more lifetime mental disorders were reported by more than one-third of respondents in five countries (Colombia, France, New Zealand, Ukraine, United States), more than one-fourth in six (Belgium, Germany, Lebanon, Mexico, The Netherlands, South Africa), and more than one-sixth in four (Israel, Italy, Japan, Spain). The remaining two countries, Metropolitan PRC (13.2%) and Nigeria (12.0%), had considerably lower prevalence estimates that are likely to be downwardly biased. Prevalence estimates for other developing countries were all above the lower bound of the inter-quartile (WHO, 2001a).

Mental and behavioral disorders are common among persons seeking care in primary healthcare settings, accounting for approximately 24% of all such individuals. The most common mental health diagnoses made in primary care settings are depression, anxiety, and substance abuse disorder. These disorders may be present either alone or in addition to one or more physical disorders. There are no consistent differences in prevalence between developed and developing countries (WHO, 2001a).

In a report commissioned by the WHO mhGAP, the vulnerability of persons with mental health conditions was addressed. The researchers found that persons with mental health conditions are likely to be subjected to stigma and discrimination on a daily basis, and they experience extremely high rates of physical and sexual victimization. Moreover, they are restricted in ability to access essential health and social care, including emergency relief services, and may also have limited access to work and schooling. Collectively, these effects result in increased likelihood of disability and premature death (WHO, 2010).

In 2009, the World Psychiatric Association (WPA), in response to global disasters, joined with WHO to initiate a series of "train the trainer" workshops to train psychiatrists from the various regions of the world to deal with the mental health consequences of disaster so that they, in turn, can become resources for their countries (WPA, 2011).

DEVELOPMENT OF MENTAL HEALTH POLICY

Health policy is always developed within the context of the larger social and political environment. All health policy is a work in progress that acknowledges the current state of health, invites discussion, focuses attention on specific issues, and at its best creates a sense of priority and encourages development of services and evaluation of effectiveness of the impact of services on human life. The *World Health Report 2001* on mental illness made available new knowledge about the understanding of mental and behavioral disorders. It also offered possible solutions and policy options to governments and policy makers that could influence strategic decision making and point toward positive changes in the acceptance and treatment of mental disorders (WHO, 2001b). It is beyond the scope of this chapter to explore all policy issues and the ramification of policy directions, but suffice it to say that policy development is a slow process that is affected by many internal and external issues, as well as by available resources and public understanding and will.

Appearing in *World Health Report 2001,* and reinforced in the mhGAP (WHO, 2002a), were broadly conceived recommendations for action as well as plans for follow-up. They included the following measures:

- *Provide treatment in primary care,* as it enables the largest number of people to get easier and faster access to services. This recommendation implies that general health personnel should be trained in the essential skills of mental health care, which in turn has implications for education and training programs.
- *Make psychotropic drugs available.* Include essential psychotropic drugs in every country's essential drugs list, as such medications can ameliorate symptoms, reduce disability, shorten the course of many disorders, and prevent relapse.
- *Give care in the community,* as community care has a better effect on quality of life of individuals with chronic mental disorders than does institutional treatment. Such care is also cost effective, respects human rights, and can lead to early interventions and limit the stigma of seeking treatment.
- *Educate the public.* Educational and awareness campaigns on mental health should be launched in all countries to reduce barriers to treatment and care by increasing awareness of the frequency of mental disorders, their treatability, the recovery process, and the human rights of people with mental disorders.

- *Involve communities, families, and consumers in the development and decision making regarding policies, programs, and services,* taking into account factors such as age, sex, culture, and social conditions.
- *Establish national policies, programs, and legislation for sustained action* based on current knowledge and human rights considerations. Mental health reforms, including budgetary allocations, should be part of larger health system reforms.
- *Develop human resources,* especially in developing countries, to increase and improve the training of mental health professionals, who will provide specialized care as well as support the primary healthcare programs. Specialist mental healthcare teams ideally should include medical and nonmedical professionals, such as psychiatrists, clinical psychologists, psychiatric nurses, psychiatric social workers, and occupational therapists, who can work together toward the total care of individuals in the community.
- *Link with other sectors.* Sectors such as education, labor, welfare, and law and nongovernmental organizations should be involved in improving the mental health of communities.
- *Monitor community mental health* through the inclusion of mental health indicators in health information and reporting systems to determine trends, detect mental health changes resulting from external events such as disasters, and assess the effectiveness of mental health prevention and treatment programs, all the while building the case for the provision of resources.
- *Support more research.* Increase research on an international basis to elucidate variations across communities; to identify factors that influence the cause, course, and outcomes of mental disorders; and to increase understanding of the biological and psychosocial aspects of mental health as a method of understanding mental disorders and the development of more effective interventions. These recommendations provided the foundation for further work in global mental health policies and programs.

Despite the recommendations, many of the barriers to care were still evident in WHO's report titled *Improving Health Systems and Services for Mental Health* which makes the case for improved laws and policies but also considers that primary care for mental health "is fundamental but must be supported by other levels of care including community-based and hospital services, informal services and self-care to meet the full spectrum of mental health needs of the population" (2009c, p. 21). Such integration of services also serves to reduce stigma and support worker training and improved access to services.

There is much work to be done in educating healthcare providers and the general population about mental illness and its effective treatment. Major policy changes related to including mental health care in primary care and providing such care in community settings will come about only when governments and individuals demand such care and see the benefit of the outcomes for individuals and populations. Opportunities are present for developing countries to apply current knowledge and the lessons of exemplar programs to their developing healthcare policies and programs. Development of culturally congruent programs illustrates that major mental disorders can be treated in an efficient and cost-effective manner with low cost and technically simple treatment. Community and primary care treatment programs need the support of philanthropic organizations as well as government entities to increase understanding of their effectiveness. WHO (2009b) has produced checklists for evaluating mental health plans, but it will take the greater community to address implementation of mental health services in a meaningful fashion.

The 2001 recommendations were addressed in WHO's *Mental Health Atlas* reports dating back to 2000 when the first assessment of mental health resources of WHO member states was conducted. The reports indicated the progress made in each area. Published reports followed in 2001, 2005, and 2011. The *2014 Mental Health Atlas* report made an assessment of mental health services and resources (WHO, 2015b).

This section will present some of the key findings of WHO's 2014 *Mental Health Atlas* related to five areas, Global Reporting on Core Mental Health Indicators, Mental Health System Governance, Financial and Human Resources for Mental Health, Mental Health Service Availability and Uptake, and Mental Health Promotion and Prevention and some change since the 2011 Atlas report. In reference to Global Reporting on Core Mental Health Indicators, 88%, or 171 out of WHO's 194 member states, completed parts of the Atlas instrument with a response rate of 80%. Of the response rate, 60% were able to provide information on the five core indicators and 33% reported regularly compiling mental health service and activity data for at least the public sector. In reference to Mental Health System Governance, 58% of those reporting have plans for a mental health or a stand-alone policy, while 51% have a stand-alone mental health law. However, in many countries, persons with mental disorders and family members have limited involvement and the implementation is weak. Financial and Human Resources for mental health in the reporting countries show levels of public distributions of funds to be very low in both low and middle-income countries and most of the funds go to inpatient care in mental hospitals. Globally the median number of mental health workers is 9 per 100,000 population; however, in low-income countries it can be from 1 per 100,000 population while high-income countries have up to and over 50 per 100,000. Relating to Mental Health Service Availability and Uptake, there are large disparities in the number of beds per 100,000 population between low- and lower-middle-income countries (five) to over 50 in high-income countries. Also, wide disparities exist among income levels for outpatient services and welfare support. Finally, in the category of Mental Health Promotion and Prevention 41% of the WHO member states report having at least two functioning mental health programs and preventions programs out of over 400 reported programs. Fifty percent of the programs were focused on improving mental health literacy or combating stigma (WHO, 2015b).

Among the WHO countries participating in the 2014 *Mental Health Atlas* report, there were some changes since the 2011 *Atlas* report. In the mental health workforce there was a slight decline of 6% in the reported number of psychiatrists. This finding may reflect under-reporting in the 2014 survey of psychiatrists working in private practice. In contrast, in the Southeast Asian and African Regions there was an increase of over 25% of psychiatrists, but the number is still low for the two regions. There was a 37% increase in the number of nurses working in mental health globally with higher increases in the American Region (63%) and Eastern Mediterranean Region (46%). Overall the number of nurses working in mental health is greatest in low-income countries and least in high-income countries. However, the absolute number of nurses working in mental health in high-income countries is still many times higher than in lower-income country groups (WHO, 2015b).

In reference to hospital beds and admissions, globally, there was a 5% decrease in the number of mental hospitals and the number of mental hospital beds decreased by almost 30% compared to 2011. Even though there was a global decrease in the number of beds, there was an increase of over 20% in the admission rate to mental hospitals, indicating a higher turnover rate.

The trends across WHO regions are varied; for example, one region (Western Pacific) showed a decline of over 50% and the Eastern Mediterranean and Southeast Asian Regions show an increase of 25% in hospital admission rates. There was an 84% increase in admission rates to general hospital facilities in three regions (American, Southeast Asian, and Western Pacific). The increases are found in middle-income countries and the rates in low-income and high-income countries have decreased (WHO, 2015b).

To better focus on regional issues, a selected review of examples of mental health programs is presented here. These examples include analysis of the scope, effectiveness, and cultural and economic issues related to such programs in various countries within larger regions. The greatest work accomplished has been in the integration of mental health care and primary care, an approach that combines financial resources, increases access, and mitigates some stigma associated with mental illness.

REGIONAL MENTAL HEALTH ISSUES AND OUTCOMES

There are no specific worldwide groups that can address all cultural and ideological issues that affect mental health care. The thrust of WHO's efforts is to focus on scientific research and good practices, while acknowledging that many cultures base local policies and programs on religious or ideological beliefs. The WHO efforts shed light on the role of stigma and exclusion, both of which represent barriers to care on an individual and population basis. The various action plans described also acknowledge the fear factor and stigma that promotes delivery of care in institutions rather than in communities. The descriptions highlight programs that have been successful when community-based care is developed. In the following sections, regional mental health policies, programs, and outcomes are examined. Exemplar programs are presented when available, and examples are used to illustrate problems as well as successes.

North America

United States

In the United States, the prevalence of self-reported mental health disability is 2 million adults, representing 2.7% of all respondents to the U.S. National Health Interview Survey (Mojtabai, 2011). Both trends are rather discouraging considering the more than 20-year history of mental health care in the United States since the 1999 publication of *Report of the Surgeon General on Mental Health*. In that report, the directors of the Substance Abuse and Mental Health Services Administration (SAMHSA), the National Institute of Mental Health (NIMH), and the Center for Mental Health Services issued a challenge to the nation as a whole, to U.S. communities, and to health and social services, policy makers, employers, and citizens to take action and collaborate on generating needed knowledge about the brain and behavior and then translating that knowledge into service systems and action by citizens. The Surgeon General at that time, Dr. David Satcher, called for a social resolve to make the needed investment to change attitudes about mental health and usher in a healthy era of mind and body for the nation (USDHHS, 1999). The fact that this 1999 report was the first Surgeon General's report ever issued on the topic of mental health and mental illness was significant. The report emphasized two main findings: (1) the well-documented efficacy of mental health treatments and the range of treatment that exists for most mental disorders and (2) the view of mental health and mental illness as points on a continuum, which suggested efforts were needed along the entire continuum.

The Surgeon General's report (USDHHS, 1999) heralded the inclusion of mental health care in the overall healthcare schema for the United States, created a vision for the future that encouraged good access to a range of mental health treatment programs, and continued to build on the scientific bases of neuroscience, molecular genetics, and pharmacotherapies. The report urged the reduction of stigma attached to mental illness by dispelling myths with accurate knowledge and improving public awareness of effective treatment. Further, it called for the supply of mental health services and providers to be developed in different venues, ensuring that state-of-the-art treatment would be delivered in a manner that considered age, gender, race, and culture by facilitating entry into treatment and by reduction of financial barriers to treatment. The report was greeted with enthusiasm by consumers and mental health advocates alike. Indeed, it did mark a major emphasis on the essential inclusion of mental health care in healthcare discussions, but unfortunately few direct-care programs resulted from the report.

In 2001, the New Freedom Commission on Mental Health was convened to conduct a comprehensive study of the U.S. mental health service delivery system and issue advice on methods to improve the system and fill the gaps in the mental health system. By 2003, the commission had issued its report, which confirmed that "recovery from mental illness is now a real possibility . . . yet for too many Americans with mental illness, the mental health services and supports they need remain fragmented and disconnected—often frustrating the opportunity for recovery. Today's mental healthcare system is a patchwork relic—the result of disjointed reforms and policies" (USDHHS, 2003, p. 4). While not painting a pretty picture, the report incorporated the views of consumers, families, and professionals.

In 2003, the New Freedom Commission focused on creating a transformed mental health system. As part of this effort, new goals were established. The commission also noted that "the system (of mental health care) was not oriented to the single most important goal of the people it serves—the hope of recovery. Even though treatments are available, they are not being transferred to community settings" (USDHHS, 2003 p. 3).

In 2008, following up on the New Freedom Commission, the Veterans Administration (VA) reported two initiatives implemented in their VA Medical Centers (VAMCs) and Community Based Outpatient Clinics (CBOCs) and in "community Living Centers" formerly called nursing homes. The first initiative relates to implementing the Primary Care–Mental Health Integration Initiative, which has three parts: (1) collocated collaborative care, (2) care management, and (3) blended models. In collocated collaborative care, mental health and primary care practitioners practice together in a clinical setting and share the responsibility of patient care, including evaluations, treatment plan, and patient outcomes. For example, in North Carolina there are three integrated care programs in Durham, Raleigh, and Fayetteville. The national office is involved with an evaluation method in collaboration with the Serious Mental Illness Treatment Research and Evaluation Center in Ann Arbor, Michigan (Post & Van Stone, 2008).

The other initiative relates to serving aging veterans in community living centers and a suicide-prevention hotline. One main focus of the VA is the integration of primary and behavioral health care with equal importance to both aspects. Twenty-three mental health providers were placed in community living centers to implement the integration of primary and mental health providers by delivering psychosocial services to manage behavioral symptoms found in dementia and other neuropsychiatric conditions. In addition, to better meet veterans' behavioral health, especially for those veterans returning from Middle East conflicts, a suicide prevention hotline (800-273-TALK; press one for veterans) was launched in 2007 and the number was active in 2015. The hotline is staffed 24/7 by VA mental health professionals who can access veteran callers' medical records. In one year the service has prevented 885 potential suicides (Douglas, 2008).

Goals: In a Transformed Mental Health System

The National Alliance on Mental Illness grades the states on a regular basis as a way to address needs and recognize achievement and to evaluate how policy is being implemented. *Grading the States: Report on America's Health Care System for Serious Mental Illness* was published in 2006 and 2009. Unfortunately, many of the states that had worked hard since the first report saw their initial gains wiped out with the economic crisis: Budget shortfalls meant cuts to mental health services. In the 2009 analysis, the states assigned "D" grades remained the same as in the first study. Fourteen states had improved their grades since 2006, but not enough to raise the national average. Twelve states had fallen back. Twenty-three states stayed the same (NAMI, 2009).

There are some areas where innovation and excellence exist in mental health care. The recovery movement has been a significant motivator toward reform and inclusiveness in care delivery. Many of the NAMI programs are designed around education and peer support. NAMI's Peer Support Center offers programs to families, providers, and peers who have experienced mental illness. Its programs also include those focused on understanding mental illness and treatment, and the importance of living a healthy life. Nationally, NAMI sponsors nine programs of education and support that address the needs of families, peer support for persons living with a mental illness, providers, parents of children and adolescents living with mental illness, and the general public (NAMI, 2011).

Many recovery-focused programs have emerged from the work conducted at Boston University, Center for Psychosocial Rehabilitation, Sargent College of Health and Rehabilitation Sciences. The center, which was founded in 1979, has been innovative in both assisting in the design of programs and evaluating their outcomes. Its Hope and Health program, Training for the Future program, individual services in recovery and research, and evaluation projects are directed toward "increasing knowledge in the field of psychiatric rehabilitation and applying the knowledge to train treatment personnel, to develop effective rehabilitation programs, and to assist in organizing both personnel and programs into efficient and coordinated service delivery systems" (Center for Psychiatric Rehabilitation, 2006, p. 4). The Center for Psychiatric

Rehabilitation has evolved into a "think tank" for the development of recovery-focused psychosocial programs. William Anthony, the center's executive director, in his book *Toward a Vision of Recovery* (2007), states emphatically that "I am more convinced than ever that recovery from severe mental illness is possible for many more people than was previously believed. I believe that much of the chronicity in severe mental illness is due to the way the mental health system and society treat mental illness and not the nature of the illness itself" (p. 3).

One such program is the St. Louis Empowerment Center, a peer-run drop-in center that emphasizes participatory decision making, self-help, and mutual assistance. Peer support workers are matched via a "buddy" system, and the pair participates in recreational and social activities. The center also operates a "friendship line" to combat feelings of social isolation. A multisite study of such programs noted specific positive effects of consumer-driven programs when compared with traditional programs (Rogers et al., 2007). In 2015, the St. Louis Empowerment Center was still operating and is open to consumers of mental health services; its services include a friendship line, support groups, classes, guidance for goal development, employment program, benefits acquisition assistance, lunches, a computer lab, and additional amenities such as cable TV, a pool table, DVD library, and a lending library. Because the center is funded by the Missouri Department of Mental Health and the Missouri Foundation of Health all services at the center are free of charge. Their website can be accessed at http://www.dbsaempowerment.org/support-groups/.

Another developing trend is integration of mental health programs with primary care services. Integrating mental health services into a primary care setting offers an efficient way of providing needed mental health services and making sure that people have access to them. Also, mental healthcare services delivered in an integrated setting can be instrumental in minimizing stigma and discrimination that has the potential to improve overall health outcomes (Collins, Hewson, Munger, & Wade, 2010). The Milbank Memorial Fund studied many programs built on various types of integration models. One such model—the unified primary care and behavioral health model—has been implemented by the Cherokee Health Systems in Tennessee, which expanded community mental health centers at 22 sites to become federally qualified general health centers. At these sites, case managers work with adults and children with serious mental illness, as well as patients with chronic physical health problems. Co-location enables collaborative practice where treatment teams can work together with those individuals who have complex problems. Brief intervention methods are used as the behavioral health model (Collins et al., 2010).

Advances in programs using recovery, peer participation, and integrated care models provide a promising direction for future development but are unlikely to compensate for the overall scarcity of programs to serve the mentally ill in the United States. However, accumulating evidence on their efficacy and efficiency may spur mental health policy to mend the mind–body schism and provide meaningful programs that are more easily accessed and acceptable to both individuals and communities.

Canada

Canada established a Mental Health Commission in 2005 "to provide leadership to make mental health a long-term priority of governments: facilitating the exchange of research and best practices, reducing fragmentation of mental health and illness policies and programs, and developing a strategy to increase awareness and reduce stigma around mental illness" (Canadian Collaborative Mental Health Initiative, 2005a). The Canadian Collaborative Mental Health Initiative was funded for two years by Health Canada's Primary Health Care Transition Fund.

As the funding model suggests, the Canadian healthcare system focused on the primary care model (Canadian Psychiatric Association [CPA]/College of Family Physicians of Canada [CFPC], 2003). When reviewing patterns of use, it was found that one in every five Canadians experience a mental illness during their lifetime, and the integration model offered the best options for greater access to mental health care. The Canadian Collaborative Mental Health Initiative addressed the complex interplay between physical and mental illnesses. It sought to maximize the shared care focus in mental health care through evaluation of various initiatives undertaken by a consortium of 12 national organizations representing mental health consumers, families, caregivers, community providers, dietitians, family physicians, nurses, occupational therapists, pharmacists, psychologists, psychiatrists, and social workers. One of the first activities of the initiative was to conduct a survey to obtain "buy-in" of the various groups, resulting in an engaged community of interest that provides ongoing advice. The initiative produced 10 research papers and 12 toolkits to ensure dissemination of the information (Canadian Collaborative Mental Health Initiative, 2006). In a follow-up report issued by the Mental Health Commission of Canada (MHCC) in 2009, efforts were directed toward recovery and well-being along the continuum of the seven goals articulated in the work of the commission and called for a social movement that puts mental health policy and programs in the forefront of health care.

Programs established continued and have since been joined by Mental Health First Aid projects, in which connections are provided for a person developing a mental health problem or experiencing a mental health crisis. This program provides a point of access and considerable training to improve mental health literacy while increasing recognition of signs and symptoms of mental health problems. The Mental Health First Aid program provides initial help and guides persons toward appropriate professional mental health services. Nearly 50,000 Mental Health First Aid personnel have been trained, thereby expanding the outreach of the healthcare system (MHCC, 2011b).

Another initiative developed a geriatric psychiatry outreach team bringing together psychiatrists, registered nurses, social workers, and a neuropsychologist to provide consultation to two family practice clinics and one community health center as well as home-based assessment when appropriate. The collaborative also sponsors a shared care conference annually (MHCC, 2011a).

In 2010, a Peer Project was launched that targeted peer-based education strategies aimed at youth in schools and adults in workplaces. The commission is developing national standards of practice but also encourages innovation in program development geared toward mental health. The concept of psychological safety in the workplace is designed to begin a conversation on occupational health that includes mental health (MHCC, 2011c).

All of these activities were based on a shared belief that Canadians are entitled to a health system with the capacity to help them meet both their physical and mental health needs, whether those needs comprise illness prevention, early detection, treatment, rehabilitation, or recovery. The consortium produced a general toolkit for providers and policy makers on planning and implementing collaboration between mental health and primary care services; additionally, the consortium produced a two-volume report on emerging trends in mental health care, including descriptions of more than 90 Canadian initiatives (Canadian Collaborative Mental Health Initiative, 2005b, p. 25). In all, 61% (55 programs) of long-term mental health initiatives were started during the years of the collaboration (2000–2004) (Canadian Collaborative Mental Health Initiative, 2005b, p. 28). The work of the Canadian Collaborative Mental Health Initiative and the MHCC laid the ground for launching a Partners of Mental Health Initiative in 2012 that is expected to spur a social movement to position mental health on the national agenda by making use of the voices of ordinary Canadians (MHCC, 2011a).

A current position paper lends support for interest in mental health in Canada. A position paper approved by the Canadian Psychiatric Association (CPA) in 2014 was aimed at supporting the mental health of people who identify as lesbian, gay, bisexual, transgender, and/or queer (LGBTQ). CPA has recognized the need for psychiatrists to increase their understanding of the mental health needs of this population. Eleven recommendations were made of which one is "The CPA encourages physician practices, medical schools, hospitals, and clinics to broaden any nondiscrimination policies or statements to include sexual orientation, gender identity and gender expression" (Veltman & Chalmowitz, 2014, p. 3). There is considerable agreement in North America on the scope of mental health problems and a growing focus on the efficacy of recovery, community, and social change as being the route forward to providing mental health services. Although outstanding examples exist, the Canadian system's main focus is on keeping the care system working with the consumer as the focus and streamlining access to care.

Latin America

The Latin American region includes many different cultural groups. In geopolitical terms, there are 13 countries in South America, 5 in Central America, Mexico, and 13 other countries in the Caribbean basin (Pan American Health Organization [PAHO], 2005).

In the 2010 *Annual Report of the Director of the Pan American Sanitary Bureau,* mental health was viewed in the context of personal security. The report noted that mental health problems continue to be a major concern in Latin America and the Caribbean. It is estimated that more than 125 million people in this region suffer from some form of mental illness but that fewer than half have access to treatment.

In Cuba, El Salvador, and Guatemala, policies on mental health have been integrated and focused on community-based care versus the traditional cure models. These policies mandated decentralization of mental health services, moving them from a hospital setting to community-level primary care (PAHO, 2010).

Chile has reported that it has experienced improvements in social indicators since the 1990s but that only 39% of persons with mental illness receive treatment. Efforts since 2000 have focused on increasing the role of primary health care in delivery of mental health services and access to psychotropic medications. There were still few mental health professionals per capita in the country, however, this is an issue for future development (WHO, 2008b). In addition, there is a lack of mental health services designed specifically for the indigenous people of Latin America despite PAHO goals (Incayawar & Maldonado-Bourchard, 2009).

The Program of Treatment for Depression in Primary Health Care (PTDPHC) was gradually introduced in 2001 and made national coverage in 2003 in Santiago, Chile, based on the recommendation of primary care interventions. Three antecedents influenced the initiation of the program. They are (1) three studies indicating the high incidence of depression in Chile that represented a most important disease burden for the population, (2) the knowledge of pharmacotherapy and psychotherapies that could be effective if applied in an organized manner by healthcare teams with special attention to the severity of persons' depression, and (3) the results of a controlled trial in primary clinics that showed positive results of a comprehensive multicomponent treatment for depression (Alvarado, Rojas, Minoletti, Alvarado, & Dominaguez, 2012).

In the program potential patients with depression are identified when seen by any provider for another health issue. If depression was suspected, the patient was referred to a physician or psychologist at the center whose responsibility was to confirm the diagnosis using the International Statistical Classification of Diseases and Related Health Problems, tenth revision (ICD-10) and to assign them to a treatment group. Patients who were diagnosed with severe depression were referred to a psychiatrist. In 10 years of functioning and several evaluation studies that show the effectiveness of the PTDPHC, over one million adults have been served. This treatment program uses evidence-based practice in caring for their patients.

In Argentina, mental healthcare reform was implemented on a state/provincial level. In the Rio Negro province, beds in a psychiatric hospital were replaced by beds in general hospitals, and a network of community-based services such as mental health centers and psychosocial rehabilitation programs was set up throughout the province (Caldas de Almeida & Horvitz-Lennon, 2010).

The Pan American Health Organization conduced a mental health assessment of the Latin American countries using the World Health Organization's Assessment Instrument for Mental Health Systems (WHO-AIMS) in 2013. Some of the findings include the burden of mental and neurological disorders that was 22.2% for the total burden of disease measured in disability-adjusted life years (DALYs), and the most common neuropsychiatric disorders are the unipolar depressive disorders (13.2%) and those disorders produced by excessive use of alcohol (PAHO, 2013).

Eight countries in South America have developed a national mental health policy and some have updated their mental health policies. In these countries the mental health budget as a percentage of the total health budget is low (0.2%–7%) with a median of 2.05%. In the six countries of Central America, Mexico, and the Latin Caribbean, the percentage ranged from 0.4% to 2.9%, with a median of 0.9%. Mental healthcare services are diverse and include primary care centers with primary care or mental health professionals or those in the community mainly by specialists. Another difference is the mental disorders treated, ranging from mild to severe mental illnesses. There is limited ability for follow-up in the community to provide continuity of patient care in the entire region. Conclusions of the report include:

Issues in the health system's capacity to respond to the needs of the populations served.
Mental hospitals continue to dominate mental health care, taking a large portion of available resources.
There is limited development of the mental health part in primary care;
workers in primary care do not have the needed skills to respond to patients with mental health disorders.

On a positive note there are innovative experiences that can be used as examples of what can be done in public health in the region (PAHO, 2013).

A feature story on the World Bank Web page supports the WHO-AIM Report of 2013 by suggesting that poor mental health is a hindrance to development in Latin America. The most common mental health illness is depression, affecting 5% of the adult population, but most of those with depression do not seek or receive treatment. Severe depression can lead to suicide and in the Americas 63,000 people kill themselves annually. Less severe depression can affect activities of daily living and relationships, and it is apparent in Latin American and the Caribbean as mental and neurological disorders account for almost a quarter of the disease burden. Interference with productivity due to depression has economic implications for individuals and can lead to poverty. There remains a stigma associated with mental illness that may hinder people from getting treatment, which may be a result of discrimination and poor treatment of people with mental disorders. One solution is to strengthen primary care and mental health care by having workers better trained and making access in the community a priority (Cruz, 2015).

Based on the broad policy recommendations and the demonstration programs, it would seem that mental health programs would most likely be effective if they addressed increasing understanding of mental health issues and treatment and if they could be provided along with mental health care as part of the primary care system. These efforts will require the development of trained healthcare workers who can identify mental health issues and direct individuals to primary care or community resources, as appropriate. There remain gaps in both stated policies and implemented programs in Latin America, especially for those addressing vulnerable groups. Recent policy initiatives have been developed that focus on the connection between mental health and economic development, but stretching limited resources will continue to be a challenge.

Europe
Countries in the WHO European Region face continued challenges with mental health problems, with 27% of persons in the European Union experiencing at least one mental disorder. Depression is the leading chronic condition in Europe, where the suicide prevalence rate is 13.9 deaths per 100,000 population. In Lithuania, this rate is 30.7 suicides per 100,000 population (WHO, 2009a).

Mental health policies and services vary greatly across the region. Community care has been shown to offer a better quality of life and greater satisfaction to consumers and family caregivers. Across Europe, the number of institutional beds is decreasing. Unfortunately, many

European countries have limited services available in the community, and more than 50% of all patients are still treated in large mental hospitals. A recent publication, *Policies and Practices for Mental Health in Europe*, noted that 42 countries have adopted or updated their mental health policies since 2005 (WHO, 2011c). However, the establishment of such policies does not necessarily mean advancement of programs given the economic constraints and reduction in public spending related to the economic crisis that started in 2007 and continues to offer a challenging atmosphere (WHO, 2011b). The United Kingdom leads in the percentage of health spending earmarked for mental health at 13.5%, with Bulgaria, Romania, and Portugal all allocating less than 4% of their health expenditures to mental health services.

Some of the ongoing policy issues relate to the availability of mental health professionals. In some countries, care is delivered by doctors and nurses in institutional settings; in others, mental health care is provided as part of primary care. This practice varies considerably. In Malta, a relatively small county, there are no community-based services and it has the highest rate of hospital beds per capita—more than 180 beds per 100,000 population. In France, in contrast, mental health services include those provided at day hospitals, part-time therapeutic welcome centers, and therapeutic workshops (WHO, 2011c). Although the Mental Health Declaration for Europe emphasized the role of primary care as part of mental health service delivery, this role remains underdeveloped in many parts of Europe. In some countries, diagnosing mental disorders or prescribing related medication is illegal for family doctors. This policy often reflects a lack of training, but also results from longstanding stigma against persons with mental health problems (WHO, 2011c).

Efforts to improve or increase training since the 2005 report have resulted in inclusion of mental health training in the education of general practitioners in Austria; additional training for family doctors in Germany; development of courses in psychiatry, protocols on disease management, and standards of providing medicine in psychiatry in Russia; and establishment of improved access to evidence-based psychological therapy focused on anxiety and depression in the United Kingdom (WHO, 2011c). Activities generally support the defined scope of mental health policy and practice related to promoting mental well-being in the population; tackling stigma, discrimination, and social exclusion; prevention of mental health problems; and providing comprehensive and effective care for those who experience mental health disorders. These services also include recovery-focused programs for caregivers and patients that involve choice, including rehabilitation (WHO, 2011c).

In the United Kingdom, a 5-year initiative was undertaken to deal with stigma and discrimination around mental health issues. Project SHIFT works with young people, public services and professional and private organizations, and the media to promote communication and disability rights. Another program, Our Choice in Mental Health, encourages the exercise of choice among people who use mental health services and their caregivers; it also provides best-practices models to be used as a basis for developing future programs (WHO, 2011c). Addressing the need for an educated mental health workforce, a 3-year program on innovations in community-based mental health nursing was developed to include sites in the United Kingdom, Germany, and Italy. The training also focused on developing noninstitutional approaches to mental health (Leonardo da Vinci Pilot Projects, 2007).

In Europe, there are islands of hope in a region that has much institutional history and stigma to overcome. Plans are well under way to make changes in the types of care provided, the accessibility of care, and delivery models for mental health care. The dissemination of evidence-based practices remains a challenge. Nevertheless, the gap is narrowing between policy and practice among some countries. The move toward greater community focus and away from institutional care is an economic issue as well as a social and political issue. Innovations and demonstrations provide a pathway to future success.

Africa

Africa is a vast land that encompasses many diverse peoples and has been the site of much strife and war. In a presentation entitled "Mental Health and Poverty: Challenges in Service Delivery in Sub-Saharan Africa" (2011), Dr. Fred Kigozi, executive director of Butabika Nation Hospital, noted that Africa is the second-largest continent in the world, with a population of more than one billion. There is a low life expectancy related to the fact that 60% of the population lives on less than $1 per day. Adding to the difficulties faced by this region are civil strife, unemployment, the HIV/AIDS epidemic, and an overall shortage of resources. There is only 0.05 psychiatrist per 100,000 population across Africa; few countries have clinical psychologists or social workers; and 79% of the African countries spend less than 1% of their health budget on mental health. Further, poverty often aggravates the stigma about mental illness and delays help-seeking. In most countries, services are limited to a central large mental hospital, a few beds in regional general hospitals, and very little community care. Generally, needs are focused on development of policies that will guide the development of services and counter stigma, as well as development of training for general health workers in the districts. The region embraces the principles of integration of mental health into primary health care and is focused on meeting structural needs to make that happen (Kigozi, 2011).

The HIV pandemic persists in some African communities, and the mental health consequences of AIDS contribute to overall psychiatric morbidity in the region, exacerbating the consequences of hunger, displacement, and lack of material resources. Compounding the fear of mental illness is the lack of mental health workers in most countries and the existence of only a limited drug formulary. Nearly half of the countries in Africa have just one hospital for the mentally ill. Further, because many families do not understand the manifestation of mental illness in their family members, they may chain or tie patients up and administer beatings (Kaplan, 2006).

Clearly, there are many challenges to providing mental health care in Africa that cannot be overcome by policy statement and goal setting. Several programs, however, provide beacons of hope for the future. In the WHO Mental Health Improvement for Nations' Development (MIND) country summary series in 2007, Ghana reported that mental health services are available at most levels of care but the majority of care is provided through specialized psychiatric hospitals with less funding for general hospital– and primary care–based services. The current laws support institutional care to keep mentally ill people off the streets and protect their assets. In Ghana, 5.74% of the total health budget is dedicated to administration and mental health services. The national healthcare system provides community psychiatric nurses who report to the coordinator of community psychiatry, and some primary healthcare workers have received on-site mental health training. In addition, Ghana has many traditional healers, with 70 to 80% of the population using traditional medicine as their primary care. Ideally, more of the traditional healers will be integrated into the formal healthcare system and provided with standard accreditation and practice guidelines to provide mental health care (WHO, 2007).

An evaluation of Ghana's mental health system using the WHO-AIMS instrument was conducted using data on the Mental Health System in Ghana for the year 2011. The hope was that the information gathered would provide planning information for the implementation of Ghana's new Mental Health Act 846 of 2012 and provide a baseline to measure progress in Ghana. The data showed both strengths and weaknesses in the six domains of the WHO-AIMS; (1) Policy and Legislative Frameworks, (2) Mental Health Services, (3) Mental Health in Primary Health Care, (4) Human Resources, (5) Public Education, and (6) Monitoring and Research. The overall main strength was the longevity of established service with staff in outpatient departments and hospitals. In contrast, the low government spending on mental health was the main weakness. The data gathered provided detailed information to make top-level priorities to implement the recommendations to be used for Ghana's new mental health act and can be used as a baseline measure of progress in the future (Roberts, Mogan, & Asare, 2014).

Elsewhere on the African continent, Zimbabwe launched mental health treatment guidelines for mental health care within its primary care system. They describe how a mentally ill patient should be managed holistically from history taking through diagnosis and delivery of the appropriate treatment and management (WHO, 2011a).

Where poverty is endemic, low-cost integrated public mental health programs are vital, as are programs that train and involve community workers. Culturally sensitive programs that include significant local involvement are important to change attitudes and offer hope to persons with mental illness. The vastness of Africa makes it important that individual countries and provinces make efforts to better the life of persons with mental illness within the constraints of few limited financial resources and much civil strife.

Asia and the Western Pacific

In 2003 in Beijing, Dr. Henk Bekedam spoke at the Second International Mental Health Development Conference and noted that even with some aspects of physical health improving in the region over the past 50 years, mental health has gotten worse. He also acknowledged that the burden of mental health goes hand-in-hand with rapid urbanization and social changes such as poverty and physical illness. To address these difficult realities, the region adopted three basic goals related to mental health: (1) Reduce the human, social, and economic burden produced by mental and neurological disorders, including intellectual disability and substance abuse and dependence, (2) promote mental health, and (3) give appropriate attention to psychosocial aspects of health care and the improvement of quality of life.

Bekedam (2003) further called for the integration of mental health into general health care and primary care systems. As in Europe and largely as the lingering result of past European colonization, mental health activities in the countries of WHO's Southeast Asia Region have been concentrated on hospital-based psychiatry. A report on the work of WHO in this region called for mental health services that could be integrated into the primary healthcare system, and the development of innovative community-based programs. As in Africa, considerable attention in Asia has been paid to crisis situations such as tsunami relief efforts, provision of basic health care, and the demands of bird flu outbreaks. Additionally, some areas in Asia have been marked by war and insurgent activities that contribute to human suffering and mental illness. Mental health has been a low priority in such circumstances. In most of the countries in Southeast Asia, mental health spending represents less than 2% of the total health budget, with 80 to 90% of those funds going to hospitals (Maramis, Nguyen, & Minas, 2011). A notable exception to the trend of hospital-based care is found in Cambodia, because of the necessity for the country to start from the beginning in creating a healthcare system following the Pol Pot regime. Cambodia has focused on the development of a primary care and community-focused care model. Capacity is still limited in these programs, but they are growing as there was no hospital-based system to disassemble before their adoption (Maramis, Nguyen, & Minas, 2011).

One project examined factors that influence Asian communities' access to mental health care and noted that both health professionals and the general public have considerable knowledge deficits regarding mental illness and mental health. Shame and stigma were commonly reported. "The sense of shame was significant, and it was noted that the shame connected with mental illness for Chinese people meant that 'you can't go out and face other people'" (Wynaden, Chapman, Org, McGowan, Zeeman, & Yeak, 2005, p. 90). Another commonly reported barrier to seeking care was the level of knowledge about mental illness, which was related to the level of education, country of origin, and religion. Karma, the law of cause and effect in Eastern spirituality, and beliefs about reincarnation are important concepts in many Eastern religions. Consequently, having a child with mental illness often results in the parents feeling as if they are being punished for conduct in their past lives. Others might believe that a mentally ill person is possessed by evil spirits, or that bad blood is passed down to the child from the mother. Even if a general practitioner asks about mental illness, concern about family reputation and shame may prohibit discussion of the illness. These beliefs often result in mental illness being hidden from the community, and family members not doing anything about the illness, or simply hoping that it will go away. Seeking help for mental illness is often seen as a last resort (Wynaden, Chapman, Org, McGowan, Zeeman, & Yeak, 2005).

On a more positive note, the Pacific Island Mental Health Network (PIMHnet) was launched in March 2007. It includes 18 members: American Samoa, Australia, Commonwealth of the Northern Mariana Islands, Cook Islands, Federated States of Micronesia, Fiji, Kiribati, Marshall Islands, Nauru, New Zealand, Niue, Palau, Papua New Guinea, Samoa, Solomon Islands, Tokelau, Tonga, and Vanuatu. There has been considerable progress made in raising awareness of mental health issues within these countries. The government of each PIMHnet member country has nominated a leader to direct national activities in collaboration with a specially designated in-country mental health team. Acknowledging the many challenges faced in providing mental health services, there has been some progress in development of human resources and expansion of the use of primary health workforce to build services for people with mental health problems. One such program that came out of the partnership was developed in Vauatu, where two Australian family physicians with expertise in mental health were engaged to provide training of local health workers, who included doctors, nurses, and community health workers. The training consisted of classroom sessions, interactive activities, and visits to hospitals. The participants were also engaged in setting up a prevalence study for mental health problems that utilized a cultural awareness tool translated into Bislama, the local language. Outcomes have included using the new skills to identify and manage mental health problems and developing a series of educational activities for young people to raise understanding of mental illness. Other activities undertaken by PIMHnet include newsletters as well as teleconferences with member countries every six months to provide updates and opportunities to request assistance. Contacts have also been established with academic organizations, professional organizations, and church and spiritual organizations to add to the network's resources (Hughes, 2009).

In response to the recent earthquakes and tsunami in Japan, physicians and research fellows went to the University of California, San Francisco, to learn how to provide mental health counseling when dealing with a crisis. They were especially focused on the response for children in the face of disaster; thus, psychologists taught the guiding principles for parents and other caregivers—listen, protect, and connect. In Japan, the stigma associated with mental health concerns often leads to guilt and shame, so training is being organized to help Japanese physicians and others improve their response to individuals who may be vulnerable to post-traumatic stress disorder (PTSD) (Norris, 2011).

To erase long-held stigma and promote delivery of mental health services in community settings, innovations such as the mood disorders center in Hong Kong were developed in 2001. When the center opened, a hotline was established to bypass the taboos about talking about depression. The center's phone lines were heavily used by people asking for help and provided a point of contact regarding reports of chronic fatigue, headaches, and poor memory, which are often correlates of depression. The mood disorders center, developed by the Chinese University of Hong Kong, also trained family doctors to better recognize and treat anxiety disorders and depression as a face-saving way for people to seek treatment. The center was still operating in 2015 and can be accessed at http://www.heart2heart.org.hk/new/en/node/237.

The government and a private organization planned to open one-stop centers in all 18 districts in Hong Kong but faced considerable community resistance linked to continued community stigma and fear (Bayron, 2010).

In China, the scope of the taboos regarding mental illness has prompted the Chinese government to draft the country's first mental health law formally recognizing that mental health care is both a legal issue and a medical matter. Often hospitalization of mentally ill persons is sought for political reasons, whereas other individuals with mental health issues avoid care because of stigma; thus, human rights issues are being discussed in the public comment period related to the law (Pumin, 2011).

A unique demonstration program known as "686" was implemented in China in 2005 to improve access to evidence-based care and promote human rights for those with severe mental disorders. The mental health initiative was focused on "unlocking" people with severe mental disorders who were found in some form of restraint in their homes without treatment, especially those living in poverty. Persons who were unlocked and did not need hospitalization entered the "686" program and received a physical exam, a psychiatric diagnosis, treatment, medication, regular follow-up visits, and community-based rehabilitation with no charge. A nationwide two-stage follow-up study was conducted to determine the effectiveness of the "686" program. Data was collected in stage one in 2009 and again in 2012. The time participants had been locked ranged from 2 weeks to 28 years and the number regularly taking medication increased from one at the time of unlocking to 74% in 2009 and 76% in 2023. Over 92% of the participants were free of restraints in 2012. Major findings were continued improvement in social functioning and significant declines in family burden (Guan et al., 2015).

Much effort is necessary to overcome centuries of cultural beliefs and political propaganda about the causes and treatment of mental illness. Small, locally developed programs delivered as part of a health system are likely to produce the best results for treatment if personal stigma and fear can be overcome by individuals and families.

SUMMARY

It is clear that considerable attention to mental health and mental illness issues needs to be paid by, and involve more, government entities and community agencies. There is increased evidence of the biopsychosocial nature of both mental illness and mental health, as well as evidence that mental illness has a profound impact on the lives of persons with such illness, their families, and their communities. The publication of such evidence has increased the global profile of international mental health, but sustained and sustainable action remains limited. Mental disorders have clear economic costs, as persons experiencing mental illness often experience reduced productivity at home and in the workplace. Mental disorders also can lead to poverty and homelessness, have a range of consequences on the course and outcomes of comorbid chronic conditions, some of which are heart disease, diabetes, and HIV/AIDS, and persons with untreated mental disorders are at heightened risk for poor health behaviors, noncompliance with prescribed medical regimens, diminished immune functioning, and unfavorable disease outcomes (WHO, 2013).

Understanding of the importance of mental health and the treatment of mental illness does not necessarily instantly produce needed resources and programs. WHO's (2015b) *2014 Mental Health Atlas,* a compendium of global data from 171 countries out of WHO's 194 member states was compared with previous data from 2011. Fifty-eight percent of those reporting have plans for mental health or stand-alone policies in their countries, while 51% have stand-alone mental health laws. However, even with these plans, policies, and laws in many countries, the family members have limited involvement and the implementation is weak. The levels of public distributions of funds is very low in both low and middle countries, and most of the funds go to inpatient care in mental hospitals, limiting funds to community efforts. In terms of global mental health workers, the median number is 9 per 100,000 population, but in low-income countries it can be as low as 1 per 1,000,000 population, and in high-income countries have up to and over 50 per 1,000,000 population.

The results also showed some changes in the 2011 results. There was a slight decline of 6% in reported numbers of psychiatrists, which may reflect underreporting of psychiatrists working in private practice. The Southeast Asian and African Regions report an increase of over 25% of psychiatrists, but the number is still low in these two regions. There was a 37% increase in the number of nurses working in mental health globally with higher increases in the American Region (63%) and Eastern Mediterranean Region (46%). The numbers of nurses working in mental health in high-income countries is still many times higher than in lower-income country groups (WHO, 2015b).

Globally, there was a 5% decrease in the number of mental hospitals and the number of mental hospital beds decreased by almost 30% compared to 2011. Even though there was a global decrease in the number of beds, there was an increase of over 20% in the admission rate to mental hospitals, indicating a higher turnover rate. The trends across WHO regions are varied: one region (Western Pacific) showed a decline of over 50% and the Eastern Mediterranean and Southeast Asian Regions showed an increase of 25% in hospital admission rates. There was an 84% increase in admission rates to general hospital facilities in three regions (American, Southeast Asian, and Western Pacific). The increases are found in middle-income countries and the rates in low-income and high-income countries have decreased (WHO, 2015b).

In keeping with the spirit of the first Global Mental Health Day, mental health needs to have a larger presence on the world health agenda. The case needs to continue to be made that good mental health care enhances overall health and the prosperity of the population. The mhGAP mental health program (WHO, 2008a) makes the case that more effort is required to change policy, practice, and services delivery systems to ensure that mental health needs are assigned the level of priority necessary to guarantee that they are addressed. There should be no more excuses for marginalizing funding and people who suffer from mental illness.

Study Questions

1. Relate the barriers to receiving mental health care as compared to physical health services, in both developed and developing countries.
2. Describe WHO policies that favor mental health services worldwide.
3. Discuss the social and economic loss of persons with mental health problems.
4. Do you believe that mental health care should be a "right" or an entitlement for all residents of a nation, within developing as well as developed countries? Why?

Case Study: Canada

As a Chinese immigrant survivor of bipolar disorder living in Toronto, I would like to highlight two issues. People with a mental health condition are subject to stigma and discrimination. It exists because of the lack of mental health education and the traditional notion that mental illness is a loss of face for the family.

I was new to Toronto and did not know of any social or mental health support services after my hospitalization. I was lost and isolated in the cold winter. Our world today has many people suffering from mental illness and it is my sincere hope that more services and programs will address our needs and those of our families.

Modified from World Health Organization (WHO). (2010). *Mental health and development: Targeting people with mental health conditions as a vulnerable group*. Mental Health and Poverty Project. Geneva, Switzerland: Author.

Case Study: China

When Sun Yuhua was 71, she began losing her memory. In addition to forgetting what she had just said or done, she would repeat the same question often and not remember the answer, and finally she could not manage to perform simple household tasks. Sun Yuhua was aware of what was happening but did not go to a doctor. Her husband, Zhou Zhensheng, knew of a caregiver support group for dementia sufferers and he convinced Sun Yuhua to make an appointment at the memory clinic. Caregiver support groups are found in bigger cities, but outside the cities resources are very limited. Sun Yuhua's and Zhou Zhensheng's lives have improved since attending the support group. "Joining the group, learning from the mini-lectures and other families' experiences, I am picking up ideas and becoming more confident that I can help my wife with her dementia and I feel more hopeful," said Zhou Zhensheng.

Modified & summarized from WHO. (2014). *China: Improving home care for dementia patients.* Retrieved from http://www.who.int/features/2014/china-dementia-patients/en/

Case Study: New Zealand

Hotorene Brown (Ngāti Pikiao, Ngāti Whakaue), age 37, was told if he didn't change his lifestyle he would not live to see his three young sons grow up. Hotorene knew he had to do something and that led him to a 3-year journey to take control of his health and his destiny. His Whānau Ora plan played a key role in this; Making a plan and detailing my goals made me look at my reality, and by doing that, I couldn't ignore my health any longer," said Hotorene. Initially, Hotorene's goal was to get off of the medication he needed to keep his blood pressure under control, but it was the medication that was keeping him from having a stroke. As a result he had to work out what key goals would enable him to get there. First thing he did was get a bike and begin to take the 32k journey from Mourea to Rotorua and back each day. He began to find the control he needed to eat a balanced diet and make healthy eating choices. "The support I got from my Paearahi was important because having someone there who understood how to navigate those initial challenges meant I could get over some of the speedbumps I encountered early on," said Hotorene. Looking back on it all, it still seems like a dream, but when he looks in the mirror he can finally *see* the effort. Something that Hotorene didn't anticipate were the many Whānau, friends, and strangers who are now looking to him for guidance, support, and inspiration.

Modified from Te Arawa Whānau Ora. (2014). *Whānau Ora = Fitness for Life.* Retrieved from http://tearawawhanauora.org.nz/2014/04/whanau-ora-fitness-for-life/

References

Alvarado, R., Rojas, G., Minoletti, A., Alvarado, F., & Dominaguez, C. (2012). Depression program in primary health care: The Chilean experience. *International Journal of Mental Health, 41*(1), 38–47.

Anthony, W. A. (2007). *Toward a Vision of Recovery for Mental Health and Psychiatric Rehabilitation Services* (2nd ed.). Boston, MA: Center for Psychiatric Rehabilitation, Boston University.

Bayron, H. (2010). Hong Kong undertakes first mental health survey in wake of violent cases. *Voice of America News: Asia.* Retrieved from http://www.voanews.com/english/news/asia/Hong-Kong-Undertakes-First-Mental-Health-Survey-in-Wake-of-Violent-Cases-102901909.html

Bekedam, H. (2003). *Speeches: WHO Representative in China on the Occasion of the Second International Mental Health Development Conference.* China: World Health Organization.

Boyle, P. (2001). Bulletin: Religion and the brain: The decade of the brain. *Park Ride Center, 19,* 1–6.

Caldas de Almeida, J., & Horvitz-Lennon, M. (2010, March). Mental health care reforms in Latin America. *Psychiatric Services, 61*(3), 218–221.

Canadian Collaborative Mental Health Initiative. (2005a). Canadian Collaborative Mental Health Initiative applauds the establishment of landmark commission. *Canada NewsWire.*

Canadian Collaborative Mental Health Initiative. (2005b). *A Review of Canadian Initiatives, Vol. I: Analysis of Initiatives.* Mississauga, Ontario, Canada: Author.

Canadian Collaborative Mental Health Initiative. (2006). Health Canada Primary Care Transition Fund, *2006 Canadian Collaborative Mental Health Initiative, final report.* Retrieved from http://www.ccmhi.ca

Canadian Psychiatric Association/College of Family Physicians of Canada. (2003). Retrieved from https://ww1.cpa-apc.org/Press_Releases/PR_Oct29_2003.asp

Carolla, B. (2015). 17 million Americans hear NAMI's message for mental health reform, *National Alliance on Mental Illness* (NAMI). Retrieved from https://www.nami.org/Blogs/NAMI-Blog/October-2015/17-Million-Americans-Hear-NAMI-s-Message-for-Menta

Centers for Disease Control and Prevention. (2011). *Public Health Action Plan to Integrate Mental Health Promotion and Mental Illness Prevention and Chronic Disease Prevention, 2011–2015.* Atlanta: U.S. Department of Health and Human Services.

Center for Psychiatric Rehabilitation. (2015). *About the Center for Psychiatric Rehabilitation.* Retrieved from http://cpr.bu.edu/about

Collins, C., Hewson, D., Munger, R., & Wade, T. (2010, May). *Evolving models of behavioral health integration in primary care, Miliband reports.* Retrieved from http://www.milbank.org/reports/10430EvolvingCare/1043EvolvingCare.html

Cruz, A. (2015). *Poor mental health, an obstacle to development in Latin America.* The World Bank. Retrieved from http://www.worldbank.org/en/news/feature/2015/07/13/bad-mental-health-obstacle-development-latin-america

Douglas, E. (2008). Transforming the VA. *Behavioral Healthcare, 28*(7), 4–7.

Guan, L., Liu, J., Wu, X., Chen, D., Wang, X., Ma, N., Wang, Y., Good, B., Ma, H., Yu, X., & Good, M. (2015). Unlocking patients with mental disorders who were in restraints at home: A national follow-up study of China's new public mental health initiatives. *PLOS ONE, 10*(4), 1–14. doi:10.1371/journal.pone.0121425

Hughes, F. (2009). Mental health in the Pacific: The role of the Pacific Island Mental Health Network. *Pacific Health Dialog, 15*(1), 177–180.

Incayawar, M., & Maldonado-Bourchard, S. (2009). The forsaken mental health of the indigenous peoples: A moral case of outrageous exclusion in Latin America. *BMC International Health and Human Rights, 9,* 27.

Kigozi, R. (2011, August). *Mental Health and Poverty: Challenges in Service Delivery in Sub-Saharan Africa.* Presentation at Mbarara University, Uganda. Retrieved from http://www.slideshare.net/jasonharlow/kigozi-mental-health-service-delivery-in-africa

Kaplan, R. L. (2006). HIV/AIDS in the Middle East and North Africa: A brief review of prevention, research, and resources. *Middle East Studies Bulletin, 40*(1), 45–51.

Leonardo da Vinci Pilot Projects. (2007). *WAP vocational training community based mental health nursing.* Retrieved from http://www.bcu.ac.uk/_media/docs/ccmh_wap_report.pdf

Lopez, A. (2005). The evolution of the global burden of disease framework for disease, injury and risk factor quantification: Developing the evidence based for national, regional and global public health action. *Globalization and Health, 1*(5), 1144–1186.

Maramis, A., Nguyen, V., & Minas, H. (2011). Mental health in Southeast Asia. *Lancet, 377*(9767), 700–702.

McNeil, T. (2005–2006, Winter). An offer of hope: A pioneering BU effort bring mental health programs to the developing world. *Bostonian,* 20–25.

Mental Health Commission of Canada. (2009). *Toward Recovery and Well-being: A Framework for a Mental Health Strategy for Canada: Summary.* Retrieved from http://www.mentalhealthcommission.ca/SiteCollectionDocuments/Key_Documents/en/2009/Mental_Health_ENG.pdf

Mental Health Commission of Canada. (2011a). *Annual Report 2010–2011.* Retrieved from http://www.mentalhealthcommission.ca/annualreport/

Mental Health Commission of Canada. (2011b). *Mental Health First Aid Canada.* Retrieved from http://www.mentalhealthfirstaid.ca/EN/about/Pages/default.aspx

Mental Health Commission of Canada. (2011c). *Mental Health in the Workplace.* Retrieved from http://www.mentalhealthcommission.ca/English/Pages/Mentalhealthintheworkplace.aspx

Mojtabai, R. (2011, September 22). National trends in mental health disability, 1997–2009. *American Journal of Public Health First Look.* Retrieved from http://ajph.aphapublications.org/cgi/content/abstract/AJPH.2011.300258v2

Murray, C., & Lopez, A. (2013). Global health: Measuring the global burden of disease. *New England Journal of Medicine, 369*(5), 448–457.

Murray, C., & Lopez, A. (Eds.). (1996). *The Global Burden of Disease: A Comprehensive Assessment of Mortality and Disability from Diseases, Injuries and Risk Facts in 1990 and Projected to 2020.* Cambridge, MA: Harvard University Press on behalf of the World Health Organization and the World Bank.

National Alliance on Mental Illness. (2006). *Grading the states report, 2006.* Retrieved from http://www.nami.org/content/navigationmenu/grading_the_states/project_overview/overview.htm

National Alliance on Mental Illness. (2009). *Grading the states report, 2009.* Retrieved from http://www.nami.org/gtsTemplate09.cfm?Section=Overview1&Template=/ContentManagement/ContentDisplay.cfm&ContentID=75090

National Alliance on Mental Illness. (2011). *Treatment and services.* Retrieved from http://www.nami.org/template.cfm?section=About_Treatments_and_Supports

Nga Kete, Te Arawa, & Whānau Ora. (2014). Whānau Ora = Fitness for life. *Health and Well Being.* Retrieved from http://tearawawhanauora.org.nz/2014/04/whanau-ora-fitness-for-life/

Norris, J. (2011). *UCSF experts aim to provide mental health services in Japan*, University of California San Francisco (UCSF). Retrieved from http://www.ucsf.edu/news/2011/04/9702/ucsf-experts-aim-provide-mental-health-services-japan

Pan American Health Organization. (2005). *Mental disorders in Latin America and the Caribbean forecast to increase* [press release]. Retrieved from http://www.paho.org/English/DD/PIN/pr051209.htm

Pan American Health Organization. (2010). *Annual report of the director of the Pan American Sanitary Bureau: Promoting health, well-being, and human security in the Americas.* Retrieved from http://scm.oas.org/pdfs/2011/PAHO/CP25544E.pdf

Pan American Health Organization. (2013). *WHO-AIMS: Report on mental health systems in Latin America and the Caribbean.* Author. Retrieved from http://www.paho.org/hq/index.php?option=com_docman&task=doc_view&gid=21325&Itemid

Patel, V., Saraceno, B., & Kleinman, A. (2005). Beyond evidence: The moral case for international mental health. *American Journal of Psychiatry, 163,* 1312–1315.

Post, E., & Van Stone, W. (2008). Veterans health administration primary care-mental health integration initiative. *North Carolina Medical Journal, 69*(1), 49–52.

Pumin, Y. (2011). A mental challenge: New law in the works to improve care for mentally ill persons. *Beijing Review.* Retrieved from http://www.bjreview.com.cn/print/txt/2011-09/30/content_395352.htm#

Roberts, M., Mogan, C., & Asare, J. (2014). An overview of Ghana's mental health system: Results from an assessment using the World Health Organization's Assessment Instrument for Mental Health Systems (WHO-AIMS). *International Journal of Mental Health Systems, 8,* 16. doi:10.1186/1752-4458-8-16

Rogers, E., Teague, G., Lichenstein, C., Campbell, J., Lyass, A., Chen, R., & Banks, S. (2007, November 6). Effects of participation in consumer-operated service programs on both personal and organizationally mediated empowerment: Results of a multisite study. *Journal of Rehabilitation Research & Development, 44,* 785–799.

U.S. Department of Health and Human Services. (1999). *Mental health: A report of the Surgeon General. Executive summary*. Retrieved from http://www.surgeongeneral.gov/library/mentalhealth/home.html

U.S. Department of Health and Human Services. (2003). *President's new freedom commission on mental health, 2001*. DHHS Publication No. SMA-03-3832.

Veltman, A., & Chalmowitz, G. (2014). Mental health care for people who identify as lesbian, gay, bisexual, transgender, and (or) queer. *Canadian Journal of Psychiatry, 59*(11), 1–7.

Weaver, M. (2015). *The first annual global peer supporter celebration day*. National Alliance on Mental Illness [NAMI]. Retrieved from https://www.nami.org/Blogs/NAMI-Blog/October-2015/The-First-Annual -Global-Peer-Supporter-Celebration

World Health Organization. (1999). *The World Health Report 1999: Making a Difference*. Geneva, Switzerland: Author.

World Health Organization. (2001a). Burden of mental and behavioural disorders. In *The World Health Report 2001: Mental Health: New Understanding, New Hope* (pp. 1–169). Geneva, Switzerland: Author.

World Health Organization. (2001b). *Mental disorders affect one in four people* [press release]. Geneva, Switzerland: Author.

World Health Organization. (2002a). *Mental health global action programme*. Retrieved from http://www.who .int/mental_health/actionprogramme/en/index.html

World Health Organization. (2002b). *Mental Health Global Action Programme mhGAP: Close the gap, dare to care*. Geneva, Switzerland: Author.

World Health Organization. (2003a). Investing in mental health. Retrieved from http://www.who.int/entity/ mental_health/media/investing_mnh.pdf

World Health Organization. (2007). *Mental Health Improvements for Nations' Development, the Country Summary Series: Ghana, October, 2007*. Geneva, Switzerland: Author.

World Health Organization. (2008a). *mhGAP Mental Health Gap Action Programme: Scaling Up Care for Mental, Neurological, and Substance Use Disorders*. Geneva, Switzerland.

World Health Organization. (2008b). *WHO Mind: Mental Health Improvement for Nations' Development: The Country Summary Series, Chile*. Geneva, Switzerland: Author.

World Health Organization. (2009a). *Europe mental health facts and figures: Prevalence of mental disorders*. Retrieved from http://www.euro.who.int/en/what-we-do/health-topics/noncommunicablediseases/ mentalhealth

World Health Organization. (2009b). Growing mental health services in the Pacific. *NZ Aid*. Retrieved from http://www.who.int/mental_health/policy/pimhnet/NZAid_PIMHnetArticle_3June2009.pdf

World Health Organization. (2009c). Improving health systems and services for mental health. Retrieved from http://whqlibdoc.who.int/publications/2009/9789241598774_eng.pdf

World Health Organization. (2010). *Mental health and development: Targeting people with mental health conditions as a vulnerable group. Mental Health and Poverty Project*. Geneva, Switzerland: Author.

World Health Organization. (2011a, April). *Health Harare: An information bulletin of the SCO Zimbabwe, Vol. 7*.

World Health Organization. (2011b). *Impact of Economic Crises on Mental Health*. Copenhagen, Denmark: Regional Office for Europe.

World Health Organization. (2011c). *Policies and Practices for Mental Health in Europe*. Copenhagen, Denmark: Regional Office for Europe.

World Health Organization. (2013). *Comprehensive mental health action plan 2013–2020*. Author. Retrieved from http://apps.who.int/gb/ebwha/pdf_files/WHA66/A66_R8-en.pdf?ua=1

World Health Organization. (2014a). *Mental Health Atlas Project*. Retrieved from http://www.who.int/ mental_health/evidence/atlasmnh/en/

World Health Organization. (2014b). *China: Improving home care for dementia patients*. Author. Retrieved from: http://www.who.int/features/2014/china-dementia-patients/en/

World Health Organization. (2015a). *World Mental Health Day 2015*. Author. Retrieved from http://www.who .int/mental_health/world-mental-health-day/2015/en/.

World Health Organization. (2015b). *Mental Health Atlas 2014*. Author. Retrieved from http://apps.who.int/iris/bitstream/10665/178879/1/9789241565011_eng.pdf?ua=1

World Psychiatric Association. (2011). *WPA contribution to the management of mental health consequences of major disasters*. Retrieved from http://www.wapnet.org/detail.php?section_id=20&conten_id=1049

Wynaden, D., Chapman, R., Org, A., McGowan, S., Zeeman, Z., & Yeak, S. (2005). Factors that influence Asian communities' access to mental health care. *International Journal of Mental Health Nursing, 14*(2), 88–92.

Footnote

1. This chapter is dedicated to the memory of Dr. Mary Ann Camann, a professor of nursing, psychiatric nurse leader, and book author.

Global Perspectives on Selected Chronic Cardiovascular Diseases

Bowman O. Davis, Jr.

Objectives

After completing this chapter, the reader will be able to:

1. Compare and contrast cardiovascular disease risks, disease screening, and treatments available within developed and developing countries.
2. Discuss metabolic syndrome and its relationship to chronic diseases in both developed and developing countries.
3. Explain why developing countries have a "double burden of disease."

INTRODUCTION

As people of the world saw their calendars roll over to a new millennium, few realized that the 21st century would be greeted differently by different groups of people around the globe. Technologically developed, industrialized countries anxiously awaited the prospect of some undetected Y2K glitches that threatened to corrupt databases on systems ranging from those of major financial institutions to individual home computers and jeopardize cherished financial security or personal convenience. By comparison, individuals in developing nations saw the day as one of continuing poverty and the struggle to acquire adequate nourishment and to survive disease. The dawn of the new millennium revealed a persistent disparity in relative prosperity among the diverse human populations of the world. Converted to U.S. dollars, people of developed nations averaged approximately 18 times the per capita gross domestic product (GDP) of their developing nation counterparts (World Health Organization [WHO], 1996).

In this age of global economic trade and global communication, the rapid spread of technology has not had equitable impact on everyone. Not only has there not been equitable sharing of technological advances and socioeconomic prosperity, but the assumption that all technological advances are good is subject to serious debate. Close examination reveals both positive and negative influences of technological advances. Paradoxically, as developed nations export beneficial advances in technology, including health care, they also export popular culture and lifestyles, such as alcohol and tobacco use, stressful work environments, sedentary lifestyles, and calorie-dense diets high in salt, sugar, and saturated fat, that can have negative effects on the health of persons influenced by these trends. Disease burdens around the world often reflect this paradox. Developing nations struggle under the burden of infectious and communicable diseases, while socioeconomically developed nations see their disease burden shift toward one involving chronic and noncommunicable diseases. This shift is primarily because infant mortality decreases as a country's economic development accelerates, allowing life expectancy at birth to increase sufficiently for chronic diseases to become prevalent. From the most developed nation to the least, the gap in average life expectancy can be as much as 37 years. Unfortunately, the path from developing to developed status leads through a transitional phase during which the disease burden on the population may be dual in nature, such that both infectious and chronic diseases have nearly equal mortality impact.

Accurately assessing the disease burden among populations around the world is a daunting task complicated by factors such as the need to account for migratory segments of the population, inaccurate diagnoses of medical conditions, and inconsistent reporting and recording of disease incidences and causes of death. Within these constraints, the United Nations' WHO agency collects and publishes in its annual World Health Report a yearly compilation of causes of death among its member states around the world. The availability of this comprehensive database reveals emerging trends in disease burdens and allows for analyses of health needs and of the effectiveness of healthcare measures, as well as for the redirection and prioritization of healthcare efforts and resources.

Specific methods are used to measure and characterize the overall health status of a given population, and specific terminology is used to reference these data. For example, prevalence of a given disease is the total number of cases, both previously existing and newly diagnosed, present within a population at any given time, whereas incidence or morbidity refers to the number of new cases of a given disease reported each year. The mortality rate reflects the actual deaths due to a specific, identifiable cause. For this discussion of chronic diseases, mortality rate is used as the index of disease burden within a population.

DEMOGRAPHIC AND SOCIOECONOMIC TRANSITION

Biologists often represent the developmental status of a population by means of graphic "age pyramids," as shown in Figure 8-1. Growing populations have fertility rates greater than basic replacement levels (more than two offspring per female of reproductive age) and exhibit a typical upright pyramid with the number of individuals declining, primarily due to mortality, as they move vertically through the various age groups. Populations with fertility

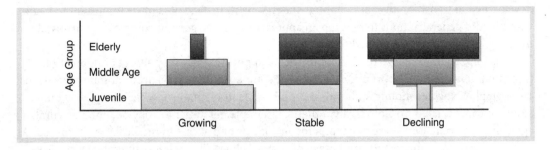

FIGURE 8-1 Population Age Structures

rates approaching replacement level show a loss of the pyramid shape as stability is reached. If fertility rates drop below replacement levels, the age structure pyramid becomes inverted as the population moves into decline. Human populations fit this model very closely, but to consider only age structure would give an incomplete picture with no insight into the other aspects of population dynamics that might be causing the growth, decline, or stability.

WHO groups its member states by geographic regions and mortality strata to give a more complete picture of population status. Mortality strata range from A, which is characterized by very low child mortality and very low adult mortality, to E, where child mortality is high and adult mortality is very high. Based on these criteria, a majority of United Nations member states fall into the "developing" category with comparatively few having attained "developed" status.

Although causes of death due to disease can be conveniently reduced to either infectious or chronic disease categories, the demographic and socioeconomic contexts within which these deaths occur are not as simply described. Demographically, a population can be described by certain characteristics such as age composition, immigration and emigration rates, fertility rate, life expectancy at birth, death rate, and so on. Although these properties are generally objective and quantifiable, they convey little about the actual lifestyles experienced by members of the population. Socioeconomic aspects of a population, such as per capita GDP, literacy rate, percent urbanization, and so on, give a better picture of the overall quality of life within the population. Interestingly, as populations transition from developing toward developed status, they undergo changes in both demographic and socioeconomic aspects that can be generally reflective of their stage of development and its characteristic causes of death.

It is important to emphasize the "generally reflective" descriptor here to avoid the pitfall of imposing stereotypic benchmarks on the progress of a population through its development. In reality, populations do undergo demographic and socioeconomic changes as they progress, but rather the characteristics of this developmental process are inevitably directed by geographical, political, cultural, and religious influences present within the population. Because these influences can be dramatically different from one population to another, each developing nation experiences this process within its own unique set of circumstances. Therefore, each nation must be considered individually if a truly accurate assessment of its developmental progress is desired. It is not the purpose of this discussion to analyze in detail every aspect influencing this developmental transition in every country undergoing it. Instead, it is more important to begin with broader generalizations to develop an appreciation of the general complexities involved in the progression toward developed status.

It is important to realize the lack of universal application of every aspect of population transition. It is equally important to realize that complex interactions occur among the various demographic, socioeconomic, cultural, and political factors, many of which are poorly understood and appreciated. In a purely hypothetical example, fertility rate may be high in a rural, agricultural population where per capita income is low and access to medical care is limited. As a result, infant mortality is high and life expectancy is low. The high fertility rate is a positive factor in this population, where large families are essential to maintain an agrarian lifestyle. In contrast, a high fertility rate in a different population might be a negative factor because it might increase child dependency stress on constituent families. Because literacy is of little perceived value in this hypothetical population, literacy rates are low. Thus, preventive healthcare measures are difficult to communicate, and resultant communicable disease avoidance is also low. Such a population would be vulnerable to infectious diseases, circuitously making high fertility even more advantageous to offset disease losses. Cultural and religious factors can figure into the equation if they permit promiscuity, impose restrictions on family planning practices, or reinforce gender preferences of offspring. Such practices could keep family size large but enforce inequitable distribution of family resources to one gender. At the same time there may be increased risk of spreading infectious sexually transmitted diseases within and among family units.

Typically, high fertility and mortality combined with low income and literacy rates are characteristic of developing states. Nevertheless, such a characterization does not address the population's stability. In fact, the population may be quite stable and in equilibrium with its geographic, demographic, cultural, and socioeconomic environment. The question then becomes one of humanitarian concern—namely, whether to intervene in an attempt to raise the standard of living of individuals at the potential risk of disturbing the population's equilibrium. Although the preceding example is purely hypothetical, it clearly illustrates that there can be no universal set of standards for assessing population development if the unique circumstances within which that group is developing are not considered as well. With those precautionary notes emphasized, the following characterization of population transition identifies major transitional phases. It also describes some of their demographic and socioeconomic characteristics, with the understanding that they may not be universally applicable.

By applying the phases of demographic transition described by Lee and Cyrus Chu (2000) as a basic framework and adding certain socioeconomic factors as appropriate, it is possible to generate a more descriptive model of population development within which the causes of death can be examined more specifically.

Beginning with a hypothetical, undeveloped population, the people are often widely dispersed in individual family units across a basically rural environment. With the primary livelihood being agriculture, the labor force is small and per capita income is low. Financial savings are virtually nonexistent because any family income is devoted to living essentials. Families often reside in primitive, unsanitary living conditions and are exposed to contaminated indoor air from fuels used for heating and cooking. Clean water for drinking and food storage capability may be inadequate, as investment in infrastructure is minimal. Fertility rate is high but perinatal health care is substandard for both mothers and their children, leading to an increased child mortality rate. Fertility rate may also be affected by the cultural preference for large families and the benefit of having large families to share the agricultural workload. Literacy levels are low, because literacy has little perceived value in this agrarian lifestyle. The status of women in the population is often low, as women have little incentive to improve either their literacy or their participation in the workforce. The combination of primitive living conditions, poor sanitation, illiteracy, and limited access to health care increases the prevalence of infectious diseases and results in a low life expectancy at birth because both child and adult mortality rates are high. With high fertility rates helping to offset the high mortality rates, the population may be transiently stable. At the same time, it is extremely vulnerable to environmental disasters such as drought or infectious disease epidemics that could tip the delicate balance toward decline.

Phase One Transition: Reducing Child Mortality

The first phase of transition usually begins with a decline in child mortality. This decline may be the result of internal healthcare measures within the population structure or attributable to external humanitarian efforts. Many developed nations export medical technology such as vaccination programs in an effort to reduce child mortality on a global basis. A decline in child mortality increases the proportion of children in a developing country's population and raises the child dependency stress on individual family units and on the population as a whole. This increased dependency stress can result in continued low per capita income with all of its consequences, including continued low expenditure on healthcare practice and infrastructure. With minimal healthcare access and continued low literacy rates, infectious diseases remain the primary cause of death among adults as life expectancy remains low. The rural, agrarian lifestyle persists, and the unsanitary living conditions and female status within the population show little change.

Phase Two Transition: Fertility Decline

In the second phase of transition, the most distinguishing feature is the beginning of a decline in fertility. A number of factors may influence this trend (Poston, 2000), and it may take two or three generations, or approximately 50 years, to go to completion. Completion is considered to be the attainment of a replacement level of about two children per reproductive female. For example, the People's Republic of China and Taiwan serve as examples of how socioeconomic and political factors can curtail fertility rate. In 1950, both China and Taiwan had fertility rates of approximately six children per reproductive female. By 1995, both countries' fertility levels had declined to fewer than two children per reproductive female. However, Taiwan's fertility decline resulted from voluntary reductions in family size as a possible result of socioeconomic development, whereas the decline in China reflected the combination of socioeconomic development and government intervention in family planning (Poston, 2000).

Socioeconomically speaking, as livelihood gradually shifts from an agricultural base to one of an industrial or service labor force, large family size is no longer an asset and, indeed, can be a liability. Under these conditions, adequate food can no longer be grown to feed a large family and most living essentials must now be purchased. To be competitive in the new work environment, literacy is of greater value than large family size. Literacy rate and educational level negatively correlate with fertility rate especially when the educational level of females is considered. Additionally, female value within the population may trend upward as more women move into the workforce, which can also negatively impact fertility rate. During this phase, the labor force grows rapidly and boosts the per capita income, assuming the economy grows sufficiently to provide jobs for the growing workforce. Because a workforce tends to locate close to a work source, migration from rural to urban environments may be evident. Urbanization of the population has a positive impact by increasing access to both education and health care and a negative impact on fertility as literacy improves. However, the shift from the physical labor of agriculture to the more stressful structured work environment can increase the mental stress on working adults. As actual work becomes more structured and less physically demanding, leisure time also increases and more sedentary lifestyles may become the norm.

Total dependency stress is low in this phase of transition, as the generally healthy, middle-aged segment of the population predominates with very few dependent children and few dependent elderly members. With low dependency stress, financial savings may increase along with consumption as labor becomes more lucrative and the overall standard of living increases. Unfortunately, exposure to popular cultural promotions also increases as businesses perceive the population with its improving standard of living as a potential market for goods and services, some of which may be accompanied by behavioral practices and lifestyles that may not be conducive to good health. The glamorization of alcohol, tobacco, and drug use have negative impacts on health and longevity, as does ready access to prepared foods that are dense in calories and high in salt, sugar, and fats; the convenience of these foods may encourage the population to substitute these widely available options for healthy diets. The resulting dietary changes can increase the prevalence of obesity within a population whose members are following an increasingly sedentary lifestyle. Such lifestyle practices can exacerbate existing risk factors for chronic diseases, especially those of a cardiovascular nature. Thus the mortality rates resulting from these chronic diseases increase at about the same time as, or even before, infectious diseases have been adequately controlled. In this case, socioeconomic improvement may simply change the nature of a population's overall disease burden instead of reducing it.

With increased per capita income, expenditure on healthcare services and infrastructure is now an affordable option. Easier access to improved health care further reduces mortality rates from infectious diseases and increases life expectancy. As life expectancy increases, individuals now live long enough to develop chronic diseases, especially if unhealthy lifestyles have become the cultural norm. In fact, the population may pass through a time period where infectious and chronic diseases have a dual impact on mortality rates. Eventually, the population may progress beyond the dual disease burden stage toward one where chronic diseases predominate as the major cause of death.

Figure 8-2 shows a global perspective of the causes of death worldwide (WHO, 2009). Examination of these data shows a shift away from an infectious disease burden and toward one characterized by chronic diseases as the mortality stratum trends from E (high child, very

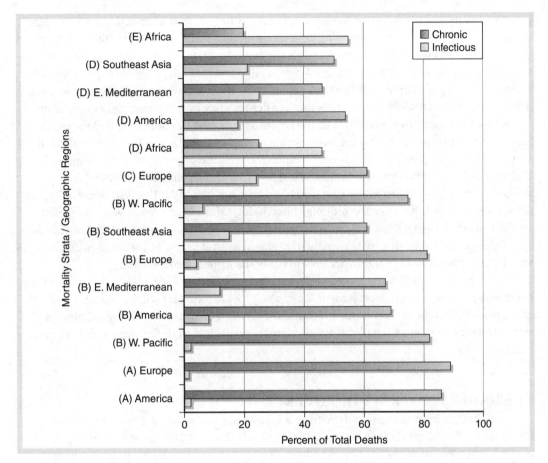

FIGURE 8-2 Comparison of Deaths Due to Infectious Versus Chronic Diseases by UN/WHO Mortality Strata and Geographic Regions for the Year 2000
Data from World Health Organization (WHO). (2001). *World Health Report 2001. Mental Health, New Understanding, New Hope.* Geneva, Switzerland: Author.

high adult) to A (very low child, very low adult). Interestingly, the D mortality stratum of the geographic regions of Southeast Asia, Eastern Mediterranean, South America, and Eastern Europe shows a significant dual disease burden. Also important is the recognition that chronic diseases now account for more deaths worldwide than infectious diseases. This point is both a testament to the effectiveness of infectious disease eradication measures and an indication of the need to direct more effort toward the emerging chronic disease problem.

Phase Three Transition: Increasing Age Dependency
To appreciate the final phase of population development, selected aspects of the second phase must be considered as contributing to the major characteristic of third-phase development— namely, emerging age dependency. Increased life expectancy combined with the declining

infant mortality and the shift to a more gender-diverse, urban labor force generates a comparatively large "balloon" of persons moving both into the labor force and into the older age strata of the population. As this ballooned middle-aged population stratum grows older, age dependency stress on the population increases. Interestingly, as this aging occurs, the total dependency stress increases on the population until the total dependency stress is now similar to that experienced during phase one. The only difference is that age dependency now replaces child dependency.

Age is a primary, irreversible risk factor for chronic disease development, and the prevalence of these diseases inevitably increases within any aging population. The extent to which they increase in prevalence depends on the number of risk factors occurring simultaneously. Unfortunately, a past history of substance abuse, tobacco and alcohol use, sedentary lifestyle, and unhealthy diet serves to exacerbate the chronic disease burden of the susceptible aging population segment. Additionally, the prolonged psychological stress of urban living and genetic predisposition, should it exist, can be contributing factors to the rise in chronic disease burden. This increase in chronic disease is particularly evident as an increase in cardiovascular disorders with ischemic heart disease and hypertension being the general manifestations.

Up to this point, hypothetical situations have been used to provide a basic awareness of the complexities of population development. They also provide a context within which to assess the importance of chronic disease burdens around the world. The next step in a logical progression is to examine in more detail the major contributing factors to this emerging global chronic disease burden.

THE UNDERLYING ROLE OF POVERTY

Although people around the world die from a variety of causes, ranging from accidental deaths and political conflicts to infectious and chronic diseases, the age at which they die is somewhat more predictable. The old adage, "The rich die old while the poor die young," appears to have a factual basis. Nations with higher per capita GDPs also have longer life expectancies. This relationship should come as no surprise, given that a higher GDP leads to greater expenditure on healthcare infrastructure and greater individual access to health care. The impact of literacy can be seen across the entire age spectrum. Infant mortality is negatively correlated with literacy level for the obvious reasons that literate parents are more likely to be aware of disease prevention measures and to have the necessary personal income to access and practice them. For example, the WHO's Global Immunization Program, begun in 1974, helped to eradicate smallpox and increase the level of child immunization globally from 5 to 80% by 1995 (WHO, 1997). Although the reduction of childhood diseases was significant by the end of the last century, efforts to achieve these goals were least effective in underdeveloped countries. This lack of child immunization combined with substandard or total absence of adequate peripartal care drives the child mortality rates high and drives life expectancy at birth low in developing nations.

In the middle and elderly age strata, the role of literacy is more individual in nature, as these age groups are less directly dependent on care from others to protect them from diseases and unhealthy practices. Their receptivity to publicly communicated health warnings and their vulnerability to unhealthy cultural and lifestyle practices depend in part on their literacy level and the ease with which sound health practices can be communicated to them.

The WHO World Health Report (1995) devoted much of its narrative to the role of poverty in global mortality rates. In 1990, it was estimated that 20% of the world's human population lived in poverty. This estimate was accompanied by an observed 37-year gap in life expectancy between richer and poorer nations.

Poverty affects longevity and subjects people to disease in a variety of ways: It destines people to drink unclean water and to live in unsanitary conditions; it forces people to breathe air polluted by industrial emissions as well as unclean fuels used for home heating and cooking; and it can be a contributing factor to mental stress, family unit disintegration, and substance abuse. More importantly, it excludes people from the educational process, thereby depriving them of the essential knowledge needed to prevent diseases that could be avoided by lifestyle changes. This educational deficiency leaves vulnerable populations with only cultural or religious practices for protection, which very often may not be adequate.

It is easy to make an erroneous leap in generalization by assuming that wealthier, developed nations are devoid of poverty. Conversely, a variant impact of poverty can be seen to be the result of industrialization. A developing industrial economy can entice people to migrate from rural to urban environments in search of higher incomes and better lifestyles. Their lack of adequate marketable skills or periods of economic depression, however, may then leave them stranded in isolated pockets of poverty within the urban environment. Similarly, it is a mistake to assume that everyone within a population will "catch the wave" of industrialization and be swept equally toward personal financial improvement. As the United States underwent industrialization during the 1800s and 1900s, some people in rural environments were not included in the transition. Although many migrated to the industrialized urban environments, others remained behind—for example, those subpopulations in pockets of central Appalachia. In this geographic area, poverty rates approach 35% compared to the U.S. national rate of 14% (Phipps, 2006). Regardless of the circumstances that produced them, these pockets of poverty are not unique to either a rural or an urban environment; indeed, they can be seen in both. Unfortunately, the people living in them, as with those in underdeveloped nations, may be subject to a dual threat from both infectious and chronic diseases.

THE CHRONIC DISEASE BURDEN

Increasing life expectancy of a population has both positive and negative effects on disease burden. Clearly, reducing child mortality and controlling infectious diseases to enable a longer life expectancy is, without doubt, a positive aspect. Nevertheless, if a longer life expectancy increases the risk of developing chronic diseases, the population's disease burden is not eliminated but rather just changed in character. Life expectancy at birth for the total world population is 67.07 years. For males, it is 65.21 years; for females, 69.05 years (2011 est.) (Infoplease, 2011). Developed nations with greater average life expectancies, however, present a different mortality profile. As individuals within a population survive to adulthood and live longer, chronic diseases, which can be age dependent, emerge and prevail as the major cause of deaths.

Chronic diseases can occur with any organ system, but typically include a variety of malignancies, as well as respiratory, cardiovascular, renal, and neuropsychiatric disorders. In recognition of the fact that renal and neuropsychiatric diseases combined account for only about 3% of
the total deaths during any one year, the major emphasis here will be on cardiovascular diseases.
Figure 8-3 illustrates the prevalence of these chronic diseases and their effects on mortality data
for the decade between 1993 and 2003.

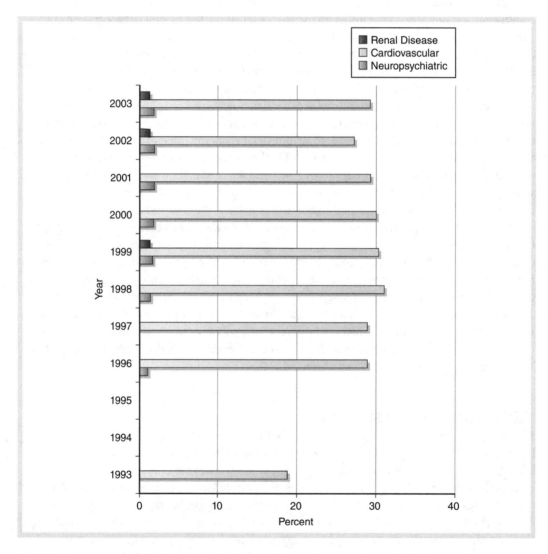

FIGURE 8-3 Percentage of Total Deaths Due to Selected Chronic Diseases Among WHO Member States
Data from WHO World Health Reports, 1995, 1996, 1997, 1998, 1999, 2000, 2001, 2002, 2003, 2004.

Cardiovascular diseases far outweigh the distant second (neuropsychiatric) and third (renal disease) causes of death. Interestingly, when available data were plotted, cardiovascular diseases could be seen to increase until the middle 1990s, then remained high but relatively stable through the remainder of the observation period. During the same time interval, renal disease remained low in prevalence and unchanging while neuropsychiatric disorders, although low in prevalence compared to cardiovascular disease, almost doubled in prevalence from 1996 to 2003. Although this point is somewhat speculative, the prevalence of neuropsychiatric disorders may prove to be an index of societal stress experienced by a population.

The Cardiovascular Disease Burden

Cardiovascular disease (CVD) is a broad category of generally chronic diseases affecting the heart and blood vessels. This category includes conditions ranging from pericardial disorders, to heart valve and rhythm abnormalities, to elevated blood pressure values, to inflammatory disease states affecting the walls of arteries. From a global health perspective, detailed and specific diagnoses are not readily available, but generalized mortality data are available. Such data are collected by the WHO and grouped categorically into ischemic heart disease (diminished blood supply to the myocardium), cerebrovascular disease (cerebrovascular accident [CVA], stroke), and rheumatic heart disease. Synonyms for ischemic heart disease are commonly used within medical literature and require notation here to avoid confusion. These synonyms are coronary heart disease (CHD or coronary artery disease) and atherosclerotic coronary heart disease (ACHD). Data pertaining to the prevalence of these three major cardiovascular disorders are summarized in Figure 8-4 for the decade ending in 2003.

A cursory examination of the data reveals that ischemic heart disease and cerebrovascular strokes far exceed the prevalence of rheumatic heart disease, and their combined percentages accounted for about 25% of the total annual deaths worldwide by the end of the 1900s. Rheumatic heart disease is an acute inflammatory disorder that follows a group A streptococcal (GAS) infection of the throat in 3 to 5% of these pharyngitis cases. During the acute inflammatory phase of the disease (rheumatic fever), valve leaflets of the heart become inflamed and thicken from scar tissue formation. The diseased valves do not close properly, leading to regurgitation (murmur) with the danger of congestive failure and death (Howson, Reddy, Ryan, & Bale, 1998; Porth, 2005). Rheumatic heart disease is epidemiologically interesting because it is a chronic disease caused by an infectious microorganism that can be successfully treated with antibiotics when and where they are available. In developed industrialized countries with access to antibiotic therapy, the prevalence of rheumatic heart disease dramatically declined in the last half of the 20th century. Although it ranked a distant third to ischemic heart disease and CVA globally, this condition was still responsible for 500,000 deaths worldwide in 1998 (WHO, 1998). Rheumatic heart disease can be part of the dual disease burden of developing nations where access to antibiotic therapy may be limited.

It is not just the prevalence of rheumatic heart disease that differs globally when the epidemiology of cardiovascular disease is examined. In fact, the mortality profile of major cardiovascular diseases differs with the particular country and its developmental status. In developed

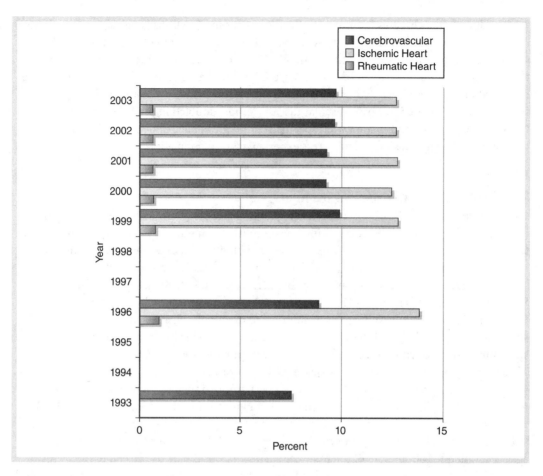

FIGURE 8-4 Percentage of Total Deaths Due to Selected Cardiovascular Diseases Among UN/WHO
Member States
Data from WHO World Health Reports, 1995, 1996, 1997, 1998, 1999, 2000, 2001, 2002, 2003, 2004.

nations, CVD is the major cause of death within the populations, but the specific ranking of
individual types of CVD shows atherosclerosis and hypertension to be the most prevalent. In
developing states, CVD can be a part of the dual disease burden along with high mortality rates
from a variety of infectious diseases. For example, rheumatic heart disease is the most prevalent
CVD in Asia, but hypertension and related ischemic heart diseases are more ubiquitous in the
Americas, in the Caribbean, and in more urbanized areas of Africa (Akinkugbe, 1990). This
trend suggests that urbanization or the exposure to Western lifestyles may correlate positively
with the prevalence of ischemic heart disease and cerebrovascular strokes.

Akinkugbe (1990) provided more supportive evidence of this trend. It has long been
observed that blood pressure tends to rise with age in human populations. However, this

age-dependent hypertension trend is not seen in developing populations of Africa that are isolated from Western influence and show relative freedom from known CVD risk factors. Among the examples cited for future study were the pygmies of northeastern Zaire, the bushmen of Botswana, and the Koma people of northeastern Nigeria. Additionally, a study of Kenyans showed a rise in blood pressure with migration into more urbanized areas of the country. Apparently, improvement in socioeconomic status along with exposure to Western lifestyle can yield a population within which the chronic disease profiles reflect an increased probability of developing cardiovascular disease.

Cardiovascular Disease Risk Factors

Factors that increase the risk of developing chronic cardiovascular disease may be demographic (age and gender), behavioral (lifestyle patterns), or genetic (familial). The presence of any given risk factor is considered to increase the likelihood of developing CVD, and the concurrence of multiple risk factors seriously compound this probability.

Chronological Age

Age, along with gender and familial inheritance, make up the irreversible risk factors predisposing individuals to develop CVD. Because CVDs are classed as chronic diseases, it is logical to expect them to increase in prevalence in the older age strata of a population. In fact, males who are older than 45 years of age are at increased risk, as are women who are older than 55 or who have undergone premature menopause without exogenous estrogen (estradiol) replacement therapy (Porth, 2005). The gender differences in age susceptibility are poorly understood but may involve dietary and/or hormonal differences. For example, testosterone in males can mobilize body lipid reserves and increase blood lipid levels, while estrogen seems to protect against early onset of CVD and increase body fat stores. Female fertility depends in part on adequate body fat stores, and the proportion of body fat to lean muscle mass increases in both sexes with advancing age.

Regardless of the underlying physiological mechanisms, phases two and three of population transition are characterized, in part, by increased life expectancy. This factor alone predisposes individuals to increased risk of CVD, as individuals may now be living long enough to develop these chronic diseases. However, many transitional populations also develop unhealthy lifestyles, which expose them to multiple other risk factors in addition to simple aging.

Genetic Predisposition and Hyperlipidemia

Because lipids, including cholesterol and triglycerides, are insoluble in the water of blood plasma, they must be transported in minute chylomicron forms and in combination with water-soluble proteins as blood lipoproteins. These blood lipoproteins include the common low-density lipoproteins (LDLs), which are high in fat and cholesterol components, and the beneficial high-density lipoproteins (HDLs), which are high in protein including the cholesterol-destroying enzyme, cholesterol esterase. Additionally, a typical blood lipid profile includes metabolic intermediates such as very-low-density lipoproteins (VLDLs) and intermediate-density lipoproteins (IDLs), which are also controlled through metabolic activity of the liver. The processing of these lipid fractions involves metabolic pathways with enzymes or receptors that are produced by inherited genes of the human genome (Porth, 2005). Consequently, familial inheritance of hyperlipoproteinemia patterns constitutes a major irreversible risk factor for CVD.

Although familial inheritance is irreversible, unhealthy lipid profiles can often be controlled by medication. Yet, because of the cost of these medications, many developing populations do not have this option. Genetic predisposition is often compounded in its risk severity by dietary intake of saturated fats, trans fats, and cholesterol. These compounding factors are reversible with education regarding sound dietary practices. Again, developing populations may not have high literacy levels or may not have access to this dietary information. Making matters worse are the existence of cultural dietary preferences and societal pressures to resort to convenience foods, which may exacerbate the lipid problem. Regardless of whether the high-risk blood lipid profile is caused by genetics or behavior, such a condition can predispose individuals to develop CVD, especially atherosclerosis.

Atherosclerosis is a type of arteriosclerosis, or "hardening of the arteries." Some arterial hardening is a normal consequence of aging. More ominously, the often premature hardening due to atheromatous, fibrofatty, inflammatory lesions developing within and beneath the inner intimal layer of arteries leads to an acceleration of the sclerotization process. This inflammatory, atheromatous reaction in arteries can weaken the artery wall while occluding the vessel lumen and providing a site for platelet aggregation. Because atherosclerosis commonly affects the aorta, arteries of coronary circulation, and the arterial supply to the brain, it can result in aneurysms as well as thromboembolic ischemic events leading to angina pectoris, myocardial infarction, transient ischemic attacks (TIA), or more serious CVAs.

Clearly, genetic predisposition and/or diets rich in saturated fats and cholesterol can lead to a variety of cardiovascular and cerebrovascular disorders. The current trend for developing populations to adopt Western lifestyles—that is, lifestyles characterized by stressful, sedentary jobs and diets consisting mainly of convenience foods that are calorie rich and contain high salt, fat, and sugar content—acts to exacerbate any genetic predisposition to develop CVD. Unfortunately, unhealthy lifestyles can act independently to increase the risk for CVD in individuals without an inherited risk.

Hypertension

Hypertension can be defined as a persistent increase in systolic and diastolic arterial pressures, and the condition can present as either essential or secondary elevation in blood pressure. Secondary hypertension results from some concurrent pathophysiological condition and is commonly seen in renal disease as a consequence of fluid and salt retention with resultant blood volume expansion. In contrast, essential hypertension is a chronic elevation of blood pressure, either systolic or diastolic, above 140/90 mm Hg with no identifiable secondary cause. The actual causes of essential hypertension are unknown, but a number of risk factors, such as age, sodium retention, and anxiety, have been identified and correlated with the condition. Mood and anxiety disorders are more prevalent in city dwellers, and urban stress has been shown to increase activity in brain regions associated with social stress processing (Lederbogen et al., 2011). In contrast, sporadic anxiety episodes seem to cause acute hypertensive events but have not been convincingly correlated with chronic hypertension (Porth, 2005).

Blood pressure is known to increase with age, rising from an average of 50/40 mm Hg at birth to about 120/80 mm Hg by adolescence (Porth, 2005). Systolic pressure continues to increase slowly throughout life, ultimately increasing the risk of cerebrovascular stroke in later life as high pulse pressure (systolic minus diastolic) stresses aging arteries. Because this phenomenon is not seen in isolated African populations distantly removed from Western influence, it is speculated that lifestyle changes during population transition may be a contributing factor to its emergence. People of African descent in developing or developed populations tend to show hypertension earlier in life, and they are statistically more susceptible to cardiovascular and renal damage compared to Caucasians. This observation is not completely understood and may have a genetic component. People of African descent do not respond readily to increased dietary sodium with an increased renal salt excretion (Porth, 2005). This tendency to retain salt may have had evolutionary survival value in a hot, sodium-deficient environment but can have negative survival value in an environment with excessive dietary salt availability, such as exists with the convenience diets of many developed and some developing nations.

Nicholas, Agodoa, and Norris (2004) reported very little difference in prevalence of early-stage chronic kidney disease (CKD) among Caucasian, Hispanic, and African people in the United States. However, people of African descent were twice as likely as Hispanics and four times more likely than Caucasians to progress to end-stage renal disease (ESRD). This racial/ethnic disparity in disease prevalence may reflect low levels of educational experience, income, and access to health care. Any or all of these factors could contribute to the observed high rates of prerenal disorders, such as hypertension and diabetes, in these minorities. These risk factors for ESRD can be controlled if detected and treated early, but both actions require educational awareness and adequate income to ensure healthcare access.

Additionally, it is not uncommon to see several risk factors for hypertension occurring in the same individual. An example of this phenomenon, the *insulin resistance syndrome* (metabolic syndrome), is a situation in which a cluster of risk factors occurs simultaneously in one individual (Porth, 2005). For example, obesity, particularly abdominal fat accumulation, and type 2 diabetes (non-insulin-dependent diabetes mellitus [NIDDM]) leads to hyperinsulinemia due to insulin insensitivity, or insulin resistance, in body cells. This elevated insulin level results in an increase in sympathetic nervous system activity, which in turn leads to an elevated heart rate and increased vasoconstriction. Because both cardiac output and peripheral resistance are increased simultaneously, blood pressure increases accordingly with hyperinsulinemia.

Dietary salt intake can affect blood pressure as well. High-sodium diets can expand blood volume through fluid retention and increase blood pressure. Because high-salt diets are usually high in either sodium or potassium, but rarely both, a high-sodium diet would likely be low in potassium. Low potassium can increase blood pressure, possibly by suppression of the renin–angiotensin–aldosterone (RAA) mechanism (Porth, 2005).

Regardless of its causative factors, chronic hypertension is extremely dangerous for the simple reason that it is often asymptomatic and can exist for years undetected in persons who do not receive regular medical exams. Uncorrected elevated arterial blood pressure has negative effects on retinal, cardiac, cerebral, and renal blood vessels, as well as a direct effect on heart workload. Specifically, high blood pressure distends flexible vessel walls, creating small lesions that predispose the individual to development of aneurysms and atheromatous plaque. Simultaneously, high systemic arterial pressure increases the workload (afterload) on the left ventricle, leading to hypertrophy and, ultimately, ischemic heart disease. Myocardial ischemia evolves gradually as the enlarged muscle mass increases in its metabolic requirements for blood oxygen and nutrient delivery beyond that which the partially occluded vessels can provide. However, a sudden cardiac ischemic event (infarction) can occur should an embolus originating from an atheromatous artery totally block a smaller arterial branch of coronary circulation.

Finally, the increased renal perfusion as a result of elevated arterial blood pressure causes a concomitant increase in glomerular filtration. Chronically elevated glomerular filtration leads to an inflammatory thickening of the glomerular membrane and subsequent renal dysfunction or failure. Failing kidneys can expand blood volume by fluid retention and constrict arteries via activation of the RAA mechanism, both of which would increase pressure further and produce an unfavorable positive feedback situation leading to more progressive damage. Unfortunately, the large renal reserve in the human requires approximately 75% loss of the total renal capacity before symptoms appear. Consequently, both hypertension and its associated renal damage can progress unnoticed until serious damage is done.

It is not difficult to see how a transitioning population, which is experiencing a changing lifestyle with longer life expectancy, would be susceptible to marketing of convenience foods and might value a more leisurely life with a sedentary type of employment. Should these lifestyle modifications be accorded a high value in the changing culture, it is easy to understand the observed high levels of CVD and CVA in populations as they progress through the phases of this demographic transition.

Obesity

Obesity has become a major public health problem of global significance, with its prevalence increasing in countries around the world regardless of their developmental status. The fact that obesity is currently responsible for twice as many deaths as malnutrition worldwide is not surprising given that the global food supply has generally increased as a result of enhanced productivity and distribution.

By definition, obesity results when excess fat accumulates in adipose cells to the extent of endangering the individual's health. It is easier to define obesity than it is to quantify it, however. More specifically, at what point does energy storage as body fat cease to be an advantage and become detrimental to health, given that there are cultural, racial, and gender differences that influence the perception of the ideal body type? In some cultures, excess body fat is viewed as an index of good health or prosperity. Strauss and Duncan (1998) found that even in the United States, earned wages increased with body mass up to a peak within the normal body mass index (BMI) range and then declined as the BMI range approached obesity. In terms of racial characteristics, populations in colder climates, for example, tend to be shorter in stature with greater amounts of body fat serving physiologically for heat energy conservation. Likewise, the human female tends to have a higher proportion of subcutaneous fat; because of its role in body contouring, this aspect of anatomy can be considered a secondary sex characteristic. Physiologically, female fertility depends on the presence of a certain amount of body fat, which may possibly be an adaptive mechanism ensuring that the mother's nutritional status is adequate to support dependent children. In the United States, minority females of African and Hispanic descent show a greater prevalence of obesity than do Caucasians (Porth, 2005). This observation suggests roles of genetics and socioeconomic status in the prevalence of obesity. Obesity is known to run in families, which indicates a genetic component of the disorder. Additionally, the diets consumed by lower-income individuals are often more dense in caloric content, which serves to increase the risk of obesity in persons in the lower socioeconomic strata. Thus, when people genetically predisposed to obesity occur in lower socioeconomic strata, the risk of developing obesity is compounded.

In light of these complicating factors, WHO has attempted to quantify obesity by means of the BMI, which is calculated by dividing an individual's weight in kilograms by his or her height in meters squared; the resulting ratio value is considered reflective of obesity level. By this standard, BMIs between 18.5 and 24.9 are considered normal, while values greater than 30 represent obesity (WHO, 1998). However, caution must be exercised when applying these standards across racial and ethnic lines, as the relationship between BMI and actual body fat varies with body build and may require adjustment for these variables. For instance, Americans of African and Polynesian descent have higher average BMIs, while Asians and Indonesians tend toward lower BMIs than Caucasians (Deurenberg, Yap, & van Staveren, 1998). Moreover, it is important to realize that central fat (abdominal or upper-torso fat) is more indicative of health risk than is subcutaneous fat. This realization has led to the use of waist circumference or waist/hip circumference ratio as a measure of unhealthy obesity levels. These alternative indices correlate more closely with increased risk for CVD, such that waist circumferences greater than 102 cm (40.2 in.) for men and 88 cm (34.6 in.) for women are associated with substantially increased risk of obesity-related metabolic complications. From a health perspective, the risk of premature death more than doubles in a population when the mean BMI increases from 25 to 35 (Antipatis & Gill, 2001).

The primary reason for the effect of obesity on premature death involves the negative impact of excessive central fat on workload of the heart and on organ perfusion in general. Obese individuals with excessive central fat deposits are at greater risk of type 2 diabetes mellitus and hypertension leading to premature ischemic heart disease. It has been estimated that 2–3 mL of blood per minute is required to perfuse every 100 g of adipose tissue. This increased workload can lead to myocardial hypertrophy and increased heart muscle metabolism. Yet, the required increased blood supply through coronary circulation to support this increased metabolism may be impaired by premature atherosclerosis resulting from chronic hypertension, type 2 diabetes mellitus, and hyperlipidemia. This medley of pathophysiological disorders, referred to as metabolic syndrome, is generally more prevalent in obese individuals. Additionally, general inflammation, as indicated by C-reactive protein (CRP) levels, is elevated with central obesity while platelet aggregation is enhanced, contributing further to vascular damage and increased risk of thrombotic events in obese individuals. CRP level has become a useful indicator of systemic inflammation and risk of myocardial infarction and can be assessed by simple blood tests. In fact, the American Heart Association has established indices of CRP levels that correlate with risk levels (less than 1 mg/L = low risk, 1–3 mg/L = average risk, and more 3 mg/L = high risk).

Central obesity with elevated BMI is a modifiable risk factor for CVD that can be controlled by nutrition education intervention (Kelly Hedgepeth et al., 2008). Furthermore, obesity in combination with hypertension might predictably increase in prevalence in aging populations who have chronically exhibited these risk factors (Tiengo & Avogaro, 2001).

The WHO/MONICA Project (Monitoring of Trends and Determinants in Cardiovascular Disease) collected data from randomly selected participants from different nations and found, with few exceptions, general increases in levels of obesity approaching epidemic status among United Nations member states over a 5-year observation interval during the 1980s. Mean BMI demonstrably increases with socioeconomic transition and is a greater problem in urban populations with more sedentary lifestyles. For each single-point increase in average BMI, obesity prevalence increases by 5% within a population (Seidell, 2001). Obesity has been known to increase with age but now shows a progressively earlier age of onset, a factor that increases the time of chronic exposure for affected individuals and poses a significant child health problem. In developing populations, women are more frequently obese than men. Interestingly, men in developed countries are more likely to be obese than are either their female cohorts or males in developing countries (Antipatis & Gill, 2001; Gutzwiller, 1994). Apparently, socioeconomic status, which is reflective of income level, occupational physical activity, educational level, and place of residence, correlates with obesity prevalence. However, the correlations are not the same across different populations. In developed countries, these socioeconomic factors correlate negatively with obesity levels. In contrast, in developing countries, the correlation is positive, with early improvements in lifestyle appearing to increase obesity levels (Antipatis & Gill, 2001). This reverse correlation in developing countries may reflect exposure to Western culture with its convenience foods and sedentary lifestyles too early in their transition and before healthy lifestyles can be adopted. This same Western popular culture places more emphasis on the stereotypic "ideal" female body type than it does on that of males, which may help account for the gender difference in obesity observed in developed countries.

Although increased BMI has been found to be the major risk factor for CVD, a recent study of premenopausal and postmenopausal women in the United States showed definite ethnic differences in risk levels as well. African American women had the highest risk of CVD, while Asian Americans had the lowest.

Because of the complex interactions among demographic, socioeconomic, cultural, and genetic factors that contribute to obesity prevalence, obesity may prove to be the most difficult CVD risk factor to control. Further complicating this challenge is the awareness that preventing obesity is easier than correcting it once it has developed. Preventing obesity requires early intervention with identification of at-risk individuals and subsequent application of preventive public health measures including educational awareness. Any control strategy becomes less likely to be effective as the number of obese individuals increases progressively over time—a relationship that is likely to occur if the condition continues to appear at progressively earlier ages. Yet, without correction, the trend will merely increase in negative economic impact through increasing healthcare costs and continued lost productivity.

Diabetes Mellitus and Metabolic Syndrome

Diabetes mellitus, or sugar diabetes, is characterized by elevated blood sugar (hyperglycemia), increased urine output (polyuria) with excessive thirst (polydipsia), and glucose in the urine (glucosuria). It may have a variety of pathophysiological causes, all related to either the availability of or the sensitivity to the hormone insulin produced by beta pancreatic islet cells. Type 1 diabetes (formerly called juvenile or insulin-dependent diabetes) is thought to result from insulin deficiency caused by autoimmune (type 1A) or idiopathic (type 1B) destruction of pancreatic beta cells. Type 2 diabetes (non-insulin-dependent diabetes [NIDDM]) exhibits a range of pathophysiology from insulin resistance to insulin deficiency, or a combination of the two.

Type 2 diabetes is the most prevalent form (accounting for approximately 95% of all diabetes cases) and is part of the metabolic syndrome risk factor for CVD. It is also the most common form of diabetes occurring with obesity. The etiology of type 2 diabetes and metabolic syndrome in obese people shows an initial resistance to insulin peripherally. Increased body fat is accompanied by increased macrophages within adipose tissue. These macrophages produce pro-inflammatory cytokines that increase generalized inflammation, as evidenced by C-reactive protein levels, and decrease cellular sensitivity to insulin. Macrophages can also produce a hormone, resistin, which further increases insulin resistance as the diabetes evolves (Maizels & Allen, 2011). This early insulin resistance raises the blood sugar level (hyperglycemia) and increases lipid lysis in adipocytes as an alternative energy source, which in turn can lead to ketosis and ketoacidosis. Also, the elevated blood sugar increases beta cells' secretion of insulin, leading to hyperinsulinemia, and can ultimately lead to loss of beta cell function. This cluster of pathophysiological signs predisposes people to atherosclerosis and ultimately to ischemic heart disease and cerebrovascular stroke (Porth, 2005).

At this point, a dangerous disease sequela emerges. Obesity leads to peripheral insulin resistance and hyperglycemia, which in turn leads to hyperinsulinemia. Excess blood insulin levels produce metabolic syndrome, culminating in CVD or CVA. Because central body fat increases with both advancing age and dietary caloric excess, it is reasonable to expect a higher prevalence of chronic cardiovascular and cerebrovascular diseases in populations during the second phase of the demographic and socioeconomic transition as improvements in life expectancy and personal income occur. This relationship would be particularly evident if changes in general lifestyle lead to unhealthy diets and more sedentary lives. Similarly, in phase three of the demographic and socioeconomic transition, in which the proportion of elderly individuals in the overall population increases, age-related obesity alone would be expected to increase the risk for CVD and CVA. When this trend is combined with an earlier onset of obesity in the population age structure, risks for CVD and CVA can be chronically exacerbated.

The risk of death among diabetics is twice that of nondiabetic people of similar age. In the United States, nearly two million people 20 years of age or older were diagnosed with diabetes in 2010 alone, with approximately 35% of that age group showing signs of prediabetes. In fact, the prevalence of diabetes has doubled globally since 1980, with the United States, Saudi Arabia, and Samoa showing the greatest increases in their populations with this disease. This epidemic increase in obesity and diabetes constitutes a significant economic burden, given that healthcare expenditures for diabetics are double those for persons without diabetes (Centers for Disease Control and Prevention [CDC], 2011).

Alcohol and Tobacco Use

Alcohol and tobacco use have long been correlated with chronic hepatic, gastrointestinal, respiratory, and cardiovascular diseases, but the detailed pathophysiology of their effects remains poorly understood. Because alcohol and tobacco use are often seen in conjunction with obesity, hypertension, and diabetes, it is often difficult to separate out the true causes and effects of these conditions. In fact, a major effect of alcohol and tobacco use is known to be the exacerbation of existing cardiovascular risk factors. Moreover, because of their addictive properties, alcohol and tobacco pose unique challenges for control efforts.

Alcohol consumption in excess of three drinks per day increases blood levels of catecholamines, leading to increased blood pressure; systolic values are more dramatically affected than diastolic pressures. This effect becomes quite serious when seen in elderly or obese individuals with sedentary lifestyles and constitutes a significant health risk in these people. Alcohol use decreases hepatic gluconeogenesis, a major mechanism of hepatic glucose production, and can lead to hypoglycemia. This effect is dangerous for people with diabetes who are on insulin therapy and at risk of hypoglycemia through their treatment regimens. Cerebrovascular stroke risk increases with alcohol consumption because of three known physiological effects. First, cardiac arrhythmias—particularly atrial fibrillation (the "holiday heart" phenomenon)—can transiently retard blood flow, causing thrombi to form on the atrial walls or heart valve leaflets. Such thrombotic events may give rise to emboli that can obstruct brain circulation and cause a thromboembolic stroke. Second, the tendency for alcohol to exacerbate existing hypertension can contribute to accelerated atherosclerosis with resultant thromboembolic events. Third, an enhanced effect on blood coagulation further increases thromboembolic risks (Massie & Amidan, 1998; Porth, 2005).

With chronic tobacco use, components of cigarette smoke may be toxic to the extent of causing inflammatory damage to vascular endothelium, increasing the likelihood of thrombotic events. Additionally, nicotine increases the incidence of vascular spasms while increasing plasma norepinephrine levels and lowering HDL levels. These effects would predispose a smoker to hypertension, atherosclerosis, and CHD (Massie, 1998; Porth, 2005). In populations with a high underlying risk for cardiovascular disease, such as in South Asia, India, and former USSR countries, tobacco consumption has been shown to exacerbate their risk levels (Howson et al., 1998). The WHO World Health Report (1999) presented disturbing statistics on the prevalence of tobacco use globally. Estimates were that at the end of the 1900s approximately four million deaths per year were caused by tobacco use. This number was extrapolated to reach 10 million per year by 2030. It is easy to speculate that this mortality rate is primarily attributable to tobacco use in more developed nations, as their per capita GDP would be high enough to permit significant tobacco use. In reality, smoking is increasing by 3.4% per year in developing countries, a level declared by the WHO to be an epidemic. Because people in these developing nations must contend with infectious diseases as well, tobacco use and related chronic diseases may prove to be a significant part of their dual disease burden.

Because chronic diseases resulting from tobacco use can also be caused by other inherent or environmental risk factors, it is difficult to single out tobacco as the solitary causative agent. Consequently, it is difficult to get a reliable estimate of the true impact of tobacco use on health. Ezzati and Lopez (2004) attempted to factor out statistically any background disease rates caused by environmental factors other than smoking. They found that in developing countries cardiovascular diseases were the major smoking-attributable causes of death, representing 27.8% of total smoking-related deaths. Contrastingly, in developed countries, the portion of cardiovascular deaths that were deemed tobacco related jumped to 42.1%. The disproportionately high percentage of tobacco-related cardiovascular deaths in developed nations may be due to the fact that, in these populations, other risk factors for chronic diseases have been minimized by their level of socioeconomic development. A corollary to this conclusion might be that developing populations have to contend with both tobacco-related risks and other chronic disease risks inherent in their developmental status.

Although tobacco use is increasing in developing nations, there is an overall decline in this habit in developed nations, led primarily by North America and Western Europe. This decline occurred after a peak in tobacco consumption in the early 1980s. It may reflect the efficacy of antismoking campaigns in developed nations in raising awareness of the hazards of smoking. Unfortunately, it may also reflect the recognition by tobacco manufacturers and marketers of the large potential market afforded by developing nations. As the per capita income in these developing nations increases and they are exposed to Western popular culture, they could be seen to represent an opportunity to extend tobacco sales.

After examining all of the risk factors for CVD, it is noteworthy that only chronological age and genetic inheritance represent irreversible risks over which individuals have no control. The remaining risks, which are considered to be behavioral in nature, can be reduced or eliminated entirely by behavioral modification. To do so, however, requires first that people be made aware of potential health risks through education and, second, that through personal choice, they avoid behaviors that predispose them to CVD. Unfortunately, these lifestyle behaviors can be acquired during adolescence or early adulthood, which further compounds the problems. Adolescents and young adults often are perceived as being more susceptible to peer pressure and mass marketing of glamorized behaviors. In addition, they may lack the experience and maturity to fully appreciate the risks that certain behaviors might pose because the immediate negative effects of these behaviors rarely appear early in their indulgence. Additionally, alcohol, tobacco, and substance use can be psychologically and physiologically addictive, making behavioral change in addicted individuals more difficult to achieve. Adopting these high-risk behaviors early in life increases the time of exposure as life expectancies increase within a population. In such situations, the unavoidable age risk factor eventually occurs in conjunction with the results of behavioral risks, leading to multiple risk factors and an increased probability of contracting chronic cardiovascular diseases.

CONCLUSIONS

At the beginning of the 21st century, only 22% of the United Nations' WHO member states had attained developed status. More than 150 nations around the globe are in some phase of demographic or socioeconomic transition. Of these developing nations, 68 countries in Africa, the Americas, Southeast Asia, and the Eastern Mediterranean regions are experiencing high mortality levels at both ends of the population age strata; that is, they are contending with high child mortality and high adult mortality with generally low average life expectancies. However, a reexamination of the infectious versus chronic disease death rates by geographic region after the first decade of the 21st century showed a definite positive trend (Table 8-1). In all geographic regions, infectious disease rates were stable or declining as chronic disease mortality increased. As expected, these increases in chronic disease mortality rates and declining infectious disease burdens were less profound in more highly developed geographic regions. Disease burdens were more stable in geographic regions that had attained developed status historically earlier and had persisted there for longer times.

Poverty is prevalent in these developing countries and is sustained by poor health and high fertility rates, both of which serve to keep per capita income low. Breaking this cycle of poverty is a meaningful goal of intervention efforts for this century. Interrupting this cycle requires an intervention stimulus to any or all of the following (Bloom, Canning, & Malaney, 2000):

- Income level
- Health status
- Fertility rate

Income Level Versus Health Status Improvements

It has long been known that economic and financial conditions affect access to food supply and have a direct impact on mortality. Child mortality is of particular concern because it

TABLE 8-1

Percent of Total Adult Deaths Globally by Geographic Region for the Decade 2000–2011

Geographic Region	2011 Infectious	2011 Chronic	2000 Infectious	2000 Chronic	Difference Infectious	Difference Chronic
Africa	36	26	45	20	−9	+6
S.E. Asia	16	52	21	41	−5	+11
E. Mediterranean	16	46	21	39	−5	+7
Americas	6	73	8	68	−2	+5
Europe	4	81	4	78	0	+3
W. Pacific	6	75	7	66	−1	+9

Data from WHO methods and data sources for global burden of disease estimates 2000–2011.

correlates positively with high fertility rates, correlates negatively with per capita income, and, where prevalent, impedes socioeconomic development. Prevalent childhood diseases and poor perinatal health care influence socioeconomic development by reducing the number of individuals surviving, thriving, and moving into the economically productive labor force of the middle-aged demographic strata. It would be logical to expect that improvements in economic status of a population would decrease child mortality and increase life expectancy through better living conditions and better access to health care. Although effective as a short-term emergency measure, financial aid alone without concomitant economic expansion is controversial and may be ineffective in some cases. Simple money infusion increases the cost burden on donor countries and carries the inherent risk of the funds being diverted by corrupt regimes away from targeted peoples. Additionally, a simple, short-term boost in economic activity can have the reverse effect of causing a surge in population growth, increasing dependency stress, and driving the population back to baseline per capita income levels. For an economic stimulus to have a long-term effect on the economic status of a population, it must involve sustainable measures that will perpetuate further economic growth.

Preston (1975) suggests that, during the 20th century, mortality became increasingly dissociated from economic level. This dissociation occurred primarily because of the tendency for advances in medical care and health technologies to spread from developed nations to their lesser-developed neighbors. As a result of this trend, underdeveloped populations benefit from a reduction in mortality without having a concomitant remarkable improvement in their per capita incomes. In these situations, mortality is more responsive to health interventions than it is to boosts in per capita income. When comparing per capita income with life expectancy in 30 countries during the 1930s and 1960s, Preston (1975) noted that average per capita incomes between $100 and $600 (in 1963 U.S. dollars) were associated with dramatic increases in life expectancy. By comparison, incomes greater than $600 resulted in little improvement in life expectancy.

It can be speculated that the observed initial economic-related improvements in life expectancy may have resulted from decreased rates of child mortality and other deaths caused by infectious disease. Because of the relative low cost of antibiotics and vaccines, child mortality and infectious diseases can be relatively inexpensively managed through minimal peripartal care, vaccination programs, and easy access to antibiotics. Thus, these initial improvements in life expectancy would require minimal financial resources. However, the chronic disease burden that inevitably occurs with an aging population created through increasing life expectancy poses a different long-term problem, and one that requires substantially more income for health management. For example, many chronic cardiovascular diseases cannot be "cured" in the traditional sense of the word. Instead, people afflicted with these diseases undergo comparatively expensive health management regimens involving costly surgical procedures or expensive, long-term drug therapy. These treatment regimens may continue or recur throughout their life spans and can extend their life expectancies only within certain limits. Consequently, it may be that slight improvements in economic status will prove effective in minimizing the mortality from infectious diseases, but significantly larger economic expansion may be required to make the extended health management of chronic diseases affordable. Additionally, the simple ability to afford chronic disease management does not always guarantee a significantly longer life expectancy when compared to that of disease-free individuals.

Developed nations can and do export antibiotics, immunization vaccines, and other health-care technologies as a humanitarian commitment to lesser-developed countries. Such exports should raise child survival rates and can give recipient populations a boost along the path of socioeconomic development. Within the context of typical population development, this practice should increase the number of people moving into the middle-aged labor force and eventually break the poverty cycle, providing sufficient income growth to manage the eventual chronic disease burden as the population ages. However, this scenario requires that the developing economy grow at a rate capable of providing jobs for the growing labor force. Should this not be the case, the danger exists that subsequent generations may slip back into a low per capita income situation.

Further complicating the preceding scenario is the fact that, in addition to the export of medical technology, cultural practices may be exported. This potential activity is enhanced by the rapid growth of global communication. In such an environment, the improving lifestyles and personal income levels of developing nations may make them targets for marketing strategies undertaken to expand business consumer bases and overall profits. The impact of exporting these marketing strategies can be mixed. It may encourage people to strive toward better lifestyles through the pursuit of jobs that lead them to safer work environments and higher educational achievements, but it can also result in the adoption of lifestyles that include less physical activity and greater dependence on convenience diets and other unhealthy behaviors. The combination of sedentary lifestyles with unhealthy diets and behaviors predisposes people to increased risk of chronic cardiovascular disease later in life as multiple risk factors begin to accrue along with normal aging. Moreover, as adoption of these unhealthy practices occurs progressively earlier in life, the likelihood of developing chronic disease will increase.

Tobacco use and obesity serve as examples of this trend. Tobacco-related deaths occur at nearly equal levels—approximately 2.4 million deaths per year—in both developed and developing countries (Ezzati & Lopez, 2004). Nearly 7% of the world's population has a BMI greater than 30, and obesity is occurring at earlier ages (Seidell, 2001). In children, increases in BMI correlate with increased blood pressure (Raj, Sundaram, Paul, Sudhakar, & Kumar, 2010); if this situation is not corrected, it will yield a generation of adult individuals with extended exposures to CVD risk factors. This increasing prevalence of obesity is occurring in both developed and developing countries and is likely related to unhealthy dietary practices in populations with increasingly more sedentary lifestyles.

Fertility Rate Improvements

Poston (2000) considered four specific factors to have influential effects on fertility:

- Advances in economic development through participation in a nonagricultural labor force
- Improvement in general health conditions with reduction in infant mortality
- Improvement in social conditions particularly in educational attainment
- Absolute and relative improvement in female status within the population

These four factors may also interact with one another. For example, movement from an agricultural to an industrial labor force can generate higher per capita income. Higher incomes relate to better access to health care and education. Better education, especially among females, leads to improved female status within the population. Better education can also lead circuitously back to improved jobs and better health conditions. More affluent and better educated populations with improved health conditions show lower fertility rates, as large families become more of a liability in a nonagrarian lifestyle. Thus, improvements in any or all of these factors should lead naturally to a decline in fertility. Such a decline in fertility correlates with elevated socioeconomic status and can contribute to breaking the poverty cycle of a developing population by relieving the child dependency stress while increasing per capita GDP.

All of these fertility influences can occur naturally in the typical developmental process of a population. However, fertility declines can be accelerated over and above the decreases that would occur naturally, such as by governmental mandate, for example, as was done in the People's Republic of China (mainland China). In the 1970s, China instituted a coercive fertility control program as discussed earlier in this chapter. Although it was successful in dropping the fertility rate below replacement levels, Taiwan was able to accomplish a similar reduction in fertility without direct government intervention. In Taiwan, the natural socioeconomic development process was effective in diminishing the fertility rate, presumably by affecting the perceived or actual economic costs and social value of children (Poston, 2000). Because both approaches were effective in reducing fertility rates below replacement levels, these examples illustrate how different social and political climates in two separate populations can produce similar outcomes.

Future Considerations

Even in developed countries, high prevalence levels of chronic diseases pose a significant economic threat through lost productivity from afflicted workers, along with increased healthcare costs. If this economic impact can be significant in developed market economies, it would be considerably more damaging to the fragile, fledgling economies of developing nations. Thus, a major problem confronting both developed and developing economies is deciding how to prioritize expenditures for chronic disease risk avoidance compared to the expenditures required for the expansion of healthcare infrastructure to sufficiently manage increasing levels of chronic disease. Both approaches require a significant, though not necessarily equal, financial commitment. Chronic health care has historically proved to be more costly than education. Regardless of the priority, the costs must come from the overall GDP generated through a population's economic activity, and its economy must be strong enough to withstand the added stress. As a larger percentage of GDP is diverted into risk management and health care for the chronically ill, less will be available for economic expansion, and the risk of economic stagnation or decline increases. The decision is not a simple one and, in reality, both probably will have to be dealt with simultaneously. Moreover, the combined actions will take a financial toll on a population's economy.

Study Questions

1. Discuss the impact of expanding technology in developing countries upon the increased burden of chronic diseases such as diabetes, cardiovascular diseases, and hypertension.
2. Explain the role of obesity and its influence on metabolic syndrome both in developed and developing countries.
3. Compare and contrast the impact of polysubstance abuse (alcohol, drugs, and tobacco) on chronic diseases within developed and developing countries.

Case Study for Global Cardiovascular Diseases

The prevalence of obesity is increasing worldwide. Obesity, the result of chronic positive energy balance, is associated with many chronic diseases, including diabetes, heart disease, hypertension, and some forms of cancer. Determining those factors that influence the prevalence of obesity in developing countries is important, as these countries generally lack the infrastructure to adequately treat the chronic diseases associated with obesity. As developing countries' economies improve and the population becomes urban, changes in dietary habits and physical activity create an environment in which a person predisposed to weight gain could become obese. Ironically, nutritional stunting early in life has been associated with obesity in later years. Those countries that have had traditionally high prevalences of undernutrition and stunting may be faced with a double burden of under- and overnutrition. These countries are already poorly equipped to handle acute and chronic diseases. In the future, they will face the increased economic burden of supporting an overweight or obese population, together with the associated and costly chronic diseases.

Case Study Questions

1. Explain why obesity in a developing country creates a "double burden" to its society.
2. How does urbanization of a population affect increased rates of obesity and more chronic diseases?
3. What are some ways that developing countries could decrease the rate of obesity while maintaining costs within a limited budget?

© FAO 2001, Hoffman, D. J. (2001). Obesity in developing countries: Causes and implications. *Food, Nutrition and Agriculture, 28*. Retrieved from http://www.fao.org/docrep/003/y0600m/y0600m05.htm#P0_0

References

Akinkugbe, O. O. (1990). Epidemiology of cardiovascular disease in developing countries. *Journal of Hypertension, 8*(7), S233–S237.

Antipatis, V. J., & Gill, T. P. (2001). Obesity as a global problem. In P. Bjorntorp (Ed.), *International Textbook of Obesity* (pp. 2–22). New York: John Wiley & Sons.

Bloom, D. E., Canning, D., & Malaney, P. N. (2000). Population dynamics and economic growth. In C. Y. Cyrus Chu & R. Lee (Eds.), *Population and Development Review: A Supplement to Volume 26* (p. 257). New York: Population Council.

Centers for Disease Control and Prevention. (2011). *National Diabetes Fact Sheet: National Estimates and General Information on Diabetes and Prediabetes in the United States.* Atlanta, GA: U.S. Department of Health and Human Services, Centers for Disease Control and Prevention.

Deurenberg, P., Yap, M., & van Staveren, W. A. (1998). Body mass index and percent body fat: A meta analysis among different ethnic groups. *International Journal of Obesity, 22,* 1164–1171.

Ezzati, M., & Lopez, A. D. (2004). Regional, disease specific patterns of smoking-attributable mortality in 2000. *Tobacco Control, 13,* 388–395.

Gutzwiller, F. (1994). Monitoring of cardiovascular disease and risk factor trends: Experiences from the WHO/MONICA project. *Annals of Medicine, 26*(1), 61–65.

Hoffman, D. J. (2001). Obesity in developing countries: Causes and implications. *Food, Nutrition and Agriculture, 28.* Retrieved from http://www.fao.org/ag/agn/publications/fna/article.jsp?lang=en&myURI=id497

Howson, C. P., Reddy, K. S., Ryan, T. J., & Bale, J. R. (1998). *Control of Cardiovascular Diseases in Developing Countries: Research, Development, and Institutional Strengthening* (p. 237). Washington, DC: National Academy Press.

Infoplease. (2011). *Profile of the World.* Retrieved from http://www.infoplease.com/ipa/A0004373.html

Kelly-Hedgepeth, A., Lloyd-Jones, D. M., Calvin, A., Matthews, K. A., Johnston, J., Sowers, M. R., . . . Chae, C. U. (2008). Ethnic differences in C-reactive protein concentrations. *Clinical Chemistry, 54,* 1027–1037.

Lederbogen, F., Kirsch, P., Haddad, L., Streit, F., Test, H., Shuch, P., . . . Meyer-Lindenberg, A. (2011). City living and urban upbringing affect neural social stress processing in humans. *Nature, 474,* 498–501. doi:10.1038/nature10190

Lee, R., & Cyrus Chu, C. Y. (2000). Introduction. In C. Y. Cyrus Chu & R. Lee (Eds.), *Population and Development Review: A Supplement to Volume 26* (pp. 1–9). New York: Population Council.

Maizels, R. M., & Allen, J. E. (2011). Eosinophils forestall obesity. *Science, 332,* 186–187.

Massie, B. M. (1998). Systemic hypertension. In L. M. Tierney, Jr., S. J. McPhee, & M. A. Papadakis (Eds.), *Current Medical Diagnosis and Treatment* (37th ed., pp. 429–447). Stamford, CT: Appleton and Lange.

Massie, B. M., & Amidan, T. M. (1998). Heart. In L. M. Tierney, Jr., S. J. McPhee, & M. A. Papadakis (Eds.), *Current Medical Diagnosis and Treatment* (37th ed., pp. 333–348). Stamford, CT: Appleton and Lange.

Nicholas, S., Agodoa, L., & Norris, K. (2004, November). Ethnic disparities in the prevalence and treatment of kidney disease. *Nephrology News and Issues,* 29–36.

Phipps, S. R. (2006). Settlement and migration. In R. Abramson & J. Haskell (Eds.), *Encyclopedia of Appalachia* (pp. 285–292). Knoxville, TN: University of Tennessee Press.

Porth, C. M. (2005). *Pathophysiology: Concepts of Altered Health States* (7th ed., p. 1582). Philadelphia: Lippincott Williams and Wilkins.

Poston, D. L., Jr. (2000). Social and economic development and the fertility transitions in mainland China and Taiwan. In C. Y. Cyrus Chu & R. Lee (Eds.), *Population and Development Review: A Supplement to Volume 26* (pp. 40–41). New York: Population Council.

Preston, S. H. (1975). The changing relation between mortality and level of economic development. *Population Studies, 29,* 213–248.

Raj, M., Sundaram, K. R., Paul, M., Sudhakar, A., & Kumar, R. K. (2010). Body mass index trend and its association with blood pressure distribution in children. *Journal of Hypertension, 24,* 652–658.

Seidell, J. C. (2001). The epidemiology of obesity. In P. Bjorntorp (Ed.), *International Textbook of Obesity* (pp. 23–29). New York: John Wiley & Sons.

Strauss, J., & Duncan, T. (1998, June). Health, nutrition and economic development. *Journal of Economic Literature, 36,* 766–817.

Tiengo, A., & Avogaro, A. (2001). Cardiovascular disease. In P. Bjorntorp (Ed.), *International Textbook of Obesity* (pp. 365–377). New York: John Wiley & Sons.

World Health Organization. (1995). *World Health Report 1995: Bridging the Gaps.* Geneva, Switzerland: Author.

World Health Organization. (1996). *World Health Report 1996: Fighting Disease, Fostering Development.* Geneva, Switzerland: Author.

World Health Organization. (1997). *World Health Report 1997: Conquering Suffering, Enriching Humanity.* Geneva, Switzerland: Author.

World Health Organization. (1998). *World Health Report 1998: Life in the 21st Century: A Vision for All.* Geneva, Switzerland: Author.

World Health Organization. (1999). *World Health Report 1999: Making a Difference.* Geneva, Switzerland: Author.

World Health Organization. (2000). *World Health Report 2000. Health Systems: Improving Performance.* Geneva, Switzerland: Author.

World Health Organization. (2001). *World Health Report 2001. Mental Health, New Understanding, New Hope.* Geneva, Switzerland: Author.

World Health Organization. (2002). *World Health Report 2002. Reducing Risks, Promoting Healthy Life.* Geneva, Switzerland: Author.

World Health Organization. (2003). *World Health Report 2003. Shaping the Future.* Geneva, Switzerland: Author.

World Health Organization. (2004). *World Health Report 2004. Changing History.* Geneva, Switzerland: Author.

World Health Organization. (2009). Chronic diseases and risk factors. Retrieved from http://www.smartglobalhealth.org/issues/entry/chronic-diseases

World Health Organization. (2013). Methods and data sources for global burden of disease estimates 2000–2011. *Global Health Estimates Technical Paper.* Retrieved from http://www.who.int/healthinfo/statistics/GlobalDALYmethods_2000_2011.pdf

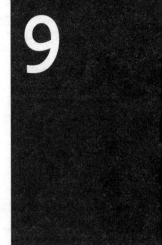

Infectious Diseases from a Global Perspective

9

Barbara J. Blake
Gloria A. Taylor

Objectives

After completing this chapter, the reader will be able to:

1. Relate the historical aspects of selected infectious diseases.
2. Discuss the need for global infectious disease surveillance.
3. Compare and contrast the causes, transference patterns, and treatments of diseases such as typhoid; tuberculosis (TB); HIV/AIDS; dengue fever; West Nile virus; hepatitis A, B, and C; avian influenza; malaria; Ebola virus disease; and seasonal influenza.

INTRODUCTION

During the 20th century, the race to combat infectious diseases made great strides in saving millions of lives as nations became more developed through industrialization, advances in prevention and health promotion education, and pharmacological innovation. Despite such gains, infectious diseases continue to cause approximately 20% of all deaths (lower respiratory infections, HIV/AIDS, and diarrheal diseases) in the worldwide ranking of the 10 leading causes of mortality. This percentage does not include deaths in resource-poor countries from malaria and tuberculosis, 35 per 100,000 and 31 per 100,000, respectively (World Health Organization [WHO], 2014a). Many complex issues surround infectious diseases, including those related to geography, environment, economics, population characteristics, infrastructure, and health conditions. From an international perspective, the lack of public health infrastructure has been identified as the primary reason for outbreaks of disease (Olson et al., 2015).

As the world becomes "smaller" as a result of air travel, population growth, and transnational commerce, existing, emerging, or reemerging infectious diseases continue to pose complex challenges and threats to systems of healthcare delivery, regional and national poli-cies, security, disease surveillance, and research. Because of the enormous variety of infectious diseases endemic (occurs every year) to some nations and regions of the world, this chapter cannot hope to describe, characterize, and define the hundreds of viral, bacterial, fungal, and parasitic diseases that coexist with humans throughout the world. Rather, this chapter selec-tively describes some of the most common infectious diseases that manifest themselves globally and discusses the challenges that nations routinely confront in their battle to coexist with their invisible neighbors.

HISTORICAL APPROACHES TO INFECTIOUS DISEASES

According to philosopher George Santayana, "Those who cannot remember the past are condemned to repeat it." This saying is quite appropriate in the context of infectious diseases. As societies evolved from hunters and gatherers and formed larger civilizations, acute infec-tious diseases became noticeable as populations expanded outward. When small, nomadic tribes began bartering resources between Asia and Europe, contact among these civilizations increased. Within the past six centuries, the Black Death (bubonic plague), killed almost half of the European population, an estimated 20 to 25 million people over a five-year period. The infectious organism that caused the plague, Yersina pestis, was carried by merchant traders from central Asia (China) to Western Europe (Italy) around 1340 (History.com.Staff, 2010; Middle Ages.net, 2011).

During the 11th and 12th centuries, Crusaders introduced smallpox into Europe and by the 15th century it was well established throughout the region. Subsequently, European explorers introduced the virus into the Americas (viral naive) and the indigenous people were devastated. By the 20th century, this disease impacted every country in the world; however, vaccination against smallpox was widely used in developed countries. In 1967, the (WHO) launched a global immunization campaign to wipe out smallpox. The Global Commission for the Certifica-tion of Smallpox Eradication concluded in 1979 that this disease had been eradicated from the world, which makes smallpox the only infectious disease to achieve this groundbreaking status (Fenner, Henderson, Arita, Ježek, & Ladnyi, 1988; WHO, 1980).

Although many historical examples can be cited to characterize the link between people and their environment, none is more telling than how cholera spread throughout London in the 1800s. In the mid-1850s, Dr. John Snow, a physician in London, spent a great deal of time trying to convince his colleagues that cholera was a waterborne disease. His assertion contra-dicted the current theory of the time, which stated that cholera was transmitted through the air in the form of mists or miasmas (noxious atmosphere). It was not until 1854, when Snow began mapping the location of all well water pumps and the location of every case of cholera, that a pattern began to emerge. Through his geospatial mapping of cholera incidence and deaths and the city's well water pumps, Snow was able to link the well on Broad Street to the cholera outbreak. Snow used this evidence to persuade officials to remove the Broad Street pump handle. Afterward, cholera was contained and decreased in London (Magner, 2009; Sherman, 2007).

Another historical snapshot that links international travel and migration to infectious diseases, people, and their environment entails the story of Mary Mallon. Mallon was an Irish immigrant to the United States at the turn of the 1900s, who eventually became known as "Typhoid Mary." She became the first documented asymptomatic carrier of the typhoid bacterium, *Salmonella typhi*, in the United States. During this time, Mallon was employed as a domestic cook. While working in this position, she infected more than 50 people with the disease, of whom three died. However, given the many years she worked as a cook in domestic settings, it was never clearly determined just how many people became infected from Mallon preparing their meals. As the typhoid bacteria were expelled through Mallon's feces, improper handwashing was probably to blame for the spread of the organism through her food preparation (Hasian, 2000).

These examples reflect the variable nature of how infectious diseases spread between people and their environment. As one continues to examine the global infectious diseases most common throughout the world, it becomes clear how the sciences of clinical and molecular epidemiology, virology, bacteriology, mycology, and public health can have global, regional, national, and local effects on the detection, prevention, or eradication of various infectious diseases. Differences within countries—such as political instability, economic unrest, and limited healthcare infrastructure—can, in turn, affect a community's response to the threat of infectious diseases.

CHOLERA

Cholera is an acute diarrheal disease caused by the bacterium *Vibrio cholerae* (serogroups O1 and O139 are responsible for the majority of outbreaks worldwide). It remains one of the most feared enteric diseases, often affecting poor and vulnerable populations. Persons are typically infected by consuming water or eating food that has been contaminated with the organism. Each year 1.4 to 4.3 million cases are identified globally and more than 100,000 deaths occur, the vast majority in Sub-Saharan Africa. This disease is endemic in many countries across Asia and Africa. A lack of basic infrastructure (access to clean water, sanitation, and hygiene) plays a predominate role in disease transmission. Once persons are infected, they continue to shed the organism in their feces for 7 to 14 days, thereby creating new opportunities for the infection to spread to others in environments that lack adequate basic hygiene (Centers for Disease Control and Prevention [CDC], 2014a; Nygren, Blackstock, & Mintz, 2014; WHO, 2015).

Persons affected may experience mild to severe symptoms characterized by profuse watery diarrhea, vomiting, and abdominal and leg cramps. Symptoms can appear as soon as two hours to as long as five days after exposure. Among persons affected, approximately 80% will develop mild to moderate symptoms, and 20% will have acute diarrhea and severe dehydration. Symptoms can develop quickly, and the disease has been known to kill healthy adults within hours. Dehydration is the primary factor contributing to mortality. When available, most people can be successfully treated with oral rehydration salts. Severely dehydrated individuals require treatment with intravenous (IV) fluids. In addition to IV fluids, antibiotics can be helpful in diminishing the duration of diarrhea and reducing the amount of IV fluids needed for recovery. Use of IV fluids and antibiotics shortens the excretion time of the organism from the body. However, in resource-poor countries access to rehydration and antibiotics is limited. If immediate response measures are instituted (e.g., safe/clean water, proper sanitation, hygiene education, and safe food handling), the mortality rate will typically remain less than 1% in an outbreak (CDC, 2014a; Nygren, Blackstock, & Mintz, 2014; WHO, 2015a).

In areas of the world where cholera is endemic, WHO recommends the use of vaccines to assist in controlling the spread of disease. In addition, vaccination is recommended in complex emergency situations such as a natural disaster, internally displaced people, or refugees due to famine or war. Currently, two vaccines are available: Dukoral® and Shanchol®. Both vaccines are administered orally, two doses. These vaccines provide protection for as long as two years in endemic settings and have demonstrated efficacy of 85% to 90%; however, such vaccines do not take the place of adequate environmental controls, access to health care, clean water, and sanitation (CDC, 2014a; Charles et al., 2014; WHO, 2010, 2015a).

Recognizing that cholera remains a global concern, WHO launched the Global Task Force on Cholera Control in 1992. The aim of this initiative was to reduce morbidity and mortality related to cholera and address the social and economic consequences of the disease. This WHO-supported group brings together government agencies and nongovernmental organizations (NGOs) and institutions from around the world to address epidemics and develop technical reports and training guidelines to minimize the spread of cholera, thereby decreasing the number of epidemics worldwide. Priority activities currently focus on improved surveillance, support to communities to reduce the risk of spread during an outbreak, and environmental controls, such as access to clean water to diminish the incidence of waterborne diseases in general (WHO, 2015a). Overall, cholera continues to be a global infectious disease, and is considered to be endemic in many parts of the world and a reemerging infectious disease where the incidence has been low.

DENGUE AND SEVERE DENGUE

Dengue is the most common mosquito-borne infection in the world and is a global public health problem. It is considered an emerging infectious disease given its spread around the world since the early 1950s and its appearance in the Americas in 1981. Four serotypes of Flaviviridae viruses cause dengue: DEN-1, DEN-2, DEN-3, and DEN-4. About one-third of the world's population lives in areas where these viruses are transmitted. Dengue is the leading cause of morbidity and mortality in tropical and subtropical areas and an estimated 390 to 400 million infections occur annually, but only 100 million clinical cases are diagnosed. Of these, a small percentage progress to severe dengue. As urban areas and newly emerging urban environments continue to extend their reach, the prevalence of dengue has expanded to more than 128 countries and is endemic in more than 100 countries throughout Africa, the Americas, the Eastern Mediterranean, Southeast Asia, and the Western Pacific (CDC, 2014b, 2015a; WHO, 2015b).

Dengue is a vector-borne illness caused by the bite of the female *Aedes aegypti* or *Aedes albopictus* mosquito, which spreads the infection from person to person. Many people who are infected may be asymptomatic or experience only a mild form of the disease. When symptoms do occur, the disease typically presents as a flulike illness with high fever, headache, exhaustion, severe joint and muscle pain, swollen lymph nodes, and rash and can affect persons of all ages. In general, symptoms of the illness usually begin 4 to 10 days after the mosquito bite and last for 2 to 7 days. Dengue can progress to severe illness: dengue hemorrhagic fever (DHF) and dengue shock syndrome (DSS). Severe disease is characterized by a decrease in body temperature, severe abdominal pain, persistent vomiting, rapid breathing, bleeding gums, and restlessness. Currently, DHF is a leading cause of morbidity and mortality among children in some Asian and Latin American countries, where the burden of disease is greatest. Severe hemorrhage can lead to DSS, which consists of increased vascular permeability along with myocardial dysfunction and dehydration leading to the development of multi-organ failure and death. There is no specific treatment for dengue; however, supportive therapy saves lives (CDC, 2014b, 2015a; Rajapakse, 2011; WHO, 2015b).

Currently, there is no vaccine for dengue, although progress is occurring on this front and three vaccines are being tested with human subjects, phase II and phase III clinical trials. A major hurdle in vaccine development is finding a preparation that is effective against all four dengue serotypes, as infection from one strain does not confer immunity to the others and consecutive infections can increase the likelihood of developing DHF and DDS (CDC, 2015a; WHO, 2015b).

Given the lack of a vaccine, the first line of defense against dengue is prevention, environmental controls, and health education. Approaches for prevention should be addressed within the context of the environment, as mosquitoes breed in different habitats based on the community. In Asia and the Americas, mosquitoes breed in human-made vessels for water storage (e.g., jars, metal drums, concrete cisterns); in contrast, in Africa, mosquitoes breed in natural habitats. Communities can benefit from the use of insecticides to help control this vector population. In addition, the community can be educated regarding proper waste disposal and water storage practices (i.e., covering containers to prevent mosquito access for breeding). During outbreaks, the broad application of insecticides can be helpful, but the effect is not long lasting. In general, active monitoring and surveillance of dengue illness and mosquito populations represent basic control measures. Their implementation allows for immediate tracking of new cases so as to strengthen and recommend prevention strategies that affect and alter the behavior of individuals, households, and community infrastructures (CDC, 2015a; WHO, 2015b).

MALARIA

A disease resembling malaria was described in ancient Chinese medical writings, making it one of the oldest-known diseases. However, the causative organism was not identified until 1880 by Charles Louis Alphonse Laveran. This protozoan parasitic, mosquito-borne disease is caused by four different forms of *Plasmodium* parasites: *falciparum, malariae, ovale,* and *vivax*. Of these, the most common types are *falciparum* and *vivax*; however, *falciparum* is associated with the highest mortality among persons affected. These organisms are transferred to humans through the bites of *Anopheles* mosquitoes, which predominantly feed at night (CDC, 2015c; WHO, 2015c). However, a fifth *Plasmodium* parasite, *knowlesi*, that naturally occurs in macaques (monkeys) found in Southeast Asia, can be transmitted to humans via the bite of an infected mosquito. This type of malaria has been identified in Malaysian Borneo (highest prevalence), Thailand, Myanmar, the Philippines, and Singapore. *Knowlesi* is very responsive to treatment but fatal cases have been identified. Incidence is increasing and *knowlesi* is now considered an emerging zoonotic malaria parasite (Antinori, Galimberti, Milazzo, & Corbellino, 2013; van Hellemond et al., 2009).

Currently, 3.4 billion people (approximately half the world's population) live in areas at risk of malaria transmission (106 countries and territories). The most vulnerable and greatest number of victims of malaria are children, especially those who have not developed protective immunity against the infection. Recent estimates indicate that worldwide in 2013, malaria was responsible for 198 million cases of illness (82% occurring in Africa) and 584,000 deaths (90% occurring in Africa). Epidemics can occur in areas where climatic conditions are favorable to the survival of mosquitoes—that is, in areas with high levels of rainfall, temperature, and humidity. Therefore, outbreaks of disease can be seasonal or occur in areas where people have little or no immunity to malaria. These same variables apply in areas where malaria is endemic. Malaria is the fourth leading cause of death in Africa and the fifth leading cause of death from infectious diseases globally (CDC, 2015c; Medicines for Malaria Venture, 2015; WHO, 2014b, 2015c).

Early symptoms of malaria include fever, headache, chills, and vomiting. Because these symptoms can be mild and resemble a flulike illness, malaria may be misdiagnosed or go undiagnosed. A delay in recognizing and initiating treatment for *falciparum* malaria can lead to death within a short period of time. Effective treatment is key; however, *P. falciparum* has become resistant to conventional (monotherapy) antimalarial drugs (chloroquine, sulfadoxine–pyrimethamine, and amodiaquine), especially in endemic areas of the world. A long history of inappropriate use of these drugs has rendered them ineffective due to resistance, especially in Africa. The best treatment is an artemisinin-based combination medication (ACT), especially for *P. falciparum*, as monotherapy contributes to the development of resistance. Also, it is recommended that all cases of suspected malaria be confirmed with diagnostic testing, microscopy, or rapid diagnostic testing (RDT). Identification of the four primary types of malaria can be made within 15 minutes using RDT. The proportion of suspected malaria cases receiving diagnostic testing has increased, especially in Africa (CDC, 2015c; WHO, 2014b, 2015c).

In high-endemic areas, mosquito control represents the best strategy to reduce malaria transmission. A two-pronged approach is best, consisting of mosquito nets and indoor spraying with residual insecticides. Insecticide-impregnated mosquito nets should be distributed communitywide so that everyone sleeps under an appropriate mosquito net. Indoor household spraying should be routine (the results last for three to six months depending on the agent used) and achieved at the 80% level within the community. This action has proved to be the most powerful way to reduce malaria transmission. For persons traveling to areas of the world where malaria is endemic, several drugs have been found to be effective prophylactic agents: chloroquine, proguanil, mefloquine, and doxycycline (CDC, 2015c; WHO, 2014b, 2015c).

Malaria continues to be a public health concern related to infectious disease. In countries where the disease is rampant, many interventions are being tried to reduce the number and severity of seasonal malaria cases (which account for 80% to 90% of all cases). A recent review of the literature regarding community-based interventions to prevent and control malaria identified that indoor residual spraying, use of nets, administration of intermittent preventive treatment with sulfadoxine-pyrimethamine during pregnancy, presumptive treatment of disease, and education were found to be effective in many African countries. These types of strategies and others are helping to lower the incidence of malaria on a broad scale (Salam, Das, Lassi, & Bhutta, 2014).

AVIAN INFLUENZA A (H5N1) AND (H7N9)

Avian influenza (H5N1), commonly referred to as "bird flu," manifests its presence primarily in birds and poultry (especially ducks and geese). In 1996, The H5N1 virus was first isolated among geese in China. In 1997, representing the first evidence of human infection, the world community saw a new virus emerge when the virus crossed over from birds to humans and caused severe respiratory disease, leading to respiratory failure in many persons. This virus was considered to be highly pathogenic, resulting in high death rates in some poultry species. Persons who became ill were in close contact with infected poultry, alive or dead. No additional cases were identified until the virus reemerged in 2003 and 2004. During this time, the virus spread and became embedded in poultry in Asia, Europe, and Africa resulting in millions of poultry infections and many human cases and human deaths. During this same period Avian H7N9 (a low pathogenic virus) infected three persons in China. Overall, both viruses cause illness in humans and have a higher case fatality rate than seasonal influenza infections. Human-to-human spread is rare and infections have been primarily associated with prolonged close contact with infected poultry. In January 2014, Canada reported its first case of H5N1; however, this case was associated with a person who had recently traveled to China. H5N1 was detected in the wild bird population of North America in November 2014. These viruses pose a threat since they have pandemic potential and can likely spread person to person. To date, both viruses have been responsible for human illness worldwide (CDC, 2015d; Flint, Pearce, Franson, & Derksen, 2015; WHO, 2014c).

Symptoms of H5N1 infection include high fever, cough, sore throat, muscle aches, diarrhea, vomiting, and abdominal pain. The illness can progress into the lower respiratory system (sometimes early in the illness) and causes shortness of breath, respiratory distress, hoarse voice, crackling on inhaling, and respiratory failure. In addition, severe cases can include neurologic changes, multiple organ dysfunction, and secondary bacterial and fungal infections. The typical incubation period is about two to eight days (CDC, 2015d; WHO, 2014c).

Effective treatment involves the use of antiviral medications: oseltamivir, peramivir, or zanamivir. For these drugs to be efficacious, they must be initiated within 48 hours of onset of symptoms. However, due to the prolonged viral replication associated with these viruses, antiviral medications can be considered for use with patients coming into care late in the illness. Since these viruses are now circulating worldwide, there have been reports of possible drug resistance. Organisms can develop resistance to such therapies by mutating to a different strain, thereby rendering the medication ineffective. Drug resistance can be very much a reality, especially since these viruses mutate frequently. Resistance is a huge concern for effectively managing future outbreaks to minimize loss of life (CDC, 2015d; WHO, 2014c).

From a prevention perspective, careful attention to handwashing and adhering to strict food-handling procedures (avoiding cross-contamination) are paramount in minimizing the spread from poultry. The aforementioned antiviral drugs can be used to prevent infection in someone who has been exposed to these influenza viruses. Of note, seasonal influenza vaccination will not prevent infection with avian influenza A viruses. Any exposed person should be carefully observed for symptoms for at least seven days following contact, and diagnostic testing is recommended on suspect cases who meet specific criteria, such as direct contact with sick or dead domestic poultry, surfaces contaminated with poultry feces, and sick or dead wild birds suspected or confirmed to have influenza H5N1 (CDC, 2015d; WHO, 2014c).

WEST NILE VIRUS

West Nile virus, a member of the Flaviviridae family, is maintained in nature in a cycle involving transmission between birds and mosquitoes. However, this virus is also known to infect humans, horses, and other mammals. Birds of many varieties serve as its primary reservoir, with mosquitoes being the transmission vector. West Nile virus is virulent enough to cross species, nations, and continents, and it has had a long history of traversing Africa, parts of Europe, west and central Asia, the Middle East, and Australia. It was first isolated in 1937 from a Ugandan woman in the West Nile province of the country—hence the name. However, it has only been in the past 50 years that the virus has been reported in many countries. This virus was imported into the United States in 1999, when it produced a large-scale outbreak for the first time; since then West Nile cases have been reported across the United States. Epidemiologically, this phenomenon represents a classic case of importation and the establishment of a pathogen outside of its normal habitat, to the point that the organism now represents a potential global threat. In the Western Hemisphere, cases of West Nile virus infection have been reported in many geographical regions since its introduction: Canada, Mexico, the Caribbean islands, Central America, Venezuela, Columbia, and Argentina (CDC, 2015e; Chakarova, Dimitrov, & Chenchev, 2011; WHO, 2011a).

West Nile virus is carried in mosquitoes' salivary glands; when they bite humans or other animals, the virus is transferred to the target. Eighty percent of persons infected with the virus will remain asymptomatic, the other 20% will become ill, and only a small percentage of these individuals will develop severe disease—neuroinvasive disease—in the form of West Nile encephalitis, West Nile meningitis, or West Nile poliomyelitis. Symptoms associated with uncomplicated West Nile infection include fever, headache, fatigue, body aches, nausea, vomiting, skin rash (occasionally), and swollen lymph glands. Neuroinvasive West Nile disease is characterized by high fever, headache, stiffness of the neck, involuntary movements, stupor, disorientation, tremors, convulsions, coma, muscle weakness, and paralysis. The areas of the brain most often affected by West Nile Virus are the cerebral cortex, thalamus, basal ganglia, brain stem, cerebellum, and spinal cord. Persons older than the age of 50 and individuals with weakened immune systems are at greatest risk for severe disease (CDC, 2013a, 2015e; Lim, Koraka, Osterhaus, & Martina, 2011; WHO, 2011a).

There is no vaccine for West Nile virus, so environmental mosquito control measures, monitoring and disease surveillance (human and veterinary), and prevention education are paramount to decreasing transmission. Mosquito control entails insecticide spraying during peak mosquito seasons, use of insecticide mosquito nets, and use of repellents. Monitoring and surveillance are best achieved by maintaining an active animal health surveillance system (birds and horses) to provide early warning of the presence of West Nile virus. It is also important to report dead birds to local authorities, as their demise may be an early warning sign. Use of insect repellents and wearing long-sleeve garments during peak mosquito seasons can also lower the risk of infection, especially in endemic environments (CDC, 2013a; WHO, 2011a).

West Nile virus is an emerging infectious disease that has made its way around the globe in just a few decades. Expansion of the virus across the Western Hemisphere within a decade indicates a rapid spread. There will be much to learn about this pathogen in the years ahead.

EBOLA VIRUS DISEASE

The Ebola virus is part of the Filoviridae family of viruses that cause hemorrhagic fever (multiple organs in the body are affected). This family of viruses include Cuevavirus, Marburgvirus, and Ebolavirus. There are five species of Ebola virus (named after the Ebola River Valley in the Democratic Republic of the Congo): Zaire, Sudan, Taï Forest, Bundibugyo, and Reston. Of these species, only Zaire, Sudan, and Bundibugyo have been associated with large outbreaks with high case fatality rates; the majority of the time greater than 50% (CDC, 2015f; WHO, 2015d).

Ebola was first identified in 1976 in two concurrent outbreaks, Nzara, Sudan and Yambuku, Democratic Republic of the Congo (formally Zaire), comprising 151 and 280 cases, respectively. The higher case fatality rate was associated with Yambuku, 88%. Since that time other large-scale outbreaks have occurred: 1995, Democratic Republic of the Congo (315 cases, mortality 81%); 2000–2001, Uganda (425 cases, mortality 53%); 2003, Democratic Republic of the Congo (143 cases, mortality 89%); and 2007–2008, Democratic Republic of the Congo (149 cases, mortality 25%). However, in March 2014, the largest and deadliest outbreak in history began in multiple countries in West Africa (Guinea, Sierra Leone, Liberia, Nigeria, and Senegal). The burden of disease has been primarily associated with Guinea, Sierra Leone, and Liberia where there was widespread transmission. What has made this outbreak extraordinary, this is the first time Ebola has been imported to other parts of the world: Spain, United States, Italy, and the United Kingdom. This outbreak continues; more than 28,000 cases have been diagnosed and the number of deaths exceeds 11,000. The number of persons affected is ongoing, as this outbreak is still active (CDC, 2015f; WHO, 2015e).

Ebola virus disease is characterized by fever, fatigue, intense weakness, muscle pain, severe headache, and sore throat. These symptoms are typically followed by vomiting, diarrhea, unexplained bleeding (internal and external) or bruising, rash, and impaired kidney and liver function. The disease has an incubation period ranging from 2 to 21 days (average 8 to 10) and persons are infectious as long as their blood contains the virus. By the tenth day of the infection, fever subsides and a person who has been infected either improves or dies. Organ necrosis is an indication of end stage disease (CDC, 2015f; WHO, 2015d).

Ebola infection is diagnosed by blood tests that can identify antigens or genes of the virus. Diagnosis cannot be made by signs and symptoms because Ebola is difficult to differentiate from other illnesses such as malaria, typhoid fever, and meningitis. New testing techniques can identify the organism using a blood or urine sample. Currently, the only treatment for this disease is supportive: electrolyte and body fluid replacement therapy, maintaining good oxygen saturation and blood pressure, and treating specific symptoms as they occur. The affected person's immune system also plays a key role. There is no evidence to support that recovery confers lifelong immunity; however, persons who do recover develop antibodies for at least 10 years. Also, there is no indication that recovering from one type/species of Ebola infection is protective against developing other types. There is no vaccine for Ebola, although two potential vaccines are in testing stages, Sierra Leone Trial to Introduce a Vaccine against Ebola (STRIVE) and Partnership for Research on Ebola Vaccines in Liberia (PREVAIL) (CDC, 2015f; U.S. Department of Health and Human Services, 2015; WHO, 2015d).

The natural reservoir of the Ebola virus and how it is transferred to humans remains a mystery. However, there have been documented cases in which persons have become infected after coming into contact with blood, secretions, organs or bodily fluids of infected animals such as gorillas, chimpanzees, fruit bats, monkeys, forest antelope, and porcupines found ill or dead in the rainforest. The disease apparently spreads through human-to-human transmission via direct contact with bodily secretions from an infected person and fomites (bedding, clothing, surfaces) contaminated with these fluids. This means that health care workers can be frequently infected if they do not adhere to meticulous use of personal protective equipment during patient care (Boone & Gerba, 2007; CDC, 2015f; WHO, 2015d).

Ebola continues to be an emerging infectious disease. Due to the high case fatality rate associated with outbreaks, preparedness is a key factor in minimizing the impact on a community. Containment is the priority, as evidenced by the following recommendations: isolation of suspected cases; strict barrier protection during care; good contact tracing; effective environmental controls—disinfection of clothing and bed linens; and careful and appropriate handling (safe burial) of the deceased (WHO, 2015d). Now that it has been documented that Ebola can be spread to other countries in the world, many nations have instituted entry screening, exit screening, or both to possibly identify active infection among travelers. This is especially true regarding international travel (CDC, 2015f; Koonin et al., 2015).

ENTEROHAEMORRHAGIC *ESCHERICHIA COLI* (EHEC)

Escherichia coli (*E. coli*) comprise a large and diverse group of bacteria that live in the intestines of healthy humans and warm-blooded animals, identified by six pathotypes: Shiga toxin-producing *E. coli* (STEC), Enterotoxigenic *E. coli* (ETEC), Enteropathogenic *E. coli* (EPEC), Enteroaggregative *E. coli* (EAEC), Enteroinvasive *E. coli* (EIEC), and Diffusely adherent *E. coli* (DAEC). Most of these bacteria are less likely to cause severe illness, but one strain creates a powerful toxin that can cause serious illness. Known as Shiga toxin-producing *Escherichia coli* (STEC), this pathogenic organism also identified as Verocytotoxin-producing *E. coli* (VTEC) and Enterohaemorrhagic *E. coli* (EHEC) has been isolated from the feces of cattle, sheep, pigs, deer, and poultry, and produces toxins (verotoxins) similar to those made by the *Shigella dysenteriae* organism. STEC was first identified in 1982 during an outbreak of diarrheal disease (*E. coli* O157:H7) in the United States. People generally become infected by consuming contaminated food or water; hence, *E. coli* is considered to be a foodborne illness. Worldwide, it is difficult to estimate the number of people affected each year by foodborne diseases, as many individuals do not see a physician. However, a recent approximation from the United States for *E. coli* O157 (63,153 cases in 2013) indicates that the total burden of this illness cost $271,418,690. This figure includes acute and chronic medical costs, lost productivity, and premature death. In resource-poor countries, the incidence is even higher and suggests there may be underlying issues with food safety in affected regions where outbreaks are frequent (Bardiau, Taminiau, Duprez, Labrozzo, & Mainil, 2012; CDC, 2015g; U.S. Department of Agriculture, Economic Research Services, 2014; WHO, 2011b).

E. coli O157:H7/STEC symptoms include abdominal cramps, diarrhea that can progress to bloody diarrhea (hemorrhagic colitis), and sometimes fever (usually less than 101°F/38.5°C) and vomiting. Most persons affected recover within five to seven days. However, a small percentage of people will develop hemolytic uremic syndrome (HUS), especially vulnerable populations such as children and the elderly. Other populations at risk include persons with compromised immune systems and multiple chronic diseases. HUS is associated with acute renal failure and can cause other problems, such as seizure, stroke, and coma (CDC, 2015g; WHO, 2011b).

The primary source for transmission of the bacteria is consumption of undercooked meats, raw milk (unpasteurized), fecal contamination of water and foods (associated with fecal polluted drinking and recreational waters), cross-contamination during food preparation (using the same food surface to prepare raw meats and uncooked foods without proper disinfection between types of food preparation tasks), and person-to-person spread (oral-fecal route). A clear example of transmission via a food source was the devastating outbreak of hemorrhagic *E. coli* (O104:H4) in Germany in 2011. This foodborne organism moved through the food chain to the dinner table and produced a large number of HUS cases and resulted in 54 fatalities. The cause was contaminated Fenugreek sprouts that were produced at a farm in Germany (Steiner, 2014; WHO, 2011b).

Prevention education related to food safety is important to prevent *E. coli* infection. Also, improving surveillance efforts can lower the response time by public health officials when new cases are identified. Controls at all stages of the food chain (agriculture, processing and manufacturing, and food preparation—commercial and domestic) can make a difference in the number of cases identified each year (CDC, 2015g; WHO, 2011b).

INFLUENZA (SEASONAL)

Influenza (flu) is a respiratory disease caused by influenza viruses that infect the nose, throat, and lungs of people and can cause serious illness, leading to hospitalization and/or death among very young and elderly persons. Three types of influenza viruses typically circulate annually: A, B, and C. Human influenza viruses A and B cause seasonal epidemics of disease almost every fall and winter. Globally, annual epidemics of A and B result in approximately three to five million cases of severe illness and 250,000 to 500,000 deaths. Influenza type C infection causes a mild respiratory illness and is not thought to lead to epidemics. Current subtypes of influenza A viruses circulating among people include influenza A(H1N1) and influenza A(H3N2). In spring 2009, influenza A (H1N1) caused the first influenza pandemic in more than 40 years (CDC, 2015h; WHO, 2014d).

The flu virus can be transmitted when someone who is infected coughs, sneezes, or talks; infected droplets travel through the air and another person inhales them. People with flu can spread the virus to others up to 6 feet away. Less often, a person might become infected from touching surfaces or objects that have the flu virus on them and then touching his or her own mouth or nose. Transmission of the virus can occur one day before symptoms become evident and as long as seven days after someone gets sick (CDC, 2015h; WHO, 2014d).

Flu cases are typically diagnosed based on clinical symptoms, but laboratory tests that confirm infection are available. Rapid testing can detect influenza viruses within 15 minutes. Some rapid tests are approved for use in outpatient settings, whereas others must be performed in a moderately complex clinical laboratory. These tests detect influenza A only or both influenza A and B viruses. However, rapid tests do not provide information about subtypes. Rapid testing during an acute respiratory disease outbreak can help determine whether influenza virus is the underlying cause of the illnesses. For surveillance purposes and development of vaccines, collecting and culturing nasal and throat specimens are important because only culture isolates can provide specific information about circulating strains and subtypes of influenza viruses (CDC, 2015h; WHO, 2014d).

Seasonal flu is characterized by a sudden onset of high fever, cough (usually dry), headache, muscle and joint pain, fatigue, sore throat, and runny nose. Most people recover from fever and other symptoms within a week without requiring medical attention, but among high-risk individuals, the flu can cause severe illness and death. The highest risks of complications occur among children younger than 2 years of age, adults age 65 or older, and people with certain medical conditions such as chronic heart, lung, kidney, liver, blood, and metabolic diseases such as diabetes, or persons with weakened immune systems. Other serious complications include bacterial pneumonia, ear infections, sinus infections, and dehydration. The time from infection to the development of symptoms (incubation period) is approximately two days (CDC, 2015h; WHO, 2014d).

The best way to prevent flu and possible severe outcomes is annual vaccination, at least by October. Safe and effective flu vaccines have been available and used for more than 60 years. Seasonal flu vaccines are updated every year based on information about which influenza viruses are causing illness and how well the previous season's vaccine protects against the newly identified virus. These recommendations are made by the WHO Global Influenza Surveillance and Response System, which monitors the influenza viruses circulating in populations. WHO recommends specific influenza vaccine compositions for vaccine production, and each country then makes a decision about licensing the vaccines. In addition to flu vaccine, antiviral medications are recommended for use as adjunct treatment for hospitalized individuals and outpatients who are at high risk for complications. There are two classes of medications: adamantanes (amantadine and rimantadine) and neuraminidase (oseltamivir, zanamivir, peramivir, and laninamivir). Ideally, antivirals should be administered within 48 hours of the onset of symptoms (CDC, 2015h; Flannery et al., 2015; WHO, 2014d).

Traditional flu vaccines are trivalent (protects against influenza A H1N1 and H3N2 and an influenza B virus) and quadrivalent (protects against two influenza A viruses and two influenza B viruses). Flu vaccines can be administered in different forms, intramuscular injection (trivalent and quadrivalent), nasal spray (quadrivalent), and intradermal (quadrivalent). For persons who have sensitivity to eggs, there is a recombinant trivalent injection that is egg free. Traditional flu vaccine contains inactivated (killed) virus and is given by injection. It is recommended for people six months of age and older and makes up the majority of the vaccine supply. A high-dose vaccine for people 65 years of age and older is also available (trivalent). The intradermal (microinjection under the skin) vaccine is only for persons 18 to 64 years of age. Nasal spray flu vaccine is made with live, weakened flu viruses and is approved for use in healthy people 2 to 49 years of age and women who are not pregnant. Pregnant women should receive flu vaccine, as studies have shown that after vaccination pregnant women have developed protective antibodies and confer immunity to their newborns. Pregnant women have been receiving flu vaccine for several decades. Antibodies that protect against influenza viruses usually develop about two weeks after receiving the vaccine. Other prevention measures to decrease transmission of the flu virus include frequent handwashing, using hand sanitizers, and covering the mouth and nose when coughing or sneezing (CDC, 2015h; Macias, Precisos, & Falsey, 2015; WHO, 2014d).

VIRAL HEPATITIS

The first WHO World Hepatitis Day was held on July 28, 2011. It was established to increase awareness and understanding of viral hepatitis and hepatitis immunization programs. Hepatitis is a general term meaning inflammation of the liver. Five main hepatitis viruses exist, referred to as types A, B, C, D, and E; however, the most common types are A, B, and C. These three types of hepatitis are of paramount concern because of the burden of illness and death they cause and the potential for outbreaks and epidemics. Worldwide, approximately 57% of liver cirrhosis cases and 78% of primary liver cancers result from being infected with hepatitis B or C (WHO, 2013a; World Hepatitis Alliance and WHO, 2015).

Hepatitis A

Hepatitis A (HAV) is the most common form of viral hepatitis. It is estimated that 1.5 million cases of HAV infection occur annually. The virus is primarily spread person to person when an uninfected individual ingests a food or beverage that has been contaminated with stool of an infected person (oral-fecal route). Waterborne outbreaks can occur when there is inadequate sanitation or water is not treated properly. Depending on the environmental conditions, HAV can live outside of the human body for months (CDC, 2015i; Franco, Meleleo, Serino, Sorbara, & Zaratti, 2012; WHO, 2015f).

Geographic patterns of HAV infection can be characterized as high, intermediate, or low. Prevalence of disease is directly associated with hygienic and sanitary conditions. In resource-poor countries with less than adequate sanitation systems and hygienic practices, the lifetime risk of infection with HAV is 90%. Most infections occur in early childhood, and symptoms of the disease are minimal or nonexistent. After infection, immunity to the virus develops and epidemics are less likely to occur. Countries with intermediate levels of infection have transitional economies and variable sanitary conditions, so young children often avoid infection. This leads to higher HAV susceptibility rates within older age groups and creates the potential for an outbreak that cannot be well controlled. In countries with good sanitary systems and hygienic practices, HAV infection rates are low (Franco, Meleleo, Serino, Sorbara, & Zaratti, 2012; WHO, 2015f).

The symptoms of HAV range from mild to severe and can include fever, fatigue, loss of appetite, diarrhea, nausea, abdominal discomfort, dark-colored urine, and a yellowing of the skin and whites of the eyes (jaundice). Adults develop symptoms more often than children, and not everyone who is infected will have all of the symptoms. The incubation period for asymptomatic and symptomatic HAV infection ranges from 15 to 50 days (average is 28 days). There is no specific treatment for HAV infection and most people recover within weeks or months without complications. A diagnosis of HAV requires laboratory testing of the blood (CDC, 2015i; WHO, 2015a).

Improved sanitation, food safety, and immunization are the most effective ways to prevent the spread of HAV. Because HAV is transmitted primarily through the oral-fecal route, good personal hygiene is important. Recommended measures include good handwashing or use of a hand sanitizer after using the bathroom, changing diapers, and before preparing or eating food. Safe and effective HAV vaccine has been available since 1992. The vaccine is recommended for all children at age one, persons at increased risk for HAV infection (immunosuppressed people and persons with chronic liver disease), and any person wishing to obtain immunity. Based on current scientific evidence, lifelong immunity occurs after a complete HAV series (two doses) is obtained (CDC, 2015i; Hendrickx, Vorsters, & Van Damme, 2012; WHO, 2015f).

Hepatitis B

Hepatitis B virus (HBV) causes a potentially life-threatening liver infection that is transmitted through contact with infected blood or other body fluids (i.e., semen, vaginal fluids, and saliva). Modes of transmission include having sex with an infected partner; sharing needles, syringes, or other drug paraphernalia; acquiring needle sticks or sharp instrument exposures; sharing items such as razors or toothbrushes with an infected person; and vertical transmission from mother to baby at birth. This virus is not transmitted through casual contact. HBV is 50 to 100 times more infectious than HIV; it can survive outside the body for seven days and still be capable of causing infection. HBV infection is considered an occupational hazard for healthcare workers (CDC, 2015j; WHO, 2015g).

HBV infection can cause both acute and chronic disease. Symptoms of acute disease include fever, fatigue, loss of appetite, nausea, vomiting, abdominal pain, jaundice, dark-colored urine, clay-colored bowel movements, and joint pain. After exposure to HBV, symptoms usually appear within 60 to 150 days (average is 90 days). Symptoms typically resolve in a few weeks, but can persist up to six months. The likelihood that HBV infection will become chronic depends on the age at which a person becomes infected. Ninety percent of infants and 25 to 50% of children aged 1 to 5 years are more likely to develop a chronic infection, whereas 95% of healthy adults who become infected with HBV will recover within the first year and not become chronically infected (CDC, 2015j; WHO, 2015g).

Complications of chronic HBV infection include cirrhosis of the liver and primary liver cancer. To diagnose HBV and determine the phase of infection (acute versus chronic), blood testing is required. For acute HBV infections, no curative medications are available; instead, treatment is supportive and based on symptoms. Persons with chronic HBV infection require long-term follow-up to assess progression of the disease, and the infection can be treated with medications that include interferon and antiviral drugs (CDC, 2015j; WHO, 2015g).

Worldwide, approximately 350 million have chronic HBV infections and more than 600,000 people die each year from the disease. HBV prevalence is highest in Sub-Saharan Africa and East Asia. High rates of chronic infection are also found in the Amazon and southern parts of eastern and central Europe. In the Middle East and Indian subcontinent, an estimated 2 to 5% of the general public is chronically infected as compared to less than 1% of the population in Western Europe and North America (Papasterfiou, Lombardi, MacDonald, & Tosochatzis, 2015; WHO, 2015g).

Vaccine is the backbone of HBV prevention. WHO recommends that all infants receive the vaccine as soon as possible after birth. After the initial dose, two or three doses are needed to complete the vaccination series. Implementation of universal vaccination for infants has lowered the prevalence of HBV in most countries. As of 2013, 93 member states from the World Health Assembly vaccinate infants against HBV at birth and 183 member states include the vaccine in their vaccination schedule. Global coverage with three doses of HBV vaccine is estimated to be at 82% and as high as 92% in the Western Pacific. In 95% of infants, children, and young adults who receive the series, protective antibody levels are attained. This protection lasts at least 20 years and may be lifelong. Any unvaccinated individual who is seeking protection from HBV should receive the vaccination, especially persons traveling to parts of the world where the virus is prevalent or working in healthcare settings where exposure to HBV-infected body fluids can occur (CDC, 2015j; WHO, 2015g, 2015h).

Hepatitis C

Similar to HBV infection, hepatitis C virus (HCV) infection is a contagious liver disease that can range in severity from a mild illness to a serious, lifelong disease. HCV is spread when blood from a person who is infected enters the body of someone who is not infected. The most common forms of transmission include receiving a contaminated blood transfusion, blood product, or organ transplant; injection with a contaminated syringe, needle-stick injuries in healthcare settings, or injection drug use; and inadequate sterilization of medical equipment. The virus is less commonly transmitted through tattooing, sexual exposure, perinatally from mother to child, and sharing of personal items contaminated with infected blood (CDC, 2015k; WHO, 2015i).

HCV can be classified as either acute or chronic. Acute HCV usually occurs within the first six months after someone is exposed to the virus. During the acute phase of HCV disease, most people (70%–80%) have no symptoms. When symptoms do occur, they can include loss of appetite, vague abdominal discomfort, nausea and vomiting, fever, fatigue, dark-colored urine, clay-colored feces, joint pain, and jaundice. Approximately 75 to 85% of people who become infected with HCV develop a chronic infection. People living with chronic HCV often go many years without having symptoms. However, when symptoms appear, it usually indicates the presence of advanced liver disease such as fibrosis, cirrhosis, or liver cancer (CDC, 2015k; WHO, 2015i).

HCV is recognized as a major global health problem. However, the true burden of disease is not well known because the ability to collect epidemiological data varies by country and region. WHO estimates that 130 to 150 million people around the world are living with chronic HCV. This represents 2 to 3% of the world's population. Annually, three to four million people are newly infected and more than 500,000 people die from HCV-related liver disease. HCV transmission in resource-poor countries usually results from exposure to contaminated blood and blood products in healthcare and community settings; whereas in countries with adequate resources, transmission is associated with injection drug use (CDC, 2015k; Gower, Estes, Blach, Razavi-Shearer, & Razavi, 2014; WHO, 2015i).

HCV testing is recommended in select populations based on demography, prior exposures, high-risk behaviors, and medical conditions. This includes people who inject drugs, recipients of infected blood products, or invasive procedures in healthcare facilities with inadequate infection control practices, persons who received long-term hemodialysis treatment, children born to mothers infected with HCV, HIV-infected individuals, individuals with signs or symptoms of liver disease, and people who have sexual partners who are infected with HCV. In the United States, it is recommended that every person born between 1945 and 1965 (baby boomers) be tested. This is because people in this birth cohort are five times more likely than other adults to be infected with HCV. In fact, 75% of adults in the United States living with HCV were born during these years. The reasons why this age group has the highest rates of HCV are not completely understood (CDC, 2013b; 2015k; WHO, 2015i).

There are six genotypes (strains) of HCV and over 50 subtypes. Their distribution varies by geographical region. Globally, genotype 1 is most common and accounts for 46% of all infections. It is primarily found in Australia, Europe, Latin America, and North America. Genotype 3 accounts for 22% of the worldwide HCV infections and 40% of the infections in Asia. In the Middle East and North Africa, genotype 4 is most common (71%) (Gower, Estes, Blach, Razavi-Shearer, & Razavi, 2014).

HCV infection can be detected through blood testing. Typically, an individual will first be screened to see if they have developed antibodies to the virus. An antibody is a protein that his produced by the body in response to a virus. If the test is antibody positive, the person has been exposed to HCV at some time in his or her life and a second test (HCV ribonucleic acid [RNA] test) to confirm that the virus is still present is needed. If the HCV RNA test is negative, no further testing is required. However, if the HCV RNA test returns positive, additional testing is needed to assess for liver damage and identify the genotype of the HCV strain. The degree of liver damage and virus genotype are used to guide treatment decisions and management of the disease (American Association for the Study of Liver Diseases, Infectious Disease Society of America & International Antiviral Society—USA, 2015; CDC, 2013; WHO, 2015i).

The treatment goal for HCV infection is to obtain a sustained virologic response (SVR), which can also be called a cure. Historically, the standard medical care was 24 to 48 weeks of treatment that required weekly injections of interferon along with oral antiviral medications. Approximately 50% of persons receiving treatment were cured, but the medications caused frequent and sometimes life-threatening side effects. In 2013, more effective and safer antiviral drugs were developed to treat HCV, and in 2014 the FDA approved interferon-free treatments. Clinical trials have shown that these new medications achieve a SVR in 80 to 95% of people after 12 to 24 weeks. Unfortunately, the cost for these newer drugs is quite high (approximately $84,000 for a 12-week regimen) and likely to make access difficult. On a more positive note, treatment for HCV continues to evolve rapidly and evidence-based guidance about HCV testing, linkage to care, and treatment is continuously being updated by the American Association for the Study of Liver Diseases and the Infectious Disease Society of America (American Association for the Study of Liver Diseases, Infectious Disease Society of America & International Antiviral Society—USA, 2015; CDC, 2015k; Graham & Swan, 2015; WHO, 2015i).

Currently, no vaccine is available that can prevent HCV infection. Therefore, prevention of HCV infection relies on education to alter risk factors and behaviors associated with contracting the disease (e.g., injection drug use) and universal HCV screening of blood and organ donors. In persons already infected, the focus should be on linkage to care and early and appropriate treatment along with changing or modifying behaviors (e.g., alcohol consumption) that contribute to liver disease and subsequent liver failure (WHO, 2015).

SYPHILIS

Despite the existence of effective prevention measures and relatively inexpensive treatment options, syphilis remains a global problem. It is estimated that 11 to 12 million adults become infected each year, mostly in resource-poor countries in Sub-Saharan Africa and Southeast Asia. There are also between 700,000 to 1.5 million congenital syphilis cases that occur annually with more than 50% resulting in an adverse event such as a miscarriage or stillbirth (Ham, Lin, Newman, Wijesooriya, & Kamb, 2015; Stamm, 2015).

Syphilis is a systemic disease that is caused by the bacterium *Treponema pallidum*. Because of the enormous variation in disease symptoms, it is sometimes called the "Great Imitator." Depending on the stage of the disease, syphilis can be characterized as primary, secondary, latent, or late. In the primary stage of syphilis, a painless, spontaneously resolving sore (called a chancre) appears. The chancre develops where the organism enters the body. If syphilis is not treated in the primary stage, it becomes a chronic disease (CDC, 2014c; Stamm, 2015).

The development of a rash on one or more parts of the body characterizes the secondary stage. The rash usually does not cause itching and may be so faint that it is not noticed. Other signs and symptoms of secondary syphilis can include fever, swollen lymph glands, sore throat, patchy hair loss, headaches, weight loss, muscle aches, and fatigue. The symptoms of secondary syphilis will also resolve without treatment (CDC, 2014c; Stamm, 2015).

Latent (hidden) syphilis begins after the primary and secondary symptoms of syphilis disappear. Early latent syphilis is when the infection occurred within the last 12 months. Late latent syphilis is when the infection occurred more than 12 months ago and can last for years. Late-stage syphilis develops in about 15% of people who have not been treated and can appear 10 to 20 years after the infection was first acquired. In late-stage syphilis, the disease can damage the brain, nervous system, blood vessels, liver, bones, and joints. Signs and symptoms of late-stage syphilis include difficulty in coordinating muscle movements, paralysis, numbness, gradual blindness, and dementia (CDC, 2014c; Stamm, 2015).

Syphilis can invade the nervous system at any stage of infection. Individuals can be asymptomatic but can also develop headaches, altered behavior, and movement disorders that resemble neurological diseases, such as Parkinson's or Huntington's. By examining material from a chancre using a special microscope or through blood testing, syphilis can be diagnosed. If an individual tests positive for syphilis, the person should also be tested for HIV and other sexually transmitted infections (CDC, 2014c; Morshed & Singh, 2015; Stamm, 2015).

Syphilis is primarily transmitted through vaginal, anal, or oral sexual contact, but a pregnant woman who is infected can transmit the infection to her fetus, causing congenital syphilis or an adverse pregnancy outcome such as low birth weight or fetal death. WHO estimates that 1.8 million pregnancies around the world are affected by syphilis annually and a large proportion go untreated. Analysis of multinational antenatal surveillance data found that two-thirds of adverse pregnancy outcomes due to syphilis occurred in women who had at least one antenatal care visit. These women were either not screened for syphilis or did not receive adequate treatment. The seroprevalence of women with syphilis attending antenatal clinics is estimated to be highest in Latin America and Africa. It is estimated that 20% of all pregnant women with syphilis do not obtain antenatal care. Ensuring universal access to early antenatal care is fundamental in eliminating congenital syphilis. Point-of-care rapid testing of pregnant women for syphilis and same-day treatment within existing antenatal care programs are cost-effective methods for reducing congenital syphilis in low-income regions of the world (Newman et al., 2013; Swartzendruber, Steiner, Adler, Kamb, & Newman, 2015; WHO, 2014e).

For the purposes of treatment, syphilis is divided into early syphilis (less than one year's duration) and late latent syphilis. A single intramuscular injection of Benzathine penicillin G (an antibiotic) will cure a person who has had syphilis for less than a year. Additional doses are needed to treat someone who has late latent syphilis. For people who are allergic to penicillin, another antibiotic, tetracycline, is available. Treatment will kill syphilis and prevent further damage, but will not repair any harm that has already been done. The best way to avoid transmission of syphilis is to abstain from sexual contact or be in a long-term mutually monogamous relationship with a partner who has been tested and is known to be uninfected. In lieu of abstinence or monogamy, using male or female condoms properly and consistently can reduce the risk of contracting syphilis (CDC, 2013c, 2014c; Stamm, 2014).

TUBERCULOSIS

Tuberculosis (TB) has often been considered a disease of poverty. This airborne illness is caused by *Mycobacterium tuberculosis* (Mtb). The acid-fast bacilli are spread through infected, aerosolized droplets from people who cough, sneeze, or talk with vigor. Other people may then breathe in the aerosolized droplets and become infected. The bacteria usually attack the lungs, but can attack other parts of the body such as the kidney, spine, or brain (CDC, 2012; WHO, 2015j).

It is important to differentiate between being infected with TB and having active disease. Someone who has been infected with TB has the bacteria in his or her body, but the immune system is protecting the person from the bacteria so the individual is not sick. This condition is called latent TB. In contrast, someone with active TB disease is sick and can spread the disease to others. Persons with active TB disease may develop a persistent cough, fatigue, weight loss, decreased appetite, fever, bloody sputum, and night sweats (CDC, 2012; WHO, 2015j).

Approximately one-third of the world's population is infected with the TB bacillus. Around 10% of people who are infected with TB become sick or infectious at some time in their lives. Between 1990 and 2013, the prevalence and mortality rates of TB decreased by 41 and 45%, respectively. Despite downward trends in disease prevalence and mortality, there were an estimated 9 million people who became ill with TB and 1.5 million died in 2013. TB is one of the top five causes of death in women 15 to 44 years of age. It is second only to HIV/AIDS as the greatest killer due to a single infectious agent (WHO, 2014f, 2015j).

Globally, more than half (56%) of the new TB cases in 2013 were in Southeast Asia and Western Pacific regions and 25% were in Africa. India and China accounted for 24% and 11% of total cases, respectively. Among the 9 million TB cases reported, approximately one million occurred in people who were also HIV positive. Persons with compromised immune systems, such as people living with HIV, malnutrition, and diabetes or people using tobacco, have a much higher risk of becoming ill from TB (WHO, 2014f).

TB infection can be detected through a skin (Mantoux) or blood test (interferon-gamma release assays or IGRAs). If someone has a positive test for TB, it means that the individual has been infected with the TB pathogen, but does not indicate that a person has an active disease. Additional tests (chest X-ray and sputum cultures) are needed to confirm a diagnosis of TB disease. In 2010, WHO endorsed the first rapid test that identifies TB infection. The test also identifies whether the bacteria is resistant to the antibiotic rifampin, a primary drug used in the treatment of TB. The test simultaneously answers both questions in about 2 hours while traditional methods to identify antibiotic-resistant TB can take one to three months. The molecular test, *Xpert MTB/RIF Assay* (Cepheid), is also simpler to perform than previous tests used for detecting TB and drug-resistant strains (CDC, 2012; WHO, 2014f).

Treatment for TB depends on whether a person has latent or active disease. The most common treatment for latent TB is six to nine months of isoniazid (INH). This regimen kills bacteria that are currently not causing any damage; if left untreated, there is potential for illness in the future. In contrast, if an individual has active TB disease, a combination of medications is used for six to nine months. The most common treatment is INH in addition to three other drugs (rifampin, pyrazinamide, and ethambutol). In 2013, 86% of all new TB cases were treated successfully (CDC, 2012; Chee, Sester, Zhang, & Lange, 2012; WHO, 2015j).

It is very important that people who have TB disease finish their medicine and take the medications exactly as prescribed. If the drugs are stopped too soon, the individual can become sick again. If the drugs are not taken correctly, the TB bacteria that are still alive may become resistant to the drugs being used for treatment. TB that is resistant to drugs is harder and more expensive to treat (CDC, 2012; WHO, 2015j).

Multidrug-resistant TB (MDR-TB) is defined as the disease caused by TB bacilli that are resistant to at least INH and rifampin, the two most powerful anti-TB medications. About 480,000 people worldwide developed MDR-TB in 2013. MDR-TB is treatable but requires extensive pharmacological treatment (up to two years) with second-line TB medications that are more expensive than the first-line drugs. Almost 50% of the global burden of MDR-TB is found in India, China, and the Russian Federation. Extensively drug-resistant TB (XDR-TB) is a subset of MDR-TB in which the strains of TB bacteria are resistant to several of the best second-line drugs. It is estimated that 9% of MDR-TB cases in 2013 had XDR-TB (WHO, 2014f, 2015j).

TB is largely a preventable disease, with adequate ventilation being the most important measure to prevent its transmission. In countries that have adequate financial resources, hospitals and clinics take precautions to prevent the spread of TB by using ultraviolet light to sterilize the air, as well as special filters, special respirators, and masks. In hospitals, people with TB are isolated in negative pressure rooms with controlled ventilation and airflow until they can no longer spread the TB bacteria. In parts of the world where TB is endemic, WHO recommends that infants receive a vaccine called bacille Calmette-Guérin (BCG), which is made from a live weakened bacterium related to Mtb. The vaccine protects children from miliary TB and TB meningitis. The United States has never used mass immunization of BCG and instead relies on the detection and treatment of latent tuberculosis. One of the highest priorities of TB research is the development of vaccines that are more efficacious for preventing TB than BCG (Pitt, Blankley, McShane, & O'Garra, 2013; WHO, 2013b, 2015j).

Directly observed treatment—short course (DOTS) is the internationally recommended strategy for TB control and is recognized as being highly efficient and cost-effective. It was launched in 1994 after WHO declared the TB epidemic to be a global public health emergency. DOTS was created based on five key elements: (1) political commitment with increased and sustained financing; (2) case detection through quality assured technology; (3) standardized treatment with supervision and patient support; (4) an effective drug supply and management system; and (5) monitoring and evaluation system and impact measurement. The fundamental goals of DOTS are to stop TB at the source, halt spread of the disease, avert development of MDR-TB, and prevent complications that occur (CDC, 2012; Frieden & Sbarbaro, 2007; Lienhardt et al., 2012; WHO, n.d.a).

The "Stop TB Partnership" is a global movement that was built on the DOTS program. It was established in 2001 to help eliminate TB as a public health problem and ultimately eradicate the disease on a worldwide basis. The mission of the organization is to ensure that every TB patient has access to effective diagnosis, treatment and cure; stop transmission of TB; reduce the inequitable social and economic toll of TB; and develop and implement new preventive, diagnostic, and therapeutic tools and strategies to stop TB. The partnership is a network of more than 1,300 international organizations, countries, donors from the public and private sectors, governmental agencies and programs, and individuals committed to achieving the program's vision and mission. An important aim of the program is to decrease the global incidence of TB disease to less than one case per million persons by 2050. If this aim is reached, TB as a global health problem will be eliminated (Stop TB Partnership, 2015; WHO, 2015k).

HUMAN IMMUNODEFICIENCY VIRUS/ACQUIRED IMMUNE DEFICIENCY SYNDROME

Human immunodeficiency virus (HIV) is a retrovirus that infects cells of the immune system, destroying or impairing their function. There are two forms of the virus: HIV-1 and HIV-2. Compared to HIV-1, HIV-2 is much less prevalent and is found primarily among people living in West Africa or countries such as France and Portugal, which have large West African immigrant populations. The most advanced stage of HIV infection is acquired immunodeficiency syndrome (AIDS). During this stage of infection, the immune system becomes extremely weak and is unable to fight off other infections and diseases. Many of these illnesses, such as pneumocystis jirovecii pneumonia, cytomegalovirus disease, and esophageal candidiasis, only occur in people who are immunocompromised and are often called opportunistic infections (CDC, 2015l; WHO, 2015l).

A type of chimpanzee in West Africa has been identified as the source of HIV infection in humans. Scientists believe that the chimpanzee version of the immunodeficiency virus (called simian immunodeficiency virus [SIV]) was transmitted to humans and mutated into HIV when these chimpanzees were hunted for their meat and people came into contact with infected blood. Over decades, the virus slowly spread across Africa and later into other parts of the world (CDC, 2015l; Maartens, Celum, & Lewin, 2014).

HIV is transmitted through unprotected sexual intercourse (anal or vaginal), contaminated blood, sharing of contaminated injecting-drug equipment, and from a mother to her infant during pregnancy, childbirth, and breastfeeding. Globally, the majority of new HIV infections occurs through sexual transmission. There is now evidence that male circumcision is associated with a reduced risk of sexual transmission because circumcised males harbor fewer bacteria after removal of the foreskin. Consequently, WHO and the Joint United Nations Programme on HIV/AIDS (UNAIDS) recommend voluntary adult male circumcision in areas where the rates of HIV infection are high and prevalence of circumcision is low. Sharing contaminated drug-injecting equipment is the primary mode of transmission in countries throughout Eastern Europe and parts of Asia. Many countries in this region do not have effective health education programs in place that help reduce the risk of acquiring the disease (CDC, 2015l; Rosario, Kasabwala, & Sadeghi-nejad, 2013; Sgaier, Reed, Thoms, & Njeuhemeli, 2014; UNAIDS, 2013; WHO, 2015l).

In 2014, there were an estimated 36.9 million people around the world living with HIV/AIDS. Approximately 2 million people were newly infected with HIV in 2014, but this is significantly less than the 3.1 million new infections in 2000. This decline represents a 35% decrease in the number of new infections worldwide. An estimated 1.2 million AIDS-related deaths occurred in 2014; however, this represents a 41% drop since 2004 (Beyrer & Karim, 2013; UNAIDS, 2014).

Despite the overall decline in the number of new HIV infections, examining the global HIV/AIDS epidemic from a regional perspective highlights areas that are experiencing declines, and areas where the numbers are rising. For example, Sub-Saharan Africa accounts for 66% of the new HIV infections; however, incidence of the disease declined by 41% between 2000 and 2014. The rate of new infections in Asia and the Pacific declined 31% between 2000 and 2014. China, Indonesia, and India account for 78% of the new infections in this region. When examining the epidemic in Western and Central Europe and North America, the United States accounts for more than half of the new HIV infections in these parts of the world. In Latin America and the Caribbean, the rate of new infections declined by 17 and 50%, respectively.

Eastern Europe and Central Asia's rate of new HIV infections rose 30% between 2000 and 2014. Sex workers and injection drug use are driving factors in the spread of HIV in this region. The Middle East and North Africa are also experiencing a rise in the number of new infections, 26% between 2000 and 2014. This region of the world has the lowest number of people receiving medications that can reduce the amount of virus in body fluids, which ultimately decreases transmission (Beyrer & Karim, 2013; Maartens, Celum, & Lewin, 2014; UNAIDS, 2014; Vermund, 2014).

To improve access to HIV prevention and care, WHO and UNAIDS issued guidance on provider-initiated testing and counseling (PITC) for HIV infection at all healthcare encounters. The recommendation for PITC was based on worldwide evidence suggesting that many opportunities to provide HIV testing and counseling (HTC) are being missed. HTC is a critical entry point to care for people infected with HIV and essential for prevention of mother-to-child HIV transmission. PITC may include either an opt-in or opt-out option. The opt-out approach, where an individual who does not want the HIV test declines it, is more common than the opt-in option. Research findings support PITC and have found that it improves HIV testing rates within healthcare settings (Kennedy et al., 2013; WHO & UNAIDS, 2007).

Over time, HIV testing has become quicker and less invasive. Rapid testing allows clients to receive results on the day of the test. This is important in situations and settings where clients do not return for test results. These tests use oral fluid, urine, and finger-stick blood samples versus the collection of blood by venipuncture. In 2013, the U.S. Preventive Services Task Force (USPSTF) recommended that healthcare providers screen and test all adolescents and adults ages 15 to 65 years for HIV infection. Younger adolescents and older adults who are at increased risk should also be screened and tested. The USPSTF also recommends testing all pregnant women for HIV, including those who present to the hospital in labor and their HIV status is unknown (CDC, 2015m; Moyer & USPSTF, 2013).

Prior to 1996, scientists estimated that half of all HIV-positive people would develop AIDS within 10 years after becoming infected with HIV. This time varied greatly from person to person and depended on many factors, including a person's health status and health-related behaviors. Since 1996, however, the introduction of antiretroviral therapy (ART) regimens has dramatically changed the progression of HIV infection to AIDS and transitioned AIDS from a death sentence to a chronic illness. More than 25 medications are currently available for treatment, although not all countries have access to these drugs. Nonetheless, the overall decline in the number of deaths reflects increased availability of ART on a worldwide basis. Medical treatments are also available that can prevent or cure some of the illnesses or opportunistic infections associated with HIV/AIDS, but these treatments do not cure HIV/AIDS. As with other diseases, early detection allows for more treatment options and implementation of preventive healthcare measures (Maartens, Celum, & Lewin, 2014; Panel on Antiretroviral Guidelines for Adults and Adolescents, 2015; UNAIDS, 2013).

An individual's viral load is the single greatest risk factor for HIV transmission. ART suppresses the HIV viral load in blood and genital fluids, which decreases the risk of transmitting the virus to others. For a number of years, there has been growing evidence about the benefits of HIV treatment as a prevention method. Treating an HIV-infected individual not only improves the person's health, it also reduces the risk of viral transmission. The current campaign to give everyone ARTs for HIV disease is known as Treatment as Prevention (TasP) (CDC, 2013d; Cohen et al., 2011; Kavanagh et al., 2015; WHO, 2012, 2015m).

Oral HIV pre-exposure prophylaxis (PrEP) is another approach being used to decrease the spread of HIV. This prevention method provides people who do not have HIV the opportunity to reduce their risk of infection by taking a pill. The pill contains two medications (tenofovir and emtricitabine) that are used to treat HIV and must be taken every day to be effective. PrEP should be considered for all HIV negative persons who are at substantial risk for becoming infected. This includes anyone who is HIV negative and is having a sexual relationship with someone who is HIV positive, people who are not in a monogamous relationship, men or women who do not regularly use condoms or have been diagnosed with a sexually transmitted disease in the last six months, and injection drug users who share their drug paraphernalia. When PrEP is combined with other prevention methods, such as consistent condom use and risk reduction, it can provide greater protection than when used alone (Cohen et al., 2015; CDC, 2014d; McMahon et al., 2014; WHO, 2015m).

Access to treatment, care, and support services has improved significantly around the world. In March 2015, an estimated 15 million people were accessing ART as compared to 13.6 million in 2014. In 2010, only 23% of all adults living with HIV were able to access ARTs, but in 2014, approximately 41% were receiving treatment. In addition, 73% of pregnant women living with HIV had access to ARTs to prevent the transmission of HIV to their babies. Between 2000 and 2014, new HIV infections among children were reduced by 58%. From 1996 to 2012, ART therapy prevented 6.6 million AIDS-related deaths worldwide. Efforts to reach universal access for HIV treatment and care are ongoing (UNAIDS, 2014; WHO, 2014g).

Preventing new HIV infections is an urgent global priority, but there is no single solution to this problem. A combination of biomedical, behavioral, and structural strategies that promote risk reduction is needed for both HIV-positive and HIV-negative individuals. These strategies must target individual, group, and societal levels of prevention. Despite global efforts to address HIV-related stigma and discrimination, these issues continue to be challenging. To address these problems, countries have been urged to scale up their stigma and discrimination laws, build the capacity of their HIV-related service providers, and empower those individuals who are infected with and/or affected by HIV. Decriminalization of sex workers, people who use drugs, men who have sex with men, and transgender individuals will also help break down obstacles to effective worldwide HIV prevention strategies (Delva & Karim, 2014; UNAIDS, 2013; WHO, 2014g).

INFECTIOUS DISEASE SURVEILLANCE

An effective and comprehensive global disease surveillance and response capability is required to identify and control infectious diseases. Global disease surveillance includes disease detection through a mature information collection system that can ensure data quality, analyze and interpret data, and get information to those individuals who can act on it and facilitate a response that will deal with the problem effectively. To achieve these goals, surveillance and response capabilities must be developed based on a foundation of skills in areas such as case detection, epidemiology, data analysis and interpretation, laboratory diagnostic confirmation, and appropriate response (Gorman, 2014; Jombart et al., 2014; Pinner et al., 2015).

The crux of infectious disease surveillance is to identify disease occurrence and undertake activities to prevent those diseases from becoming a threat to global health. Disease surveillance is an essential prerequisite for establishing local, national, regional, and global priorities; planning, mobilizing, and allocating resources; detecting epidemics early; and monitoring and evaluating disease prevention and control programs. WHO has long-term data on numerous infectious disease epidemics and has the mandate to lead and coordinate the international effort in global surveillance and response (Louis, 2012; Troppy, Haney, Cocoros, Cranston, & DeMaria, 2014; WHO, n.d.b.).

SUMMARY

This chapter provided an overview of the more common infectious diseases that are found around the world. These descriptive summaries serve as a foundation for understanding how infectious diseases fit into the context of global health. Learning about infectious diseases can potentially improve global health and better prepare the world to cope with future epidemics.

Study Questions

1. Discuss, giving examples of how infectious diseases can spread in a rapid manner.
2. How do the diagnoses and treatments of infectious diseases differ globally and culturally within different regions of the world?
3. How does economics affect a country's ability to prevent and treat infections?
4. Why is it necessary for developed countries to share their knowledge and technology with developing countries?
5. Relate the role of climate and the global spread of infectious diseases.

Case Study 1 on Infectious Disease

Mr. S., a recently retired 67-year-old male living in an urban area, has decided to become more involved in his passion, home renovations. This summer he has been spending many hours on several external home projects, repairing siding, and performing other home-related tasks. The weather had been unusually hot and wet this year, so, he was really grateful for the bright sunny days. To feel comfortable while working, Mr. S. wore short-sleeve shirts and on many occasions removed his shirt while working. In late September, he started to feel fatigued for no apparent reason but kept this information from his wife. One Saturday afternoon while his friend was visiting for his birthday, he noticed that he was having difficulty walking and was experiencing some involuntary movements. Mr. S. admitted that he had a stiff neck and occasionally had headaches. His friend offered to take him to the hospital, where he was evaluated and admitted. After two days, the doctors concluded that Mr. S. probably had a stroke as evidenced by problems with walking and involuntary movements; however, the diagnostic data did not clearly support this conclusion. What was suspicious was that Mr. S. had a low-grade fever. Two days later, an infectious disease specialist was consulted; additional tests were ordered and a diagnosis of West Nile virus was confirmed.

Case Study 1 Questions

1. What may have put this 67-year-old male at risk for West Nile virus infection?
2. Which preventive measures could Mr. S. have taken to decrease his risk of disease?
3. What are some important facts about the epidemiology of West Nile disease?

Case Study 2 on Infectious Disease

Parsi is 25-year-old Indian female working on a graduate degree at the local university in southern India. She is upset because recently she has been recovering from a second bout of diarrhea illness within the past two months. Her doctor recommended over-the-counter medications for the diarrhea. Parsi was feeling frustrated because she really needed to return to her studies. During her most recent episode of illness, she experienced a weight loss of 15 pounds. Also, she had a low-grade fever and was feeling fatigued most of the time. In the past week she noticed neck pain and some swelling of the glands in her neck. At night she had a slight cough, which she found annoying. Parsi became exasperated and returned to the doctor, who did a chest X-ray and noted the swelling in her neck. The X-ray was positive for a problem in the upper portion of the left lung and a tuberculin skin test was administered. Two days later, the skin test was positive. Active tuberculosis (TB) disease was confirmed by the laboratory, which found tuberculosis organisms in Parsi's sputum specimens. Parsi was started on medication.

Case Study 2 Questions

1. What is important for Parsi and her family to be aware of now that she has been diagnosed with TB?
2. Why is it likely that Parsi developed TB?
3. What are some important facts related to taking TB medication?

Case Study 3 on Infectious Disease

Myra, a 26-year-old female, has been working in advertising at a local firm for the past two years and recently moved from her parents' home to a small apartment. She is delighted at finally being on her own. A male colleague at work had been asking her for a date for several weeks and she finally consented. Myra was very impressed with this young man and felt they had a lot in common. Over the next few months, the relationship became very serious and there was talk of marriage in the near future. Their relationship progressed to a sexual level. Myra felt that she had found her soul mate. Discussions about marriage became more serious, with the couple talking about starting a family soon after getting married.

Myra was having lunch with her best friend recently, when her friend informed Myra that she had seen Myra's boyfriend with another woman, and even disclosed the person's name. That evening Myra searched Facebook and discovered that her boyfriend and the other person were sharing intimate information with each other. Myra was devastated. She called her best friend and revealed that her relationship with the boyfriend had reached a sexual level but noted that they were not using condoms. Her friend encouraged her to see a doctor, as she had heard rumors that Myra's boyfriend was also having a sexual relationship with the other woman. Taking her friend's advice, Myra saw her doctor immediately. Following the exam, the doctor informed Myra that syphilis was suspected because of a small lesion near Myra's vaginal opening. A blood sample was taken and the diagnosis of syphilis confirmed. Myra was immediately treated.

Case Study 3 Questions

1. What should Myra keep in mind when engaging in a sexual relationship in the future?
2. What could have been the possible long-term consequences for Myra if her syphilis had not been diagnosed?
3. If Myra had not been diagnosed and had become pregnant, would there be concerns regarding the health of the unborn child?

References

American Association for the Study of Liver Diseases, Infectious Disease Society of America & International Antiviral Society—USA. (2015). *HCV Guidance: Recommendations for Testing, Managing, and Treating Hepatitis C*. Retrieved from http://hcvguidelines.org/full-report-view

Antinori, S., Galimberti, L., Milazzo, L., & Corbellino, M. (2013). Plasmodium knowlesi: The emerging zoonotic malaria parasite. *Acta Tropica, 125*, 191–201. doi:10.1016/j.actatropica.2012.10.008

Bardiau, M., Taminiau, B., Duprez, J., Labrozzo, S., & Mainil, J. G. (2012). Comparison between a bovine and a human enterohaemorragic Escherichia coli strain of serogroup 026 by suppressive subtractive hybridization reveals the presence of atypical factors in EHEC and EPEC strains. *FEMS Microbiology Letters, 330*, 132–139. doi:10.1111/j.1574-6968.2012.02542.x

Beyrer, C., & Karim, Q. A. (2013). The changing epidemiology of HIV in 2013. *Current Opinion in HIV/AIDS, 8*(4), 306–310. doi:10.1097/COH.0b013e328361f53a

Boone, S. A., & Gerba, C. P. (2007). Significance of fomites in the spread of respiratory and enteric viral disease. *Applied Environmental Microbiology, 73*, 1687–1696. doi:10.1128/AEM.02051-06

Campbell-Yesufu, O. T., & Gandhi, R. (2011). Update on human immunodeficiency virus (HIV) -2 infection. *Clinical Infectious Diseases, 52*(6), 780–787. doi:10.1093/cid/ciq248

Centers for Disease Control and Prevention. (2012). *Tuberculosis*. Retrieved from http://www.cdc.gov/tb/topic/basics/default.htm

Centers for Disease Control and Prevention. (2013a). *West Nile Virus in the United States: Guidelines for Surveillance, Prevention and Control*. Retrieved from http://www.cdc.gov/westnile/resources/pdfs/wnvguidelines.pdf

Centers for Disease Control and Prevention. (2013b). Testing for HCV infection: An update for clinicians and laboratories. *Morbidity and Mortality Weekly Report (MMWR), 62*(18), 362–365. Retrieved from http://www.cdc.gov/mmwr/preview/mmwrhtml/mm6218a5.htm?s_cid=mm6218a5_w

Centers for Disease Control and Prevention. (2013c). *Condoms and STDs: Fact sheet for public health personnel.* Retrieved from http://www.cdc.gov/condomeffectiveness/latex.html

Centers for Disease Control and Prevention. (2013d). *Prevention benefits of HIV treatment.* Retrieved from http://www.cdc.gov/hiv/prevention/research/tap/

Centers for Disease Control and Prevention. (2014a). *Cholera—Vibrio cholerae infection.* Retrieved from http://www.cdc.gov/cholera/index.html

Centers for Disease Control and Prevention. (2014b). *Clinical guidance: Dengue virus.* Retrieved from http://www.cdc.gov/dengue/clinicalLab/clinical.html

Centers for Disease Control and Prevention. (2014c). *Syphilis—CDC fact sheet (Detailed).* Retrieved from http://www.cdc.gov/std/syphilis/stdfact-syphilis-detailed.htm

Centers for Disease Control and Prevention. (2014d). *Preexposure prophylaxis for the prevention of HIV infection in the United States—2014.* Retrieved from http://www.cdc.gov/hiv/pdf/PrEPguidelines2014.pdf

Centers for Disease Control and Prevention. (2015a). *Division of vector-borne diseases.* Retrieved from http://www.cdc.gov/ncezid/dvbd/

Centers for Disease Control and Prevention. (2015b). *Dengue.* Retrieved from http://www.cdc.gov/Dengue/

Centers for Disease Control and Prevention. (2015c). *Malaria.* Retrieved from http://www.cdc.gov/malaria/

Centers for Disease Control and Prevention. (2015d). *Highly pathogenic Asian avian influenza A (H5N1) virus.* Retrieved from http://www.cdc.gov/flu/avianflu/h5n1-virus.htm

Centers for Disease Control and Prevention. (2015e). *West Nile virus.* Retrieved from http://www.cdc.gov/westnile/

Centers for Disease Control and Prevention. (2015f). *Ebola (Ebola virus disease).* Retrieved from http://www.cdc.gov/vhf/ebola/

Centers for Disease Control and Prevention. (2015g). *E. Coli (Escherichia coli).* Retrieved from http://www.cdc.gov/ecoli/

Centers for Disease Control and Prevention. (2015h). *Influenza (Flu).* Retrieved from http://www.cdc.gov/flu/

Centers for Disease Control and Prevention. (2015i). *Hepatitis A questions and answers for health professionals.* Retrieved from http://www.cdc.gov/hepatitis/hav/havfaq.htm#general

Centers for Disease Control and Prevention. (2015j). *Hepatitis B FAQs for health professionals.* Retrieved from http://www.cdc.gov/hepatitis/hbv/hbvfaq.htm

Centers for Disease Control and Prevention. (2015k). *Hepatitis C FAQs for health professionals.* Retrieved from http://www.cdc.gov/hepatitis/hcv/hcvfaq.htm#section1

Centers for Disease Control and Prevention. (2015l). *About HIV/AIDS.* Retrieved from http://www.cdc.gov/hiv/basics/whatishiv.html.

Centers for Disease Control and Prevention. (2015m). *HIV testing.* Retrieved from http://www.cdc.gov/hiv/testing/index.html

Chakarova, S. R., Dimitrov, K. M., & Chenchev, I. I. (2011). Etiology, epidemiology, clinical features and laboratory diagnostics of West Nile fever: A review. *Bulgarian Journal of Veterinary Medicine, 14*(2), 71–79. Retrieved from http://tru.uni-sz.bg/bjvm/BJVM%20June%202011%20p.71-79.pdf

Charles, R. C., Hilaire, I. J., Mayo-Smith, L. M., Teng, J. E., Jerome, J. E., Frank, M. F., . . . Harris, J. B. (2014). Immunogenicity of a killed bivalent (O1 and O139) whole cell oral Cholera vaccine, Shanchol, in Haiti. *PLOS Neglected Tropical Diseases, 8,* e2828. doi:10.1371/journal.pntd.0002828.

Chee, C. B., Sester, M., Zhang, W., & Lange, C. (2013). Diagnosis and treatment of latent infection with Mycobacterium tuberculosis. *Respirology, 18*(2), 205–216. doi:10.111/resp.12002

Cohen, M. S., Chen, Y. Q., McCauley, M., Gamble, T., Hosseinipour, M. C., Kumarasamy, N. H., . . . Fleming, T. R. (2011). Prevention of HIV-1 infection with early antiretroviral therapy. *New England Journal of Medicine, 365*(6), 493–505. doi:10.1056/NEJMoa1105243

Cohen, S. E., Vittinghoff, E., Bacon, O., Doblecki-Lewis, A., Postle, B. S., Feaster, D. J., . . . Liu, A. Y. (2015). High interest in preexposure prophylaxis among men who have sex with men at risk for HIV infection: Baseline data from the US PrEP demonstration project. *Journal of Acquired Immune Deficiency Syndromes, 68*(4), 439–448. doi:10.1097/QAI.0000000000000479

Delva, W., & Karim, Q. A. (2014). The HIV epidemic in southern Africa: Is an AIDS-free generation possible? *Current HIV/AIDS Reports, 11*(2), 99–108. doi:10.1007/s11904-014-0205-0

Fenner, F., Henderson, D. A., Arita, I., Ježek, Z., & Ladnyi, I. D. (1988). *Smallpox and its eradication.* Geneva, Switzerland: World Health Organization. Retrieved from http://citeseerx.ist.psu.edu/viewdoc/download?doi=10.1.1.382.6617&rep=rep1&type=pdf

Flannery, B., Clippard, J., Zimmerman, R. K., Nowalk, M. P., Jackson, M. L., Jackson, L., . . . Fry, A. M. (2015). Early estimates of seasonal influenza vaccine effectiveness—United States, January 2015. *Morbidity and Mortality Weekly Report (MMWR), 64*(1), 10–15. Retrieved from http://www.cdc.gov/mmwr/pdf/wk/mm6401.pdf

Flint, P. L., Pearce, J. M., Franson, J. C., & Derksen, D. V. (2015). Wild bird surveillance for highly pathogenic avian influenza H5 in North America. *Virology Journal, 12*(151). doi:10.1186/s12985-015-0377-2

Frieden, T. R., & Sbarbaro. (2007). Promoting adherence to treatment for tuberculosis. The importance of direct observation. *Bulletin of the World Health Organization, 85*(5), 407–409. doi:10.2471/BLT.06.038927

Gorman, S. (2013). How can we improve global infectious disease surveillance and prevent the next outbreak? *Scandinavian Journal of Infectious Diseases, 45*(12), 944–947. doi:10.3109/00365548.2013.826877

Gower, E., Estes, C., Blach, S., Razavi-Shearer, K., & Razavi, H. (2014). Global epidemiology and genotype distribution of the hepatitis C virus infection. *Journal of Hepatology, 61*(1 Supp), S45–S57. doi:10.1016/j.jhep.2014.07.027

Graham, C. S., & Swan, T. (2015). A path to the eradication of hepatitis C in low- and middle-income countries. *Antiviral Research, 119*, 89–96. doi:10.1016/j.antiviral.2015.01.004

Ham, D. C., Lin, C., Newman, L., Wijesooriya, N. S., & Kamb, M. (2015). Improving global estimates of syphilis in pregnancy by diagnostic test type: A systematic review and meta-analysis. *International Journal of Gynecology and Obstetrics, 130*(Supp 1), S10–S14. doi: 10.1016/j.ijgo.2015.04.012.

Hasian, M. A. (2000). Power, medical knowledge, and the rhetorical invention of "Typhoid Mary." *Journal of Medical Humanities, 21*(3), 123–139. doi:10.1023/A:1009074619421

Hendrickx, G., Vorsters, A., & Van Demme, P. (2012). Advances in hepatitis immunization (A, B, E): Public health policy and novel vaccine delivery. *Current Opinion in Infectious Diseases, 25*(5), 578–583. doi:10.1097/QCO.0b013e328357e65c

History.com staff. (2010). Black death. *A & E Networks.* Retrieved from http://www.history.com/topics/black-death

Joint United Nations Programme on HIV/AIDS. (2013). *UNAIDS global report on the global epidemic: 2013.* Retrieved from http://www.unaids.org/sites/default/files/media_asset/UNAIDS_Global_Report_2013_en_1.pdf

Joint United Nations Programme on HIV/AIDS. (2014). *Fact sheet: 2014 Global statistics.* Retrieved from http://www.unaids.org/sites/default/files/en/media/unaids/contentassets/documents/factsheet/2014/20140716_FactSheet_en.pdf

Jombart, T., Aanensen, D. M., Baguelin, M., Birrell, P., Cauchemez, S., Camacho, . . . Wallinga, J. (2014). OutbreakTools: A new platform for disease outbreak analysis using the R software. *Epidemics, 7*, 28–34. doi:10.1016/j.epidem.2014.04.003

Kavanagh, M. M., Cohn, J., Mabote, L., Meier, B. M., Williams, B., Russell, A., . . . & Baker, B. K. (2015). Evolving human rights and the science of antiretroviral medicine. *Health and Human Rights Journal, 17*(1). Retrieved from http://www.hhrjournal.org/2015/06/04/evolving-human-rights-and-the-science-of-antiretroviral-medicine/

Kennedy, C. E., Fonner, V.A., Sweat, M.D., Okero, F.A., Baggaley, R., & O'Reillly, K. R. (2013). Provider-initiated HIV testing and counseling in low- and middle-income countries: A systematic review. *AIDS Behavior, 17*(5), 1571–1590. doi:1007/s10461-012-0241-y

Koonin, L. M., Jamieson, D. J., Jernigan, J. A., Van Beneden, C. A., Kosmos, C., Harvey, M. C., . . . Damon, I. (2015). Systems for rapidly detecting and treating persons with Ebola virus disease—United States. *Morbidity and Mortality Weekly Report (MMWR), 64*(8), 222–225. Retrieved from http://www.cdc.gov/mmwr/preview/mmwrhtml/mm6408a5.htm

Lienhardt, C., Glaziou, P., Uplekar, M., Lönnroth, K., Getahun, H., & Raviglione, M. (2012). Global tuberculosis control: Lessons learnt and future prospects. *Nature Reviews. Microbiology, 10*(6), 407–416. doi:10.1038/nrmicro2797

Lim, S. M., Koraka, P., Osterhaus, A. D., & Martina, B. E. (2011). West Nile virus: Immunity and pathogenesis. *Viruses, 3,* 811–828. doi:10.3390/v3060811

Louis, M. S. (2012). Global health surveillance. *Morbidity and Mortality Weekly Report (MMWR), 61*(3), 15–19. Retrieved from http://www.cdc.gov/mmwr/preview/mmwrhtml/su6103a4.htm?s_cid=su6103a4_x

Maartens, G., Celum, C., & Lewin, S. R. (2014). HIV infection: Epidemiology, pathogenesis, treatment, and prevention. *Lancet, 384*(9939), 258–271. doi:10.1016/S0140-6736(14)60164-1

Macias, A. E., Precisos, A. R., & Falsey, A. R. (2015). The Global Influenza Initiative recommendations for the vaccination of pregnant women against seasonal influenza. *Influenza and Other Respiratory Viruses*, Suppl 1, 30–37. doi:10.1111/irv.12320

Magner, L. N. (2009). *A History of Infectious Diseases and the Microbial World*. Westport, CT: Praeger.

McMahon, J. M., Myers, J. E., Kurth, A. E., Cohen, S. E., Mannheimer, S. B., Simmons, J., . . . Haberer, J. E. (2014). Oral pre-exposure prophylaxis (PrEP) for prevention of HIV in serodiscordant heterosexual couples in the United States: Opportunities and challenges. *AIDS Patient Care and STDs, 28*(9), 462–474. doi:10.1089/apc.2013.0302

Medicines for Malaria Venture. (2015). *Malaria facts and figures*. Retrieved from http://www.mmv.org/malaria-medicines/malaria-facts-figures.

Morshed, M. G., & Singh, A. E. (2015). Recent trends in the serologic diagnosis of syphilis. *Clinical and Vaccine Immunology, 22*(2), 137–147. doi:10.1128/CVI.00681-14

Moyer, V. A., & U.S. Preventative Services Task Force (2013). Screening for HIV: U.S. Preventive Services Task Force recommendation statement. *Annals of Internal Medicine, 159*(1), 51–60. doi:10.7326/0003-4819-159-1-201307020-00645

Newman, L., Kamb, M., Hawkes, S., Gomez, G., Say, L., Seuc, A., & Broutet, N. (2013). Global estimates of syphilis in pregnancy and associated adverse outcomes: Analysis of multinational antenatal surveillance data. *PLOS Medicine, 10*(2). doi:10.1371/journal.pmed.10011396

Nygren, B. I., Blackstock, A. J., & Mintz, E. D. (2014). Cholera at the crossroads: The association between endemic cholera and national access to improved water sources and sanitation. *American Journal of Tropical Medicine and Hygiene, 91,* 1023–1028. doi:10.4269/ajtmh.14-0331

Olsen, S. H., Benedum, C. M., Mekaru, S. R., Preston, M. N., Mazet, J. A., Joly, D. O., & Brownstein, J. S. (2015). Drivers of emerging infectious disease events as a framework for digital detection. *Emerging Infectious Diseases, 21,* 1285–1292 doi:10.1371/journal.pmed.1001354

Panel on Antiretroviral Guidelines for Adults and Adolescents. (2015). *Guidelines for the use of antiretroviral agents in HIV-1-infected adults and adolescents*. Retrieved from http://www.aidsinfo.nih.gov/ContentFiles/AdultandAdoles- centGL.pdf

Papastergiou, V., Lombardi, R., MacDonald, D., & Tsochatzis, E. A. (2015). Global epidemiology of hepatitis B (HBV) infection. *Current Hepatology Reports, 14*(3), 171–178. doi:10.1007/S11901-015-0269-3

Pinner, R. W., Lynfield, R., Hadler, J. L., Schaffner, W., Farley, M. M., Frank, M. E., & Schuchat, A. (2015). Cultivation of an adaptive domestic network for surveillance and evaluation of emerging infections. *Emerging Infectious Diseases, 21*(9), 1499–1509. doi:10.3201/eid2109.150619

Pitt, M., Blankley, S., McShane, H., & O'Garra, A. (2013). Vaccination against tuberculosis: How can we get better BCG? *Microbial Pathogenesis, 58,* 2–16. doi:10.1016/j.micpath.2012.12.002

Rajapakse, S. (2011). Dengue shock. *Journal of Emergencies, Trauma, and Shock, 4*(1), 120–127. doi:10.4103/0974-2700.76835

Rosario, I. J., Kasabwala, K., & Sadeghi-Nejad, H. (2013). Circumcision as a strategy tominimize HIV transmission. *Current Urology Reports, 14*(4), 285–290. doi:10.1007/s11934-013-0343-8

Salam, R. A., Das, J. K., Lassi, Z. S., & Bhutta, Z. A. (2014). Impact of community-based interventions for the prevention and control of malaria on intervention coverage and health outcomes for the prevention and control of malaria. *Infectious Diseases of Poverty, 3*(25), 1–15. doi:10.1186/2049-9957-3-25

Sgaier, S. K., Reed, J. B., Thomas, A., & Njeuhmeli, E. (2014). Achieving the HIV prevention impact of voluntary medical male circumcision: Lessons and challenges for managing programs. *PLOS Medicine, 11*(5). doi:10.1371/journal.pmed.1001641

Sherman, I. W. (2007). *Twelve Diseases That Changed Our World*. Washington, DC: American Society of Microbiology Press.

Stamm, L. V. (2015). Review article. Syphilis: Antibiotic treatment and resistance. *Epidemiology and Infection, 143*(8), 1567–1574. doi:10.1017/S0950268814002830

Steiner, T. S. (2014). The worst of both worlds: Examining the hypervirulence of the Shigatoxigenic/ Enteroaggregative Escherichia coli O104:H4. *Journal of Infectious Diseases, 210*, 1860–1862. doi:10.1093/infdis/jiu400

Stop TB Partnership. (2015). Retrieved from http://www.stoptb.org

Swartzendruber, A., Steiner, R. J., Adler, M. R., Kamb, M. L., & Newman, L. M. (2015). Introduction of rapid syphilis testing in antenatal care: A systematic review of the impact on HIV and syphilis testing uptake and coverage. *International Journal of Gynecology and Obstetrics, 130*(Supp 1), S15–S21. doi.org/10.1016/ j.ijgo.2015.05.002

The Middle Ages.net. (2011). The black death: Bubonic plague. *The Middle Ages.Net*. Retrieved from http:// www.themiddleages.net/plague.html

Troppy, S., Haney, G., Cocoros, N., Dranston, K., & DeMaria, Jr., A. (2014). Infectious disease surveillance in the 21st century: An integrated web-based surveillance and case management system. *Public Health Reports, 129*(2), 132–138. Retrieved from http://www.publichealthreports.org/issueopen.cfm?articleID=3148

United States Department of Agriculture, Economic Research Services. (2014). *Cost estimates of foodborne illnesses*. Retrieved from http://www.ers.usda.gov/data-products/cost-estimates-of-foodborne-illnesses .aspx#48448

United States Department of Health and Human Services, United States Food and Drug Administration. (2015). *Licensure of Ebola vaccines: Demonstration of effectiveness*. Retrieved from http://www.fda.gov/downloads/ AdvisoryCommittees/CommitteesMeetingMaterials/BloodVaccinesandOtherBiologics/VaccinesandRelated-BiologicalProductsAdvisoryCommittee/UCM445819.pdf

van Hellemond, J. J., Rutten, M., Koelewijn, R., Zeeman, A. M., Verweij, J. J., Wismans, P. J., . . . van Genderen, J. J. (2009). Human Plasmodium knowlesi infection detected by rapid diagnostic tests for malaria. *Emerging Infectious Diseases, 15*, 1478–1480. doi:10.3201/eid1509.090358

Vermund, S. H. (2014). Global HIV epidemiology: A guide for strategies in prevention and care. *Current HIV/ AIDS Reports, 11*(2), 93–98. doi:10.1007/s11904-014-0208-x

World Health Organization. (n.d.a). *Tuberculosis: The five elements of DOTS*. Retrieved from http://www.who .int/tb/dots/whatisdots/en/

World Health Organization. (n.d.b). *Global infectious disease surveillance [Fact Sheet No. 200]*. Retrieved from http://www.who.int/mediacentre/factsheets/fs200/en/

World Health Organization. (1980). *The global eradication of smallpox: The final report of the Global Commission for the Certification of Smallpox Eradication*. Retrieved from http://apps.who.int/iris/ bitstream/10665/39253/1/a41438.pdf

World Health Organization. (2010). Cholera vaccines, WHO position paper. *Weekly Epidemiologic Record (WER), 13*, 117–128. Retrieved from http://www.who.int/immunization/cholera_PP_slides_20_Mar_2010.pdf

World Health Organization. (2011a). *West Nile virus [Fact Sheet No. 354]*. Retrieved from http://www.who.int/ mediacentre/factsheets/fs354/en/

World Health Organization. (2011b). *Enterohaemorrhagic Escherichia coli [Fact Sheet No. 125]*. Retrieved from http://www.who.int/mediacentre/factsheets/fs125/en/

World Health Organization. (2012). *Antiretroviral treatment as prevention (TasP) for HIV and TB*. Retrieved from http://apps.who.int/iris/bitstream/10665/70904/1/WHO_HIV_2012.12_eng.pdf

World Health Organization. (2013a). *Hepatitis*. Retrieved from http://www.who.int/immunization/topics/ hepatitis/en/#

World Health Organization. (2013b). *Biologicals: BCG (Tuberculosis)*. Retrieved from http://www.who.int/biologicals/areas/vaccines/bcg/Tuberculosis/en/

World Health Organization. (2014a). *The top 10 leading causes of death [Fact Sheet No. 310]*. Retrieved from http://www.who.int/mediacentre/factsheets/fs310/en/index2.html

World Health Organization. (2014b). *World malaria report 2014*. Retrieved from http://www.who.int/malaria/publications/world_malaria_report_2014/en/

World Health Organization. (2014c). *Avian influenza [Fact Sheet]*. Retrieved from http://www.who.int/mediacentre/factsheets/avian_influenza/en/

World Health Organization. (2014d). *Influenza (Seasonal) [Fact Sheet No. 211]*. Retrieved from http://www.who.int/mediacentre/factsheets/fs211/en/

World Health Organization. (2014e). *Global guidance on criteria and processes for validation: Elimination of mother to child transmission of HIV and syphilis*. Retrieved from http://apps.who.int/iris/bitstream/10665/112858/1/9789241505888_eng.pdf?ua=1&ua=1

World Health Organization. (2014f). *Global tuberculosis report 2014*. Retrieved from http://www.who.int/tb/publications/global_report/en/

World Health Organization. (2014g). *Global update on the health sector response to HIV, 2014*. Retrieved from http://www.who.int/hiv/pub/global-update.pdf

World Health Organization. (2015a). *Cholera [Fact Sheet No.107]*. Retrieved from http://www.who.int/mediacentre/factsheets/fs107/en/

World Health Organization. (2015b). *Dengue and severe dengue [Fact Sheet No. 117]*. Retrieved from http://www.who.int/mediacentre/factsheets/fs117/en/

World Health Organization. (2015c). *Malaria [Fact Sheet No. 94]*. Retrieved from http://www.who.int/mediacentre/factsheets/fs094/en/

World Health Organization. (2015d). *Ebola virus disease [Fact Sheet No.103]*. Retrieved from http://www.who.int/mediacentre/factsheets/fs103/en/

World Health Organization. (2015e). *Ebola virus disease outbreak*. Retrieved from http://www.who.int/csr/disease/ebola/en/

World Health Organization. (2015f). *Hepatitis A [Fact Sheet No. 328]*. Retrieved from http://www.who.int/mediacentre/factsheets/fs328/en/

World Health Organization. (2015g). *Hepatitis B. [Fact Sheet No. 204]*. Retrieved from http://www.who.int/mediacentre/factsheets/fs204/en/

World Health Organization. (2015h). *Immunization coverage [Fact Sheet No. 378]*. Retrieved from http://www.who.int/mediacentre/factsheets/fs378/en/

World Health Organization. (2015i). *Hepatitis C. [Fact Sheet No. 164]*. Retrieved from http://www.who.int/mediacentre/factsheets/fs164/en/

World Health Organization. (2015j). *Tuberculosis. [Fact Sheet No. 104]*. Retrieved from http://www.who.int/mediacentre/factsheets/fs104/en/

World Health Organization. (2015k). *Stop TB partnership*. Retrieved from http://www.who.int/workforcealliance/members_partners/member_list/stoptb/en/

World Health Organization. (2015l). *HIV/AIDS. [Fact Sheet No. 360]*. Retrieved from http://www.who.int/mediacentre/factsheets/fs360/en/

World Health Organization. (2015m). *Guidelines on when to start antiretroviral therapy and on pre-exposure prophylaxis*. Retrieved from http://apps.who.int/iris/bitstream/10665/186275/1/9789241509565_eng.pdf

World Health Organization & Joint United Nations Programme on HIV/AIDS. (2007). *Guidance on HIV testing and counseling in health facilities*. Retrieved from http://whqlibdoc.who.int/publications/2007/9789241595568_eng.pdf

World Hepatitis Alliance & World Health Organization. (2015). *World Hepatitis Day*. Retrieved from http://worldhepatitisday.org

10

HIV/AIDS, Stigma, and Disclosure: A Need for a Human Rights Perspective

Richard L. Sowell
Kenneth D. Phillips

Objectives

After completing this chapter, the reader will be able to:

1. Define stigma.
2. Discuss the historical evolution of the concept of HIV/AIDS stigma.
3. Identify the consequences of stigma on persons with HIV/AIDS and on society.
4. Identify the effects of prevention efforts on stigma and discrimination for HIV/AIDS.
5. Discuss the phenomenon of multiple stigma or layer stigma.
6. Discuss the relationships among stigma, discrimination, and disclosure in HIV/AIDS.
7. Compare the manifestations of HIV/AIDS stigma in resource-rich and resource-limited countries and regions.
8. Discuss HIV/AIDS stigma and discrimination in the context of a human rights framework.

INTRODUCTION

In the past decade, there has been a significant decrease in the number of new cases of HIV/AIDS, AIDS-related deaths, and HIV infections in children. Much of this success has been attributed to greater global access to antiretroviral drugs (UNAIDS, 2013). Yet, despite these encouraging statistics, HIV/AIDS remains at pandemic levels worldwide (UNAIDS, 2014). It is clear that the spread of HIV/AIDS is multifaceted, and antiretroviral medications will not be able to stop the spread of HIV/AIDS alone. AIDS is the final stage of a protracted illness caused by the human immunodeficiency virus (HIV). HIV selectively attacks the immune system and, if unchecked, it completely destroys the T-helper lymphocytes, resulting in severe cellular immune deficiency. These lymphocytes are important in defending the body against a variety of pathogens, virally infected cells, and malignant cells.

Since it was first identified in the early 1980s (Centers for Disease Control and Prevention [CDC], 1981a, 1981b), HIV/AIDS has been associated with fear, progressive physical deterioration, and suffering resulting in death (Feller & Lemmer, 2007). Yet, despite the devastating physical manifestations for individuals infected with the virus, the consequences of HIV/AIDS are far more complex and far-reaching. Closely tied to HIV/AIDS is a secondary pandemic of stigma and discrimination that negatively affects persons with HIV/AIDS, their families and communities, and the global society (Bogart, Cowgill, Kennedy, Ryan, Murphy, Elijah, & Schuster, 2008; Hatzenbuehler Phelan, & Link, 2013; Mahajan, Saylers, Patel, Remien, Ortiz, Szekeres, & Coates, 2008). Even in resource-rich countries where access to advanced treatments has resulted in HIV/AIDS becoming a more chronic disease, HIV/AIDS stigma and varying degrees of discrimination remain pervasive (Block, 2009; Chandra, Deepthivarma, & Manjula, 2003; Dlamini et al., 2007; Kohi et al., 2006; Sengupta, Strauss, Miles, Roman-Isler, Banks, & Corbie-Smith, 2010; Zukoski & Thorburn, 2009). Persons with HIV/AIDS, as well as persons associated with HIV-infected individuals, are routinely subjected to fear, rejection, ostracism, hostility, and potential physical and economic violence (Balabanova, Coker, Atun, & Drobniewski, 2006; Galvin, Davis, Banks, & Bing, 2008; Holtz & Sowell, 2014; Ogunmefun, Gilbert, & Schatz, 2011; Sterken, 2010; Surkan et al., 2010).

The stigma associated with HIV/AIDS can have severe consequences both physically and psychologically for the person with the HIV infection. Fear of rejection and social isolation are frequent outcomes of a known HIV/AIDS diagnosis (Gilbert & Walker, 2010; Mukolo, Blevins, Victor, Vaz, Sidat, & Vergara, 2013; Visser, Makin, Vandormael, Sikkema, & Forsyth, 2009). Individuals can lose their housing, their employment, and social relationships if their HIV-infected status becomes known (Kohi et al., 2006; Lee, Wu, Rotheram-Borus, Detels, Guan, & Li, 2005). Research has demonstrated that HIV-related stigma and the discrimination that follows decrease one's quality of life (Fuster & Molero, 2010; Varni, Miller, McCuin, & Solomon, 2012). In countries where health insurance exists, insurance and access to treatment are often linked to employment. Because of HIV/AIDS stigma and its related discrimination, there are great incentives for one to keep an HIV/AIDS diagnosis secret. A reluctance to disclose being HIV-infected in both resource-rich and resource-limited countries, as well as across cultures, has been well documented (Akani & Erhabor, 2006; Chandra, Deepthivarma, & Manjula, 2003; Kebaabetwe, 2007; Visser, Neufeld, de Villiers, Makin, & Forsyth, 2008). Such nondisclosure can have dire consequences for both the individual and society. When individuals are not willing to disclose their infection or even be tested for HIV infection, that factor limits their ability to access treatment and support (Allen et al., 2006; Greeff & Phetlhu, 2007; Lee, Li, Iamsirithaworn, & Khumtong, 2013; Li, Murry, Suwanteerangkul, & Wiwatanadate, 2014). Additionally, lack of willingness to disclose the presence of HIV infection can negatively affect HIV/AIDS prevention efforts both on individual and community levels (Babalola, 2007; Buseh & Stevens, 2006; Genberg et al., 2008; UNAIDS, 2012). Therefore, HIV/AIDS-related stigma and its related actions represent a psychosocially based pandemic that profoundly affects individuals and communities across cultures and feeds the ever-increasing global HIV/AIDS pandemic.

STIGMA

Stigma is a social phenomenon that has been defined as "an attribute that is deeply discrediting" (Goffman, 1963, p. 3). The standards by which individuals or groups are categorized as ordinary in the course of daily interactions are established by society and its related culture (Goffman, 1963). Stigma results when there is the presence of attributes that are not viewed as being within acceptable norms for an individual or a group. It denotes a difference or departure from the norm in a negative context. Such variance from normal expectations is frequently met with prejudice, discrimination, stereotyping, and distancing (Goffman, 1963; Jones, Farina, Hastorf, Markus, Miller, & Scott, 1984). Jones and associates (1984, p. 6) define individuals who are stigmatized as "the bearer of the 'mark' that indicates they are somehow deviant, flawed, spoiled, or generally undesirable." The ancient Greeks used the term "stigma" to refer to bodily signs designed to expose something unusual and bad about the moral status of the signifier. The sign (mark) was cut or burned into the body and advertised that the bearer was a slave, a criminal, or a traitor—that is, a blemished person, ritually polluted, to be avoided, especially in public places (Goffman, 1963, p. 1). Therefore, the basic concept of bearing the mark or being stigmatized has its origin in the very term "stigma."

The negative responses to individuals who are assessed as different or unworthy remain a reality and can be identified globally transcending cultures and geographic borders. The act of stigmatizing focuses on assigning blame to an individual or group, which not only allows for the discrediting and devaluing of an individual or a group, but also provides the basis for behaviors that would otherwise be unacceptable. By stigmatizing the individual or group, it becomes acceptable to blame the individual or group for processing the stigmatizing attribute, which, in turn, supports the concept of punishment (Abler, Henderson, Wang, & Avery, 2010; Laryea & Gien, 1993). Ekstrand, Bharat, and Ramakrishna (2010) report that blame and inaccurate information concerning HIV/AIDS transmission were found to be associated with coercive public policies and intent to discriminate targeted persons living with HIV/AIDS (PLWHA).

Stigma is often rooted in fear, and it can validate avoidance, discrimination, and economic and social violence toward the stigmatized. Individuals and groups can be stigmatized for a variety of reasons, including lifestyle choices, physical characteristics, ethnic or racial group membership, socioeconomic status, and medical conditions. In examining stigma within the context of HIV/AIDS, it becomes clear that HIV/AIDS stigma is complex and multifaceted. HIV/AIDS stigma not only results from fear of a contagious, life-threatening illness, but also is layered with negative attitudes and beliefs toward groups or lifestyles believed to be associated with the disease (Logie, James, Tharao, & Loutfy, 2010).

HIV/AIDS STIGMA

Stigma and discrimination have been closely related with HIV infection since HIV/AIDS was first identified. Homosexual men, intravenous drug users, hemophiliacs, and people of color were the groups in whom HIV/AIDS was first recognized (CDC, 1981a, 1981b). These groups represent individuals who were the targets of stigma and discrimination even before the advent of HIV/AIDS. Prior to the identification of its causative virus, HIV/AIDS was initially referred to by many as gay-related immune deficiency (GRID) or the "gay plague"

(Shilts, 1987). The GRID designation for a new and deadly syndrome serves as evidence that individuals in the general society sought to place blame for the disease on a stigmatized group, as well as distance themselves from the disease and the "deviant behavior" that was proposed as the source of its spread. Sontag (1998) suggests that the term "plague" represents a metaphor that indicates that an illness is inflicted on a group and often is a "punishment from God." This idea that HIV/AIDS is a punishment from God transcends religions and represents a threat that facilitates discrimination against persons with HIV/AIDS and also acts as a barrier to HIV/AIDS prevention efforts (Blumberg, 2014; Hess & McKinney, 2007; Huy, Johansson, & Long, 2007; Obermeyer & Osborn, 2007; Svensson, 2014; Varas-Diaz, Neilands, Cintron-Bou, Santos-Figueroa, Marzan-Rodriguez, & Marques, 2014; Varas-Diaz, Neilands, Malave-Rivera, & Betancout, 2010). The role of stigmatizing behaviors and attitudes is to distance oneself from the illness and its associated negative consequences and attributes, thereby supporting the contention that "those individuals with HIV/AIDS are different from me."

Although those individuals who contracted HIV infection through blood or blood component transfusions were not viewed as directly responsible for their infection (i.e., guilty of immoral behavior), these persons—especially hemophiliacs—were viewed as being flawed or were considered imperfect. Having a chronic health condition or illness predisposed these individuals to some level of stigma that was further compounded by a diagnosis of HIV/AIDS. Further, the rapid spread of HIV/AIDS among ethnic and racial minorities, people of color, and the poor continues to support the global stereotyping of persons with or at risk for HIV/AIDS as individuals and groups that are immoral, unworthy, devalued, and responsible for their disease (Balabanova, Coker, Atun, & Drobniewski, 2006; Kelso, Cohen, Weber, Dale, Cruise, & Brody, 2014; Mustanski, Newcomb, DuBois, Garcia, & Grov, 2011; Muthuswamy, 2005). Such stigma can be so strong and pervasive that individuals who are HIV infected or who engage in high-risk behaviors may accept and internalize negative feelings and stereotypes, resulting in feelings of unworthiness and shame (Goffman, 1963; Jones, Farina, Hastorf, Markus, Miller, & Scott, 1984).

Petros and colleagues (2006) identified the concept that they called "othering" among South Africans. It was noted that blame for HIV/AIDS was most often imputed based on race, culture, homophobia, and xenophobia. Black Africans blamed whites, and whites blamed black Africans (Petros, Airhihenbuwa, Simbayi, Ramlagan, & Brown, 2006). HIV-infected women are viewed by some as sexually promiscuous, as loose, as prostitutes, and as dirty and immoral. Through this process of "gender othering," men absolve themselves from blame (Petros, Airhihenbuwa, Simbayi, Ramlagan, & Brown, 2006). Another means of distancing oneself from HIV/AIDS is by blaming "outsiders." In the Petros study, for example, South African participants held people from Zimbabwe, Mozambique, and Botswana responsible for bringing HIV/AIDS disease to the people of South Africa.

The phenomenon of othering has been described in other cultures as well, and is often based on racism, sexism, or homophobia (Gilmore & Somerville, 1994; Logie, James, Tharao, & Loutfy, 2011). Attributing negative attributes to others, as well as to individuals with HIV/AIDS, provides an excuse for majority groups, those with economic resources, and local, national, and international leaders to not fully engage in responding to the ever-growing HIV/AIDS pandemic.

Although specific groups, lifestyles, and individual attributes may carry varying degrees of stigma within different cultures and geographic regions, HIV/AIDS stigma, in most cases, has an additive effect to stigma already experienced by individuals and groups experiencing the highest rates of HIV infection. This situation makes HIV/AIDS stigma and the resultant discrimination a complex phenomenon that can drastically increase the social isolation, physical pain, and psychological distress of individuals fighting to survive after a HIV/AIDS diagnosis. The complexity of such layered stigma and potential discrimination, in turn, influences the type and level of healthcare and support services that is required to adequately respond to the individual's situation and needs.

CHARACTERISTICS OF THE ILLNESS AND STIGMA

Jones and colleagues (1984) described six dimensions of stigma that determine the degree of stigma that is associated with a particular characteristic, as well as the ability to conceal or minimize stigma resulting from the characteristic. These dimensions are *concealability* (the degree to which the characteristic is hidden or obvious), *course* (the degree to which the change occurs over time and the ultimate outcome), *disruptiveness* (the degree to which the characteristic hampers communication), *aesthetic qualities* (the degree to which the characteristic makes the person repellent, ugly, or upsetting), *origin* (the degree to which the person is to blame for the characteristic), and *peril* (the degree of danger that results from the characteristic).

HIV/AIDS progresses through several stages, which over time, increasingly limits the person's ability to conceal the disease. *Stage 1,* the primary infection, may begin weeks or months after infection and lasts for approximately 1 to 2 weeks. This first stage of illness is characterized by flulike or mononucleosis-like symptoms. Often HIV is overlooked as the diagnosis. Because no major symptoms are apparent during *Stage 2,* this phase is called the asymptomatic stage; it lasts for an average of 10 years. During the first two stages, HIV-infected persons may not know that they are infected. Moderate unexplained weight loss, recurrent respiratory infections, shingles, skin and nail lesions, and oral conditions may occur in this phase. Persistent generalized lymphadenopathy may begin in this phase as well.

In *Stage 3,* the symptomatic stage, immunity progressively declines and the person may begin to experience a variety of symptoms, such as severe weight loss (more than 10% of the total body weight), diarrhea, persistent fever, thrush, oral hairy leukoplakia, skin lesions, or mouth conditions that worsen over the course of time. Even during this stage, however, it is often possible for a person to hide the fact that he or she has HIV/AIDS, although nondisclosure becomes more difficult in the symptomatic stage. Thus, for the majority of the time that a person is living with HIV/AIDS, it is possible to conceal his or her illness.

In *Stage 4,* with a decline of the T-helper lymphocyte count to less than 200 cells/mm^3, the person advances to the stage known as AIDS, in which he or she suffers from a variety of opportunistic infections (e.g., *Pneumocystis jiroveci* pneumonia) and malignancies (e.g., Kaposi's sarcoma) that are very difficult to hide (AIDS Education and Training Center [AETC], 2014; Weeks & Alcamo, 2008).

Not only does the increasing symptomatology of HIV infection identify an individual as having HIV/AIDS, thereby subjecting the person to the overall stigma associated with the disease, but many of the symptoms exhibited (wasting syndrome, profound diarrhea, and open lesions) can, in themselves, also result in distancing and social isolation. Examining the continuum of symptoms and opportunistic infections resulting from HIV/AIDS in relation to Jones and colleagues' (1984) dimensions that determine the degree of stigma, it is easily seen that characteristics of HIV/AIDS support the severe stigmatization of individuals contracting the illness. HIV progression and its resultant symptoms makes *concealing* HIV/AIDS almost impossible. A number of physical symptoms cause a change in physical appearance, making the individual *unattractive or repellent*. HIV/AIDS remains a life-threatening illness that across its *course* adversely affects physical and psychological well-being, *disrupting* social relationships and quality of life. Individuals with HIV/AIDS are in *peril* of facing psychological stress and physical deterioration.

Collectively, these factors make HIV/AIDS one of the most stigmatizing illnesses in history. HIV/AIDS is an illness that has devastating consequences for PLWHA, their families, communities, and society.

CONSEQUENCES OF HIV/AIDS STIGMA

The global response to HIV/AIDS can be said to represent discrimination and devaluing of the "humanness" of the poor and the disenfranchised. HIV/AIDS is most frequently transmitted through heterosexual sex and places the greatest hardship on women and children (UNAIDS, 2008b; UNICEF, 2006).

The diminished rights of women and young girls is a major factor in fueling the continued spread of HIV/AIDS on a worldwide basis (Kehler, 2010; Kehler & Crone, 2010; Moreno, 2007; Nyanzi, 2010; UNAIDS, 2012). In some regions, women can be considered property and are subjected to the will of men (Familusi, 2012; Mendenhall, Muzizi, Stephenson, Chomba, Ahmed, Haworth, & Allen, 2007; Nwaebuni, 2013; Seeley, Grellier, & Barnett, 2004). In some African cultures, a woman becomes the property of a male member of her husband's family if her husband dies. She has no rights to her husband's property and is often expected to become sexually active with the male relative who inherits her (Nyanzi, 2010). The U.S. Department of State estimates that up to 900,000 people are trafficked across international borders each year; trafficking occurs in almost every country (Kloer, 2010) In countries such as Nepal, Bhutan, and India, the spread of HIV/AIDS can be related to the trafficking of young girls to Indian brothels (Kloer, 2010; Sarkar, Bal, Mukherjee, Chakraborty, Saha, Ghosh, & Parsons, 2008), while African girls frequently become HIV infected between the ages of 15 and 19 years of age. In both of these examples, young girls become HIV infected as a result of sexual exploitation, gender-based violence, and economic insecurity (Goldberg, Silverman, Engstrom, Bojorquez-Chapela, Usita, Rolon, & Strathdee, 2015).

Globally, more than 17 million children are believed to have been orphaned by HIV/AIDS and at least 3.4 million children under 15 years of age are living with HIV (UNAIDS, 2014). These children live in a variety of settings, ranging from the streets of large cities to orphanages. Children who have been orphaned as a result of their parents dying from AIDS suffer the triple stigma of having an association with parents who died because of their "immoral behavior," the fear that the children may carry HIV infection, and their status as "the poorest of the poor" (Coursen-Neff, 2004; UNAIDS, 2004; UNICEF, 2006). The result of such stigma and discrimination is that the vast majority of AIDS orphans are viewed as "throwaway children" and are left to fend for themselves. This situation promotes sexual exploitation of both young boys and girls and the further spread of HIV infection within communities (Sowell & Phillips, 2010, pp. 395–396;

Wenani, 2010). A major goal of the U.S. President's Emergency Plan for AIDS Relief Orphans and Vulnerable Children Program (PEPFAR) is to improve the health and well-being of children by mitigating the impact of HIV/AIDS on children and their families (UNAIDS, 2014).

In Latin cultures, a major influence in the lives of women is machismo, which refers to male dominant behavior and excessive masculinity. In Mexico, machismo essentially defines the father of the family as the head of the household, who is often feared by both the wife and children. The wife is expected to handle childrearing and household responsibilities without questioning her husband's authority (Galanti, 2003; Moreno, 2007). A study of Mexican migrant workers (Sowell, Holtz, & Velasquez, 2008; Holtz, Sowell, VanBrackle, Velasquez, & Hernandez 2012) found that women were willing to accept unrealistic explanations of how their husbands contracted HIV as a strategy to maintain their families and avoid conflict. In many resource-limited countries, women's dependence on men is formalized in culture and/or law (Familusi, 2012; UNAIDS, 2004). Of course, this dominance of men over their female partners is not limited to Latin cultures. The societal view of women as family caregivers and as submissive to their husbands is prevalent in many cultures and regions of the world (Anderson, 2010; Beaulleu, Adrien, & Lebounga Vouma, 2010; Pharris, Tishelman, Huyen, Chuc, & Thorson, 2010). Research findings revealed that even in the United States women often remain in relationships where their partners put them at risk for HIV/AIDS. Women reported feelings of dependence on the male partner and needing him to provide for them and/or their children (Moser, Sowell, & Phillips, 2001; Sowell, Phillips, Seals, Murdaugh, & Rush, 2002). Nevertheless, despite the lack of status of many women and the unequaled hardship that HIV/AIDS has placed on women, women have frequently been the innovators in taking leadership in community development efforts around HIV/AIDS care and prevention (Campbell & Cornish, 2010; Green, Halperin, Nantulya, & Hogle, 2006; McGovern, 2006; Romero, Wallerstein, Lucero, Fredine, Keefe, & O'Connell, 2006).

A growing number of individuals aged 55 and over are living with HIV/AIDS in the United States and in other Western countries. In 2010, individuals aged 55 and older accounted for almost one-fifth (19%, 217,000) of the estimated 1.1 million people living with HIV/AIDS in the United States (CDC, 2013). This increasing number of people 55 and older who are HIV infected has resulted both in persons living longer with HIV/AIDS and in a growing number of new infections. These individuals represent a group that may have unique issues and concerns, and face an additional layer of stigma related to age (Slater, Moneyham, Vance, Raper, Mugavero, & Childs, 2015). Further, researchers have found that older women may experience feelings of greater shame and reluctance to seek support due to their age (Grodensky, Golin, Jones, Mamo, Dennis, Abernethy, & Patterson, 2015). Many symptoms of HIV infections can be confused or overlap with the physical results of normal aging, which ca potentially make treatment more complex (AIDS.gov, 2015).

Globally, fear, prejudice, and misinformation related to HIV/AIDS and the way in which the infection is transmitted and prevented, continue to be widespread and form the basis for stigma, discrimination, and punitive behaviors (Ekstrand, Bharat, Ramakrishna, & Heylen, 2012; Kehler & Crone, 2010; Mykhalovskiy, 2010). In Western countries, stigma and discrimination associated with HIV/AIDS have generally become somewhat more subtle, but remain a significant challenge for PLWHA and those associated with HIV/AIDS (Anderson, 2009; Blake, Taylor, Reid, & Kosowski, 2008; Valdiserri, 2002). Both the United States and Canada have enacted legislative protections for person with HIV/AIDS (Elliott & Gold, 2005). Nevertheless, such legislative actions were not instigated until a number of high-profile cases occurred in which individuals experienced extreme consequences because they were believed to have HIV/AIDS or were at high risk for the disease (Botnick, 2000; Sowell & Phillips, 2010, p. 396).

Even where such protection has been enacted, punitive sanctions or restrictions have often been placed on persons with HIV/AIDS (CDC, 2014; Chang, Prytherch, Nesbitt, & Wilder-Smith, 2013; Lambda Legal, 2009; Yager, 2012). For example, it was not until 2010 that the United States lifted travel restrictions targeting potential visitors with HIV/AIDS (Oh, 2010). Despite WHO's declaration that travel restrictions and sanctions against persons with HIV/AIDS are not effective, 66 countries maintain their restrictions on HIV-infected persons entering and/or residing in their countries, thereby targeting noncitizens with HIV/AIDS. Additionally, migrants and refugees who test HIV seropositive frequently face governmental-level discrimination and deportation (Chang, Prytherch, Nesbitt, & Wilder-Smith, 2013; Dang, Giordano, & Kim, 2012; Human Rights Watch, 2009). Governments that take immigration detainees into custody have the obligation to ensure that those detainees receive adequate medical care that is equivalent to the care available to the general population during the resolution of their cases. For detainees who have HIV/AIDS, evidence indicates that systems are not in place to ensure adequate treatment of their disease (Human Rights Watch, 2004, 2007). Migrant workers and refugees fleeing political persecution or war, for example, represent not just the most vulnerable members of society, but also the groups at high risk for HIV infection and/or need for treatment.

In reality, HIV/AIDS stigma and discrimination are not limited to noncitizens. Verbal and physical abuse (beatings), including denial of food and basic care, remain a consequence of being identified as having HIV/AIDS in a number of countries (Abler, Henderson, Wang, & Avery, 2010; Tran Huy & Nguyen, 2010). Since HIV/AIDS was first identified, there has been an increase in the criminalization of groups or behaviors associated with HIV/AIDS (Dej & Kilty, 2012; Galletly & Pinkerton, 2004; Weait, 2013), even though there is no evidence that criminalization of behaviors is an effective deterrent to the spread of HIV/AIDS (Jurgens, Cohn, Cameron, Burris, Clayton, Elliott, Pearshouse, Gathumbi, & Cupido, 2009; Lazzarini, Galletly, Mykhalovoskiy, Harsono, O'Keefe, Simter, & Levine, 2013). Numerous international groups have expressed human rights concerns about the effects of such criminalization and efforts to prevent the spread of HIV/AIDS (Kazatchkine, 2010; UNICEF, 2010). It is likely that such criminalization will disproportionately affect women, including sex workers, drug users, and men who have sex with men, resulting in these marginalized groups retreating further underground—thereby decreasing their access to prevention efforts, leading them to avoid HIV testing and treatment, and increasing the likelihood of the spread of HIV infection (Baral et al., 2010; Horter, Nkhoma, Baradaran, Baggaley, & Stedwick, 2010; Molina & Lainez, 2010; Poteat et al., 2010; Thomas, Lalu, Mukambetov, Odhiambo, & Williams, 2010).

DISCLOSURE

HIV testing has been touted as one of the most important strategies in the prevention of HIV transmission (Thompson et al., 2010). Nevertheless, a raft of consequences must be considered in "testing," including the ability to keep test results confidential and manage the disclosure of an HIV seropositive result. Knowing one's HIV status and sharing an HIV seropositive status is important for a number of reasons, including the need to access health care and social support services. The advances made in treatment of HIV infection in recent years allow individuals who have access to appropriate antiretroviral therapy to remain healthy and slow the progression of their illness (Thompson et al., 2010). Additionally, research findings indicate that persons with HIV/AIDS who receive social support and/or mental health services have more positive outcomes (Moneyham, Hennessy, Sowell, Demi, Seals, & Mizuno, 1998; Smith, Rossetto, & Peterson, 2008; Vyavaharkar, Moneyham, Corwin, Tavakoli, Saunders, & Annang, 2011). A second potential outcome that supports the value of disclosure is the ability to negotiate with potential sex partners, thereby making the implementation of "safe sex" strategies more likely and preventing HIV transmission. For individuals who have decided to publicly disclose their HIV status, such disclosures can provide the foundation for an open dialogue within communities that can support a change of social norms that demonize and discriminate against persons with HIV/AIDS (Macintyre, Rutenberg, Brown, & Karim, 2004).

Disclosure of an HIV seropositive status is a serious step, and one that should be thoughtfully considered and based on factual information. The stigma and potential discrimination associated with HIV/AIDS make the disclosure of being HIV positive a complex and risky decision. Factors that may influence the decision to disclose and the response to such disclosure can include culture, access to HIV/AIDS treatment, region, community size, beliefs about HIV/AIDS, and economic considerations (Hossain, Islam, Islam, & Kabir, 2010; Ibekwe & Agbo, 2010; Muchenje et al., 2010; Pedrotti, Bishop, & Dunhma, 2010; Tenkorang, Obeng-Gyimah, Maticka-Tyndale, & Adjei, 2010). Numerous researchers have documented that the fear of being stigmatized and facing discrimination is a primary factor that prevents many individuals from accessing HIV testing and counseling services, as well as disclosing their status when HIV infection is identified (Abaynew, Deribew, & Deribe, 2011; Akani & Erhabor, 2006; Chinkonde, Sundby, & Martinson, 2009; Duff, Kipp, Wild, Rubaale, & Okech-Ojony, 2010; UNAIDS, 2003). For women, this fear may be compounded by concerns that their families, especially children, will be stigmatized or face discrimination (Moneyham, Hennessy, Sowell, Demi, Seals, & Mizuno, 1998; UNAIDS, 2004). Until HIV/AIDS stigma and its consequences are effectively addressed, it is likely that the secrecy surrounding an HIV/AIDS diagnosis will continue to fuel the pandemic.

One of the key concepts related to disclosure of HIV infection is that of damage control. As well as managing the disease itself, individuals with HIV/AIDS have to manage their concern of who knows their HIV infection (Bairan, Taylor, Blake, Akers, Sowell, & Mediola, 2007; Sowell, Seals, Phillips, & Julious, 2003). Disclosure of an HIV/AIDS diagnosis is not an "all or nothing" decision, but rather a series of decisions about how to disclose, to whom, and when to disclose. Trust issues and concerns about confidentiality are paramount in deciding to whom to disclose this status. Lazarus and Folkman's (1984) theory of stress and coping provides a framework for HIV/AIDS disclosure decision making. In this framework, HIV-infected individuals cognitively assess the potential value of disclosing their HIV-positive status against the potential negative consequences that may result from disclosure. Based on the outcome of this evaluation, disclosure either will or will not occur. It is well documented that PLWHA frequently disclose their HIV infection to some groups, such as healthcare workers and sex partners, while not disclosing this information to some members of their family, friends, and casual acquaintances (Bairan, Taylor, Blake, Akers, Sowell, & Mediola, 2007; Sowell & Phillips, 2010, p. 397; Sowell, Seals, Phillips, & Julious, 2003).

Sowell and associates (2003), in a study of women with HIV/AIDS, found that participants in their study had specific criteria for deciding to whom to disclose their infection. These criteria were based on one or more factors that included the following: (1) their relationship to the individuals to whom they disclosed (healthcare provider, sex partner, or family member); (2) the quality of their relationship with the individual (accepting versus rejecting); and (3) the perceived ability or likelihood of the other person to keep the information confidential. Even then, many individuals report that disclosing their HIV infection is based on a "need to know" basis. This can result in partial disclosure to healthcare providers, employers, and family, based on the assessment of whether there is any reason for that individual to know about their HIV infection. Therefore, an individual with an HIV infection who is seeing a healthcare provider who is not treating him or her for an HIV-related condition and/or will not be placed at risk of contracting the virus as a result of the care delivered, may not be informed that the individual is HIV infected. Likewise, insisting on condom use during casual sexual encounters may be used by PLWHA to prevent HIV transmission rather than telling the sex partner that he or she is HIV infected. This selective disclosure is an important aspect of managing the disclosure experience and limiting the negative consequences that can result from becoming known as having HIV/AIDS (Sowell & Phillips, 2010, p. 398).

Bairan and associates (2007) proposed a model of selective disclosure of HIV status based on the quality of relationships. This model identifies two primary types of relationships that influence disclosure decisions: sexual relationships and nonsexual relationships. The second tenet of the model is the concept that the attributes of the relationship (quality of the relationship, the level of intimacy in the relationship, and the length of the relationship) significantly influence the likelihood of disclosure or nondisclosure. This model may be useful in understanding factors that influence disclosure, thereby helping healthcare and social services providers to assist and support PLWHA in their disclosure decisions. Nevertheless, a question remains about the responsibility of healthcare and social services providers who are aware of an individual's nondisclosure of his or her HIV infection to inform or protect those who are being placed at risk. There is obviously no easy answer to this ethical dilemma. The obligation to maintain confidentiality must be weighed against the potential harm that may result from nonintervention, as well as the question of whether breaking confidentiality will actually prevent harm or result in even greater negative consequences. A harm reduction framework may be helpful to healthcare and social services providers in determining the most effective way to meet their professional standards while maintaining the confidentiality and trust of clients. The philosophical perspective of that framework supports actions that decrease the negative outcomes of a situation without having to eliminate all negative results, which is often unrealistic (Collins, Clifasefi, Logan, Samples, Somers, & Marlatt, 2012; Hasnain, 2005).

Clearly, supportive strategies that assist HIV-infected individuals to disclose their status, as well as community development efforts that change attitudes related to HIV stigma and discrimination, offer the greatest promise for positive outcomes. Despite the continued pandemic of stigma and discrimination targeting PLWHA, a limited number of research-based interventions have proved successful in decreasing HIV/AIDS stigma and facilitating dialogue concerning HIV/AIDS, including personal disclosure of HIV status. Table 10-1 provides an overview of interventions that have been tested to reduce stigma and promote disclosure at the individual level, the specific group level, and the community/societal level (Sowell & Phillips, 2010, pp. 398–400).

TABLE 10-1

Examples of Interventions and Strategies to Reduce the Stigma of HIV/AIDS

Type and Levels of the Intervention/ Strategy	Intervention/Strategy Description	Results	Reference
Issue Addressed: Stigma among hospital service providers. **Type:** Random control study, Intervention—Small group participatory activities and testimonials by HIV advocate **Primary Level:** Individual **Secondary Level:** Group	**Sample:** 138 service providers from four county hospitals in Yunnan, China. **Purpose:** To compare reduction in HIV stigma in intervention and control groups at three and six months.	Members of the intervention group reported significantly better protection of patients' confidentiality and right to HIV testing, lower levels of negative feelings toward PLWH, and more accurate understanding and practice of universal precautions.	Wu, Li, Wu, Liang, Cao, Yan, & Li, 2008
Issue Addressed: Stigma **Type:** Media simulation **Primary Level:** Individual **Secondary Level:** Group	**Sample:** 96 young women enrolled in an introductory psychology course. **Purpose:** To test whether a mock pilot radio broadcast could increase empathy toward PLWHA. The broadcast consisted of testimonials by a female PLWHA who had acquired HIV through either a blood transfusion (victim not responsible) or through sexual behavior (victim responsible).	The empathy scores were higher in the high-empathy group than in the low-empathy group. The empathy scores were higher for the victim-not-responsible group than for the victim-responsible group. The results demonstrated that inducing empathy for a stigmatized individual can also induce empathy for a stigmatized group.	Batson et al, 1997
Issue Addressed: Stigma and empowerment **Type:** Comprehensive community intervention with PLWH and persons close to PLWH (PCL). **Primary Level:** Individual	**Sample:** 18 PLWH (10 urban; 8 rural). PLC included partners; children close to family, close friends, spiritual leaders, and community members. **Purpose:** To increase knowledge of stigma, empower individuals and community, and wellness enhancement.	Participants gained greater knowledge about stigma and how to cope with stigmatizing behavior. Participants ready to educate community members. Increased disclosure skills.	MCur, DuCur, Watson, & Doak, 2015

(continues)

TABLE 10-1 (Continued)

Examples of Interventions and Strategies to Reduce the Stigma of HIV/AIDS

Type and Levels of the Intervention/Strategy	Intervention/Strategy Description	Results	Reference
Issue Addressed: Stigma **Type:** Multimethod educational intervention. An HIV/AIDS education intervention was delivered in six weekly sessions. Each session included lectures, film, role-plays, stories, songs, debates, and essays. **Primary Level:** Individual **Secondary Level:** Group	**Sample:** 240 secondary school students in urban Ibadan, Nigeria. **Purpose:** To improve knowledge, attitudes, and behaviors of secondary school students.	Students in the intervention group were more likely to be tolerant of PLWHA when compared to controls.	Fawole, Asuzu, Oduntan, & Brieger, 1999
Issue Addressed: Stigma **Type:** Multimethod intervention. The intervention combined factual information, student-created posters, songs, poetry, small-group discussions, plays, and role-play. **Primary Level:** Individual **Secondary Level:** Group	**Sample:** 814 students who were recruited from two school districts in Tanzania. **Purpose:** The purpose was to test the effectiveness of an educational program to reduce children's risk of HIV infections and to improve their tolerance of and willingness to care for a PLWHA.	Attitudes toward PLWHA significantly improved in the treatment group, when compared to the control group.	Klepp, Ndeki, Leshabari, Hannan, & Lyimo, 1997
Issue Addressed: Stigma **Type:** Acceptance by high-profile individuals. **Primary Level:** Societal	**Target Population:** The country of Cambodia. **Purpose:** Cambodian Prince Ranariddh gave flowers to a PLWHA at a national AIDS conference to demonstrate care and compassion for a PLWHA.	Anecdotal evidence shows a reduction in stigma.	Busza, 2001
Issue Addressed: Stigma **Type:** Emotional writing disclosure **Primary Level:** Individual	**Sample:** 11 HIV-positive women living in a large metropolitan area. **Purpose:** The researchers tested the effects of an emotional writing disclosure intervention on stigma and other health outcomes. Participants were asked to write for 20 minutes on three consecutive days about their deepest thoughts and feelings about the most traumatic event they ever experienced.	This pilot study tested the feasibility and acceptability of this intervention. In this small sample, the researchers found that stigma scores increased for the control group and decreased for the experimental group. The changes did not achieve significance.	Abel, Rew, Gortner, & Delville, 2004

Issue Addressed: Stigma **Type:** Community participatory intervention **Primary Level:** Community/societal	**Sample:** 199 PLWHA, 31 caregivers, and 195 randomly selected community members who were heads of household. **Purpose:** To test an intervention developed from a community participatory perspective and process.	A significant reduction in HIV/AIDS stigma scores was observed for the intervention group when compared to the control group.	Apinundecha, Laohasiriwong, Cameron, & Lim, 2007
Issue Addressed: Stigma **Type:** Sex workers were trained as peer educators and workshops were offered on self-care **Primary Level:** Individual **Secondary Level:** Group	**Sample:** The sample included women, men, and transsexual sex workers. **Purpose:** To describe educational interventions presented in two programs: "In the Battle for Health" and "Get Friendly with Her."	Anecdotal evidence shows a reduction in stigma	Chacham, Diniz, Maia, Galati, & Mirim, 2007
Issue Addressed: Stigma **Type:** Diffusion of positive messages about HIV/AIDS such as (1) advocating for universal precautions, (2) advocating that PLWHA receive the same level of care as everyone else, (3) advocating that PLWHA should not be discriminated against, and (4) advocating for protecting the confidentiality of PLWHA. **Primary Level:** Group **Secondary Level:** Community/society	**Sample:** Healthcare providers currently working at 89 general healthcare facilities. **Purpose:** To describe characteristics of popular opinion leaders and investigate factors associated with the diffusion of AIDS care messages by healthcare providers.	Female providers, members of the Han ethnic group, providers with less education, personnel at larger provincial hospitals, and personnel with HIV training were more likely to diffuse positive messages about HIV/AIDS.	Li, Cao, Wu, Wu, & Xiao, 2007
Issue Addressed: Stigma **Type:** Training/Education **Primary Level:** Individual **Secondary Level:** Community/group	**Sample:** Community-based organization in Tanzania trained staff and volunteers (n=56), PLWH (n=24), and community leaders (n=10) to recognize stigma and integrate stigma reduction into their routine work and carry out community sensitization and mobility activities.	Recognition of HIV-related stigma significantly increased over a two-year period. Statistically significant difference in stigmatizing attitudes associated with shame and blame at end-line evaluation among those exposed and not exposed to the intervention. However, the intervention did not reduce stigma communitywide. Stigma-reduction training had a profound effect on those trained, particularly the community leaders who visibly changed their behavior and leadership.	Pulerwitz, Michaelis, Weiss, Brown, & Mahendra, 2010

Data from Brown, L., Macintyre, K., & Trujillo, L. (2003). Interventions to reduce HIV/AIDS stigma: What have we learned? *AIDS Education and Prevention, 15*(1), 49–69. Retrieved from PM:12627743; Busza, J. R. (2001). Promoting the positive: Responses to stigma and discrimination in Southeast Asia. *AIDS Care, 13*(4), 441–456. Retrieved from PM:11454265.

HUMAN RIGHTS FRAMEWORK

There is a growing call for the response to HIV/AIDS as well as other public health issues to be addressed within the context of a human rights framework. This perspective was highlighted by the theme of the 2010 International AIDS Conference: "Rights Here, Right Now." This titling of the conference represented the explicit declaration of the International AIDS Society of the global need to bring attention to the disregard for basic human rights that fuels the spread of HIV/AIDS, as well as issues related to the allocation of resources, access to preventive education, access to treatment, and ability of PLWHA to live their lives with dignity, free of stigma and discrimination. Worldwide, PLWHA or those who represent groups at high risk for HIV infection (i.e., males having sex with males, sex workers, drug users, migrants, refugees) have not just faced stigma and discrimination, but have actually been criminalized. Criminalizing behaviors (and individuals) that are viewed as immoral has frequently been a strategy applied to control the spread of HIV/AIDS. In reality, however, evidence consistently shows that such strategies have not been effective in promoting public health, but instead have fueled the spread of HIV infection by driving such behaviors underground and decreasing potential access to HIV prevention information and programs (Poteat, Diouf, Baral, Ndaw, Drame, Traore,.. Beyrer, 2010; UNAIDS, 2008a).

In the closing session of the 2010 International AIDS Conference, Barrett (2010), in summarizing the research and programmatic presentation related to human rights and HIV/AIDS, proposed that human rights represent a necessary framework to inform any effective public health program. Some have argued that, to protect the masses, individual rights may have to be suspended (Human Rights Watch, 2008). We would propose that the suspension of individual rights is a shortsighted strategy, and that the appropriate approach is based on a respect of individual and group human rights. This view challenges practitioners and policy makers to find a balanced approach that engages at-risk individuals or targeted groups in determining effective solutions. It is important to be clear about the public health objective that is trying to be achieved. The goal of public health is to decrease the spread of disease in populations; it is not to stigmatize, disenfranchise, or criminalize individuals or groups. The failure of such a punitive approach can easily be seen in the failure of criminalization of drug use, sex work, and same-sex sexual relationships to deter or eliminate these behaviors or the negative health risks associated with these behaviors. To the contrary, research shows that positive health and societal outcomes can be effectively achieved by respecting the individual's right to self-determination and engaging individuals in finding solutions to negative outcomes such as the spread of HIV/AIDS (UNAIDS, 2010). Jonathan Mann, WHO Director (as cited in Beyrer & Pizer, 2000), proposed that health and human rights (incorrectly) have rarely been linked in an explicit manner. Building on the framework of explicitly linking human rights and public health provided by Mann, there has been recognition that human rights and the concept of human dignity must be at the center of any response to any major public health challenge (Cohen & Ezer, 2013; Rubenstein, 2000).

It may be important for the reader of this chapter to engage in values clarification. Do individuals have the right to self-determination, the right to have access to health education and medical treatment and/or nursing care? Is freedom to live without fear of stigma, discrimination, and violence a right that should be expected and protected? What, if any, obligation do resource-rich countries and governments have to respond to disease and poverty in resource-limited regions? Acknowledging the overwhelming data that link HIV/AIDS-related stigma, discrimination, and punitive sanctions to the spread of HIV infection (Abaynew, Deribew, & Deribe, 2011; UNAIDS, 2007b, 2008b), does the need to stigmatize and isolate those who are viewed as "other" serve the global public health? When prejudice, moral intolerance, and fear interfere with public policy, the result will consistently be increased morbidity and mortality. The HIV/AIDS pandemic may well have provided the definitive exemplar of this linkage and underscores the need for a reconceptualization of the relationship between human rights, human dignity, and health policy and practice.

SUMMARY

In this chapter, the authors have provided a global overview of stigma and discrimination and the devastating consequences of stigma at both individual and societal levels. While the focus of the chapter is on HIV/AIDS-related stigma and its consequences, it provides insight into the sources and effects of stigma that can be applied internationally to a large number of stigmatizing conditions, including illness, economic status, gender, sexual orientation, and any physical or psychological trait or characteristic that makes a person different or deviates from the norm. HIV/AIDS can be seen as representing a model case of stigma and resulting discrimination that, in reality, encompasses a variety of conditions. HIV/AIDS-related discrimination is a complex phenomenon that is rooted in the fear of a life-threatening disease and deviation from social standards or codes.

This chapter has also provided an overview of selected strategies that have been used globally to combat HIV/AIDS stigma and to support appropriate HIV/AIDS disclosure across a variety of cultures and settings. The authors propose that HIV/AIDS and its related stigma and discrimination may best be viewed in a human rights context. They challenge the reader to explore how HIV/AIDS stigma can be layered on other stigmatizing traits or conditions to form the basis for discrimination. Additionally, the authors suggest that freedom from stigma and discrimination and access to health care are basic human rights; public health strategies should be based on a balance between social welfare and respect for individual human rights.

Study Questions

1. Why do stigma and discrimination continue to be a challenge for HIV/AIDS patients and their families?
2. What remedies do you suggest for decreasing HIV/AIDS stigma and discrimination?
3. Name five reasons why HIV/AIDS patients hesitate to disclose their diagnosis.

Case Study 1: Stigma and Discrimination

The XIII International AIDS Conference was held in Durban, South Africa, during July 2000. This conference was significant for a number of reasons, including the fact that it marked the first time that the International AIDS Conference had been held in the southern hemisphere in a region that has been disproportionately affected by the HIV/AIDS epidemic. As delegates (scientists, HIV/AIDS care/service providers, researchers, educators, political and public figures, and persons living with HIV/AIDS) arrived in Durban, a renewed sense of challenge surrounded this conference that hosted more than 12,000 delegates. I (Sowell) had the privilege of being one of those delegates. There was an understanding that the conference would profoundly affect the region by focusing attention on HIV/AIDS, bringing it out of the shadows and confronting the devastating stigma and discrimination associated with HIV/AIDS in much of the world. To that end, the theme of the XIII International AIDS Conference was "Breaking the Silence." This theme sought to encourage persons infected and affected with HIV/AIDS to speak out and educate their communities concerning persons with HIV/AIDS and the transmission of the virus. Testing and counseling have long been important strategies in preventing the spread of HIV infection. However, being diagnosed with HIV/AIDS carries many social consequences that can be increased if this diagnosis becomes known. To openly admit to being HIV infected in many regions of the world can lead to physical danger from violence, as well as social isolation, rejection, and discrimination. This situation weighed heavy on the minds of the delegates to the XIII International AIDS Conference, in light of the murder of a South African woman in December 1998 after she publicly revealed she was HIV infected.

Gugu Dlamini was a 36-year-old, single mother living in KwaMashu, KwaZulu Natal. Unlike the conference delegates, who enjoyed the nice hotels and conference center of Durban, Gugu lived in a poor township in KwaZulu Natal. Wilson (2000) reported that "the poverty in KwaMashu attacks the soul" (p. 1). It is a place of pain and despair where the devastation and silence surrounding HIV/AIDS add to the misery of the people. The vast majority of black South Africans live in poverty and in townships that surround major urban centers. While Gugu Dlamini was honored as a hero in the fight to decrease the ignorance and fear surrounding HIV/AIDS in resource-limited regions of the world, her brutal murder provided evidence that the stigma of HIV/AIDS can be fatal.

In 1998, the South African National Association of People Living with HIV or AIDS and the KwaZulu Natal Department of Health encouraged persons with HIV/AIDS to disclose their HIV infection and urged local communities to become informed and to accept their neighbors. Gugu Dlamini became a volunteer in the provincial Department of Health Campaign (Beat It, 2011; McNeil, 1998). She publicly acknowledged her HIV infection to the press and worked to support others to disclose their own illness in an acceptance campaign in her township. She was one of the brave individuals who were willing to break the silence surrounding HIV/AIDS in an effort to try to make things better (South African Government Information, 1998). It is often women who step to the forefront in responding to HIV/AIDS, both by disclosing their own HIV status and by working to support and educate their communities. Over time, Gugu evolved into an outspoken AIDS activist. She began to meet and support other persons with HIV/AIDS in her township and believed that disclosure would be beneficial to her and to her community. She did not receive the support of her neighbors, however, but became the target of threats. Her family reported that Gugu often called them crying, saying that she was being threatened and people were coming for her. Many people in the community believed that she had brought shame on them and that her openness about her HIV status would negatively affect the community, as other community members would be viewed as likely to have the disease. Jabulani, Gugu's boyfriend, reported that people did not like her and were afraid for her to touch them or even drink with them (Beat It, 2011).

Gugu reported that she was threatened repeatedly. On December 12, 1998, she was attacked twice. In the afternoon, a man struck her and threatened her. Witnesses to the assault reported the incident to the local police, who did nothing. Gugu reportedly was afraid to go home alone and went to a local *shebeen* (tavern) to tell people about the incident and to publicly identify the man who had attacked her. Later that evening, Gugu was confronted by a man about her disclosure of her HIV status in the *shebeen*. She was dragged outside and beaten to unconsciousness by men from the community (McNeil, 1998). It was reported that after the men had beaten Gugu to unconsciousness, they sent a note to her boyfriend saying, "You can come fetch your dog. We are finished with her." It took four hours for an ambulance to arrive to take Gugu to the hospital where she died (Beat It, 2011). Even though many members of the community know who attacked and killed Gugu Dlamini, there has been little police follow-up. Her family has been threatened, and many who might speak out about this murder fear for their own safety (Beat It, 2011; Wilson, 2000).

However, Gugu's legacy did not end in KwaMashu, KwaZulu Natal, on the evening of December 12, 1998. Gugu has become a symbol of the potential extreme psychosocial and physical consequences related to the stigma and discrimination associated with HIV/AIDS. Her murder forced AIDS activists both in South Africa and globally to reevaluate their strategies in addressing HIV/AIDS stigma and related discrimination. Gugu represents only one of the many individuals who have suffered and died due to the ignorance and stigma related to HIV/ AIDS globally. Her death underscored and provided new urgency to the XIII International AIDS Conference theme of time to *Break the Silence*.

Case Study 1 Questions

1. Was Gugu Dlamini's public disclosure of her HIV-positive status worth the outcome for herself, her family, her community, and her country? Why or why not?
2. What responsibility do the organizations and groups that encouraged Gugu Dlamini to disclose her HIV-positive status have in her death?
3. Is disclosure of stigmatizing conditions always the best step to take? What are the advantages and disadvantages of such disclosure?
4. Discuss why women are more likely to respond to educate and address HIV/AIDS in their communities than men. Why was it men in this case study who instituted the violence against Gugu Dlamini?
5. Could (has) such terrible violence seen in the Gugu case study occur (occurred) in more resource-rich countries such as the United States and Europe?
6. Which types of discrimination and stigmatizing acts do persons living with HIV/AIDS continue to encounter today in different regions of the world?

7. What are the human rights implications of a woman being killed by her neighbors for disclosing her HIV/AIDS status? Why was no one willing to protect her? Would this situation have been different if Gugu had been a man?

8. What have you done in your community to ensure that persons with stigmatizing conditions do not face discrimination, including violence?

References

Some content included in this chapter was previously published in: Sowell, R. L., & Phillips, K. D. (2010). Understanding and responding to HIV/AIDS stigma and disclosure: An international challenge for mental health nurses. *Issues in Mental Health Nursing, 31*, 394–402. Referenced and used with permission.

Abaynew, Y., Deribew, A., & Deribe, K. (2011). Factors associated with late presentation to HIV/AIDS care in South Wollo Zone Ethiopia: A case-control study. *AIDS Research and Therapy 8*(8). Retrieved from http://www.ncbi.nlm.nih.gov/pmc/articles/PMC3058009/. doi:10.1186/1742-6405-8-8

Abel, E., Rew, L., Gortner, E. M., & Delville, C. L. (2004). Cognitive reorganization and stigmatization among persons with HIV. *Journal of Advanced Nursing, 47*(5), 510–525. PMID:15312114 DOI:10.1111/J.1365-2648.2004.03134.X

Abler, L., Henderson, G., Wang, X., & Avery, M. (2010). Factors associated with HIV stigma in an urban area in China: Results from the 2008 population survey [Abstract TUPE0565]. *Proceedings of the XVIII International AIDS Conference: Rights Here, Right Now.* Vienna, Austria.

AIDS Education and Training Center. (2014). HIC classification: CDC and WHO staging systems. Retrieved from http://aidsetc.org/guide/hiv-classification-cdc-and-who-staging-systems.

AIDS.gov. (2015). *Newly diagnosed: Older adults.* Retrieved from https://www.aids.go v/hiv-aids-basic/just-diagnosed-with-hiv-aids/overview/aging-population/

Akani, C. I., & Erhabor, O. (2006). Rate, pattern and barriers of HIV serostatus disclosure in a resource-limited setting in the Niger delta of Nigeria. *Tropical Doctor, 36*(2), 87–89. Retrieved from PM:16611440

Allen, C. F., Edwards, M., Williamson, L. M., Kitson-Piggott, W., Wagner, H. U., Camara, B., & Hospedales, C. J. (2006). Sexually transmitted infection service use and risk factors for HIV infection among female sex workers in Georgetown, Guyana. *Journal of Acquired Immune Deficiency Syndromes, 43*(1), 96–101. PMID:16885774

Anderson, B. J. (2009). HIV stigma and discrimination persist, even in health care. *AMA Journal of Ethics, 11*(12), 998–1001.

Anderson, E. L. (2010). How gender leaves women vulnerable to HIV infection: Lessons from Malawi [Abstract TUPE 0670]. *Proceedings of the XVIII International AIDS Conference: Rights Here, Right Now.* Vienna, Austria.

Apinundecha, C., Laohasiriwong, W., Cameron, M. P., & Lim, S. (2007). A community participation intervention to reduce HIV/AIDS stigma, Nakhon Ratchasima Province, Northeast Thailand. *AIDS Care, 19*(9), 1157–1165. PMID:18058400

Babalola, S. (2007). Readiness for HIV testing among young people in northern Nigeria: The roles of social norm and perceived stigma. *AIDS and Behavior, 11*(5), 759–769. DOI:10.1007/s10461-006-9189-0

Bairan, A., Taylor, G. A., Blake, B. J., Akers, T., Sowell, R., & Mediola, R. Jr. (2007). A model of HIV disclosure: Disclosure and types of social relationships. *Journal of the American Academy of Nurse Practitioners, 19*(5), 242–250. Retrieved from PM:17489957

Balabanova, Y., Coker, R., Atun, R. A., & Drobniewski, F. (2006). Stigma and HIV infection in Russia. *AIDS Care, 18*(7), 846–852. doi:W614R5550L10MJ00 [pii]; doi:10.1080/09540120600643641. Retrieved from PM:16971297

Baral, S., Semugoma, P., Diouf, D., Trapence, G., Poteat, T., Ndaw, M., . . . Beyrer, C. (2010). Criminalization of same sex practices as a structural driver of HIV risk among men who have sex with men (MSM): The cases of Senegal, Malawi, and Uganda [Abstract MOPE0951]. *Proceedings of the XVIII International AIDS Conference: Rights Here, Right Now.* Vienna, Austria.

Barrett, D. (2010). Track F rapporteur report. *Proceedings of the XVIII International AIDS Conference: Rights Here, Right Now.* Vienna, Austria.

Batson, C. D., Polycarpou, M. P., Harmon-Jones, E., Imhoff, H. J., Mitchener, E. C., Bednar, L. L., . . . Highberger, L. (1997). Empathy and attitudes: Can feeling for a member of a stigmatized group improve feelings toward the group? *Journal of Personality & Social Psychology, 72*(1), 105–118. Retrieved from PM:9008376

Beat It. (2011). Special report: Gugu Dlamini. *Siyayinoqoba: Beat It.* Retrieved from http://www.beatit.co.za/archive-events/1-december-1998-gugu-dlamini

Beaulleu, M., Adrien, A., & Lebounga Vouma, J. I. (2010). How gender roles influence HIV-STI risk among young Quebecers of Haitian origin [Abstract TUPE0670]. *Proceedings of the XVIII International AIDS Conference: Rights Here, Right Now.* Vienna, Austria.

Beyrer, C., & Pizer, H. F. (2000). *Public Health and Human Rights: Evidence-based Approaches.* Baltimore, MD: Johns Hopkins University Press.

Black, M. M., Nair, P., & Harrington, D. (1994). Maternal HIV infection: Parenting and early child development. *Journal of Pediatric Psychology, 19*(5), 595–615. Retrieved from PM:7807292

Blake, B. J., Taylor, G. A., Reid, P., & Kosowski, M. (2008). Experiences of women in obtaining human immunodeficiency virus testing and healthcare services. *Journal of the American Academy of Nurse Practitioners, 20*(1), 40–46. Retrieved from PM:18184164

Block, R. G. (2009). Is it just me? Experiences of HIV-related stigma. *Journal of HIV/AIDS & Social Services. 8*(1), 1–19.

Blumberg, A. (2014) Fourteen percent of Americans believe AIDS might be God's punishment: Survey. *Huffington Post.* Retrieved from http://www.huffingtonpost.com/2014/02/28/aids-hiv-ods-punishment-n-4876381.html

Bogart, L. M., Cowgill, B. O., Kennedy, D., Ryan, G., Murphy, D. A., Elijah, J., & Schuster, M. A. (2008). HIV-related stigma among people with HIV and their families: A qualitative analysis. *AIDS and Behavior, 12*(2), 244–254. Retrieved from PM:17458691

Botnick, M. R. (2000). Part 1: HIV as "the line in the sand." *Journal of Homosexuality, 38*(4), 39–76. Retrieved from PM:10807028

Buseh, A. G., & Stevens, P. E. (2006). Constrained but not determined by stigma: Resistance by African American women living with HIV. *Women & Health, 44*(3), 1–18. Retrieved from PM:17255063

Busza, J. R. (2001). Promoting the positive: Responses to stigma and discrimination in Southeast Asia. *AIDS Care, 13*(4), 441–456. Retrieved from PM:11454265

Campbell, C., & Cornish, F. (2010). Toward a "fourth generation" of approaches to HIV/AIDS management: Creating context for effective community mobilization. *AIDS Care, 22* (Supp 2), 1569–1579. doi:10.1080/09540121.2010.525812

Centers for Disease Control and Prevention. (1981a). Kaposi's sarcoma and *Pneumocystis* pneumonia among homosexual men—New York City and California. *Morbidity and Mortality Weekly Report, 30*, 305–308.

Centers for Disease Control and Prevention. (1981b). *Pneumocystis* pneumonia—Los Angeles. *Morbidity and Mortality Weekly Report, 30*, 250–252.

Centers for Disease Control and Prevention. (2013). HIV among older adults. Retrieved from http://www.cdc.gov/hiv/risk/age/olderamericans/

Centers for Disease Control and Prevention. (2014). *HIV-specific criminal laws.* Retrieved from http://www.cdc.gov/hiv/policies/law/states/exposure.html

Chacham, A. S., Diniz, S. G., Maia, M. B., Galati, A. F., & Mirim, L. A. (2007). Sexual and reproductive health needs of sex workers: Two feminist projects in Brazil. *Reproductive Health Matters, 15*(29), 108–118. Retrieved from PM:17512382

Chandra, P. S., Deepthivarma, S., & Manjula, V. (2003). Disclosure of HIV infection in south India: Patterns, reasons and reactions. *AIDS Care, 15*(2), 207–215. Retrieved from PM:12856342

Chang, F., Prytherch, H., Nesbitt, R. C., & Wilder-Smith, A. (2013). HIV-related travel restrictions: Trends and country characteristics. *Global Action Health, 6.* Retrieved from http://.globalhealthaction.net/index.php/gha/article/view/20472. doi:10.3402/gha.v6i0.20472

Chinkonde, J., Sundby, J., & Martinson, F. (2009). The prevention of mother-to-child HIV transmission programme in Lilongwe, Malawi: Why do so many women drop out? *Reproductive Health Matters, 17*(33), 143–151. doi:10.1016/S986-8080(09)33440-0

Cohen, J., & Ezer, T. (2013). Human rights in patient care: A theoretical and practical framework. *Health and Human Rights Journal.* Retrieved from http://www.hhrjournal.org/2013/human-rights-in-patient-care-a-theoritical-and-practical-framework/

Collins, S., Clifasefi, S., Logan, D., Samples, L., Somers, J., & Marlatt, G. A. (2012). Current status, historical highlights and basic principles of Harm reduction. In G. A. Marlatt, M. Lanimer, & K. Witkiewitz (Eds.), *Harm Reduction, Pragmatic Strategies for Managing High-Risk Behaviors* (2nd ed., pp. 3–35). New York: The Gilford Press.

Coursen-Neff, Z. (2004). Future forsaken: Abuses against children affected by HIV/AIDS in India. *Human Rights Watch.* Retrieved from http://hrw.org/reports/2004/india0704

Dang, B., Giordano, T., & Kim, J. H. (2012). Sociocultural and structural barriers to care among undocumented Latino immigrants with HIV infection. *Journal of Immigrant and Minority Health, 14*(1), 124–131. doi:10.1007/s10903-011-9542-x

Dej, E., & Kilty, M. (2012). Criminalization creep: A brief discussion of HIV/AIDS non-disclosure in Canada. *Canadian Journal of Law and Society, 27*(1), 55–66. doi:10.3138/cjs27.1.055

Dlamini, P. S., Kohi, T. W., Uys, L. R., Phetlhu, R. D., Chirwa, M. L., Naidoo, J. R., . . . Makoae, L. N. (2007). Verbal and physical abuse and neglect as manifestations of HIV/AIDS stigma in five African countries. *Public Health Nursing, 24*(5), 389–399. Retrieved from PM:17714223

Duff, P., Kipp, W., Wild, C., Rubaale, T., & Okech-Ojony, J. (2010). Barriers to accessing highly active antiretroviral therapy by HIV-positive women attending an antenatal clinic in a regional hospital in western Uganda. *Journal of the International AIDS Society, 13*(37). Retrieved from http://archive.biomedcentral.com/1758-2652/13/37. doi: 10.1186/1758-2652-13-37

Ekstrand, M., Bharat, S., & Ramakrishna, J. (2010). Blame and HIV misconceptions are associated with endorsement of coercive policies and intent to discriminate against PLHAs in two urban sites in India: Implications for stigma reduction interventions [Abstract TUPE0556]. *Proceedings of the XVIII International AIDS Conference: Rights Here, Right Now.* Vienna, Austria.

Elliott, R., & Gold, J. (2005). Protection against discrimination based on HIV/AIDS status in Canada: The legal framework. *HIV/AIDS Policy & Law Review, 10*(1), 20–31. Retrieved from PM:15991367

Familusi, O. O. (2012) African culture and the status of women: The Yoruba example. *Journal of Pan African Studies, 5*(1), 299–313.

Fawole, I. O., Asuzu, M. C., Oduntan, S. O., & Brieger, W. R. (1999). A school-based AIDS education programme for secondary school students in Nigeria: A review of effectiveness. *Health Education Research, 14*(5), 675–683. Retrieved from PM:10510075

Feller, L., & Lemmer, J. (2007). Aspects of immunopathogenic mechanisms of HIV infection. *Journal of the South African Dental Association, 62*(10), 432–434, 436. Retrieved from PM:18500104

Fuster, M. J., & Molero, F. (2010). The relationship between HIV related stigma and quality of life among people with HIV. [Abstract TUADO203]. *Proceedings of the XVIII International AIDS Conference.* July 18–23, 2010, Vienna, Austria.

Galanti, G. A. (2003). The Hispanic family and male–female relationships: An overview. *Journal of Trans-cultural Nursing, 14*(3), 180–185. Retrieved from PM:12861920

Galletly, C. L., & Pinkerton, S. D. (2004). Toward rational criminal HIV exposure laws. *Journal of Law Medicine & Ethics, 32*(2), 327–337. Retrieved from PM:15301197

Galvin, F., Davis, M., Banks, D., & Bing, E. (2008). HIV stigma and social support among African Americans. *AIDS Patient Care and STDs, 22*(5), 423–436.

Genberg, B. L., Kawichai, S., Chingono, A., Sendah, M., Chariyalertsak, S., Konda, K., & Clentano, D. D. (2008). Assessing HIV/AIDS stigma and discrimination in developing countries. *AIDS and Behavior, 12*, 772–780. doi:10.1007/s10461-007-9340-6

Gilbert, L., & Walker, L. (2010). My biggest fear was that people would reject me once they knew my status: Stigma as experienced by patients in an HIV/AIDS clinic in Johannesburg, South Africa. *Health and Social Care in the Community, 18*(2), 139–146. doi: 10.1111/j.1365-2524.2009.00881.x

Gilmore, N., & Somerville, M. A. (1994). Stigmatization, scapegoating and discrimination in sexually transmitted diseases: Overcoming "them" and "us." *Social Science and Medicine, 39*(9), 1339–1358. Retrieved from PM:7801170

Goffman, E. (1963). *Stigma: Notes on the Management of Spoiled Identity*. Englewood Cliffs, NJ: Prentice-Hall.

Goldberg, S. M., Silverman, J. G., Engstrom, D., Bojorquez-Chapela, I., Usita, P., Rolon, M. L., & Strathdee, S. (2015). Exploring the context of trafficking and adolescent sex industry involvement in Tijuana, Mexico: Consequences for HIV risk and prevention. *Violence Against Women, 21*(4), 478–499. doi:10.1177/1077801215569079

Greeff, M., & Phetlhu, R. (2007). The meaning and effect of HIV/AIDS stigma for people living with AIDS and nurses involved in their care in the North West Province, South Africa. *Curationis, 30*(2), 12–23. Retrieved from PM:17703819

Green, E. C., Halperin, D., Nantulya, V., & Hogle, J. (2006). Uganda's HIV prevention success: The role of sexual behavior change and the national response. *AIDS and Behavior, 10*(94), 335–346. doi:10.1007/s10461-006-9073-y

Grodensky, C. A., Golin, C. E., Jones, C., Mamo, M., Dennis, A., Abernethy, M., & Patterson, K. B. (2015). "I should know better": The role of relationships, spirituality, disclosure, stigma, and shame for older women living with HIV seeking support in the South. *Journal of the Association of Nurses in AIDS Care (JANAC), 26*(1), 12–23. Retrieved from http://dx.doi.org/10.1016/j.jana.2014.01.005

Hasnain, M. (2005). Cultural approach to HIV/AIDS harm reduction in Muslim countries. *Harm Reduction Journal, 2*(23). Retrieved from PM:16253145

Hatzenbuehler, M. L., Phelam, J. C., & Link, B. G. (2013). Stigma as a fundamental cause of population health inequalities. *American Journal of Public Health, 103*(5), 813–821. doi:10.2105/AJPH.2012.301069

Hess, R. F., & McKinney, D. (2007). Fatalism and HIV/AIDS beliefs in rural Mali, West Africa. *Journal of Nursing Scholarship, 39*(2), 113–118. Retrieved from PM:17535310

Holtz, C., Sowell, R., VanBrackle, L., Velasuez, G., Hernandez-Alonso, V. (2014). A quantitative study of factors influencing quality of life in rural Mexican women diagnosed with HIV. *Journal of the Association of Nurses in AIDS Care, 5*(6), 555–567. doi: 10.1016/j.jana.2014.03.002

Holtz, C., Sowell, R. L., Van Brackle, L., Velasquez, G., & Hernandez-Alonso, V. (2012). Oaxacan women with HIV/AIDS: Resiliency in the face of poverty, stigma, and social isolation. *Women and Health, 52*(6), 517–535. doi:10.1080/03630242.2012.690839

Horter, S., Nkhoma, H., Baradaran, S., Baggaley, R., & Stedwick, R. (2010). Proposed HIV and HIDSS bill in Malawi: Benefit or barrier to improving the HIV response? [Abstract THPE0903]. *Proceedings of the XVIII International AIDS Conference: Rights Here, Right Now*. Vienna, Austria.

Hossain, M. B., Islam, M. R., Islam, M. A., & Kabir, M. A. (2010). HIV-related stigmatized attitude and its predictors among the general population in Bangladesh [Abstract TUPE 0554]. *Proceedings of the XVIII International AIDS Conference: Rights Here, Right Now*. Vienna, Austria.

Human Rights Watch. (2004). Bad dreams: Exploitation and abuse of migrant workers in Saudi Arabia. *Human Rights Watch, 16*(5E).

Human Rights Watch. (2007). Chronic indifference: HIV/AIDS services for immigrants detained by the United States. *Human Rights Watch, 19*(5G).

Human Rights Watch. (2008). A testing challenge. *Human Rights Watch*. Retrieved from http://www.hrw.org/en/node/75974/section/5

Human Rights Watch. (2009). *2009 a bad year for migrants: Deaths, labor exploitation, violence, and poor treatment in detention*. Retrieved from http://www.hrw.org/news/2009/12/16/2009-bad-year-migrants

Huy, T. Q., Johansson, A., & Long, N. H. (2007). Reasons for not reporting deaths: A qualitative study in rural Vietnam. *World Health and Population, 9*(1), 14–23. Retrieved from PM:18270497

Ibekwe, N., & Agbo, L. (2010). HIV and AIDS related stigma and discrimination in the rural Eastern Nigeria [Abstract TUPE0550]. *Proceedings of the XVIII International AIDS Conference: Rights Here, Right Now.* Vienna, Austria.

Jones, E. E., Farina, A., Hastorf, A. H., Markus, H., Miller, D. T., & Scott, R. A. (1984). *Social stigma: The psychology of marked relationships.* New York: W. H. Freeman.

Jurgens, R., Cohn, J., Cameron, E., Burris, S., Clayton, M., Elliott, R., Pearshouse, R., Gathumbi, A., & Cupido, D. (2009). Ten reasons to oppose the criminalization of HIV exposure or transmission. *Reproductive Health Matters, 17*(34), 163–172. doi:10.1016/S0968-8080(09)34462-6

Kazatchkine, C. (2010). Criminalizing HIV transmission or exposure: The context of francophone West and Central Africa. *HIV/AIDS Policy & Law Review, 14*(3), 1–11.

Kebaabetswe, P. (2007). Barriers to participation in the prevention of mother-to-child transmission programme in Gaborone, Botswana. A qualitative approach. *AIDS Care, 19*(3), 355–360.

Kehler, J. (2010). Women's sexual and reproductive rights in national strategic plans: Are women's rights at the centre of the AIDS response? [Abstract THPE0996]. *Proceedings of the XVIII International AIDS Conference: Rights Here, Right Now.* Vienna, Austria.

Kehler, J., & Crone, E. T. (2010). Addressing the implications of HIV criminalization for women [Abstract THPE1024]. *Proceedings of the XVIII International AIDS Conference: Rights Here, Right Now.* Vienna, Austria.

Kelso, G. A., Cohen, M. H., Weber, K. M., Dale, S. K., Cruise, R. C., & Brody, L. R. (2014). Critical consciousness, racial and gender discrimination, and HIV disease markers in African American women with HIV. *AIDS & Behavior, 18*(7), 1237–1246.

Kirton, C. A. (2010). The HIV disease trajectory. In J. Durham & F. Lashley (Eds.), *The Person with HIV/AIDS* (pp. 71–92). New York: Springer.

Klepp, K. I., Ndeki, S. S., Leshabari, M. T., Hannan, P. J., & Lyimo, B. A. (1997). AIDS education in Tanzania: Promoting risk reduction among primary school children. *American Journal of Public Health, 87*(12), 1931–1936. Retrieved from PM:9431279

Kloer, A. (2010). Sex trafficking and HIV/AIDS: A deadly junction for women. *Human Rights Magazine Home, 37*(2). Retrieved from http://www.americanbar.org/publications/human_rights-magazine_home/human_rights_vol37_2010/Spring2010/sex_trafficking_and_hiv_aids_a_deadly_junction_for_women_and_girls.html

Kohi, T. W., Makoae, L., Chirwa, M., Holzemer, W. L., Phetlhu, D. R., Uys, L., . . . Greeff, M. (2006). HIV and AIDS stigma violates human rights in five African countries. *Nursing Ethics, 13*(4), 404–415. Retrieved from PM:16838571

Lambda Legal. (2009). *State criminal statutes on HIV exposure.* Retrieved from http://www.lambdalegal.org/our-work/publications/general/state-criminal-statutes-hiv.html

Laryea, M., & Gien, L. (1993). The impact of HIV-positive diagnosis on the individual, Part 1: Stigma, rejection, and loneliness. *Clinical Nursing Research, 2*(3), 245–263, discussion. Retrieved from PM:8401240

Lazarus, R. S., & Folkman, S. (1984). *Stress, appraisal, and coping.* New York: Springer.

Lazzarini, Z., Galletly, C., Mykhalovskiy, E., Harsono, D., O'Keefe, E., & Singer, M. (2013). Criminalization of HIV transmission adexposure: Research and policy agenda. *American Journal of Public Health, 103*(8), 1350–1353. doi: 10.2105/AJPH.2013.301267

Lee, M. B., Wu, Z., Rotheram-Borus, M. J., Detels, R., Guan, J., & Li, L. (2005). HIV-related stigma among market workers in China. *Health Psychology, 24*(4), 435–438. Retrieved from PM:16045380

Lee, S., Li, L., Iamsirithaworn, S., & Khumtong, S. (2013). Disclosure challenges among people living with HIV in Thailand. *International Journal of Nursing Practice, 19*, 374–380. doi:10.1111/ijn.12084

Li, L., Cao, H., Wu, Z., Wu, S., & Xiao, L. (2007). Diffusion of positive AIDS care messages among service providers in China. *AIDS Education and Prevention, 19*(6), 511–518. Retrieved from PM:18190275

Li, M. J., Murry, J. K., Suwanteerangkul, J., & Wiwatanadate, P. (2014). Stigma, social support, and treatment adherence among HIV-positive patients in Chiang Mai, Thailand. *AIDS Education and Prevention, 26*(5), 471–483.

Logie, C., James, L., Tharao, W., & Loutfy, M. (2010). The intersection of race, gender, sexual orientation, and HIV: Understanding multi-dimensional forms of stigma and discrimination experienced by women living with HIV in Ontario, Canada [Abstract WEAD0102]. *Proceedings of the XVIII International AIDS Conference: Rights Here, Right Now.* Vienna, Austria.

Macintyre, K., Rutenberg, N., Brown, L., & Karim, A. (2004). Understanding perceptions of HIV risk among adolescents in KwaZulu-Natal. *AIDS and Behavior, 8,* 237–250.

Mahajan, A. P., Saylers, J., Patel, V., Remien, R., Ortiz, D., Szekeres, G., & Coates, T. J. (2008). Stigma in the HIV/AIDS epidemic: A review of the literature and recommendations for the way forward. *AIDS, 22* (suppl 2): S67–S79. doi: 10.1097/01.aids.0000327438.13291.62

McGovern, T. M. (2006). Models of resistance: "Victims" lead. *Health and Human Rights, 9*(2), 234–255. Retrieved from PM:17265762

McNeil, D. J., Jr. (1998, December 28). Neighbors kill an HIV-positive AIDS activist in South Africa. *New York Times,* p. 28.

MCur, H. F., DCur, M. G., Watson, M. J., & Doak, C. M. (2015). A comprehensive HIV stigma-reduction and wellness-enhancement community intervention: A case study. *Journal of the Association of Nurses in AIDS Care (JANAC), 26*(1), 81–96. http://dx.doi.org/10.1016/j.jana.2014.03.007

Mendenhall, E., Muzizi, L., Stephenson, R., Chomba, E., Ahmed, Y., Haworth, A., & Allen, S. (2007). Property grabbing and will writing in Lusaka, Zambia: An examination of wills of HIV-infected cohabiting couples. *AIDS Care, 19*(3), 369–374. Retrieved from PM:17453571

Molina, E., & Lainez, H. (2010). Criminalization of sex work as an obstacle for access to integral attention on HIV/AIDS [Abstract TUPE1004]. *Proceedings of the XVIII International AIDS Conference: Rights Here, Right Now.* Vienna, Austria.

Moneyham, L., Hennessy, M., Sowell, R., Demi, A., Seals, B., & Mizuno, Y. (1998). The effectiveness of coping strategies used by HIV-seropositive women. *Research in Nursing & Health, 21*(4), 351–362. Retrieved from PM:9679811

Montaner, J., & Schmied, B. (2010). Rights here, right now. *Human Rights Magazine Home, 37.* Retrieved from http://www.americanbar.org/publications/human_rights_magazine_home/human_rights_vol37/spring2010/rights_here_right_now.html

Moreno, C. L. (2007). The relationship between culture, gender, structural factors, abuse, trauma, and HIV/AIDS for Latinas. *Qualitative Health Research, 17*(3), 340–352. Retrieved from PM:17301342

Moser, K. M., Sowell, R. L., & Phillips, K. D. (2001). Issues of women dually diagnosed with HIV infection and substance use problems in the Carolinas. *Issues in Mental Health Nursing, 22*(1), 23–49. Retrieved from PM:11885060

Muchenje, M., Tharao, W., Mehes, M., Njeri, R., Ndungu, M., Hove, P.,... Hintzen, D. (2010). To disclose or not to disclose? The factors influencing HIV disclosure among African and Caribbean women [Abstract WEPE0602]. *Proceedings of the XVIII International AIDS Conference: Rights Here, Right Now.* Vienna, Austria.

Mukolo, A., Blevins, M., Victor, B., Vaz, L. M., Sidat dat, M., & Vergara, A. (2013). Correlates of social exclusion and negative labeling and devaluation of people living with HIV/AIDS in rural settings: Evidence from a general household survey in Zambezia Province, Mozambique. *PLOS One, 8*(10). Retrieved from Http://www.ncbi.nlm.nih.gov/pbumed/24146771 doi:10.1371/journal.pone.00744

Mustanski, B. S., Newcomb, M. E., DuBois, S., Garcia, S., & Gov, C. (2011). HIV in young men who have sex with men: A review of epideminology risk and protective factors, and interventions. *Journal of Sex Research, 48*(2–3), 218–253. doi:10.1080/00224499/2011.558645

Muthuswamy, V. (2005). Ethical issues in HIV/AIDS research. *Indian Journal of Medical Research, 121*(4), 601–610. Retrieved from PM:15817966

Mykhalovskiy, E. (2010). HIV non-disclosure and the criminal law: Effects of Canada's significant risk test on people living with HIV/AIDS and health and social services providers [Abstract THLBF102]. *Proceedings of the XVIII International AIDS Conference: Rights Here, Right Now.* Vienna, Austria.

Nwaebuni, R. (2013, November 27). Nigeria: A different place to be widow. *The Africa Report, 19*(1). Retrieved from http://www.theafricareport.com/west-africa/nigeria-a-difficult-place-to-be-widow.html

Nyanzi, S. (2010). Contesting diverse widow inheritance customs in Uganda, Kenya, and Tanzania [Abstract MOAD0104]. *Proceedings of the XVIII International AIDS Conference: Rights Here, Right Now.* Vienna, Austria.

Obermeyer, C. M., & Osborn, M. (2007). The utilization of testing and counseling for IV: A review of the social and behavioral evidence. *American Journal of Public Health, 97*(10), 1762–1774. doi:10.2105/AJPH.2006.096263

Ogunmefun, C., Gilbert, L., & Schatz, E. (2011). Older female caregivers and HIV/AIDS-related secondary stigma in rural South Africa. *Journal of Cross Cultural Gerontology, 26*(11), 85–102. doi:10.1007/s10823-010-9129-3

Oh, K. (2010). The past, present and future of HIV-related travel restrictions in the United States and the Republic of Korea [Abstract WEPE0884]. *Proceedings of the XVIII International AIDS Conference: Rights Here, Right Now.* Vienna, Austria.

Pedrotti, C., Bishop, A., & Dunham, S. (2010). HIV, human rights and social inclusion: The experience of HIV oost-clubs over the life of the "reducing community vulnerability to HIV and AIDS program" in Kenya, Zambia, and Zimbabwe [Abstract MOPE0640]. *Proceedings of the XVIII International AIDS Conference: Rights Here, Right Now.* Vienna, Austria.

Petros, G., Airhihenbuwa, C. O., Simbayi, L., Ramlagan, S., & Brown, B. (2006). HIV/AIDS and "othering" in South Africa: The blame goes on. *Culture, Health, & Sexuality, 8*(1), 67–77. Retrieved from PM:16500826

Pharris, A., Tishelman, C., Huyen, D. T., Chuc, N. T. K., & Thorson, A. (2010). The "infected innocent": Gender roles and stigma among women living with HIV in Vietnam [Abstract WEPE0656]. *Proceedings of the XVIII International AIDS Conference: Rights Here, Right Now.* Vienna, Austria.

Poteat, T., Diouf, D., Baral, S., Ndaw, M., Drame, F., Traore, C., . . . Beyrer, C. (2010). The impact of criminalization of same-sex practices on HIV risk among men who have sex with men (MSM) in Senegal: Results of a qualitative rapid assessment [Abstract TUPE0709]. *Proceedings of the XVIII International AIDS Conference: Rights Here, Right Now.* Vienna, Austria.

Poteat, T., Diouf, D., Drame, F. M., Ndaw, M., Traore, C., Dhaliwal, M., Beyrer, C., & Baral, S. (2014). HIV risk among MSM in Senegal: A qualitative rapid assessment of the impact of enforcing laws that criminalize same-sex practices. *PLOS One.* Retrieved from http://journals.plosone/article?id=10.1371/journal. pone.0028760. doi:10.1371/journal.pone.0028760

Pulerwitz, J., Michaelis, A., Weiss, E., Brown, L., & Mahendra, V. (2010). Reducing HIV-related stigma: Lessons learned from Horizons research and programs. *Public Health Reports, 125*(2), 272–281. PMID:20297756

Romero, L., Wallerstein, N., Lucero, J., Fredine, H. G., Keefe, J., & O'Connell, J. (2006). Woman to woman: Coming together for positive change—using empowerment and popular education to prevent HIV in women. *AIDS Education and Prevention, 18*(5), 390–405. Retrieved from PM:17067251

Rubenstein, L. S. (2000). Foreword. In C. Beyrer & H. F. Pizer (Eds.), *Public Health and Human Rights: Evidence-Based Approaches.* Baltimore, MD: Johns Hopkins University Press.

Sarkar, K., Bal, B., Mukherjee, R., Chakraborty, Saha, S., Ghosh, A., & Parsons, S. (2008). Sex-trafficking, violence, negotiating skills, and HIV infection in brothel-based sex workers of eastern India, adjoining Nepal, Bhutan, and Bangladesh. *Journal of Health, Population, and Nutrition, 26*(2), 223–231.

Seeley, J., Grellier, R., & Barnett, T. (2004). Gender and HIV/AIDS impact mitigation in sub-Saharan Africa: Recognising the constraints. *Journal of Social Aspects of HIV/AIDS Research Alliance, 1*(2), 87–98. Retrieved from PM:17601014

Sengupta, S., Strauss, R. P., Miles, M. S., Roman-Isler, M., Banks, B., & Corbie-Smith, G. (2010). A conceptual model exploring the relationship between HIV stigma and implementing HIV clinical trials in rural communities of North Carolina. *North Carolina Medical Journal, 71*(2), 113–122. Retrieved from http://www.ncbi.nlm .nih.gov/pmc/articles/PMO3037544/

Shilts, R. (1987). *And the Band Played On: Politics, People, and the AIDS Epidemic.* New York: St. Martin's Press.

Slater, L. Z., Moneyham, L., Vance, D. E., Raper, J. I., Mugavero, M. J., & Childs, G. (2015). The multiple stigma experienced and quality of life in older gay men with HIV. *Journal of the Association of Nurses in AIDS Care (JANAC), 26*(1), 24–35. http://dx.doi.org/10.1016/j.jana.2014.06.007

Smith, R., Rossetto, K., & Peterson B. L. (2008). A meta-analysis of disclosure of one's HIV-positive status, stigma and social support. *AIDS Care, 20*(10), 1266–1275. doi:10.1080/09540120801926977

Sontag, S. (1998). *AIDS and Its Metaphors*. New York: Vintage Books.

South African Government Information. (1998). Press release issued by the Department of Health on the killing of Ms. Gugu Dlamini (AIDS campaign worker).

Sowell, R. L., Holtz, C., & Velasquez, G. (2008). Bringing HIV/AIDS home to Mexico: Perspectives of migrant workers and their wives. *Journal of the Association of Nurses in AIDS Care, 19*(4), 267–282.

Sowell, R. L., & Phillips, K. D. (2010). Understanding and responding to HIV/AIDS stigma and disclosure: An international challenge for mental health nurses. *Issues in Mental Health Nursing, 31*(6), 394–402. Retrieved from PM:20450341. doi:10.3109/01612840903497602

Sowell, R. L., Phillips, K. D., Seals, B., Murdaugh, C., & Rush, C. (2002). Incidence and correlates of physical violence among HIV infected women at risk for pregnancy in the southeastern United States. *Journal of the Association of Nurses in AIDS Care, 13*(2), 46–58.

Sowell, R. L., Seals, B. F., Phillips, K. D., & Julious, C. H. (2003). Disclosure of HIV infection: How do women decide to tell? *Health Education Research, 18*(1), 32–44. Retrieved from PM:12608682

Sterken, D. J. (2010). Living with HIV/AIDS. In J. Durham & F. Lashley (Eds.), *The Person with HIV/AIDS: Nursing Perspectives* (4th ed., pp. 205–219). New York: Springer.

Surkan, P. J., Mukherjee, J. S., Williams, D., Eustache. E., Louis, E., Jean-Paul, T., Lambert, W., Scanlan, F., Oswald, C., & Smith Fawzi, M. C. (2010). Perceived discrimination and stigma toward children affected by HIV/AIDS and their HIV-positive caregivers in central Haiti. *AIDS Care, 22*(7), 803–815. doi:10.1080/09540120903443392

Svensson, J. (2014). God's rage: Muslim representation of HIV/AIDS as divine punishment from the perspective of the cognitive science of religion. *NVMEN, 61*(5–6), 569–593. Retrieved from http://booksandjournals. brillonline.com/content/journals/10.1163/15685276-12341343. doi:10.1163/15685276-12341343

Tenkorang, E., Obeng-Gyimah, S., Maticka-Tyndale, E., & Adjei, J. (2010). Superstition, witchcraft, and HIV/AIDS prevention in Sub-Saharan Africa: The case of Ghana [Abstract MOPE 0508]. *Proceedings of the XVIII International AIDS Conference: Rights Here, Right Now*. Vienna, Austria.

Thomas, R., Lalu, V., Mukambetov, A., Odhiambo, T., & Williams, J. (2010). Arrest the violence and halt HIV: Strategies for reducing police abuse against sex workers [Abstract TUAF0401]. *Proceedings of the XVIII International AIDS Conference: Rights Here, Right Now*. Vienna, Austria.

Thompson, M. A., Aberg, J. A., Cahn, P., Montaner, J. S., Rizzardini, G., Telenti, A., . . . Schooley, R. T. (2010). Antiretroviral treatment of adult HIV infection: 2010 recommendations of the International AIDS Society—USA panel. *Journal of the American Medical Association, 304*(3), 321–333. Retrieved from PM:20639566. doi:304/3/321 [pii]; 10.1001/jama.2010.1004

Tran Huy, D., & Nguyen, T. H. (2010). Discrimination: A major barrier in Vietnam [Abstract WEBP0663]. *Proceedings of the XVIII International AIDS Conference: Rights Here, Right Now*. Vienna, Austria.

Joint United Nations Programme on HIV/AIDS. (2003). UNAIDS report for 2003: Most deaths and new infections ever; some good news. *AIDS Treatment News, 396,* 3. Retrieved from PM:14717110

Joint United Nations Programme on HIV/AIDS. (2004). *2004 report on the global AIDS epidemic* (4th ed.). Geneva, Switzerland: UNAIDS Joint United Nations Programme on HIV/AIDS.

Joint United Nations Programme on HIV/AIDS. (2007). *Reducing HIV stigma and discrimination: A critical part of national AIDS programmes*. Geneva, Switzerland: UNAIDS Joint United Nations Programme on HIV/AIDS.

Joint United Nations Programme on HIV/AIDS. (2008a). *International consultation on the criminalization of HIV transmission*. Retrieved from http://data.unaids.org/pub/Report/2008/20080919_hivcriminalization_ meetingreport_en.pdf

Joint United Nations Programme on HIV/AIDS. (2008b). *Stigma and discrimination*. Retrieved from http:// www.unaids.org/en/PolicyAndPractice/StigmaDiscrim/default.asp

Joint United Nations Programme on HIV/AIDS. (2010). *Human rights and HIV*. Retrieved from http://www .unaids.org/en/PolicyAndPractice/HumanRights/default.asp

Joint United Nations Programme on HIV/AIDS. (2012). Key programmes to reduce stigma and discrimination and increase access to justice in national HIV responses. Retrieved from www.unaids.org/sites/default/files/ media_asset/Key_Human_Rights_Programmes_en_May2012_0.pdf

Joint United Nations Programme on HIV/AIDS. (2013). *AIDS by the numbers*. Retrieved from http://www .unaids.org/en/media/unaids/contentassets/documents/unaidspublications/2013/JC2571_aids_by_the_ numbers_en.pdf

Joint United Nations Programme on HIV/AIDS. (2014). *Global statistics*. Retrieved from http://www.aids.gov/ hiv-aids-basic/hiv-aids-101/global-statistics/

The United Nations Children's Fund. (2006). *Africa's orphaned and vulnerable generations: Children affected by AIDS*. Retrieved from http://www.unicef.org/publications/index_35645.html

The United Nations Children's Fund. (2010). *Blame and banishment: The underground HIV epidemic affecting children in Eastern Europe and Central Asia*. Retrieved from: http://lastradainternational.org/ doc-center/2453/blame-and-banishment-the-underground-hiv-epidemic-affecting-children-in-eastern- europe-and-central-asia

Valdiserri, R. O. (2002). HIV/AIDS stigma: An impediment to public health. *American Journal of Public Health, 92*(3), 341–342.

Varas-Diaz, N., Neilands, T., Cintron-Bou, F., Santos-Figueroa, A., Marzan-Rodriguez, M., & Marques, D. (2014). Religion and HIV/AIDS stigma in Puerto Rico: A cultural challenge for training future physicians. *Journal of the International Association of Providers of AIDS Care 13*(4), 305–308. doi:10.1177/2325957412472935

Varas-Diaz, N., Neilands, T. B., Malave-Rivera, S., & Betancourt, E. (2010). Religion and HIV/AIDS stigma: Implications for health professionals in Puerto Rico. *Global Public Health, 5*(3), 295–312. Retrieved from http://www.tandjonline.com/doi/abs/10.1080/17441690903436581

Varni, S. E., Miller, C. T., McCuin, T., & Solomon, S. E. (2012). Disengagement and engagement coping with HIV/AIDS stigma and psychological well-being of people with HIV/AIDS. *Journal of Social and Clinical Psychology, 31*(2), 123–150.

Visser, M. J., Makin, J. D., Vandormael, A., Sikkema, K. J., & Forsyth, B. W. (2009). HIV/AIDS stigma in a South African community. *AIDS Care, 21*(9), 197–206. doi:10.1080/09540120801932157

Visser, M. J., Neufeld, S., de Villiers, A., Makin, J., & Forsyth, B. (2008). To tell or not to tell: South African women's disclosure of HIV status during pregnancy. *AIDS Care, 20*(9), 1138–1145. doi:10.1080/0954012070184779

Vyavaharkar, M., Moneyham, L., Corwin, S., Tavakoli, A., Saunders, R., & Annang, L. (2011). HIV-disclosure, social support, and depression among HIV-infected African American women living in the rural southeastern United States. *AIDS Education and Prevention 23*(1), 78–90. doi: 10.1521/aeap.2011.23.1.78

Weait, M. (2013). Unsafe law: Health, rights, and the legal response to HIV. *International Journal of Law in Context, 9*(4), 535–564. doi:10.1017/S1744552313000293

Weeks, B. S., & Alcamo, I. E. (2008). Defining and recognizing AIDS. In B. S. Weeks & I. E. Alcamo (Eds.), *AIDS: The Biologic Basis* (4th ed., pp. 84–113). Sudbury, MA: Jones and Bartlett Publishers.

Wenani, T. (2010). Violence, neglect and abuse of children affected by AIDS at the Dandora Dumping Site, Nairobi, Kenya [Abstract TUPE0578]. *Proceedings of the XVIII International AIDS Conference: Rights Here, Right Now*. Vienna, Austria.

Wilson, P. (2000). Perspective: Seeing the true surroundings. *HIV Plus*. Retrieved from http://aidsinfonyc.org/ hivplus/issue10/columns/perspective.html

Wu, S., Li Li, Wu, Z., Liang, L., Cao, H., Yan, Z., & Li, J. (2008). A brief HIV stigma reeducation intervention for service providers in China. *AIDS Patient Care and STDs, 22*(6), 513–520. doi: 10.1089/apc/2007.0198

Yager, A. (2012). License denied: Professional and vocational licensing restrictions affecting people living with HIV in the United States. [Abstract TUPDD0102]. *Proceedings of the XIX International AIDS Conference*, Washington, D.C.

Zukoski, A. P., & Thorburn, S. (2009). Experiences of stigma and discrimination among adults living with HIV in a low HIV-prevalence context: A qualitative analysis. *AIDS Patient Care and STDs, 23*(4), 267–276. doi:10.1089/apc.2008.0168

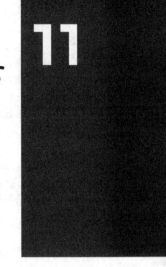

Global Use of Complementary and Integrative Health Approaches

Ping Hu Johnson

Objectives

After completing this chapter, the reader will be able to:

1. Describe complementary and integrative health (CIH) and its main categories.
2. Discuss the trends of complementary and integrative health approach use in both developing and developed countries, and explain the reasons behind the increased popularity of CIH use.
3. Identify the predictors, reasons, patterns, and cost of complementary and integrative health approach use in the United States.
4. Discuss the theories and practices of different types of complementary and integrative health approaches being used in the United States today.
5. Discuss the current status and challenges of CIH research.
6. Identify the impact of technology on the use of and research in CIH.
7. Discuss the legal and ethical issues surrounding CIH treatments and research.
8. Describe the influence of politics, economics, culture, and religion on complementary and integrative health approaches.
9. Compare the use of complementary and integrative health approaches between developing and developed societies.

INTRODUCTION

In recent years, we have seen an increased interest in complementary and integrative health (CIH) and treatments in the United States and worldwide. It appears to be a trend that more people are seeking holistic healthcare approaches and using natural products to treat their health problems, prevent diseases, and promote wellness. Although CIH is becoming increasingly popular, the conventional modern Western medicine remains predominant in the developed world, and the majority of those people continue to seek conventional medical care most of the time (Eisenberg, Kessler, Van Rompay, Kaptchuk, Wilkey, Appel, & Davis, 2001). In contrast, what Americans and others in the developed world label as CIH treatments and practices are considered traditional medicine and have been used by the majority of the global population for hundreds to thousands of years. In the past decade, CIH treatments and practices have spread rapidly in the developed countries (World Health Organization [WHO], 2011a). More recently, the term "integrative medicine" has been used to describe healthcare practices that bring together the CIH and conventional approaches. "Complementary and integrative health (CIH) approaches" is the term currently used by the National Center for Complementary and Integrative Health (NCCIH) to describe the use of non-mainstream approaches together with conventional treatment approaches (NCCIH, 2015a).

According to the U.S. National Center for Complementary and Integrative Health (NCCIH, 2015a), CIH refers to a broad set of diverse medical and healthcare systems, practices, and products that are not part of that country's own tradition and are non-mainstream approaches. Based on this definition, it is clear that the conventional modern Western medicine and treatments are considered *traditional* in the United States and other developed countries. Also, those entities that Americans and others in the Western world consider to be CIH treatments and practices have mostly originated from other countries and cultures and are considered traditional medicine in those countries. WHO (2015) defines traditional medicine as "the sum total of the knowledge, skills, and practices based on the theories, beliefs, and experiences indigenous to different cultures, whether explicable or not, used in the maintenance of health as well as in the prevention, diagnosis, improvement or treatment of physical and mental illness." Therapies and practices included in traditional medicine vary significantly based on geographic region and country of origin.

Although the terms "complementary medicine" and "alternative medicine" have been used interchangeably in the literature, they mean different practices. According to NCCIH (2015a), complementary and integrative medicine is used *together with* conventional medicine, and alternative medicine is used *in place of* conventional medicine, which is used far less often. An example of complementary medicine is using aromatherapy to help lessen a patient's discomfort following surgery. Using a special diet to treat cancer *instead of* the surgery, radiation, or chemotherapy that was recommended by a conventional doctor is an example of alternative medicine; this is *not* recommended by NCCIH. It is their view that using any form of treatments or products that have not been scientifically proven to be safe or effective to replace conventional treatments can have serious consequences (NCCIH, 2015b).

In this chapter, "CIH" refers to the medical and healthcare systems, practices, and products that are not part of or used together with the dominant conventional Western healthcare system in the United States and other developed countries. The term "traditional medicine" is used to denote the indigenous medical and healthcare systems, practices, and products that are used in developing countries.

CIH IN THE UNITED STATES

Unlike many countries in the world, allopathic medicine is the mainstream medical practice and is regarded as conventional medicine in the United States, even though Native American folk medical practices existed long before the early settlers from Europe migrated to the United States. In the past decade, there has been an upsurge of CIH use in the United States due to the increasing demand for such therapies from U.S. consumers. According to the 2005 *Institute of Medicine Report on Complementary and Alternative Medicine in the United States,* the use of CIH will continue to be present in the United States (Institute of Medicine, 2005). Several surveys of nationally representative samples of U.S. adults have revealed that the proportion of adults who used at least one CIH therapy in a given year increased from 33.8% in 1990 to 42.1% in 1997 (Eisenberg, Davis, Ettner, Appel, Wilkey, Van Rompay, & Kessler, 1998) and again to 62% in 2002 (Barnes, Powell-Griner, McFann, & Nahin, 2004). CIH usage seems even more prevalent among health educators and patients. When daily vitamins excluding megavitamins or vitamins prescribed by a doctor and exercise not for the purpose of weight management were included as forms of CIH therapy, nearly 90% of health educators in the United States reported having used at least one form of CIH in the 12 months prior to the survey (Johnson, Priestly, Porter, & Petrillo, 2010). Similarly, as many as 85% of cancer patients reported having used at least one form of CIH (Morris, Johnson, Homer, & Walts, 2000).

A recent report of a nationally representative sample of U.S. adults found that nearly 38.3% had used some form of CIH therapy in the past 12 months (Clarke et al., 2015). It is not that the use of CIH among the general population has declined so significantly in the past decade: The previous higher estimates of overall CIH use are due to broader definitions and categorizations used to describe CIH practices. The frequencies of CIH use by category are as follows, in order of prevalence:

- Nonvitamin, nonmineral dietary supplements (18.9% in 2002, 17.7% in 2007 and 2012).
- Deep breathing exercises (11.6% in 2002, 12.7% in 2007, 10.9% in 2012).
- Yoga, tai chi, qi gong (5.8% in 2002, 6.7% in 2007, 10.1% in 2012).
- Chiropractic care or chiropractic and osteopathic manipulation (7.5% in 2002, 8.6% in 2007, 8.4% in 2012).
- Meditation (7.6% in 2002, 9.4% in 2007, 8.2% in 2012).

Table 11-1 compares the age-adjusted percentages of U.S. adults who used the most commonly used complementary health approaches from 2002 (Barnes, Powell-Griner, McFann, & Nahin, 2004) to 2007 (Barnes, Bloom, & Nahin, 2008) and 2012 (Clarke et al., 2015). Based on these data, it seems that the overall complementary health approaches used decreased over the five-year period between 2002 and 2007 and remain unchanged between 2007 and 2012. The "drop" in the prevalence of complementary health approach use since 2002 is due to the narrower definition of CIH used in later years. Some forms of therapies included in complementary health approaches in the past, such as prayer for health reasons, daily vitamins, and exercise not for the purpose of weight management, are no longer considered complementary health approaches and are not included in the more recent study on complementary health approaches use among general U.S. population.

TABLE 11-1 Comparison of Commonly Used Complementary Health Approaches in the Past 12 Months Among U.S. Adults

Complementary Health Approach Use in the Past 12 Months	Age-Adjusted Percent[1]			Percentage Point Change		
	2002	2007	2012	2002–2007	2007–2012	2002–2012
Used at least one form	62[2]	35.5	33.2	3.2*	−2.3*	0.9
Nonvitamin, nonmineral, natural products	18.9	17.7	17.7	**	0.0	**
Deep breathing exercises[3]	11.6	12.7	10.9	1.1*	**	**
Yoga, tai chi, qi gong	5.8	6.7	10.1	0.9	2.5*	3.4*
Chiropractic or osteopathic manipulation[4]	7.5	8.6	8.4	**	−0.2	**
Meditation[5]	7.6	9.4	8.0	1.8*	**	**
Massage	5.0	8.3	6.9	3.3*	−1.6*	1.9*

*Difference between both years is statistically significant at $p < 0.05$.
**Direct comparisons are not available.
[1]The denominator used in the calculation of percentages was all sample adults.
[2]The prevalence was 32.3% when prayer for health reasons was excluded (Barnes, Bloom, & Nahin, 2008).
[3]In 2012, the category "deep breathing exercises" included deep breathing exercises as part of hypnosis; biofeedback; Mantra meditation (including Transcendental Meditation, Relaxation Response, and Clinically Standardized Meditation); mindfulness meditation (including Vipassana, Zen Buddhist meditation, mindfulness-based stress reduction, and mindfulness-based cognitive therapy); spiritual meditation (including centering prayer and contemplative meditation); guided imagery; progressive relaxation; yoga; tai chi; or qi gong. In 2002 and 2007, the use of deep breathing exercises was asked broadly and not if used as part of other complementary health approaches. No trend analyses were conducted on the use of deep breathing exercises.
[4]In 2002, the use of chiropractic care was asked broadly, and osteopathic approach was not specified on the survey. No trend analyses were conducted on the use of chiropractic or osteopathic manipulation.
[5]In 2012, meditation included Mantra meditation (including Transcendental Meditation, Relaxation Response, and Clinically Standardized Meditation); mindfulness meditation (including Vipassana, Zen Buddhist meditation, mindfulness-based stress reduction, and mindfulness-based cognitive therapy); spiritual meditation (including centering prayer and contemplative meditation); and meditation used as a part of other practices (including yoga, tai chi, and qi gong). In 2002 and 2007, the use of meditation was asked broadly and not if practiced as part of other complementary health approaches.
Data from Clarke, T. C., et al. (2015). Trends in the use of complementary health approaches among adults: United States, 2002–2012. *National Health Statistics Reports, 79*. Hyattsville, MD: National Center for Health Statistics.

Figure 11-1 shows the 10 most commonly used complementary health approaches by U.S. adults in 2012 (Clarke et al., 2015).

The increased popularity of CIH therapies has been accompanied by increased out-of-pocket expenditures on CIH therapies and services. Based on the most current estimates (Nahin, Barnes, Stussman, & Bloom, 2009), U.S. adults spent a total of $33.9 billion on an out-of-pocket basis on visits to CIH providers and purchases of CIH products and services. Almost two-thirds of these expenses ($22.0 billion) were devoted to self-care CIH products and services during the past 12 months, whereas the rest ($11.9 billion) were spent by 38.1 million adults on more than 354 million visits to CIH providers.

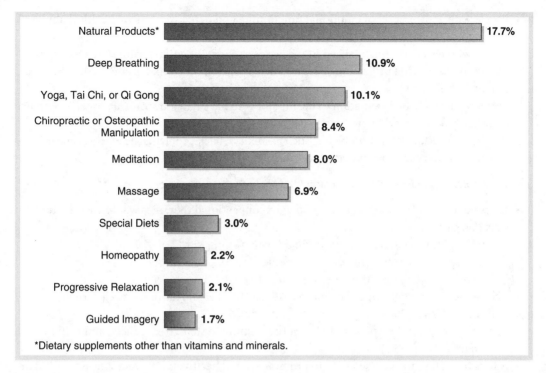

Natural Products*	17.7%
Deep Breathing	10.9%
Yoga, Tai Chi, or Qi Gong	10.1%
Chiropractic or Osteopathic Manipulation	8.4%
Meditation	8.0%
Massage	6.9%
Special Diets	3.0%
Homeopathy	2.2%
Progressive Relaxation	2.1%
Guided Imagery	1.7%

*Dietary supplements other than vitamins and minerals.

FIGURE 11-1 Use of Complementary Health Approaches in the United States
Data from Clarke, T. C., et al. (2015). Trends in the use of complementary health approaches among adults: United States, 2002–2012. *National Health Statistics Reports, 79.* Hyattsville, MD: National Center for Health Statistics.

With the increasing popularity and use of CIH, it is crucial to understand the nature and extent of CIH use. Studies have identified the following people as being more likely to use CIH:

- Women (AARP & NCCAM, 2011; Barnes, Powell-Griner, McFann, & Nahin, 2004; Barnes, Bloom, & Nahin, 2008; Eisenberg, Davis, Ettner, Appel, Wilkey, Van Rompay, & Kessler, 1998).
- People with higher household income, almost certainly attributable to the reality that most CIH therapies are not covered by health insurance policies and require cash payments at the time of service (Eisenberg, Davis, Ettner, Appel, Wilkey, Van Rompay, & Kessler, 1998; Palinkas & Kabongo, 2000).
- People with higher levels of education, private health insurance, more health conditions, and more visits to the doctor's office (AARP & NCCAM, 2011; Barnes, Bloom, & Nahin, 2008).
- Older adults (AARP & NCCAM, 2011; Barnes, Bloom, & Nahin, 2008; Barnes, Powell-Griner, McFann, & Nahin, 2004).
- Ethnic minorities (Barnes, Powell-Griner, McFann, & Nahin, 2004) and low-income individuals (Barnes, Bloom, & Nahin, 2008; Dessio, Wade, Chao, Kronenberg, Cushman, & Kalmuss, 2004).

- People with a lower level of emotional functioning and perceived general health (Palinkas & Kabongo, 2000).
- People who have been hospitalized in the last year, indicating that health status is a significant predictor of CIH utilization (Barnes, Powell-Griner, McFann, & Nahin, 2004; Barnes, Bloom, & Nahin, 2008).
- People with a holistic orientation to health and who have had a transformational experience that changed their worldview.
- People with certain health problems, such as anxiety, back problems, headaches, chronic pain, and urinary tract problems (Astin, 1998).

The most common reasons cited for using CIH include the following:

- Users believed CIH therapies integrated with conventional therapies would yield better results (54.9%).
- They thought trying CIH therapies would be interesting (50.1%).
- CIH therapies were recommended by a medical professional (26%).
- Individuals felt allopathic therapies were not effective (28%).
- They felt CIH therapies would be more cost-effective (13%) (Barnes, Powell-Griner, McFann, & Nahin, 2004).
- They believed CIH therapies could boost the immune system, treat cancer, and help them live longer (Astin, 1998).
- Adults over 50 years old used CIH to promote overall health and prevent illnesses (77%), to treat painful conditions or reduce pain (73%), to treat a specific health problem (59%), or to supplement conventional treatments (53%) (AARP & NCCAM, 2011).

Results from those studies indicate that the high prevalence of CIH use in the United States cannot be attributed solely to the perceived dissatisfaction with conventional medical care or caregivers, or to a societal rejection of allopathic medical care (Eisenberg, Kessler, Van Rompay, Kaptchuk, Wilkey, Appel, & Davis, 2001). Instead, such trends may indicate that more Americans have taken personal responsibility for their health and appreciate the choices they have between conventional and CIH care.

Although a large proportion of the U.S. adult population uses at least one of the CIH therapies, only 28 to 37% communicated such use to their doctors (Eisenberg, Kessler, Van Rompay, Kaptchuk, Wilkey, Appel, & Davis, 2001), whereas those aged 50 years and older who had ever used CIH were more likely to discuss CIH with a healthcare provider (AARP & NCCAM, 2011). The most common reason for nondisclosure of CIH use was that patients believed "it was not important for their doctor to know," followed by "the doctor never asked," "it was not the doctor's business," and "the doctor would not understand." These views reveal a trend within the broader society toward increased individual autonomy and taking greater personal responsibility for one's own health. In addition, among the U.S. adults who reported seeing both a conventional doctor and a CIH provider in a given year, the majority (70%) saw a conventional doctor before or concurrent with their visits to a CIH provider, whereas only 15% saw a CIH provider before seeing a conventional medical care provider. Such a visit presents an excellent opportunity for the conventional medical care provider to advise patients on the use or avoidance of certain CIH therapies. It also presents a challenge, however, in that conventional healthcare providers need to understand what the common CIH therapies are and whether they are safe or effective.

CIH IN THE WORLD

Throughout history, different cultures in different parts of the world have developed and used various types of traditional medicine or CIH. People residing in Africa, Asia, and Latin America, for example, have used traditional medicine for hundreds and thousands of years to meet their primary healthcare needs. In African countries, as much as 80% of the population uses traditional medicine for primary health care. In recent years, many forms of traditional medicine have been adapted by more and more developed countries and are considered "complementary" or "integrative" medicine (CIH) depending on how the traditional medicine is used (WHO, 2015b).

In the last decade, we have seen a global increase in the use of both traditional medicine and CIH in both developed and developing countries. Many types of traditional, complementary, and alternative medicines are playing a more important role in health care and healthcare reform worldwide. Several countries—for example, China, the Democratic People's Republic of Korea, the Republic of Korea, and Vietnam—have fully integrated traditional medicine into their formal healthcare systems (Robinson & Zhang, 2011). Several other countries, such as the United States, are collecting standardized data on CIH therapies and encourage the integration of CIH into their mainstream medical care system. Many other countries, however, have yet to collect and integrate standardized evidence on this type of health care.

The following facts provide a better view of CIH's increased use and popularity:

- In China, traditional herbal preparations account for 30 to 50% of the total medicinal consumption.
- In Ghana, Mali, Nigeria, and Zambia, the first line of treatment for 60% of children with high fever resulting from malaria is the use of herbal medicines at home.
- WHO estimates that traditional birth attendants in several African countries assist in the majority of births.
- In Canada, 70% of the population has used complementary medicine at least once.
- In the United Kingdom, annual expenditures on alternative medicine total $230 million.
- The global market for herbal medicines currently stands at more than $60 billion annually and is growing steadily (WHO, 2005).
- More than 100 million Europeans currently use traditional and/or complementary medicine and there are more people who currently use traditional and/or complementary medicine in Australia and countries in Africa, Asia, and North America.
- Traditional medicine is becoming increasingly popular in many developed countries. For example, 41% people in Spain, 70% in Canada, and 82% in Australia have used complementary health approaches.

- In China, a total of 907 million people visited traditional Chinese medicine doctors in 2009, which accounts for 18% of all medical visits.
- Of the 129 WHO member states that participated in the 2012 WHO Global Survey, 69 have established a national policy on traditional medicine/CIH since 2012.
- Of the 129 WHO member states that participated in the 2012 WHO Global Survey, 119 have established herbal medicines law or regulation.
- Accupuncture, which originated from China, has been used by 80% of the 129 WHO member states that participated in the 2012 WHO Global Survey.
- In 2012, the estimated output of Chinese medical materials was US$83 billion, a more than 20% increase from the 2011 level.
- The annual expenditures of traditional medicine in the Republic of Korea increased from US$4.4 in 2004 to US$7.4 in 2009 (WHO, 2015b).
- Approximately 80% of the world population uses traditional systems of medicines for primary health care, with plants (rather than other natural resources) being the dominant components of such medicines (Mukherjee & Wahile, 2006).
- There are more than 800 Chinese medicine pharmaceutical factories with an annual production of over 400,000 tons, spread among more than 5,000 drug varieties (Johnson & Johnson, 2002).
- An estimated $83 billion was spent on traditional medicine in 2008, with an exponential rate of increase being observed worldwide (Robinson & Zhang, 2011).
- In Singapore, more than 80% of the population has used some form of CIH in their lifetime (Koh, Ng, & Teo, 2004).
- In Brazil, as many as 89% of cancer patients use CIH (Samano et al., 2005).

It is clear that traditional medicine has maintained its popularity in developing countries and is used more frequently in developed countries. The global expansion of traditional medicine and CIH use in the developed world can in part be explained by these modalities' holistic approach to health and life; their belief in equilibrium between the mind, body, and environment; their emphasis on health rather than on disease; and their treatment focus on the overall condition of the individual patient, rather than on the ailment or disease (WHO, 2005).

MAJOR FORMS OF COMPLEMENTARY AND INTEGRATIVE HEALTH

In response to the increasing demand for CIH, the U.S. Congress passed legislation in 1992 to establish an office within the National Institutes of Health (NIH), known as the Office of Alternative Medicine (OAM), to investigate and evaluate potentially beneficial unconventional medical practices (NIH, 2015). In 1999, this office was elevated to a center within NIH, as the National Center of Complementary and Alternative Medicine (NCCAM). In December 2014, President Obama signed the Consolidated and Further Continuing Appropriation Act of 2015 that included a provision to change to its current name, the National Center for Complementary and Integrative Health (NCCIH). The new name, NCCIH, reflects more accurately the commitment of the center to researching promising health approaches that have already been used by the U.S. general population (NIH, 2015).

As the understanding of various unconventional health practices and therapies increases, the categorization of such practices and therapies have been evolving as well. When this text was initially published, those practices and therapies were categorized into alternative medical systems, biologically based therapies, manipulative and body-based methods, mind–body interventions, and energy therapies with five domains (Johnson, 2008). By the time of the second edition of this text, NCCAM grouped those practices and therapies into natural products, mind and body medicine, manipulative and body-based practices, and other CIH practices (Johnson, 2013). Currently, not only has the categorization of such practices and therapies changed, the overall term for the same practices and therapies is changed to "complementary and integrative health approaches (CIHA)," which are grouped into natural products, mind and body practices, and other complementary health approaches (NCCIH, 2015a). Generally speaking, approaches in each category were developed over different time periods in different places and have been used to deal with different health problems. Their therapeutic effects, efficacy, and side effects have been studied to different extents as well. While some CIH therapies are backed by scientific evidence of their safety and effectiveness, most need to be examined for their safety, effectiveness, and efficacy.

Natural Products

In the past, NCCAM referred to this area of CIH as "biologically based therapies," and defined it as including natural and biologically based practices, interventions, and products such as herbs, whole diets, functional foods, animal-derived extracts, vitamins, minerals, fatty acids, amino acids, proteins, prebiotics and probiotics, and other dietary supplements. When the second edition of this text was published (Johnson, 2013), taking a multivitamin to meet daily nutritional requirements or taking calcium to promote bone health was not considered to be using CIH. At that time, natural products only included a variety of herbal products (i.e., botanicals), and beneficial microorganisms (i.e., probiotics) that are similar to those normally found in the human digestive tract. Today, vitamins and minerals are included back in the natural products category while herbal products and probiotics remain in the category (NCCIH, 2015a). As we have seen in various forms of commercials, natural products have been widely advertised and can be found on the shelves of supermarkets, grocery stores, and specialty nutritional supplement stores.

Before manufactured drugs came into widespread use, herbal medicines played an important role in human health. A review of the history of the development of medicines reveals that many herbal medicines were originally derived from foods and that many manufactured drugs were developed from medicinal plants. A single medicinal plant may be defined as a food, a functional food, a dietary supplement, or an herbal medicine in different countries, depending on the regulations applied to foods and medicines in each country. The influences of culture and history on the use of herbal medicines differ from country to country and from region to region, and these factors continue to have a major impact on the use of herbal medicines in modern societies (WHO, 2005). For example, the novel malaria therapy was discovered and developed from a Chinese herb by Youyou Tu and her colleagues in the 1970s when the Chinese government encouraged scientists to develop effective treatments to combat malaria. The Nobel Prize committee recognized this as a significant contribution to medicine over 40 years later and awarded Youyou Tu half of the 2015 Nobel Prize in Medicine (Nobelprize.org, 2015).

In the past two decades, we have seen a considerable increase in the interest in and use of dietary supplements. In 2014, overall sales of dietary supplements increased to $36.7 billion, and the revenue is projected to top $60 billion in 2021 (*Nutrition Business Journal*, 2015). According to a recent national survey, nearly 18% of U.S. adults used at least one nonvitamin, nonmineral, natural product in a given year for health reasons. Of those natural products, fish oil (also known as omega-3 or DHA) was the most commonly used product (46.4%) among the U.S. adult population, followed by glucosamine and/or chondroitin (15.9%), probiotics/prebiotics (9.5%), melatonin (7.6%), coenzyme Q-10 (8.0%), Echinacea (5.6%), cranberry (pills or capsules) (4.8%), garlic supplements (4.7%), ginseng (4.3%), and ginkgo biloba (4.0%) (Clarke et al., 2015).

Because of their widespread use and long history (often spanning several centuries), and because the products are "natural," many people assume that dietary supplements are harmless. Unfortunately, this is not always the case. Some herbal products have proved to be quite harmful. For example, the herb "ma huang" (ephedra) has been used in traditional Chinese medicine in very small amounts to treat respiratory congestion and certain illnesses for thousands of years. In the United States, however, ma huang was marketed as a dietary aid whose inappropriate use led to at least a dozen deaths, heart attacks, and strokes. On April 12, 2004, the Food and Drug Administration (FDA) banned the sale of dietary supplements that contain ephedra after it determined that this product posed an unreasonable risk to those who used it (FDA, 2004). One FDA consumer update, "Beware of Fraudulent 'Dietary Supplements,'" informs consumers that nearly 300 fraudulent dietary supplements that have been promoted mostly for weight loss, body building, or sexual enhancement contain hidden or deceptively labeled ingredients. So far, the FDA has received numerous reports of harm caused by consuming those products, including heart palpitations, stroke, liver injury, kidney failure, and even death (FDA, 2011). One recent *New England Journal of Medicine* special report revealed that adverse events caused by dietary supplement use contribute to an estimated 23,000 emergency room visits in the United States each year. The common reasons for those ER visits include cardiovascular conditions such as chest pain, palpitations, or tachycardia among young adults from using weight-loss or energy products and choking or pill-induced dysphagia or globus among older adults from taking micronutrients (Geller et al., 2015).

It is important to recognize that many plants are poisonous, some are toxic if ingested in large doses, others are dangerous when used with prescription or OTC drugs, and still others decrease the effectiveness of the prescription or OTC drugs. One good example is the popular herbal remedy known as St. John's wort. This supplement has a significant negative interaction with Indinavir, a protease inhibitor used to treat HIV infection, and may also potentially interact with prescription drugs used to treat conditions such as heart disease, depression, seizures, and certain cancers. St. John's wort may also potentially interact with prescription drugs used to prevent conditions such as transplant rejection or pregnancy (i.e., oral contraceptives) (FDA, 2000). For dietary supplement safety information, go to NCCIH's Safe Use of Complementary Health Products and Services page at https://nccih .nih.gov/health/safety.

Unlike prescription or OTC drugs, which are all regulated by the FDA, dietary supplements are largely free of FDA oversight (FDA, 2015). The 1994 Dietary Supplement Health and Education Act (DSHEA) allows dietary supplement manufacturers to produce and promote their products without going through the stringent FDA approval process. Thus, it is up to consumers to decide which products they will use or not use. Given this fact, it is important that healthcare consumers talk to their healthcare providers and/or obtain information from reliable websites sponsored by the FDA, NCCIH, or other nonprofit health organizations before taking any dietary supplements.

Mind and Body Practices

Mind and body practices focus on the interactions among the brain, mind, body, and behavior as well as the powerful ways in which emotional, mental, social, spiritual, and behavioral factors directly affect health. The importance of mind in the development and treatment of diseases has been reflected in the diagnostic and healing approaches employed in traditional Chinese medicine and Ayurveda for thousands of years. The moral and spiritual aspects of healing were noted by Hippocrates, who believed that attitude, environmental influences, and natural remedies must be considered in treating patients (Johnson, 2013).

Mind and body practices employ different techniques to enhance the mind's capacity to affect bodily function and symptoms. They include a wide range of techniques or procedures received or learned from a trained practitioner or instructor. The most popular mind–body practices include yoga, chiropractic and osteopathic manipulations, meditation, and massage therapy. Other practices in this category include acupuncture, breathing exercises, guided imagery, progressive relaxation, tai chi, qi gong, healing touch, hypnotherapy, Pilates, and other movement therapies (NCCIH, 2015a). Comparing the surveys of national representative samples of U.S. adults in 2002, 2007, and 2012, we can see that the use of yoga, tai chi, and qi gong increased significantly, while other body and mind practices such as chiropractic or osteopathic manipulation, meditation, and massage increased from 2002 to 2007 and decreased somewhat in 2012 but were still higher than those in 2002. The practice of deep breathing exercises was highest in 2007 and lowest in 2012 (see Table 11-1) (Clarke et al., 2015).

Yoga

Yoga originated in India and has been used for health and fitness purposes for thousands of years. Although various styles of yoga are available, they all typically include physical postures, breathing techniques, and meditation to help the individual reach a state of increased relaxation and balanced mind, body, and spirit. The proportion of U.S. adults who practice yoga increased significantly from 5.1% in 2002 to 6.1% in 2007 and 9.5% in 2012 (Clarke et al., 2015). One recent review study suggests that yoga may be as effective as or better than exercise at improving a variety of health-related outcomes among populations with and without (Ross & Thomas, 2010). Other studies have found that yoga seems to be effective in relieving menopause symptoms (Lee, Kim, Ha, Boddy, & Ernst, 2009), helping children through the rehabilitation process (Galantino, Galbavy, & Quinn, 2008), improving subjective and objective outcome in bronchial asthma patients (Vempati, Bijlani, & Deepak, 2009), improving mood and reducing anxiety (Streeter et al., 2010), alleviating pain (Posadzki, Ernst, Terry, & Lee, 2011), increasing one's sense of well-being, reducing stress, decreasing heart rate and blood pressure, increasing lung capacity, improving overall physical fitness, and positively influencing certain brain or blood chemicals (NCCIH, 2015b).

Although yoga is generally considered safe in healthy individuals when practiced properly, people with certain medical conditions should not use certain types of yoga. Instead, they should consult with their healthcare provider first if they are considering yoga. In addition, yoga should not be used as a replacement for conventional medical care or to postpone seeing a doctor about a health problem (Johnson, 2013). Because certain types of yoga require a minimum physical fitness level, not everyone can practice all types of yoga. Most importantly, one should use a well-trained and experienced yoga instructor.

Tai Chi and Qi Gong

Tai chi and qi gong are also considered types of energy therapy that supposedly can restore health. It has been practiced widely in China for more than 2,000 years. Moving the body gently and having certain postures while focusing on breathing are the key characteristics of tai chi and qi gong (NCCIH, 2015c). One study examined more than 2,000 records in qi gong therapy and found that this modality has health benefits for conditions ranging from high blood pressure to asthma (Sancier & Holman, 2004). Several small randomized clinical trials have revealed the therapeutic effects of qi gong in improving psychological measures (Hui, Wan, Chan, & Yung, 2006), reducing pain and long-term anxiety (Wu et al., 1999), implementing heroin detoxification (Li, Chen, & Mo, 2002), and improving heart rate variability (Lee, Kim, & Lee, 2005). A recent meta-analysis of 77 published peer-reviewed articles that reported the results of randomized controlled trials of qi gong or tai chi interventions found that these practices are associated with consistent, significant results demonstrating a number of positive health benefits in the areas of bone density, cardiopulmonary effects, physical function, falls and related risk factors, quality of life, self-efficacy, patient-reported outcomes, psychological symptoms, and immune function (Jahnke, Larkey, Rogers, Etnier, & Lin, 2010). A review of 36 clinical trials of qi gong and tai chi in older adults found that qi gong and tai chi may help older adults improve their physical function, lower blood pressure, reduce fall risk, and decrease depression and anxiety (Rogers, Larkey, & Keller, 2009).

Chiropractic or Osteopathic Manipulation

Chiropractic and osteopathic manipulation were developed within the last 150 years. As noted in Table 11-1, the proportion of U.S. adults who had used chiropractic or osteopathic manipulation in the past 12 months increased from 7.5% in 2002 to 8.6% in 2007, and decreased slightly to 8.4% in 2012 (Clarke et al., 2015). Chiropractic is a form of spinal manipulation, which is one of the oldest healing practices. Spinal manipulation was described by Hippocrates in ancient Greece. In 1895, Daniel David Palmer founded the modern profession of chiropractic in Davenport, Iowa. Based on his observations, he developed a chiropractic theory that describes the nervous system as the most important determinant of health and posits that most diseases are caused by spinal subluxations that respond to spinal manipulation (Ernst, 2008). In turn, manipulation or adjustment of the spine is the core procedure used by chiropractic doctors, who are also called chiropractors or chiropractic physicians. Manipulation is the passive joint movement beyond the normal range of motion; chiropractic medicine prefers the term "adjustment" for this practice (NCCIH, 2012).

Chiropractic training is a four-year academic program consisting of both classroom and clinical instruction. At least three years of preparatory college work is required for admission to chiropractic schools. Students who graduate receive a doctor of chiropractic (DC) degree and are eligible to take the state licensure board examinations to practice in this field. Some schools also offer postgraduate courses, including two- to three-year residency programs in specialized fields (NCCIH, 2012).

In addition to manipulation, most chiropractors use other treatments such as mobilization, massage, and nonmanual therapies. Examples of nonmanual chiropractic treatments include the following:

- Heat and ice
- Ultrasound
- Electrical stimulation
- Rehabilitative exercise
- Magnetic therapy
- Mobilization, a technique in which a joint is passively moved within its normal range of motion
- Counseling (i.e., counseling about diet, weight loss, and other lifestyle factors)
- Dietary supplements
- Homeopathy
- Acupuncture

Meditation

Several meditation techniques exist, including mindfulness meditation, Transcendental Meditation, mantra meditation, relaxation response, and Zen Buddhist meditation, with the first two being the most commonly practiced forms. Meditation has been used for many reasons. For example, it has been employed to enhance health and well-being, to reduce stress and anxiety, and to cope with pain and certain illnesses such as depression, insomnia, heart disease, HIV/AIDS, and cancer. Recent studies have confirmed the effects of meditation in altering intrinsic functional brain connectivity after eight weeks of mindfulness meditation training (Kilpatrick et al., 2011), along with functional changes in brain regions related to internalized attention as a result of long-term meditation (Jang, Jung, Kang, Byun, Kwon, Chio, & Kwon, 2011). It has been reported that practicing Transcendental Meditation may lower the blood pressure of young adults at risk of developing hypertension (Nidich et al., 2009), while practicing mindfulness meditation for eight weeks could reduce the severity of irritable bowel syndrome (Gaylord et al., 2011). Several recent NCCIH-funded studies are examining the effects of meditation in reducing stress and improving weight management, relieving emotional distress in people with type 2 diabetes, regulating emotions, reducing the risk of heart disease through relieving stress, and improving sleep and emotional well-being (NCCIH, 2014). Once those studies are completed, the role of meditation in improving health and well-being should be clearer. Although meditation is believed to be safe for healthy individuals in general, you should not use meditation to replace conventional care for a health problem. It is important that you ask the meditation instructor about his or her training and experience beforehand.

Massage

Massage therapies manipulate muscle and connective tissue to enhance the function of those tissues and promote relaxation and well-being. Massage was first practiced thousands of years ago in ancient Greece, ancient Rome, Japan, China, Egypt, and the Indian subcontinent. In the United States, massage therapy first became popular and was promoted for a variety of health purposes starting in the mid-1800s; interest in this modality has greatly increased since the 1970s (NCCIH, 2015d).

The term "massage therapy" covers a group of more than 80 types of massage therapy practices and techniques. In all of them, therapists press, rub, and otherwise manipulate the muscles and other soft tissues of the body, often varying pressure and movement. They most often use their hands and fingers but may use their forearms, elbows, or feet. Typically, the intent is to relax the soft tissues, increase delivery of blood and oxygen to the massaged areas, warm them, and decrease pain. Based on firsthand experience of receiving Chinese massage, a massage therapist trained in the United States indicated that massage therapies practiced in the United States today are much milder in their forces and different as compared to those practiced in traditional Chinese medicine.

To learn massage, most therapists attend a school or training program, and a much smaller number receive training from an experienced practitioner. After they complete 500 hours of training from an accredited training program, they can be certified to be massage therapists—even though there is a great variation in training requirements and standards for massage therapists in different states or even cities or counties. Massage therapists are regulated in the District of Columbia, 44 states, and some cities and counties in the United States (NCCIH, 2015d).

Massage therapy appears to have few serious risks if appropriate cautions are followed and is given by a trained massage therapist. Although many scientific research studies on the effects of massage therapy are preliminary and conflicting, there is evidence that massage therapy may improve the quality of life among people living with HIV/AIDS, cancer, and depression. Such benefits are short term and ongoing massage therapy is needed to continue the benefits. People with certain conditions, such as pregnant women or those with a bleeding disorder or bleeding tendency should avoid receiving massage. Areas over a tumor or cancer should avoid receiving deep or intense pressure (NCCIH, 2015d).

Therapeutic Touch

Therapeutic touch is derived from the laying on of hands. It is founded on several ancient healing practices. Since its introduction in 1972 by Dr. Dolores Krieger and Dora Kunz (The Nurse Healers, 2006), the use of therapeutic touch has increased significantly. A 1997 national survey found that approximately 4% of the U.S. adults used therapeutic touch in a given year and that nearly 40 million visits were made to therapeutic touch practitioners, ranking it fifth among the 16 CIH therapies assessed (Eisenberg, Davis, Ettner, Appel, Wilkey, Van Rompay, & Kessler, 1998).

According to advocates of therapeutic touch, each person has a unique energy field (sometimes visible as an "aura") that is simultaneously inside and surrounding the person's physical body. For an individual to be healthy, his or her energy field must be flowing freely or balanced. One or more blockages in a person's energy field will prevent the free flow of energy, causing illness. Therapeutic touch is used to balance or retain the free flow of life energy in an individual, thereby restoring good health (Brewer, 2006).

Therapeutic touch is a deliberately directed process during which a therapeutic touch practitioner moves his or her hands approximately 4 inches above the patient's body to detect the energy imbalance and repair any "holes" where the energy escapes from the body. During the process of restoring the energy balance, the practitioner assists the healing process.

To date, there has been little rigorous scientific research in this area, with few high-quality articles on this modality having been published. A meta-analysis of 11 controlled therapeutic touch studies found that eight controlled studies demonstrated positive outcomes from such treatment, and three showed no effect (Winstead-Fry & Kijekm, 1999). Another meta-analysis of research-based literature on therapeutic touch published in a 10-year period found that although therapeutic touch appears to have a positive, medium effect on physiological and psychological variables, no substantive claims can be made because of the limited published studies and problems with research methods that could seriously bias the reported results (Peters, 1999). A review of 30 studies on therapeutic touch did not yield any generalizable results (Wardell & Weymouth, 2004).

Due to the lack of well-designed research on the effects of therapeutic touch, the efficacy of this therapy cannot be determined until sufficient scientific evidence becomes available. However, the therapist's individual attention and the passing of his or her hands over the patient's body may lead the patient to feel a sense of well-being (Brewer, 2006).

Other Complementary and Integrative Health Practices

Practices that fall under this category include whole medical systems that are based on complete systems of theory and practice and often evolved prior to, and independently of, the conventional biomedical approach used in the United States (NCCIH, 2015a). They can be categorized into systems developed in Asian (Oriental), Western, and other cultures. Systems developed in Asian cultures include traditional Chinese medicine and Ayurveda (traditional Indian medicine). Systems developed in Western cultures include homeopathic medicine and naturopathic medicine. Systems developed in other cultures include Native American, aboriginal, Middle

Eastern, Tibetan, and South American medicine. This section briefly introduces the more commonly practiced whole medical systems.

Ayurvedic Medicine

Ayurvedic medicine (or Ayurveda) originated in India and has been practiced primarily in the Indian subcontinent for more than 5,000 years (Mukherjee & Wahile, 2006). Ayurveda medicine literally means "the science of life," with *ayur* meaning "life" and *veda* meaning "science" (White, 2000). This branch of medicine is based on the Hindu belief that everyone is born in a state of balance within themselves and in relation to the universe (interconnectedness). Thus, a person will experience good health if he or she has an effective and wholesome relationship with the immediate universe, whereas disease occurs when the person is out of harmony with the universe. Ayurveda also emphasizes the importance of the body's constitution. "Constitution" is thought to be a unique combination of physical and psychological features and the way in which the body functions. Its characteristics are determined by three *doshas* (*vata*, *pitta*, and *kapha*). Each *dosha* is associated with a certain body type, a certain personality type, and a greater chance of certain types of illnesses. Therefore, the imbalance of *doshas*, the state of physical body, and mental or lifestyle factors increases a person's chances of developing certain types of diseases (NCCIH, 2015e).

To determine what is wrong with the person, an Ayurvedic practitioner seeks to identify the primary *dosha* and the balance of *doshas* by asking the person about his or her diet, behavior, lifestyle practices, and the reasons for the most recent health problem and symptoms the patient had; by observing the person's teeth, tongue, eyes, skin, and overall appearance; by checking the person's bodily sounds, urine, and stool; and by feeling the person's pulse. The practitioner may prescribe diagnostic treatment to restore the balance of one particular *dosha*. Because of the emphasis on removing the cause of the disease, Ayurvedic doctors prescribe many changes in diet and lifestyle of the patient. After these changes have been made, the doctor will then prescribe a combination of therapies that may include herbs, metals, massage, yoga, breathing exercises, and meditation to balance the body, mind, and spirit (Sharma, Chandola, Singh, & Basisht, 2007).

In India, Ayurvedic doctors are trained in a formal academic setting that includes 4½ years of coursework, a one-year internship in Ayurveda, and advanced postgraduate training. Ayurvedic practitioners in the United States have various types of training. Some study Ayurveda after they are trained in Western medical or nursing schools. Others may undergo training in naturopathy either before or after their Ayurvedic training. Still others receive training in India. Students who complete their Ayurvedic training in India receive either a bachelor's or a doctoral degree and may go to the United States or other countries to practice. Some practitioners are trained in a particular aspect of Ayurvedic practice such as massage or meditation (NCCIH, 2015e).

Some Ayurvedic medications have the potential to be toxic because of the high level of heavy metals (lead, mercury, and arsenic) used in these preparations (Saper, Kales, Paquin, Burns, Eisenberg, Davis, & Phillips, 2004; van Schalkwyk, Davidson, Palmer, & Hope, 2006). There is also a potential for interactions between Ayurvedic treatments and other medicines.

For patients, it is important to tell their healthcare providers if they are using Ayurveda therapy and any associated dietary supplements or medications. Patients who plan to use Ayurvedic remedies should do so under the guidance of an experienced Ayurvedic practitioner. In the United States, there is no national standard for certifying Ayurvedic practitioners at the present time, although several states have approved Ayurvedic schools as educational institutions (NCCIH, 2015e). Consumers interested in Ayurveda should be aware that many persons claiming to practice Ayurvedic medicine have had little formal training in this modality (White, 2000). For example, Ayurvedic services offered at spas and salons may not be provided by well-trained Ayurvedic practitioners. Anyone who is interested in Ayurvedic treatment should ask about the practitioner's training and experience and inform his or her healthcare provider about these Ayurvedic medications to ensure there is no conflict with medications or treatments prescribed by the conventional healthcare provider (NCCIH, 2015e).

Homeopathic Medicine

Homeopathic medicine, also known as homeopathy, was developed in Germany during the late 1700s by Samuel Hahnemann, a physician, chemist, and linguist. It was introduced to the United States in 1825 by a Boston-born doctor, Hans Burch Gram. Homeopathy is based on the similia principle ("Like cures like"), "potentialization," and the concept that treatment should be selected based on a total picture of the patient including the patient's physical symptoms, emotions, mental state, lifestyle, nutrition, and other aspects (Ballard, 2000; Merrell & Shalts, 2002; Tedesco & Cicchetti, 2001).

The principle of "Like cures like" considers that the symptoms are part of the body's attempt to heal itself, such that an appropriately selected homeopathic remedy will support this self-healing process (Scheiman-Burkhardt, 2001). According to this concept, the symptoms caused by a large dose of a substance can be alleviated by the extremely diluted small amount of the same substance. The concept of "potentialization" holds that systematically diluting a substance, with vigorous shaking at each step of dilution, makes the remedy more effective by extracting the vital essence of the substance. Homeopathy believes that even when the substance is diluted to the point where no single molecule exists in the remedy, the remedy may still be effective because the substance's molecules have exerted their effects on the surrounding water molecules (NCCIH, 2015f).

To select the appropriate homeopathic remedies, a homeopathic provider conducts an in-depth assessment of the patient during the patient's first visit. Based on how the patient responds to the remedy or remedies, the practitioner determines whether to prescribe any additional treatment.

In the United States, training in homeopathy is offered through diploma programs, certificate programs, short courses, and correspondence courses. Medical education in naturopathy includes homeopathic training. Most homeopathy in the United States is practiced along with another health practice for which the practitioner is licensed, such as conventional medicine, naturopathy, chiropractic, dentistry, acupuncture, or veterinary medicine when homeopathy is used to treat animals. In Europe, training in homeopathy is usually pursued as a primary professional degree completed after three to six years of formal training or as a postgraduate training for doctors.

Homeopathic remedies do not have to undergo any testing or review by the FDA, so some researchers question their effectiveness. Because they are extremely diluted solutions of natural substances that come from plants, mineral, or animals, and are given under the supervision of trained professionals, homeopathic remedies are considered safe and unlikely to cause severe adverse reactions (Dantas & Rampes, 2000). Although homeopathic remedies are not known to interfere with conventional drugs, patients should discuss with their healthcare providers that they are considering using these therapies. As when taking any medications, if patients are taking a homeopathic remedy, they should contact the healthcare provider if their symptoms have not improved in five days and keep remedies out of reach for children. Pregnant women and women who are nursing a baby should consult a healthcare provider before using any homeopathic remedies.

Naturopathic Medicine

Naturopathic medicine, or naturopathy, is an eclectic system of health care originating in Germany. Although many of its principles have been used in various healing traditions such as Chinese, Ayurvedic, Native American, and Hippocratic medicine for thousands of years, the term "naturopathy" was coined by a German-born doctor, John Scheel, in 1895 and was popularized by Dr. Benedict Lust, a hydrotherapist from Germany who in 1905 founded the American School of Naturopathy in New York. Because of the influence of various traditional healing principles, naturopathy has elements of complementary and conventional medicine that are used to support and enhance self-healing processes and works with natural healing forces within the body (NCCIH, 2015g).

The term "naturopathy" literally means "nature disease." Naturopaths seek to treat disease by stimulating an individual's innate healing capacities through the use of organic, nontoxic therapies such as fresh air, pure water, bright sunlight, natural food, proper sleep, water therapies, homeopathic remedies, herbs, acupuncture, spinal and soft-tissue manipulation, hydrotherapy, lifestyle counseling, and psychotherapy to heal ailments of body and mind (White, 2000). Naturopaths strive to treat the underlying cause of the condition and see illness as an opportunity to educate and empower patients to develop healthy lifestyles and to take responsibility for their lives.

Today, naturopathic medicine is practiced throughout Europe, Australia, New Zealand, Canada, and the United States. Naturopathic physicians are trained in the art and science of natural health care at accredited naturopathic medical schools. Five major naturopathic schools in the United States and Canada award naturopathic doctor (ND) degrees to students who have completed a four-year graduate program that focuses on holistic principles, natural therapies, and an orientation to patients as partners in their own healing (NCCIH, 2015g).

Traditional Chinese Medicine

Traditional Chinese medicine (TCM) has gained worldwide popularity. Although it sometimes seems to be foreign and mysterious to many in the Western world, more Westerners are now embracing it. TCM is a complete medical system that has been used to diagnose, treat, and prevent illness for more than 2,500 years. Inscriptions on bones and tortoise shells outline TCM treatments for health problems dating from 1500 to 1000 BC. The earliest TCM books date back to 221 BC (Johnson & Johnson, 2002). Korea, Japan, and Vietnam have developed their own unique versions of traditional medicine based on practices originated from China.

TCM is based on the ancient Chinese philosophical theory of *yin* and *yang*. In this view, all of creation is born from the marriage of the two polar principles in the body, yin and yang, which are opposing forces. These forces stand for earth and heaven, winter and summer, night and day, inner and outer, cold and hot, wet and dry, body and mind. Human beings, like everything else in the universe, have two opposite aspects, yin and yang, that are interrelated and interdependent (White, 2000). Interactions of yin and yang regulate the flow of qi (vital energy) throughout the body. Qi is believed to regulate a person's mental, physical, spiritual, and emotional, balance. If yin and yang become imbalanced, the flow of qi is disrupted and disease occurs (NCCIH, 2013).

TCM diagnosis involves taking a history; inspecting facial complexion, body build, posture, and motion; examining the tongue and its coating; listening to the sound of voice, respiration, and cough; smelling the odor of the patient; interrogating the patient; and palpating the pulses. The TCM interrogation includes the "ten askings": Question 1 asks about chill and fever, question 2 about perspiration, question 3 about the head and trunk, question 4 about stool and urine, question 5 about food intake, and question 6 about the chest. Deafness and thirst are covered in questions 7 and 8, question 9 asks about past history, and question 10 covers causes. Experienced TCM practitioners can make a diagnosis based solely on the examination of the tongue and palpation of the pulse (Johnson & Johnson, 2002).

Based on the philosophy of TCM, the purpose of treatment is to restore yin and yang harmony. The TCM doctor uses acupuncture, *tui na* (Chinese massage, a more powerful and stronger form of massage than that practiced in the United States), herbal therapy, moxibustion (applying cones of herbal substances to the skin and igniting them to make smoke, or igniting prepared strip of herbs to cause smoke and holding the smoking strip of herbs close to certain parts of the body), cupping (attachment of a small cup to the skin of the patient that creates a vacuum after the heated air inside the cup cools), energetic exercises (e.g., tai chi, qi gong), and diet (adjusting the food based on its yin and yang properties) to recover and sustain the patient's health (Johnson & Johnson, 2002).

Traditionally, TCM practitioners are trained within the family. Typically, the father would train the son to be a TCM practitioner, who would then carry on the family tradition and extend the rich first-hand experiences in TCM diagnosis and practices. Many such experiences were to be kept secret and within the family. Since 1949, the Chinese government has encouraged many of such family-trained TCM practitioners to share their secret experiences. Many of them have been employed as clinical faculty members in various TCM colleges, passing on their rich experiences in TCM to their students. A modern TCM doctor typically receives five years of academic training in one of the TCM colleges in China or several Western countries. After four years of coursework in basic science and TCM subjects, the student completes a one-year internship in a TCM hospital or a TCM department in a major comprehensive teaching hospital. Students who complete the formal academic training receive a bachelor's or doctoral degree. After they graduate from a TCM college, the TCM doctors can be employed by TCM hospitals or TCM departments in any comprehensive teaching hospitals where they receive advanced clinical training. Many TCM colleges in China also offer postgraduate training in TCM.

TCM is generally safe if it is administered under the supervision of a well-trained and experienced TCM practitioner. It is important that you tell your healthcare provider if you are using any TCM treatments, as some herbal preparations may interact with other medications you are taking.

RESEARCH AND TECHNOLOGY

Scientific evidence from randomized clinical trials is strong for many uses of acupuncture, for some herbal medicines, and for some of the manipulative therapies (such as chiropractic and massage therapy) (Robinson & Zhang, 2011). For most CIH approaches, however, there is an insufficient amount of valid and reliable randomized controlled data to demonstrate their mechanisms of action, efficacy, and applicability. In addition, many studies in CIH are flawed by insufficient statistical power, poor controls, inconsistent treatment, or lack of comparisons (Nahin & Straus, 2001).

Nevertheless, there exist significant challenges in applying research methods for CIH. The current model of research evaluation of CIH is based on the methodology of Western medicine (i.e., quantitative research methods), which cannot quantify the impact of profound traditional philosophy, culture, and religion. In this regard, qualitative research may be more appropriate. In the Western world, many researchers question the efficacy of many CIH therapies because "science has not provided sufficient evidence." However, history reveals that several traditional healing systems (e.g., traditional Chinese medicine and Ayurveda) have been practiced and used in treating diseases and promoting health for thousands of years. The long history of field-tested human experiments, long-term observations, and clinical trials may have proved the value of those ancient healing systems.

Perhaps the currently available science and technology are simply unable to measure the effects of many CIH therapies, or perhaps we do not have the appropriate research methodologies available to perform such studies. As new knowledge is discovered and technologies are developed, it may become possible to detect the effects of many CIH therapies, especially those that have been practiced for thousands of years. The historical process of discovering the mind–body connection best illustrates this possibility. For example, the connection between the mind and the body was first believed to be in existence in ancient times. Early technological advances (e.g., microscopy, the stethoscope, the blood pressure cuff, and refined surgical techniques) separated the mind from the physical body. The discovery of bacteria and antibiotics further dispelled the notion of belief influencing health. Later science discovered the link between the mind and the body. Nowadays, with functional connectivity magnetic resonance imaging (fMRI) and other modern technologies, we are able to confirm the connection between mind and body.

The U.S. government has placed significant emphasis on CIH research. In recent years, NCCIH has supported studies in various therapies in each of the major categories to different extents. It regularly examines and redefines its research priorities to fill gaps in the research, capitalize on emerging opportunities, and leverage resources. The NCCIH *Third Strategic Plan:*

2011–2015 presents the following five objectives to guide NCCAM in determining future research priorities in CIH (NCCIH, 2015g):

1. Advance research on mind and body interventions, practices, and disciplines
2. Advance research on CIH natural products
3. Increase understanding of "real-world" patterns and outcomes of CIH use and its integration into health care and health promotion
4. Improve the capacity of the field to carry out rigorous research
5. Develop and disseminate objective, evidence-based information on CIH interventions

Although NCCIH funds a wide range of research topics, the current areas of special interest focus on CIH interventions used often by the public and on health conditions in which CIH modalities are most frequently used, including investigations of the impact of CIH interventions in relieving chronic pain syndromes and inflammatory processes, and improving health and wellness (NCCIH, 2015h). Figure 11-2 illustrates NCCIH funding priorities.

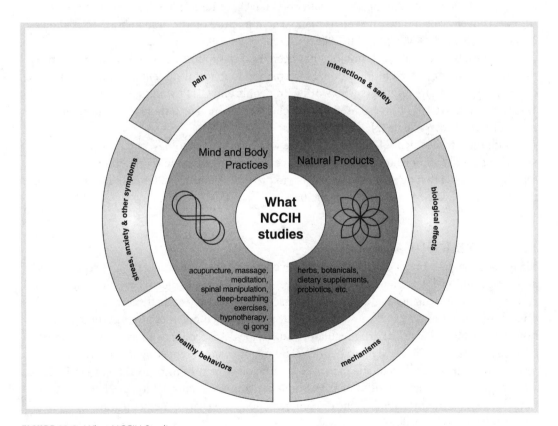

FIGURE 11-2 What NCCIH Studies
Reproduced from NCCIH. (2016). *Overview: What NCCIH funds.* Retrieved from https://nccih.nih.gov/grants/whatnccihfunds/overviewfunds.htm. Page last modified January 27, 2016. Accessed October 22, 2015.

To develop skilled investigators in CIH research, NCCIH offers funding to support predoctoral, postdoctoral, and career awards through several funding channels. To encourage clinicians interested in pursuing careers as investigators, NCCAM offers them Clinical Research Curriculum Awards and training in the skills needed for conducting rigorous research in CIH (NCCIH, 2015h). With the support from the U.S. government and many professional organizations along with the commitment and contributions from the scientists, significant progress in CIH research has been made in the last decade.

Biomedical science and technology have advanced CIH treatment and research significantly. For example, standardizing the "dose" of acupuncture through the use of an electrical apparatus to simulate the acupuncture needles makes quantitative research on acupuncture possible. Cells isolated and cultured in the laboratory have been used to study the effect of qi in TCM. Biomedical laboratory techniques have been used to assess the benefits of music (Chikahisa et al., 2006) and humor (Christie & Moore, 2005). Biopharmacology has contributed to the research on the effects of various herbal therapies on cancer (Richardson, 2001). fMRI has been used to study the effects of acupuncture on the human brain among normal persons (Li et al., 2006) and among stroke patients (Li, Jack, & Yang, 2006), as well as to measure the effects of electroacupuncture versus manual acupuncture on the human brain (Napadow, Makris, Liu, Kettner, Kwong, & Hui, 2005).

In addition, information technology has been used to support collaborative research, monitor clinical trials, and provide educational information to medical students, fellows, faculty, and community-based care providers who work with people and CIH (Monkman, 2001; Whelan & Dvorkin, 2003). NCCIH has also used the Internet to disseminate authoritative information to the public and professionals (NCCIH, 2015h).

With the advancement of biomedical science, computer technology, and human genome, we can expect to see more applications of science and technology in CIH treatment and research. It is hoped that one day we will be able to provide scientific evidence that demonstrates the effects of the ancient traditional medicines.

LEGAL AND ETHICAL ISSUES

Many countries face major challenges in the development and implementation of regulations aimed at traditional, complementary, alternative, and herbal medicines. These challenges are related to these treatments' regulatory status, assessment of safety and efficacy, quality control, safety monitoring, and lack of knowledge about traditional, complementary, alternative, and herbal medicines by national drug regulatory authorities. According to a recent WHO report (Robinson & Zhang, 2011), the number of WHO member states reporting to have regulations or laws governing herbal medicine increased significantly from 14 prior to 1986 to 110 in 2007, while slightly more than one third of WHO member countries reported to have laws or regulations focused on traditional medicine or complementary alternative medicine (38% or 54 of 141 countries) (WHO, 2005).

Currently, the United States does not have a regulatory process to ensure the safety and efficacy of various CIH practices except for homeopathic remedies and dietary supplements.

In 1938, the U.S. Congress passed a law allowing homeopathic remedies to be regulated by the FDA in the same manner as nonprescription, OTC drugs. As a consequence, people can purchase homeopathic remedies in any drugstore without a prescription from a doctor. In addition, homeopathic remedies do not need to meet the FDA's requirements for conventional prescription drugs and other OTC drugs. Specifically, the FDA requires that all conventional prescription drugs go through thorough testing and systematic review that proves their safety and effectiveness before they can be licensed for sale as prescription drugs. Only those prescription drugs that have been marketed as prescription medications for at least three years, have a relatively high use, and have not had any alarming adverse drug reactions and increased side effects during the time they were available as prescription drugs can be switched from prescription to OTC status. However, the FDA does require homeopathic remedies to meet certain legal standards for strength, quality, purity, and packaging (Junod, 2000).

The FDA regulates dietary supplements under a different set of regulations than those that apply to conventional prescription and OTC drugs. Under the Dietary Supplement Health and Education Act of 1994 (DSHEA), dietary supplements are considered products (other than tobacco) intended to supplement the diet and are not "drugs" from an official standpoint. Dietary supplement manufacturers are responsible for ensuring that a dietary supplement is safe and the product label information is truthful and not misleading before it is marketed. They are required by the Bioterrorism Act of 2002 to register with the FDA before they can make or sell supplements. However, these manufacturers do not have to prove the safety and effectiveness of any dietary supplements, nor do their products need FDA approval before they are marketed. The FDA is responsible for monitoring product information (such as package inserts and labeling claims) and taking action against any unsafe dietary supplement products after they reach the market (FDA, 2015).

A large proportion of patients who use CIH practices do not inform their conventional doctors about their use of such products and services. This omission, combined with the possibility of adverse reactions with prescription drugs, is placing the lives of many Americans in danger. Ethically, consumers have the right to use CIH practices as a matter of autonomy, but they also have the duty not to harm themselves. Ethically, manufacturers must ensure that their products are not harmful and have the claimed effect(s), but there are no laws or regulations that require manufacturers to prove that their products work as stated. When patients are experiencing problems related to health and illness, ineffective products, although not necessarily harmful on their own, may mask the signs and symptoms that would allow for accurate diagnosis, delay appropriate treatment, and jeopardize patients' lives. This, in effect, not only causes physical and emotional harm to patients, but also brings added costs to patients and society in terms of money and resources.

To ensure patients' safety, CIH practices must be evaluated with regard to safety and efficacy. The FDA has the ethical responsibility to take the lead in this area. To protect the common good, there is a need to know not only what CIH practices can do *for* us, but also what it can do *to* us. In addition, the U.S. government has the ethical responsibility to develop specific regulations that require manufacturers of CIH devices, remedies, and dietary supplements to follow the requirements for devices and prescription drugs used in conventional medicine. Unless a device or remedy is proved to be safe and effective, no products with the potential to alter health should be allowed in the market. Achieving this goal may take a long time, however. Since its passage, the 1994 DSHEA has been intensely debated in the U.S. Congress. Until such regulations are developed, approved, and implemented, we need to educate consumers on how to select qualified CIH practitioners and therapies and how to evaluate CIH information from the Internet and other sources. Tables 11-2, 11-3, and 11-4 provide useful information offered by the NCCIH.

TABLE 11-2 Are You Considering a Complementary Health Approach?
• Take charge of your health by being an informed consumer. Find out and consider what scientific studies have been done on the safety and effectiveness of any health approach that is recommended to or interests you.
• Discuss the information and your interests with your healthcare providers before making a decision.
• Choose a complementary health practitioner, such as an acupuncturist, as carefully as you would choose a conventional healthcare provider.
• Before using any *dietary supplement* or herbal product, make sure you find out about potential side effects or interactions with medications you may be taking.
• Only use treatments for your condition that have been proven safe. Do not use a product or practice that has not been proven to be effective to postpone seeing your healthcare provider for your condition.
• Tell all your healthcare providers—complementary and conventional—about all the health approaches you use. Give them a full picture of what you do to manage your health. This will help ensure coordinated and safe care.
Reproduced from NCCIH. (2014). *Are You Considering a Complementary Health Approach?* Retrieved from https://nccih .nih.gov/health/decisions/consideringcam.htm. Page last updated August 2014. Accessed October 20, 2015.

TABLE 11-3 Six Things to Know When Selecting a Complementary Health Practitioner
1. If you need names of practitioners in your area, first check with your doctor or other healthcare provider.
2. Find out as much as you can about any potential practitioner, including education, training, licensing, and certifications.
Once you have found a possible practitioner, here are some tips about deciding whether he or she is right for you:
1. Find out whether the practitioner is willing to work together with your conventional healthcare providers.
2. Explain all of your health conditions to the practitioner, and find out about the practitioner's training and experience in working with people who have your conditions.
3. Don't assume that your health insurance will cover the practitioner's services.
4. Tell all your healthcare providers about all complementary approaches you use and about all practitioners who are treating you.
Modified from NCCIH. (2015). *6 Things to Know When Selecting a Complementary Health Practitioner.* Retrieved from https:// nccih.nih.gov/health/tips/selecting. Page last modified September 24, 2015. Accessed October 20, 2015.

TABLE 11-4 Questions to Ask When Evaluating a Health-Related Website

Your search for online health information may start on a known, trusted site, but after following several links, you may find yourself on an unfamiliar site. Can you trust this site? Here are some key questions you need to ask.

Who runs and pays for the website?	Any reliable health-related website should make it easy for you to learn who's responsible for the site. Web addresses that end in ".gov" mean it's a government-sponsored site; ".edu" indicates an educational institution, ".org" is a noncommercial organization, and ".com" is a commercial organization. Sites with ".gov" and ".edu" can be trusted except that an ".edu" site produced by an individual at an educational institution may not be trustworthy. The ".org" sites are not always reputable and/or legitimate and may promote a specific agenda.
How is the site supported?	The funding source can affect what content is presented, how it's presented, and what the site owners want to accomplish. Does it sell advertising? Is it sponsored by a company that sells dietary supplements, drugs, or other products or services?
What is the purpose of the site?	The About This Site page should include a clear statement of purpose. To be sure you're getting reliable information, you should confirm information that you find on sales sites by consulting other, independent sites where no products are sold.
What is the source of the information?	If the person or organization in charge of the site didn't create the material, the original source should be clearly identified.
What is the basis of the information?	The site should describe the evidence (such as articles in medical journals) that the material is based on. Opinions or advice should be clearly set apart from information that's "evidence-based" (i.e., based on research results). Look for references to scientific research that clearly support what's said. Keep in mind that testimonials, anecdotes, unsupported claims, and opinions aren't the same as objective, evidence-based information.
Is the information reviewed?	You can be more confident in the quality of medical information on a website if people with credible professional and scientific qualifications review the material before it's posted.
How current is the information?	Some types of outdated medical information can be misleading or even dangerous. Responsible health websites review and update much of their content on a regular basis. Look for a date on the page (it's often near the bottom).
What is the site's policy about linking to other sites?	Some sites take a conservative approach and don't link to any other sites. Some link to any site that asks or pays for a link. Others only link to sites that have met certain criteria. Unless the site's linking policy is strict, don't assume that the sites that it links to are reliable. Evaluate the linked sites just as you would any other site that you're visiting for the first time.
How does the site handle personal information?	Many websites track visitors' paths to determine what pages are being viewed. A health website may ask you to "subscribe" or "become a member." Any credible site asking for this kind of information should tell you exactly what it will and will not do with it. Be sure to read any privacy policy or similar language on the site, and don't sign up for anything you don't fully understand.

(continues)

TABLE 11-4 Questions to Ask When Evaluating a Health-Related Website (*Continued*)

How does the site manage interactions with users?	You should always be able to contact the site owner if you run across problems or have questions or feedback. If the site hosts online discussion areas (forums or message boards), it should explain the terms of using this service. Spend some time reading what has been posted before joining in to see whether you feel comfortable with the environment.
Are you reading real online news or just advertising?	You should suspect that a news site may be fake if it: • Endorses a product. Real news organizations generally don't do this. • Only quotes people who say good things about the product. • Presents research findings that seem too good to be true. (If something seems too good to be true, it usually is.) • Contains links to a sales site. • Includes positive reader comments only, and you can't add a comment of your own.
How to protect yourself	If you suspect that a news site is fake, look for a disclaimer somewhere on the page (often in small print) that indicates that the site is an advertisement. Don't rely on Internet news reports when making important decisions about your health. If you're considering a health product described in the news, discuss it with your healthcare provider.

Modified from NCCIH. (2014). *Finding and Evaluating Online Resources on Complementary Health Approaches.* Retrieved from https://nccih.nih.gov/health/webresources. Page last updated September 2014. Accessed October 20, 2015.

Ethical issues related to CIH research remain to be resolved. The current clinical trials of acupuncture have examined its efficacy by administering a fixed course of treatment sessions based on biomedical diagnosis. This standardized approach conflicts with the traditional means of delivering holistic TCM treatments that are customized to the individual's level of strength or weakness of yin and yang (Hammerschlag, 1998). A similar ethical challenge exists in evaluating the effects of Ayurvedic therapies that are determined, based on the individual's constitution (Sharma, Chandola, Singh, & Basisht, 2007). Likewise, homeopathic remedies are highly individualized (White, 2000). Because many traditional medicines are deeply rooted in cultural traditions and religion, the interactions between the practitioner and the patient, and the influence of the family, religion, cultural, and personal belief systems are important factors in the success of those traditional therapies. When patients are taken out of their traditional, social, and cultural context, and placed in a scientifically controlled treatment environment, the question becomes, "Are we serving the best interests of our patients?"

With the current scientific research methods available, researchers continue to debate which research mythologies are most appropriate. Some researchers argue against the use of placebo and sham controls (patients in the control group receive no treatment or fake treatment), while others favor wait lists (patients receive the treatment once the study is completed) and standard care (patients receive routine care) designs. The former group believes withholding treatment to be inappropriate, and the latter group considers testing a treatment prior to demonstrating its efficacy against a placebo to be just as inappropriate.

From these examples, we can see that there are many legal and ethical challenges in CIH practices and research. It is hoped that we will be able to meet these challenges as we learn more about CIH practices and develop more appropriate research methods.

INFLUENCES OF POLITICS, ECONOMICS, CULTURE, AND RELIGION

Politics: The Role of Government

Government has always played a major and an important role in CIH practices and research. For example, the Indian government has undertaken systematic research of Ayurvedic practices since 1969. In China, TCM has gone through several waves of challenges and has a long history of regulation. Between 1911 and 1949, the Chinese government embraced Western medicine with the goal of modernizing the Chinese medical care system. This movement forced TCM to go underground and nearly wiped it out. Since 1949, however, the Chinese government has promoted the integration of Western and Chinese medicine, established major colleges of TCM, reprinted many older TCM-related works, and worked with WHO and other interested organizations and countries to promote TCM globally. In the last three decades, international training centers have been established in Beijing, Shanghai, Guangzhou, Nanjing, and Xiamen to train TCM personnel from all over the world. Multiple TCM colleges have been established in many Western countries, and many cooperative research projects have been conducted between China and developed countries (Johnson & Johnson, 2002).

The influence of politics and government is significant in the United States as well. One politician, U.S. Senator Tom Harkins, played a key role in the establishment of the Office of Alternative Medicine (OAM) within the National Institutes of Health (NIH) in 1992 and the National Center for Complementary and Alternative Medicine (NCCAM) in 1999. Since the establishment of OAM and NCCAM, whose name was changed to NCCIH in 2015, government funding for NCCIH has increased from $2 million in 1990 to $128.8 million in 2010 and to $124.1 million in 2015. Figure 11-3 shows the funding appropriated for each fiscal year. The support by the U.S. government has allowed NCCIH to explore CIH practices in the context of rigorous science, training of CIH researchers, and dissemination of authoritative information to the public and professionals (NCCIH, 2015i).

Worldwide, however, only slightly over half of the countries that participated in a WHO survey on national policy on traditional medicine and regulations of herbal medicines reported having a traditional medicine policy (53%, or 69 of 129 countries) whereas over 1 out of 10 of those countries reported having a national policy regulating herbal medicine (92%, or 119 of 129). Based on the definition provided by WHO (2015a), a national policy on traditional medicine or CIH may include a definition of traditional medicine/CIH, provision for the creation of laws and regulations, consideration of intellectual property issues, and strategies for achieving the objectives of the policy.

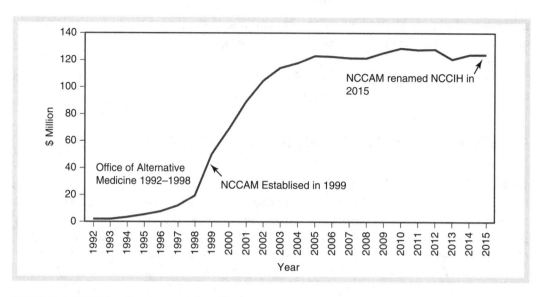

FIGURE 11-3 NCCIH Funding Appropriations History
Data from NCCIH. (2015). *NCCIH funding: Appropriations history.* Retrieved from https://nccih.nih.gov/about/budget/appropriations.htm. Page last modified March 10, 2015. Accessed October 28, 2015.

The limited scientific evidence regarding the safety and efficacy of traditional medicine/CIH and the widespread use of traditional medicine/CIH worldwide makes it important for governments to certain steps. WHO (2015a) developed three strategic objectives, the corresponding strategic directions, expected outcomes, and clinical indicator for its member states (Table 11-5).

Economics

The widespread use of traditional medicine and CIH in developing countries partly reflects the impact of each country's economy. Because traditional and herbal medicines are less expensive and more widely accessible than Western medicine, many developing countries, especially those in Africa, Asia, and Latin America, use traditional medicine to help meet some of the primary healthcare needs of their citizens. For example, 80% of Lao's population healthcare services is provided by the Lao's traditional medicine professionals. There are significantly more traditional healers than conventional medical doctors in Africa (one traditional healer per 500 people versus one conventional doctor per 40,000 people) (WHO, 2015b). The poorer economic conditions in developing countries limit their residents' access to modern Western medicine, which is typically characterized by expensive consultations provided by doctors who are expensively trained and using expensive procedures, laboratory equipment, and pharmaceuticals. One of WHO's priorities is to promote safe and effective traditional medicine/CIH therapies to increase access to health care in developing countries (WHO, 2015b).

TABLE 11-5 Traditional Medicine Strategy Key Performance Indicators

Strategic Objective		Strategic Direction		Expected Outcomes	Critical Indicator
4.1	To build the knowledge base for active management of T&CM through appropriate national policies	4.1.1	Understand and recognize the role and potential of T&CM	• T&CM practices and practitioners identified and analysed by Member State and country profile devised for T&CM. • T&CM policies and programmes established by government.	• Number of Member States reporting a national/provincial/state T&CM policy. • Number of Member States reporting increased governmental/public research funding for T&CM
		4.1.2	Strengthen the knowledge base, build evidence and sustain resources	• Strengthened knowledge generation, collaboration and sustainable use of TM resources.	
4.2	To strengthen quality assurance, safety, proper use and effectiveness of T&CM by regulating products, practices and practitioners	4.2.1	Recognize the role and importance of product regulation	• Established and implemented national regulation for T&CM products including registration. • Strengthened safety monitoring of T&CM products and other T&CM therapies. • Technical guidelines and methodology developed for evaluating safety, efficacy and quality of T&CM.	• Number of Member States reporting national regulation for T&CM products • Number of Member States reporting national/provincial/state regulation for T&CM practice • Number of Member States reporting national/provincial/state regulation/registration for T&CM practitioners

(continues)

TABLE 11-5 **Traditional Medicine Strategy Key Performance Indicators (*Continued*)**

Strategic Objective		Strategic Direction		Expected Outcomes	Critical Indicator
		4.2.2	Recognize and develop practice and practitioner regulation for T&CM education and training, skills development, services and therapies	• Standards for T&CM products, practices and practitioners developed by government. • Established education/ training programme, benchmarks and implementation capacities for T&CM practitioners • Improved safe and effective use of T&CM	
4.3	To promote universal health coverage by integrating T&CM services into health care service delivery and self-health care	4.3.1	Capitalize on the potential contribution of T&CM to improve health services and health outcomes.	• Integration of T&CM into the health system. • Improved T&CM services and accessibility. • Improved communication between conventional medicine practitioners, professional bodies and T&CM practitioners concerning the use of T&CM.	• Number of Member States reporting national plan/ programme/ approaches for integrating T&CM service into the national health service delivery • Number of Member States reporting consumer education project/ programme for self-health care using T&CM
		4.3.2	Ensure consumers of T&CM can make informed choices about self-health care.	• Better awareness of and access to information about the proper use of T&CM. • Improved communication between conventional medicine practitioners and their patients about T&CM use.	

In contrast, the economic conditions in developed countries have actually promoted the use of CIH practices. In developed countries, most CIH practices are not covered by health insurance plans. Because of the better economies found in developed countries, however, the people who live there are generally better off and are financially able to pay for various CIH services and treatments on an out-of-pocket basis (Eisenberg, Davis, Ettner, Appel, Wilkey, Van Rompay, & Kessler, 1998; Palinkas & Kabongo, 2000).

Culture and Religion

The evolution of traditional medicines has been influenced by different religious, cultural, and historic conditions in which they were first developed (WHO, 2005). For example, traditional Chinese medical care and practice are strongly influenced by Chinese tradition and religion including Confucius principles, Taoism, the theory of yin and yang, and Buddhism (Chen, 2001; Zhang & Cheng, 2000). The ideas from Hinduism, one of the world's oldest and largest religions, as well as ancient Persian thoughts about health and healing shaped the core principles of Ayurveda. Mexican American folk medicine, curanderismo, mainly draws from the combination of Mayan and Aztec teachings and the Mexican heritage of Spanish Catholicism (Krippner, 1995).

Religious and cultural beliefs also influence the practice and use of traditional medical healings. Mexican American healers often attribute an illness to an agent whose existence must be taken on faith because it cannot be detected with medical instruments. For instance, Mexican American healers use prayers and songs to treat an illness caused by an inappropriate salute to an owl. This illness is characterized by heart palpitations, anxiety, sweating, and shaking. It is believed that this disease can lead to suicide if left untreated. Many Native American healings are considered spiritual in nature and, in turn, rituals and magic such as medicine wheels and sand paintings are used to treat these supernatural disorders. Native Americans' imitative magic treatment is based on the belief that what happened to an image or drawing of a person did happen in reality (Krippner, 1995). Such beliefs were also prevalent among Chinese in the old times and still exist among many older Chinese.

Cultural beliefs significantly predict the use of traditional medical practices. For instance, in Chinese culture, it is believed that the mother loses a significant amount of *yang* during the delivery of a baby and must preserve any yang left so that her yin will not be too strong. Therefore, a new mother must stay indoors for an entire month, regardless of the season, after delivering the baby; cannot touch or eat anything cold; cannot take a bath; and cannot go outdoors without covering all of the exposed body parts to avoid cold air. Because all of those activities are considered yin, the traditional practices are believed to help promote the yang and maintain yin–yang balance. It is believed that if the new mother failed to follow those practices, her yang could not be restored and her yin would be too strong, which would cause joint pain, lower back pain, lost teeth, and headaches later in her life. Also, ancient Chinese beliefs hold that animal organs correspond to human organs. If a particular human organ is weak, the same organ of an animal should be consumed. For example, a new mother is believed to have "weakened" blood caused by losing blood during and after the delivery, so she might eat cooked pig's blood to strengthen her own blood. Such practice does have merit because the new mother could have anemia due to loss of blood, the iron and other nutrients in pig's blood would provide the nutrients needed to produce red blood cells and correct anemia.

CIH PRACTICES IN DEVELOPING VERSUS DEVELOPED SOCIETIES

Traditional medicine and CIH use is more prevalent in developing countries as compared to developed countries. In the developing world, traditional medicine has been used largely for primary health care. In India, Ayurveda has been the main healthcare system and is still used today by 80% of the population (NCCIH, 2015e). A 2008 WHO report revealed that as much as 90% of African populations use traditional medicine to meet their primary care needs, and TCM is available to 75% of the areas in China and has been fully integrated into its healthcare system.

In contrast to the developing countries, the developed world perceives traditional medicine and CIH practice as a choice because the number of well-educated and well-informed patients is increasing. These individuals are often attracted by the holistic and natural approaches employed by various CIH practices. Well-educated and well-informed healthcare consumers want to become more involved in their overall health care, take a more natural and holistic approach to achieving personal well-being, and are willing to pay for CIH therapies out of pocket (Astin, 1998; Eisenberg, Davis, Ettner, Appel, Wilkey, Van Rompay, & Kessler, 1998; Palinkas & Kabongo, 2000).

SUMMARY

This chapter presented definitions, types, and utilization of complementary and integrative health approaches from a global perspective. Current statistics regarding the varieties, utilization, cultural backgrounds and implications; current research and technology; and legal and ethical issues were also included.

Study Questions

1. What are some of the potential benefits and risks of traditional medicine/CIH practices? Why do you think these practices and products have maintained their popularity in the developing countries and are becoming so popular in the Western world?
2. What role do you believe governments should play in promoting traditional medicine/CAM?
3. Should the use of CIH practices in the United States and other developed countries be regulated? If use of CIH practices should be regulated, how should it be regulated and by whom? If the use of CIH should not be regulated, why and what would be the consequences?
4. What do you believe to be the major challenges in CIH practices and research? What would you do to address such challenges?

Case Study 1: Homeopathic Remedy Treating Anxiety and Depression After Conventional Therapies Failed

John had a relatively long history of depression. In the past, his anxiety and depression would dissipate over time after he took psychotropic drugs. His present depression started a year ago, in the wake of an incident at work where he felt betrayed. Even after John had taken six different antidepressant and antianxiety drugs and suffered from the side effects of the drugs, his depressive symptoms remained. He became more and more dysfunctional at work, to the point where he was on sick leave for the month prior to seeking homeopathic care. At the time he saw the homeopathic practitioner, he was extremely upset and still angry and aggressive. He received a single dose of Staphysagria lM. At the next appointment, three weeks later, John said he was "much better." His appetite had returned, and he had started to gain back the weight he had lost. He was calmer and sleeping better. He was working full time at home and would go back to the office that next week. He said, "I decided to change my priorities. I will do more things for myself and enjoy life a little more."

Data from D. Wember. (1997). The heart and soul of homeopathy. *Journal of the American Institute of Homeopathy, 90,* 36–40.

Case Study 2: Homeopathy Treating Postpartum Depression

A 28-year-old woman with postpartum depression revealed to her psychologist fantasies and impulses of throwing her 14-week-old daughter off of a cliff. Envying her friends without children and feeling distant and angry toward her husband as well as her infant, she was mired in a severe clinical depression that had been unresponsive to two trials of antidepressant medication. The psychologist referred the patient to a homeopath, a practitioner of the German-born form of medicine that uses a minute dose of an herb, plant, or other substance to effect healing, reportedly by stimulating a patient's "vital force." Within four days of beginning treatment with a remedy called sepia, the woman's depression lifted, and she began bonding with her infant. Homeopaths explain such rapid cures by saying that the energy of the remedy repairs the "leakage" in the patient's "energy balloon" that has been created by particular traumas or life events. The specific remedy used in this case, sepia, is made from the ink of the cuttlefish. It reportedly is indicated when a woman is exhausted physically and emotionally from a myriad of responsibilities and work or from too many pregnancies, abortions, or miscarriages. A classic sign of its indication, according to homeopaths, is a person's indifference or aversion to loved ones. "The change was astounding!" her psychologist told the homeopath. "Now she loves the baby and is taking all kinds of photographs and videotapes of her child, and her marital relationship has improved considerably."

Reproduced from K. P. White. (2000). Psychology and complementary and alternative medicine. *Professional Psychology: Research and Practice, 31,* 671–681.

Case Study 3: Traditional Chinese Medicine Treating Infertility

A Chinese couple in their early 30s went to see a TCM doctor, hoping the practitioner could help them conceive a child. This couple had been married for three years and had gone through extensive clinical examinations and laboratory tests, including ultrasound. Nothing appeared to be wrong with their reproductive organs and functions, but they just could not conceive a child. The TCM doctor checked the pulse, examined the tongue, and took the history from the couple. The TCM diagnosis was that both the husband and the wife had *yin xu* (meaning weak yin) caused by weak "kidney"; the TCM doctor prescribed Chinese herbal medicine for the couple to strengthen the kidney, which would enhance yin and balance the yin–yang harmony. After three months of treatment, the wife was pregnant. The TCM doctor checked the wife's pulse at five weeks' gestation and informed the wife that she was carrying a boy. Nine months later, a healthy baby boy was born to the couple. Now the baby boy is in his third year in a medical school in China.

Case Study 4: Qi Therapy Used to Relieve Symptoms of Cancer in a Terminally Ill Cancer Patient

Jane suffered from late-stage ovarian cancer and was experiencing unbearable abdominal discomfort and pain, depression, and fatigue. Four sessions of qi therapy on alternate days was given to Jane over a seven-day period. After 20 minutes of qi therapy, she experienced improvements in mood and alertness, and a reduction in pain, anxiety, depression, discomfort, and fatigue, on both the first and last days of the interventions. Furthermore, the scores recorded on the last day for most symptoms were improved relative to those recorded on the first day. Although the result of this case study does not constitute conclusive evidence, the data suggest that qi therapy may have some beneficial effects on some symptoms of cancer.

Data from M. S. Lee & H. S. Jang. (2005). Two case reports of the acute effects of qi therapy (external qigong) on symptoms of cancer: Short report. *Complement Therapy in Clinical Practice, 11*, 211–213.

Case Study Questions

1. Why do you think that CIH practices can be highly effective in these case studies when Western medicine was not able to produce positive results?
2. What are the reasons that many people will not believe in, nor try to use CIH practice as a first intervention for a health problem?
3. What are the legal/ethical issues (if they exist) for prescribing CIH practices in your area of residence?

References

American Association of Retired Persons & National Center for Complementary and Alternative Medicine Survey Report (2011). *Complementary and Alternative Medicine: What People Aged 50 and Older Discuss with Their Health Care Providers*. Retrieved from https://nccih.nih.gov/research/statistics/2010.

Astin, J. A. (1998). Why patients use alternative medicine. *Journal of the American Medical Association, 279*, 1548–1553.

Ballard, R. (2000). Homeopathy: An overview. *Australian Family Physician, 29*, 1145–1148.

Barnes, P. M., Bloom, B., & Nahin, R. (2008). *Complementary and alternative medicine use among adults and children: United States, 2007*. CDC National Health Statistics Report No. 12. Retrieved from http://nccam .nih.gov/news/2008/nhsr12.pdf

Barnes, P. M., Powell-Griner, E., McFann, K., & Nahin, R. L. (2004). *Complementary and alternative medicine use among adults: United States, 2002. Advance data from vital and health statistics, No. 343*. National Center for Health Statistics. Retrieved from http://www.cdc.gov/nchs/data/ad/ad343.pdf

Brewer, A. V. (2006). Energy healing. In J. Brewer & K. King (Eds.), *Complementary and Alternative Medicine: A Physician Guide* [Electronic book]. Retrieved from http://medicine.wustl.edu/~compmed/cam_toc.htm

Chen, Y. C. (2001). Chinese values, health and nursing. *Journal of Advanced Nursing, 36,* 270–273.

Chikahisa, S., Sei, H., Morishima, M., Sano, A., Kitaoka, K., Nakaya, Y., . . . Morita, Y. (2006). Exposure to music in the perinatal period enhances learning performance and alters BDNF/TrkB signaling in mice as adults. *Behavioral Brain Research, 169,* 312–319.

Christie, W., & Moore, C. (2005). The impact of humor on patients with cancer. *Clinical Journal of Oncology Nursing, 9,* 211–218.

Clarke, T. C., et al. Trends in the use of complementary health approaches among adults: United States, 2002–2012. *National Health Statistics Reports, 79.* Hyattsville, MD: National Center for Health Statistics, 2015.

Dantas, F., & Rampes, H. (2000). Do homeopathic medicines provoke adverse effects? A systematic review. *British Homeopathic Journal, 89,* S35–S38.

Dessio, W., Wade, C., Chao, M., Kronenberg, F., Cushman, L. E., & Kalmuss, D. (2004). Religion, spirituality, and healthcare choices of African-American women: Results of a national survey. *Ethnicity & Disease, 14,* 189–197.

Eisenberg, D. M., Davis, R. B., Ettner, S. L., Appel, S., Wilkey, S., Van Rompay, M., & Kessler, R. C. (1998). Trends in alternative medicine use in the United States, 1990–1997: Results of a follow-up national survey. *Journal of the American Medical Association, 280,* 1569–1575.

Eisenberg, D. M., Kessler, R. C., Van Rompay, M. I., Kaptchuk, T. J., Wilkey, S. A., Appel, S., & R. B. Davis. (2001). Perceptions about complementary therapies relative to conventional therapies among adults who use both: Results from a national survey. *Annals of Internal Medicine, 135,* 344–351.

Ernst, E. (2008). Chiropractic: A critical evaluation. *Journal of Pain and Symptom Management, 35*(5), 544–562.

Food and Drug Administration. (2000). *Risk of drug interactions with St John's wort and Indinavir and other drugs.* Retrieved from http://www.fda.gov/Drugs/DrugSafety/PostmarketDrugSafetyInformationforPatient-sandProviders/ucm052238.htm

Food and Drug Administration. (2004). *FDA announces rule prohibiting sale of dietary supplements containing ephedrine alkaloids effective April 12.* Retrieved from http://www.fda.gov/NewsEvents/Newsroom/PressAnnouncements/2004/ucm108281.htm

Food and Drug Administration. (2011). *Beware of fraudulent "dietary supplements."* Retrieved from http://www.fda.gov/ForConsumers/ConsumerUpdates/ucm246744.htm

Food and Drug Administration. (2015). *Dietary supplements.* Retrieved from http://www.fda.gov/Food/Dietary-Supplements/default.htm

Galantino, M. L., Galbavy, R., & Quinn, L. (2008). Therapeutic effects of yoga for children: A systematic review of the literature. *Pediatric Physical Therapy, 20*(1), 66–80.

Gaylord, S. A., Palsson, O. S., Garland, E. L., Faurot, K. R., Coble, R. S., Mann, J. D., Frey W., Leniek K., Whitehead, W. E. (2011, June 21). Mindfulness training reduces the severity of irritable bowel syndrome in women: Results of a randomized controlled trial, *Am J Gastroenterol 106*(9), 1678–1688. doi:10.1038/ajg.2011.184

Geller, A. I., Shehab, N., Weidle, N. J., Lovegrove, M. C., Wolpert, B. J., Timbo, B. B., Mozersky, R. P., and Budnitz, D. S. (2015). Emergency department visits for adverse events related to dietary supplements. *New England Journal of Medicine, 373,* 153–154. doi:10.1056/NEJMsa1504267

Hammerschlag, R. (1998). Methodological and ethical issues in clinical trials of acupuncture. *Journal of Alternative and Complementary Medicine, 4,* 159–171.

Hui, P. N., Wan, M., Chan, W. K., & Yung, P. M. (2006). An evaluation of two behavioral rehabilitation programs, qigong versus progressive relaxation, in improving the quality of life in cardiac patients. *Journal of Alternative and Complementary Medicine, 12,* 373–378.

Institute of Medicine. (2005). *Institute of Medicine Report on Complementary and Alternative Medicine in the United States.* Washington, DC: National Academies Press.

Jahnke, R., Larkey, L., Rogers, C., Etnier, J., & Lin, F. (2010). A comprehensive review of health benefits of qigong and tai chi. *American Journal of Health Promotion, 24*(6), e1–e25. Retrieved from http://www.ncbi .nlm.nih.gov/pmc/articles/PMC3085832/?tool=pubmed

Jang, J. H., Jung, W. H., Kang, D. J., Byun, M. S., Kwon, S. J., Chio, C. H., & Kwon, J. S. (2011). Increased default mode network connectivity associated with meditation. *Neuroscience Letter, 487*(3), 358–362.

Johnson, H. P. (2008). Global use of complementary and alternative medicine (CAM) and treatments. In C. Holtz, *Global Health*. Sudbury, MA: Jones & Bartlett Publishing.

Johnson, H. P. (2013). Global use of complementary and alternative medicine (CAM) and treatments. In C. Holtz, *Global Health* (2nd ed.). Sudbury, MA: Jones & Bartlett Publishing.

Johnson, P. H., & Johnson, R. D. (2002). *Looking to the East: The Theory and Practice of Traditional Chinese Medicine*. Paper presented at the 130th American Public Health Association (APHA) Annual Meeting, Philadelphia, PA.

Johnson, P. H., Priestley, J., Johnson, K. M., & Petrillo, J. (2010). Complementary and alternative medicine: Attitudes and use among health educators in the United States. *American Journal of Health Education, 41*(3), 167–177.

Junod, S. W. (2000). Alternative drugs: Homeopathy, Royal Copeland, and federal drug regulation. *Pharmacy in History, 42*, 13–35.

Kilpatrick, L. A., Suyenobu, B. Y., Smith, S. R., Bueller, J. A., Goodman, T., Creswell, J. D., . . . Naliboff, B. D. (2011). Impact of mindfulness-based stress reduction training on intrinsic brain connectivity. *Neuroimage, 56*(1), 299–308.

Koh, H. L., Ng, H. L., & Teo, H. H. (2004). A survey on knowledge, attitudes and usage of complementary and alternative medicine in Singapore. *Asia Pacific Biotech News, 8*, 1266–1270.

Krippner, S. (1995). A cross-cultural comparison of four healing models. *Alternative Therapies in Health and Medicine, 1*, 21–29.

Lee, M. S., & Jang, H. S. (2005). Two case reports of the acute effects of qi therapy (external qigong) on symptoms of cancer: Short report. *Complement Therapy in Clinical Practice, 11*, 211–213.

Lee, M. S., Kim, J. I., Ha, J. Y., Boddy, K., & Ernst, E. (2009). Yoga for menopausal symptoms: A systematic review. *Menopause, 16*(3), 602–608.

Lee, M. S., Kim, M. K., & Lee, Y. H. (2005). Effects of qi-therapy (external qigong) on cardiac autonomic tone: A randomized placebo controlled study. *International Journal of Neuroscience, 115*, 1345–1350.

Li, G., Jack, C. R., Jr., & Yang, E. S. (2006). An fMRI study of somatosensory-implicated acupuncture points in stable somatosensory stroke patients. *Journal of Magnetic Resonance Imaging, 24*(5), 1018–1024.

Li, K., Shan, B., Xu, J., Wang, W., Zhi, L., Li, K., . . . Tang, X. (2006). Changes in fMRI in the human brain related to different durations of manual acupuncture needling. *Journal of Alternative and Complementary Medicine, 12*, 615–623.

Li, M., Chen, K., & Mo, Z. (2002). Use of qigong therapy in the detoxification of heroin addicts. *Alternative Therapies in Health and Medicine, 8*, 50–54, 56–59.

Merrell, W. C., & Shalts, E. (2002). Homeopathy. *Medical Clinics of North America, 86*, 47–62.

Monkman, D. (2001). Educating health professionals about how to use the Web and how to find complementary and alternative medicine (CAM) information. *Complementary Therapies in Medicine, 9*, 258.

Morris, K. T., Johnson, N., Homer, L., & Walts, D. (2000). A comparison of complementary therapy use between breast cancer patients and patients with other tumors. *American Journal of Surgery, 179*, 407–411.

Mukherjee, P. K., & Wahile, A. (2006). Integrated approaches towards drug development from Ayurveda and other Indian system of medicines. *Journal of Ethnopharmacology, 103*, 25–35.

Nahin, R. L., Barnes, P. M, Stussman, B. J., & Bloom, B. (2009). Costs of complementary and alternative medicine (CAM) and frequency of visits to CIH practitioners: United States, 2007. *CDC National Health Statistics Report No. 18*. Retrieved from https://nccih.nih.gov/sites/nccam.nih.gov/files/nhsrn18.pdf

Nahin, R. L., & Straus, S. E. (2001). Research into complementary and alternative medicine: Problems and potential. *British Journal of Medicine, 322*, 161–163.

Napadow, V., Makris, N., Liu, J., Kettner, N. W., Kwong, K. K., & Hui, K. K. (2005). Effects of electroacupuncture versus manual acupuncture on the human brain as measured by fMRI. *Human Brain Mapping, 24,* 193–205.

National Center for Complementary and Integrative Health. (2012). *Chiropractic: An Introduction.* Retrieved from https://nccih.nih.gov/health/chiropractic/introduction.htm

National Center for Complementary and Integrative Health. (2013). Traditional Chinese medicine. *NCCIH Publication No. 428.* Retrieved from https://nccih.nih.gov/health/whatiscam/chinesemed.htm

National Center for Complementary and Integrative Health. (2014). *Meditation: What you need to know.* Retrieved from https://nccih.nih.gov/health/meditation/overview.htm

National Center for Complementary and Integrative Health. (2015a). *Complementary, alternative, or integrative health: What's in a name?* Retrieved from https://nccih.nih.gov/health/integrative-health

National Center for Complementary and Integrative Health. (2015b). *Yoga.* Retrieved from https://nccih.nih.gov/health/yoga

National Center for Complementary and Integrative Health. (2015c). *Tai chi and qi gong.* Retrieved from https://nccih.nih.gov/health/taichi/introduction.htm

National Center for Complementary and Integrative Health. (2015d). *Massage therapy for health purposes: What you need to know.* Retrieved from http://nccam.nih.gov/health/massage/massageintroduction.htm

National Center for Complementary and Integrative Health. (2015e). Ayurvedic medicine: An introduction. *NCCIH Publication No. D287.* Retrieved from https://nccih.nih.gov/health/ayurveda/introduction.htm

National Center for Complementary and Integrative Health. (2015f). Homeopathy: An introduction. *NCCAM Publication No. D439.* Retrieved from https://nccih.nih.gov/health/homeopathy

National Center for Complementary and Integrative Health. (2015g). *Naturopathy.* Retrieved from https://nccih.nih.gov/health/naturopathy

National Center for Complementary and Integrative Health. (2015h). *NCCAM third strategic plan: 2011–2015—Exploring the science of complementary and alternative medicine.* Retrieved from https://nccih.nih.gov/about/plans/2011

National Institutes of Health. (2015). *The NIH Almanac: National Center for Complementary and Integrative Health.* Retrieved from http://www.nih.gov/about/almanac/organization/NCCIH.htm

Nidich, S. I., Rainforth, M. V., Haaga, D. A., Hagelin, J., Salerno, J. W., Travis, F., Tanner, M., Gaylord-King, C., Grosswald, S., & Schneider, R. H. (2009, December 22). A randomized controlled trial on effects of the Transcendental Meditation program on blood pressure, psychological distress, and coping in young adults. *Am J Hypertens, 12,* 1326–1331. doi:10.1038/ajh.2009.184

Nobelprize.org. *The Nobel Prize in Physiology or Medicine 2015. Youyou Tu—Facts.* Retrieved from http://www.nobelprize.org/nobel_prizes/medicine/laureates/2015/tu-facts.html

Nutrition Business Journal. NBJ's Supplement Business Report 2015. Penton Media, Inc., 2015.

Palinkas, L. A., & Kabongo, M. L. (2000). The use of complementary and alternative medicine by primary care patients. *Journal of Family Practice, 49,* 1121–1130.

Peters, R. M. (1999). The effectiveness of therapeutic touch: A meta-analytic review. *Nursing Science Quarterly, 12,* 52–61.

Posadzki, P., Ernst, E., Terry, R., & Lee, M. S. (2011). Is yoga effective for pain? A systematic review of randomized clinical trials. *Complementary Therapies in Medicine, 19*(5), 281–287.

Richardson, M. A. (2001). Biopharmacologic and herbal therapies for cancer: Research update from NCCAM. *Journal of Nutrition, 131,* 3037S–3040S.

Robinson, M. M., & Zhang, X. R. (2011). *The world medicines situation 2011: Traditional medicines: Global situations, issues, and challenges.* Geneva, Switzerland: World Health Organization. Retrieved from http://www.who.int/medicines/areas/policy/world_medicines_situation/WMS_ch18_wTraditionalMed.pdf

Rogers, C. E., Larkey, L. K., & Keller, C. (2009). A review of clinical trials of tai chi and qigong in older adults. *Western Journal of Nursing Research, 31*(2), 245–279.

Ross, A., & Thomas, S. (2010). The health benefits of yoga and exercise: A review of comparison studies. *Journal of Alternative and Complementary Medicine, 16*(1), 3–12.

Samano, E. S. T., Ribeiro, L. M., Campos, A. S., Lewin, F., Filho, E. S. V., Goldenstein, P. T., . . . Del Giglio, A. (2005). Use of complementary and alternative medicine by Brazilian oncologists. *European Journal of Cancer Care, 14*, 143–148.

Sancier, K. M., & Holman, D. (2004). Commentary: Multifaceted health benefits of medical qigong. *Journal of Alternative and Complementary Medicine, 10*, 163–165.

Saper, R. B., Kales, S. N., Paquin, J., Burns, M. J., Eisenberg, D. M., Davis, R. B., & Phillips, R. S. (2004). Heavy metal content of Ayurvedic herbal medicine products. *Journal of the American Medical Association, 292*, 2868–2873.

Scheiman-Burkhardt, Z. (2001). Homeopathic treatment in a polluted world. *Natural Life, 81*, 10–11.

Sharma, H., Chandola, H. M., Singh, G., & Basisht, G. (2007). Utilization of Ayurveda in health care: An approach for prevention, health promotion, and treatment of disease. Part 1—Ayurveda, the science of life. *Journal of Alternative and Complementary Medicine, 13*(9), 1011–1019.

Streeter, C. C., Whitfield, T. H., Owen, L., Rein, T., Karri, S. K., Yakhkind, A., . . . Jensen, J. E. (2010). Effects of yoga versus walking on mood, anxiety, and brain GABA levels: A randomized controlled MRS study. *Journal of Alternative and Complementary Medicine, 16*(11), 1145–1152.

Tedesco, P., & Cicchetti, J. (2001). Like cures like: Homeopathy. *American Journal of Nursing, 101*, 43–49.

The Nurse Healers: Professional Associates International. (2006). *Therapeutic touch facts.* Retrieved from http://www.therapeutic-touch.org/newsarticle.php?newsID=18

van Schalkwyk, J., Davidson, J., Palmer, B., & Hope, V. (2006). Ayurvedic medicine: Patients in peril from plumbism. *New Zealand Medical Journal, 119*, U1958.

Vempati, R., Bijlani, R. L., & Deepak, K. K. (2009). The efficacy of a comprehensive lifestyle modification programme based on yoga in the management of bronchial asthma: A randomized controlled trial. *BMC Pulmonary Medicine, 9*, 37.

Wardell, D. W., & Weymouth, K. F. (2004). Review of studies of healing touch. *Journal of Nursing Scholarship, 36*, 147–154.

Wember, D. (1997). The heart and soul of homeopathy. *Journal of the American Institute of Homeopathy, 90*, 36–40.

Whelan, J. S., & Dvorkin, L. (2003). HolisticKids.org: Evolution of information resources in pediatric complementary and alternative medicine projects: From monographs to Web learning. *Journal of the Medical Library Association, 91*, 411–417.

White, K. P. (2000). Psychology and complementary and alternative medicine. *Professional Psychology: Research and Practice, 31*, 671–681.

Winstead-Fry, P., & Kijekm, J. (1999). An integrative review and meta-analysis of therapeutic touch research. *Alternative Therapies in Health and Medicine, 5*, 58–67.

World Health Organization. (2005). *National policy on traditional medicine and regulations of herbal medicines: Report of a WHO global survey.* Geneva, Switzerland: Author. Retrieved from http://apps.who.int/medicinedocs/en/d/Js7916e/

World Health Organization. (2015a). *Traditional medicine.* Geneva, Switzerland: Author. Retrieved from http://www.who.int/medicines/areas/traditional/definitions/en/

World Health Organization. (2015b). *WHO Traditional Medicine Strategy 2014–2023.* Geneva, Switzerland: Author. Retrieved from http://www.who.int/medicines/publications/traditional/trm_strategy14_23/en/

Wu, W. H., Bandilla, E., Ciccone, D. S., Yang, J., Cheng, S. C., Carner, N., . . . Shen, R. (1999). Effects of qigong on late-stage complex regional pain syndrome. *Alternative Therapies in Health and Medicine, 5*, 45–54.

Zhang, D., & Cheng, Z. (2000). Medicine is a humane art: The basic principles of professional ethics in Chinese medicine. *Hastings Center Report, 30*, S8–S12.

Global Perspectives on Diabetes, Respiratory Diseases, and Orthopedic Chronic Diseases

12

Janice Long

Objectives

Upon completion of this chapter, the reader will be able to:

1. Recognize the impact of globalization on health.
2. Discuss three of the top chronic noncommunicable diseases affecting global population health.
3. Recognize the major risk factors for chronic noncommunicable diseases.
4. State the major implications of chronic noncommunicable diseases related to social and economic demographics of various regions of the world.
5. Identify global and local strategies for prevention and treatment of chronic noncommunicable diseases.

INTRODUCTION: THE GLOBAL BURDEN OF CHRONIC (NONCOMMUNICABLE) DISEASES

Globalization, the increasing interdependency of countries and the openness of borders to ideas, people, commerce, and finances, has both beneficial and harmful effects on the health of people worldwide. Historically, globalization impacted the control and treatment of infectious diseases in addition to national security threats, provision of affordable medicines, and public policy changes for international trade and financial agreements. In contrast, noncommunicable diseases (NCDs), such as cardiovascular disease, cancers, chronic respiratory diseases, and diabetes, were neglected. Today, the global impact of NCDs is evident as we are faced with a growing prevalence of chronic, long-term, debilitating, and costly diseases. The growth of NCDs is fueled in part by population growth, aging, and unhealthy lifestyle behaviors. As the world's greatest cause of mortality, NCDs result in an estimated 38 million deaths annually (World Health Organization [WHO], 2010).

In 2008, of the estimated 57 million deaths worldwide, 60% were caused by chronic NCD illnesses. Deaths caused by chronic diseases are expected to increase by 17% over the next decade with an increase from 38 million deaths to 44 million deaths by 2020 (WHO, 2010). This increase in mortality for lifestyle dependent diseases, such as diabetes, cancers, cardiovascular and respiratory diseases is projected to affect people from all countries in the world as the impact may be felt to the greatest extent among the poorest populations.

Eighty percent of NCD deaths occur in low- and middle-income countries placing the burden of chronic disease disproportionately higher on low income countries (WHO, 2011). The age of those affected by NCDs is younger in developing countries than in developed countries yet people of all ages and in all countries suffer from chronic NCDs. The poorer populations of the world tend to bear the greatest risk for chronic illnesses paralleling social determinants. This creates a cycle of poverty and chronic disease that poor families and communities may be powerless to break. The impact of the increase of NCDs in the disadvantaged populations of the world contributes to the global widening gap in health.

CAUSES OF NCDs

While genetics contribute to chronic diseases, the primary cause of chronic NCDs is thought to be related to four behavioral risk factors that are secondary to economic changes, urbanization, and lifestyles (WHO, 2011). Tobacco use, unhealthy diets, inactivity, and excessive alcohol use are suggested factors that contribute to the lifestyle behavior risks.

Tobacco Use

The World Health Organization estimates that by 2030 an estimated 8 million tobacco-related deaths will occur each year. If current trends continue, more than 80% of these lives will be lost in developing countries. While tobacco companies have had increasing difficulty in marketing their products in developed countries, they have aggressively promoted the use of tobacco products in developing countries. "Tobacco is the only consumer product, that when used as recommended by its manufacturers, eventually kills half of its regular users" (Beaglehole & Yach, 2003, p. 904).

Despite what we know about tobacco use today, the use of tobacco products continues to increase worldwide and especially in low- and middle-income countries. In these countries, the tobacco industry has a large potential market that is not rigidly governed allowing for a great number of new customers (WHO, 2006). An example of the impact of tobacco marketing and use can be seen in India where death rates from tobacco use are estimated to rise from 1.4% in 1990 to 13.3% by 2020 (Sinha, Gupta, & Pednekar, 2006), and in China during the same time frame, from 9.2% to 16%. Families in China where smoking was practiced spent less money on education, food, housing, education, and clothing than on tobacco products.

Unhealthy Diets

Unhealthy diets are the second factor contributing to the burden of NCDs on the world. Global trade and marketing promote diets with higher proportions of saturated fats and sugars, placing consumers at risk for atherosclerosis and other cardiovascular illnesses. Even though inadequate nutrition or malnutrition remains a problem for some developing countries, the major nutritional risk factors for NCDs are increasing due to diets high in fats and carbohydrates. Diets with saturated fats and less natural carbohydrates, such as fruits and vegetables may be more readily accessible at a cost that is affordable.

Successful marketing campaigns by fast-food chains provides influence for the products to people of all ages and, reaches a young population where the result can change a lifestyle of eating habits. In 2009, the fast-food industry spent over $4.2 billion on television media and other marketing to children. Children of all ethnic groups in developed countries, where television is available, are target audiences for these campaigns; however, African American and Hispanic children are more likely to view the television ads (Rudd Center, 2011). While popular fast-food chains now offer healthier options on the menus and include them in their advertising, the ads do not encourage consumption of healthier options. The sales of the healthier choice products remain lower than sales of the historically more popular food options that are higher in saturated fats. The impact of campaigns such as those in the fast-food industry reaches children and adults across the world. In the United States, approximately 84% of parents report taking their child to a fast-food restaurant at least once a week (Rudd Center, 2011). These eating habits that are learned early in life can have a long-standing and profound effect across the lifespan. One impact of unhealthy eating habits that leads to several chronic illnesses is obesity.

The worldwide prevalence of obesity has been found to range from less than 5% in rural China, Japan, and some African countries to levels as high as 75% of the adult population in urban Samoa. Childhood obesity in the United States was approximately 32% in 2008 (Ogden, Carroll, Curtin, Lamb, & Flegal, 2010) with increasing rates of prevalence seen in the second generation immigrants or native born African American or Hispanic children. In China the obesity rates in children under the age of 15 years increased from 15% in 1982 to 27% in 2004 (Lau, 2004). Although the overall prevalence of obesity in China is low compared with Western countries such as the United States, a rapid increase of obesity is now seen among children. Data from the China national surveys on the constitution and health in school children showed that the prevalence of overweight and obesity in children aged 7 to 18 years increased 28 times and obesity increased four times between 1985 and 2000 (Wu, 2006). One explanation for the obesity increase in China is related to culture. Some Chinese cultures believe that excess body fat represents health and prosperity, which may be due in part to the history of famine and chronic malnutrition that resulted in millions dying in China in the 1950s.

By 2020, with chronic diseases becoming the leading contributors to early death and disability in many areas of the world, the obesity epidemic parallels the development of NCDs. With over 1.1 billion of the world's adults overweight, the incidence of cardiovascular disease and diabetes is expected to double over the period of 2000 to 2030. The impact of this increase will be felt across all countries; however, 70% of the burden will be borne by developing countries (Nikolic, Stanciole, & Zaydman, 2011). The factors contributing to the epidemic are related in large part to a lack of exercise and physical activity.

Physical Inactivity

In addition to tobacco use and poor nutrition, decreased physical activity has placed many people of the world at risk for obesity and its accompanying health challenges. Physical inactivity is associated with increased risk for chronic diseases, including cardiovascular disease, diabetes, and osteoporosis. Physical inactivity is estimated to cause almost one-third of diabetes and cardiovascular diseases. Despite the benefits of physical activity, inactivity, and sedentary lifestyles are seen in more than 50% of adults in the United States. This trend can be seen among most developed and developing countries. One difference across high- and low-income countries is seen in the timing of physical activity and may have a lot to do with the type and number of occupations where either high or low physical activity is required. For people living in high-income countries most of their activity occurs during leisure time, while people in low-income countries are more active during working hours.

Physical activity reduces the risk of cardiovascular disease, some cancers, and type 2 diabetes. It can also improve musculoskeletal health, control body weight, and overall improve life quality. As a result, WHO has included increasing physical activity for all countries as a challenge and responsibility.

THE COST OF NCDs

Because of the increasing burden of chronic diseases, the world faces a continuing financial and health crisis. According to the World Health Organization, about 80% of premature cardiovascular and diabetes cases could be prevented by three interventions: smoking cessation, a healthy diet, and adequate physical activity.

Over the past few decades, global alliances and funding have helped in research and treatment of many communicable diseases, particularly HIV/AIDS, malaria, tuberculosis, and vaccine-preventable diseases. Now, similar attention is provided to the challenge and global response for NCDs. "As the response to NCDs matures and the number of global initiatives and partnerships increases, it becomes increasingly important to map their respective functions, to identify gaps, and to evaluate progress overall" (Magnusson, 2010, p. 491).

Increases in funding with investments in public health prevention programs are necessary to combat the ever-increasing numbers of people with chronic illnesses (Katz, 2004). In 2004 the World Health Organization published a global strategy on diet, physical activity, and health (WHO, 2004). This was a comprehensive approach to chronic disease prevention and control directed at governments and several years later was followed by the Global Recommendations on Physical Activity for Health (WHO, 2010). In 2010, WHO published its Global Status Report on Non-Communicable Diseases to call all countries to action to prevent or control NCDs.

Few chronic diseases take the toll on the world's population as seen in the burden of cardiovascular, musculoskeletal, diabetes, and asthma disorders. These conditions are common chronic conditions affecting adults and children in every country. Lifestyles, environmental and social risk factors, many of which are controllable, contribute to the development or worsening of these chronic conditions despite advances in science and technology that make the conditions avoidable or controllable. Expert panels have made recommendations for diagnosis and treatment with guidelines and protocols available over the Internet in many languages for each of the conditions. Although there are numerous chronic global health issues that have significant worldwide concern, this chapter addresses the common global chronic diseases of these three NCDs: musculoskeletal disorders, asthma, and diabetes.

MUSCULOSKELETAL DISORDERS

In both developed and developing countries the most frequent cause of disability severely affecting people's daily lives is musculoskeletal conditions. Although diseases that cause the greatest mortality get the most public attention, musculoskeletal diseases are the major cause of morbidity throughout the world. Longer life expectancy, and the effect of increasing age of the population in all countries, has caused the corresponding increase in prevalence of disease of the musculoskeletal system.

Not only are diseases of the musculoskeletal system a problem for the elderly, but musculoskeletal conditions are responsible for more functional limitations in the adult population than any other group of disorders. They are responsible for loss of days of work, loss of years of life quality, for disability, and rising costs in all continents. Studies from Canada, the United States, and Western Europe indicate the prevalence of physical disabilities caused by musculoskeletal disorders in the past was estimated at 4 to 5% of the adult population (Woolf & Pfleger, 2003). In 2000 in both Europe and the United States combined, the point prevalence of musculoskeletal disorders involving low back pain, osteoarthritis, or tendonitis in the population over 45 was greater than 5.5% (Felson, 2000). In 2001, approximately 33% of U.S. adults were thought to be affected by musculoskeletal signs or symptoms, including limitation of motion or pain in a joint or extremity (Helmick et al., 2008). While the disorders occur in all race/ethnicities and in men and women, the prevalence of musculoskeletal disorders is higher among women particularly with increased age.

Musculoskeletal conditions are common worldwide and include more than 150 diseases and syndromes. It is believed that musculoskeletal disorders account for a major cause for loss of work and life quality. The European Occupational Safety and Health (2010) reported that musculoskeletal disorders were responsible for most of the occupational diseases in the European Union and workers from all sectors and occupations were affected. Reports from Austria, Germany, and France indicate that musculoskeletal disorders have a considerable impact on costs. Not only are wages lost when workers miss days of work due to chronic illnesses, such as musculoskeletal disorder, losses incurred from workers who are unable to work may be passed on to consumers, causing an increase in consumer goods and products.

The primary types of musculoskeletal disorders include rheumatoid arthritis, osteoarthritis, osteoporosis, spinal disorders, major limb trauma, gout, and fibromyalgia. Limb trauma is increasing rapidly, especially in developing countries, due to road traffic accidents. Rheumatoid arthritis leads to work disability and limitation of movement after approximately 10 years from disease onset. Those diagnosed with musculoskeletal diseases frequently have difficulty with activities of daily living, such as eating, walking, toileting, and bathing. Forty percent of people over 70 years old suffer from osteoarthritis of the knee, and of those having this disease, 80% have some degree of limitation of movement. Treatment and recovery are often unsatisfactory especially for more chronic causes. The end result can even be permanent disability, chronic pain, and loss of employment. These disorders are the second most common reason for consulting a doctor in many countries and result in up to 10 to 20% of all medical consultations (Health Safety Executive [HSE], 2010).

The cost as reflected in treatment and loss of work resulting from musculoskeletal diseases can be staggering. Musculoskeletal diseases were the most expensive disease category in a Swedish cost-of-illness study, representing 22.6% of the total cost of illness. Within the United Kingdom work-related musculoskeletal disorders were responsible for 11 million days lost from work in 1995, while in 2009 to 2010, an estimated 9.3 million working days were lost through work-related musculoskeletal disorders (HSE, 2010).

Pain is the most prominent symptom in people with musculoskeletal disorders. Low back pain has reached worldwide epidemic proportions. A 2005 European survey revealed that 25% of workers reported work-related lower back pain and another 23% experienced other types of muscular pain (De Broeck & Verjans, 2010). In the United States almost everyone in the workforce experiences back pain at some point in time. Back pain is the second most common neurological complaint after headaches. Americans spend over $50 billion dollars annually on treatment for back pain (National Institute of Neurological Disorders and Stroke [NINDS], 2011).

In 1990 an estimated 1.7 million people had hip fractures caused by osteoporosis, and by 2050 the number of people affected will exceed 6 million worldwide. The greatest incidence of musculoskeletal disease is expected to be found in countries such as Brazil, Chile, China, Pakistan, the Philippines, India, Indonesia, Malaysia, Mexico, and Thailand. In the developed countries of the world, the United States, European countries, Japan, New Zealand, and Australia all have high rates (WHO, 2008).

The following are types of musculoskeletal disorders of chronic noncommunicable diseases:

- *Rheumatoid arthritis*: A chronic systemic disease that affects the joints, connective tissue, muscle, tendons, and fibrous tissue, with an onset mainly in the 20- to 40-year age range. It is a chronic disability causing pain and deformity.
- *Osteoarthritis*: A noninflammatory joint disease affecting the articular cartilage, associated with aging, and attacking stressed joints such as the knees, hips, finger joints, and lower back.
- *Osteoporosis*: A disease with reduction in bone mass resulting in fractures. This may be caused by genes, inadequate intake of calcium and vitamin D, physical inactivity, or decrease in ovary function at menopause in women.
- *Spinal disorders*: Specific diseases of the spine, including trauma, mechanical injury, spinal cord injury, inflammation, infection, or tumors. These disorders may involve muscles, nerves, intervertebral disks, joints, cartilage, tendons, and ligaments.

- *Severe limb trauma*: Results from permanent disability from fractures, crushing injuries, dislocations, open wounds, amputation, and blood and nerve vessel injuries.

Rheumatoid Arthritis

Rheumatoid arthritis is the most frequent disability in the United States affecting more than 70 million people, or one out of every three adults. Costs in the United States include more than $16 billion annually. Another $80 billion is lost in productivity and wages as a result of pain and disability from this condition. Pain, together with functional limitations and dependence on others, is an increasing problem. It is a chronic, autoimmune, inflammatory disease of the joints with unknown etiology and no cure, characterized with periods of exacerbation (very active state) to remission (inactive state). Besides the physiological problems, it also may include psychological outcomes such as depression and anxiety (Chui, Lau, & Yau, 2004).

Twice as many women as men are affected by this disease. It occurs most often in the United States and northern European countries, and more rarely in developing countries. Very few cases are found in Africa, but of those in African countries, more are found in urban areas. Smoking and obesity as well as family genetics are known risk factors (Woolf & Pfleger, 2003).

Many self-management programs have been established worldwide including in the United States, Australia, Canada, and England. These include relaxation techniques, exercise, joint protection, pain and stress coping strategies, and self-management skills. In Hong Kong, PRC, a community-based rehabilitation program, offers knowledge and skill information. In a study examining a rheumatoid arthritis self-management program in Hong Kong, researchers found that the program of exercise, self-management skills, and communication with doctors enhanced positive self-help behavior and reduced visits to the general physician (Chui, Lau, & Yau, 2004).

Acupuncture therapy for rheumatoid arthritis is currently being tested in studies in Tel Hashomer, Israel. Acupuncture is a method of therapy in which thin needles are inserted into specific points (assisting energy flow), and for each treatment specific ones are manipulated. According to traditional Chinese medicine philosophy, illness results from an imbalance of energy flow and the acupuncture needle insertions are connected to precise locations or "meridians" that are certain sites for channels of energy. In spite of the use of medications for treatment of rheumatoid arthritis, complementary medicine has been found to be useful as a treatment for many patients. In the United States, 26.7% of the population uses some form of complementary medicine, such as acupuncture, for treatment for rheumatoid arthritis in addition to seeing a medical doctor for treatment (Zan-Bar, Aron, & Shoenfeld, 2004).

Many patients with rheumatoid arthritis who have muscle and joint pain are able to reduce their pain by doing physical exercise in heated pools. Since the 1960s Swedish patients with inflammatory joint disease have been prescribed intensive physiotherapy in a subtropical climate, called "climate therapy." The patients were treated in the Mediterranean regions with warmer climates and found to have significant improvement over earlier treatments in Sweden. In a study in 1996, patients treated in Tiberias, Israel's hot springs, for four weeks returned to Sweden significantly improved. The improvements were short-lived, however, as the symptoms returned after three and six months of returning (Hafstrom & Hallengren, 2003).

Osteoarthritis

Osteoarthritis is a disease in which there is a loss of articular cartilage within the synovial joints, which is associated with hypertrophy (thickening) of the bone. People with this disease often have joint pain, tenderness, limitation of movement, crepitus, and local inflammation. It can occur in any joint, but most often occurs in the hip, knee, joints of the hand, foot, and spine. This disease causes great pain and also loss of height as well as significant amount of bone fractures. Worldwide estimates for this disease are 9.6% for men and 18% for women, both genders being age 60 or greater. Research reveals that this condition is most prevalent in the United States and other European countries than elsewhere in the world, and the most commonly affected area is the knee (Chui, Lau, & Yau, 2004).

In Western Ontario, Canada, a medical study using leech therapy was found to be helpful in treating arthritis of the knee. Leech therapy was widely used in ancient times but declined rapidly in Europe and the United States with the use of modern surgery and medicine. Polypeptide hirudin, an active substance in leech saliva, was found to be effective for relieving pain in the knee caused by osteoarthritis (Michalsen, Klotz, Ludtke, Moebus, Spahn, & Dobos, 2003).

Osteoporosis

Osteoporosis is a disease characterized by low bone mass and a deterioration of the bone tissue. This results in bone fragility and vulnerability to bone fractures. In osteoporosis, the bone mineral density is greater than 2.5 standard deviations below the mean bone mineral density of young women. In addition, osteopenia (low bone mass) is between 1 to 2.5 standard deviations below the mean bone mass of young adult women. Those affected often have hip, vertebrae, and forearm bone fractures. This disease often occurs in postmenopausal Caucasian women, living in the northern parts of the United States. In the United Kingdom, 23% of women age 50 or older have osteoporosis. This disease affects more than 75 million people in Europe, Japan, and Latin and North America. In the United States alone, about 15% of the people have osteoporosis. The prevalence increases with age, and the condition is not reversible. Physical activity and adequate diet intake of especially calcium and vitamin D are vital for maintaining healthy bones and preventing this disease (Chui, Lau, & Yau, 2004).

Hip Fracture

The National Center for Injury Prevention and Control states that 3 to 4% of older adults fall, causing greater than 400,000 hip fractures in the United States each year. Within this group 4% die during their initial hospitalization, and 10 to 35% die within the first year. Of those who do survive, many never regain their prefracture level of functioning. Most hip fractures result from underlying chronic musculoskeletal conditions, such as arthritis, osteoporosis, or a bone malignancy (Centers for Disease Control and Prevention [CDC], 2004).

DIABETES

Diabetes derives its name from the Greek word meaning "going through" and the Latin word, *mellitus*, which means "honey" or "sweet." This disease can be traced to the first century AD, when Aretaeus the Cappadocian described the disorder as a chronic affliction characterized by intense thirst and voluminous, honey-sweet urine (Porth, 2009). It is a devastating disease that affects nearly every system of the body. As a disorder of the metabolism of carbohydrates, proteins, and fats, diabetes mellitus results from alterations in insulin development and use in the body. Uncontrolled diabetes results from the inability of the body to affect the way glucose is transported into fat and muscle cells. Without the ability to move the glucose to the cells where it can be broken down into energy, the body is starved and fat and proteins are broken down. As a result, the effects of the disease can be seen across nearly all organs and functions of the body.

Types of Diabetes Mellitus

Diabetes is classified as type 1 diabetes, type 2 diabetes, or gestational diabetes. Types 1 and 2 affect both genders and gestational diabetes occurs only in pregnant women. Each type of diabetes has the characteristic of glucose elevation, but each differs in the type of population affected and treatment protocols.

Type 1 Diabetes

Type 1 diabetes is characterized by the destruction of the beta cells of the pancreas and is thought to be mediated by immune factors or may be idiopathic (National Institute of Diabetes, and Digestive and Kidney Disorders [NIDDK], 2011). Type 1 diabetes is rare in occurrence, affecting only about 5 to 10% of people within the United States and Europe. Most individuals with type 1 diabetes are thought to have the immune-mediated form of the condition (Porth, 2009). Type 1 diabetes has also been referred to as juvenile diabetes and occurs most often in young persons, but can occur at any age. The condition is characterized by the complete inability of the pancreas to produce insulin with resulting high blood glucose and muscle and fat cell catabolism. Without insulin administration, body cells will starve and die.

Type 2 Diabetes

Type 2 diabetes occurs when there is a decreased amount of insulin or the cells of the body are resistant to the insulin produced and a relative loss of insulin is present. Type 2 diabetes accounts for 90 to 95% of all persons with diabetes. Most people with type 2 diabetes are adults older than 40 years of age and have some degree of obesity. The symptoms of type 2 diabetes—fatigue, frequent urination, and slow healing sores—can be difficult to detect and often develop years before a person is diagnosed. As a result, persons with type 2 diabetes often learn they have the condition when they are diagnosed with a diabetes complication. Complications often found in type 2 diabetes include microvascular disorders that can cause vision loss, renal disease, or peripheral vascular disease.

In addition to affecting the small vessels in the body, the disease also impedes the larger vessels, creating macrovascular diseases that can cause stroke or heart attacks. All diabetes complications are serious; however, recent studies have shown that the prevalence of vision complications (diabetic retinopathy) occur globally among individuals with diagnosed diabetes from a low of 10% in Norway to a high of 61% in Singapore (Ruta, Magliano, LeMesurier, Taylor, Zimmet, & Shaw, 2013). Prevalence of diabetic retinopathy was found to be higher in developing countries along with Hispanics in the United States; diabetic retinopathy was listed as the leading cause of adult onset blindness among Hispanics (48.1% prevalence). In France the rate was much lower in 2011, with approximately 10.8% of individuals diagnosed with type 2 diabetes having retinopathy (Ruta, Magliano, LeMesurier, Taylor, Zimmet, & Shaw, 2013). Preventing type 2 diabetes and its complications becomes a high priority for populations as the risk of blindness in all age groups increases.

Although obesity and physical activity are recognized as the chief factors contributing to type 2 diabetes, genetic links are also implicated.

Age of Onset and Prevalence of Type 2 Diabetes

A younger population has more recently been identified with type 2 diabetes and is increasing in prevalence. It is thought that over the next 10 years, type 2 diabetes will become the predominant form of diabetes in the young in some ethnic groups worldwide (International Diabetes Federation Consensus Workshop, 2004). Mohan and colleagues (2006) reported that in 2005, in Chennai, India, the age-standardized prevalence of diabetes increased 72% from 1989 to the present. Of those who were 40 to 49 years of age, 20% now have diabetes (Mohan et al., 2006). A study conducted by Tseng and colleagues (2006) found that incidences of diabetes in Taiwan increased across all age groups but was highest in the youngest groups (less than 35 years of age and including children). The study reported that obesity was an increasing problem particularly in the school children.

A study of more than 10,000 in one region of the United Kingdom also found a rising prevalence of diabetes by age, with the prevalence of diabetes in females increasing above that of males, beginning at age 30. Also noted in the study was a decrease of diabetes in those over 80 years old (Morgan, Currie, Stott, Smithers, Butler, & Peters, 2000). Another study conducted in Fukuoka, Japan, found that in men and women changes in lifestyle to a more Western diet and increases in dietary fat consumption were contributing factors to the increased prevalence of diabetes (Ohmura et al., 1993).

A study conducted in Italy was similar in results with increases in prevalence of type 2 diabetes, particularly in the over 44 age groups, and was associated with increased rates of obesity. This suggests a lifestyle-related contribution to the burden of diabetes (Garancini et al., 1995). As a result of lifestyle behaviors that lead to obesity, many people worldwide are at high risk for the cascade of symptoms that often follows overweight and obesity and leads to diabetes. Obesity is one of the most difficult risk factors to change once it is present, so intervening before overweight occurs is the best measure for preventing diabetes in all age groups.

In 1995 the WHO estimated the prevalence rate of diabetes (all types) in participating countries to be approximately 135 million. The International Diabetes Federation (IDF) found a much higher increase in 2003 when the organization reported global estimates of 194 million people living with diabetes. Of those with diabetes, approximately 85 to 95% have type 2 diabetes in developed countries and an even higher rate of people in developing countries have the disease (IDF, 2009). Although type 1 diabetes is less frequent in global occurrence, there are variations among the patterns of prevalence of the condition. The prevalence of type 1 diabetes is higher in North America (0.25%), followed by Europe (0.19%). The IDF findings reported an even more worrisome fact that public awareness about diabetes is quite low (IDF, 2009).

At the current global growth rate of diabetes mellitus, the prevalence of the condition will increase to much more serious levels over the next two decades. The IDF reports projections for the global prevalence of diabetes by the year 2025 to approach 6.3% for adults between 20–79 years of age (IDF, 2009). Education and care interventions are needed to forestall the disease, most of which is influenced by lifestyle (IDF, 2009).

The highest regional prevalence of diabetes is seen in North America followed by Europe (EU) both in 2003 and as projected for 2025. The Southeast Asian (SEA) region has the highest prevalence of impaired glucose tolerance over all regions.

Gestational Diabetes Mellitus

Defined by its name, gestational diabetes mellitus (GDM), occurs during pregnancy. It involves an intolerance to glucose that may be found in 2 to 14% of pregnancies and, in particular, those who have had a prior history of gestational diabetes, with a family history, are obese, had a high-birth-weight baby in the past, or have had more than five pregnancies. With gestational diabetes, early diagnosis is critical in addition to early intervention with careful medical management to prevent maternal and fetal complications (Masharani, Karam, & German, 2004). Treatment of GDM includes close monitoring for the mother and fetus and maintenance of low blood glucose levels in the mother with frequent maternal glucose monitoring.

Treatment Recommendations

The cornerstone of treatment for diabetes has been the active participation in care by the individual who has the condition (Funnell et al., 2011). To assume responsibility for one's own care, a diagnosis must be made. With the findings of the IDF suggesting that one of the greatest barriers to treatment is the lack of the public's awareness of the disease, campaigns to educate the public must become the priority global intervention. Education on diabetic symptoms in concert with screening campaigns for those at risk for diabetes could offer a first stage of awareness to the populations of the world where diabetes or impaired glucose tolerance is most prevalent.

Early intervention with diabetes education and dietary and lifestyle adjustments before complications are present could provide for improved overall outcomes of the disease. Self-monitoring for blood glucose, a process that can easily be performed in the home, offers promise for individuals to manage their disease on a daily basis by knowing their blood sugar levels. Tests for the average blood glucose level over a three-month period (hemoglobin A_1c or HbA_1c) are also available, though more costly. Research in the United Kingdom indicates that for type 2 diabetes, every 1 point reduction of the hemoglobin A_1c toward normal levels brings reductions in the risk for many of the complications that lead to the morbidity and mortality of diabetes (Stratton, Cull, Adler, Matthews, Neil, & Holman, 2006).

The ADA and the European Union-International Diabetes Federation (EUIDF) recognize that lifestyle changes alone are inadequate in the long term to achieve and maintain weight loss. Exercise and medical and nutrition adjustments are needed to attain the HbA_1c levels sought (Nathan et al., 2006). The American Diabetes Association (ADA) recommends that individuals try to maintain HbA_1c levels below 7.0%, and the EUIDF recommends a level at or below

6.5%, which is closer to the normal level. Even with global advances in pharmacologic therapy included in current-day management, reduction and maintenance of near normal levels of glycemia have not been possible. The consensus of the ADA and the EUIDF supports the position that any reduction of HbA$_1$c offers a reduction in risk for the complications of diabetes. The complex nature of diabetes makes treatment quite problematic, and morbidity is particularly high in relationship to cardiovascular disease.

The United Kingdom Prospective Diabetes Study (Stratton, Cull, Adler, Matthews, Neil, & Holman, 2006), found that hypertension and glycemia have additive effects in the development of cardiovascular mortality, and that by treating both together, the cardiovascular risk for complications could be markedly reduced. Nonetheless, studies suggest that hypertension control is not consistently well achieved (Liebl, Mata, & Eschwege, 2002). Many factors must be considered in the treatment of diabetes, from socioeconomic implications and lifestyle factors to complex comorbid conditions that may accompany diabetes. Research is constantly under way to prevent diabetes and to reduce the seriousness of the complications. The greatest effect on diabetes outcome is thought to be in the prevention of the condition with changes in lifestyles that predispose individuals to the disease.

Cost of Diabetes Care

The concern for the world is not only in the human cost and loss of life, but also in the economic burden the disease causes. The evidence of this burden was reported by Koster, von Ferer, Ihle, Schubert, and Hauner (2006) as diabetes mellitus is a "public health issue of significant economic importance with a globally increasing prevalence . . . And one that has complications that contribute to long-term disease duration" (p. 1498). Studies from the United States and Europe suggest that the economic burden of diabetes is high (Liebl, Neiß, Spannheimer, Reitberger, Wagner, & Gortz, 2001). Age and type of treatment contribute to the overall cost of treatment, with the highest costs seen in the treatment of the complications of diabetes. As one of the most common global noncommunicable diseases, diabetes ranks as the fourth or fifth cause of death in developed countries (International Diabetes Federation [IDF], 2009). Complications from diabetes range from coronary artery and peripheral vascular disease, stroke, neuropathy, renal failure, and visual impairment to increased disability and reduced life quality and expectancy. This health issue "results in enormous health costs for virtually every society" (International Diabetes Federation , 2009 p. 7). Although it is important to remember that prevention of diabetes would contribute the greatest cost savings, prevention of complications through tight glycemic control and hypertension management is needed to reduce the economic burden of costly complications once diabetes is diagnosed.

Diabetes Prevention

With advances in transportation and technology, survival in the modern world is much different than that of years ago. Exercise has little by little been taken out of the daily life of the world's population. "In their struggle for longevity, modern-day humans are dying because of lack of physical exercise" (Erikssen, 2001, p. 571). Automobiles carry people directly from the interior of their home to their destination, and parking lots for work and school often offer convenience for parking near the building entrances. Technology also has offered more advances in communication so that children and adults alike have access to friends and family via phones or the Internet, so the need to physically meet may be lessened. Even recreational activities in a virtual environment makes playtime something that occurs in a chair or on a sofa in the confines of the private residence, and running and playing are less often chosen as alternates as compared to the appeal of an online game or TV show. Fast food and vending machines with high-calorie, high-fat drinks and foods offer quick treats to all age groups and increase the diabetes risk, particularly for those who infrequently exercise.

Overweight in children is a growing worldwide concern gaining the attention of the World Health Organization (WHO) as the implications and severity of obesity are assessed in member countries (Schoenborn, Adams, & Barnes, 2002). In the United States, the CDC has placed the problem of obesity in the forefront of national efforts after studies, and trends reveal that the burden of the condition on the U.S. population is growing (Ogden, Carroll, Curtain, Lamb, & Flegal, 2010). The National Health and Nutrition Examination Survey (NHANES) from 1988 to 1994 showed rates of overweight in children and adolescents at about 10%, rising to 14.4% by 1999 to 2000 and finally, the 2001 to 2002 survey findings indicated that 16% of children between 6 and 11 years of age were overweight (Hedley, Ogden, Johnson, Carroll, Curtin, & Flegal, 2004). The childhood overweight impact varies by U.S. region, as evidenced by one study conducted in a rural region of a southern U.S. state where risk for overweight was found to be 36.2% as compared to the national rate at 31.2% (Lewis et al., 2006). These trends indicate a rapid growth in the prevalence of overweight in the United States and found that overweight is paralleled by a growing rate of chronic health conditions, particularly diabetes (Hedley, Ogden, Johnson, Carroll, Curtin, & Flegal, 2004).

Since 1990, physical inactivity has been among the leading risk factors for the global burden of disease, according to the Global Burden of Disease Study (Murray & Lopez, 1996). While many governments around the world are implementing laws to legislate smoking in public places as a deterrent to one of the health risks, legislating exercise would be very difficult to conceive and enforce in any country (Erikssen, 2001). In a unique move in the United States, a new law implemented in July 2006 charges public school systems with the responsibility of improving outcomes in child health through healthy food options in cafeterias and vending machines and through physical exercise programs while the child is in school. The hopes are that through interventions in public schools, children can learn many healthy messages, and the future of diabetes in the United States will not be so grim.

ASTHMA

Asthma is a serious public health problem that affects the lives of people from all countries, races, and ages. As a condition that causes loss of life, life quality, and productivity when it is not controlled, asthma limits daily life activities and can be fatal (Global Initiative for Asthma [GINA], 2010). Asthma is a significant global burden sparing no region or country.

Despite new knowledge, treatments, and environmental innovations, asthma continues to take its toll on the lives of the people of the world. The National Heart Lung and Blood Institute of the NIH, Expert Panel Report 3, suggests that in the United States the number of deaths due to asthma have declined, even though the prevalence of asthma is still on the increase (National Health Interview Survey [NHIS], 2007).

Definition

Asthma is a chronic episodic inflammatory disease of the airways that causes recurrent episodes of wheezing, breathlessness, chest tightness, and coughing, particularly at night or in the early morning (National Heart, Lung, and Blood Institute [NHLBI], 2010). It is one of the most common diseases of childhood and continues to afflict individuals throughout the lifespan. Asthma's symptoms result from the inflammation that occurs from environmental factors and results in airway hyperresponsiveness and airflow limitation (NHLBI, 2010). The asthmatic lung seems to overreact to stimuli such as airborne allergens and cold, dry air. Over time, the airways, or bronchial tubes, become inflamed and sensitive and if not treated may lead to an asthma "attack." Three major factors occur in the airways that contribute to the symptoms of asthma. These symptoms may occur alone or in combination. The frequency and complexity of symptoms determine the degree of severity of asthma:

- *Mucus plug formation*: Changes in the airways occur once a trigger occurs and an immediate complex inflammatory response follows, resulting in a hypersecretion of mucus from the lining of the airway. The mucus formation also may form plugs of mucus that limit airflow further.
- *Acute bronchoconstriction*: Immune complexes are released as a result of the allergen/trigger that activates the asthmatic exacerbation. These immune complexes directly contract the smooth muscle of the airways. As a result of the narrowing of the airways from the smooth muscle contraction, the airways are narrowed and airflow limited (Park, Kim, Kim, & Lee, 2010).
- *Airway edema*: Airway wall edema limits the airflow through the airways even further, resulting in diminished flow of air in asthma. The mucosa of the airway walls swell and become less compliant to changes in airflow.

Symptoms of asthma can range from mild to severe. In severe cases, the attack may be fatal if no treatment is available. Although asthma symptoms cannot be completely avoided, they can for the most part be controlled. The symptoms of asthma are usually recognizable in advance of an impending exacerbation through the use of a peak flow meter that can be purchased and used in the home. Peak flow meters are available from several manufacturers and are marketed worldwide.

Diagnosis

To diagnose asthma, a thorough history and physical assessment is performed. A spirometer is used to measure the amount of air inhaled and exhaled with each breath. The spirometer readings provide data on the level of pulmonary function and airway obstruction (NHLBI, 2010). Using the history, assessment, and spirometry readings, asthma is categorized into three levels—mild, moderate, and severe—and treatment recommendations address each level.

Asthma Prevalence

Asthma is one of the most common NCDs in the world with an estimated 300 million people affected by the condition. The pattern of asthma prevalence in the world is not explained by the current knowledge of causation. Asthma has become more common in both children and adults in recent decades as communities become increasingly urbanized. Projections from the WHO suggest that the urban population will increase from 45 to 59% by 2025 (NHLBI, 2010). Given this increase, a corresponding increase in asthma worldwide can be anticipated.

The prevalence of asthma has increased globally, affecting the people of disadvantaged groups, urban, poorly educated, low socioeconomic status, and those who live in large cities. While asthma accounts for about 1 in 250 deaths worldwide (GINA, 2010), countries in which the prevalence is the highest, such as Scotland (prevalence 18.4%, mortality 3.0%), England (prevalence 15.3%, mortality 3.2%), New Zealand (prevalence 15.1%, mortality 4.6%), Costa Rica (prevalence 11.9%, mortality 3.9%), and the United States (prevalence 10.9%, mortality 5.2%), the mortality rate is much lower. On the other hand, countries with lower prevalence rates of asthma have higher mortality, such as China (prevalence 2.1%, mortality 26.7%), Russia (prevalence 2.2%, mortality 28.6%), and Mexico (prevalence 3.3%, mortality 14.5%). Asthma is less common in low-income countries than in high-income countries (Stewart, Mitchell, Pearce, Strachan, & Weilandon, 2001). The reasons for these gaps in prevalence and mortality may be accounted for by the lack of available resources, treatments, and pharmaceutical agents available in countries where poverty and poor access to care is present.

Triggers

Factors that create an exacerbation of asthma are known as triggers. Numerous environmental factors or triggers contribute to the development of asthma. They may be from an inhaled irritant or other sources or factors. The following includes some of these triggers.

Inhaled Factors

More than 50% the world's population still cooks with wood, coal, or dung on simple stoves or open fires. Because adequate ventilation is not always present, the risk for inhalation irritants is high especially in women and children. Exposure to indoor air pollutants is responsible for over 1.6 million premature worldwide deaths, accounting for about 3% of the global burden of disease (Ezzati, 2004). Biomass-type fuels (wood, charcoal, crop residues, animal dung, and coal) are primary sources for cooking, heating, and other household needs, such as food preservation, in most developing countries. More than 3 billion people use these sources of energy, and the resulting pollutants cause chronic and acute conditions such as asthma and other respiratory conditions that affect the poor more often than individuals with higher socioeconomic conditions. Emissions of the pollutants are most worrisome when solid fuels are used in open or poorly ventilated stoves (Smith, Mehta, & Maeusezahl-Feuz, 2004; Zhao, Zhang, Wang, Ferm, Liang, & Norback, 2008).

Residents of China bear a high risk for asthma, as coal is the major source of energy, providing about 75% of all energy sources. From the coal smoke, respiratory contaminants of suspended particulate matter and sulfur dioxide pose a trigger for asthma and other respiratory conditions (Chen, Hong, & Kan, 2004).

Although stoves with improved ventilation have been developed to reduce the risk posed by burning the biomass type fuels, their use has not been widely accepted. Preprocessing of biomass fuels poses hope for reductions in risk as it offers cleaner burning of the fuels (Barnes, Openshaw, Smith, & van der Plas, 2002).

Tobacco smoke exposure ranks highest as an indoor air irritant that can trigger worsening symptoms of asthma. People with known asthma should not smoke or be exposed to environmental smoke in any form because smoking reduces lung function, increases the need for medications, and increases missed days from work. Infants of mothers who smoke have higher rates of infant and childhood asthma (Arshad, Bateman, & Matthews, 2003).

In 2003, the World Health Organization reported that 1 in 10 adult deaths could be related to tobacco smoke and estimated that by the year 2030 the number might be closer to 1 in 6. Health promotion activities and smoking cessation treatments for tobacco dependence are needed in most developing and developed countries. Although more than 30% of smokers try to quit at least annually, studies show that only 1 to 3% succeed without the help of smoking cessation programs or pharmaceutical support (Shafey, Dolwick, & Guindon, 2003).

Other Environmental Factors

Other factors that contribute to the triggers for asthma include indoor dampness and humidity. At present, indoor dampness occurs within Nordic countries at a rate of 17 to 24%, within the Netherlands at a rate of 25%, and within Canada at a 37% rate. Home indoor dampness can often be detected from signs of water leakage or visible mold on walls, floors, or ceilings (Masoli, Fabian, Holt, & Beasley, 2004). Molds and fungi are produced by the humid indoor environment and are present in homes that have dampness problems. Children who live in homes where these high humid conditions exist are at greater risk for respiratory conditions such as asthma (Tham, Zurainmi, Koh, Chew, & Ooi, 2007).

Other factors that must be considered are the common house dust mites and animal and cockroach allergens that are triggers that can cause an exacerbation of asthma. House dust mites are universal in areas of high humidity (most areas of the United States are included), but are not usually present at high altitudes or dry climates unless moisture is added to the indoor atmosphere (NHLBI, 2010). Dust mites can be found in high concentrations in pillows, mattresses, carpets, upholstered furniture, clothes, and stuffed toys. Pet dander comes from all warm-blooded pets including small rodents and birds. These animals produce dander, urine, and feces that can cause allergic reactions.

Factors where individuals have regular exposure to allergens or asthma triggers, such as in a work setting, may worsen the condition. Exposure to fluorides and other respiratory irritants are suggested as environmental agents that can result in asthma (Taiwo et al., 2006). In Australia and New Zealand asthma was found among workers in aluminum smelters and is referred to as "potroom" asthma. Individuals who had exposure improved in pulmonary function once they were removed from the potroom worksite; however, the longer the worker had been exposed, the lower the level of improvement. Studies offer hope as preventive measures are identified and implemented in the worksite (Arnaiz, Kaufman, Daroowalla, Quigley, Farin, & Checkoway, 2003).

Asthma Treatment

The treatment of asthma includes controlling the environmental factors (triggers) that make asthma worse, pharmacologic therapy geared toward quick relief, and long-term control of symptoms using a stepwise approach with self-management. By reducing the environmental factors that trigger an asthma episode and use of essential medications, control of asthma attacks is possible. For example, data from the World Health Organizations Access to Essential Drugs report (GINA, 2010), suggests that countries with greater than 95% of the population with access to the essential drugs for NCDs fare better than countries with less. The United States, Canada, New Zealand, and Ireland reported that over 95% of their population had access to essential drugs for asthma while Russia, China, and Mexico reported that between 50 and 80% of the population had access (GINA, 2010). Having access to the essential treatment for asthma can save the lives of the individuals who suffer with the disease and can offer improved quality of life.

Pharmacologic Treatments for Asthma

Pharmacologic management of asthma is broken into two components—relievers and controllers. Medications for relieving the symptoms of asthma through inhalers include products that relax and open the airway to improve the movement of air and are short term in their action. Controller medications are long term in action and include steroids and nonsteroidal medications that must be taken on a regular basis to be effective. Medications for treating asthma can be costly, and they may not be available in developing countries. Immunotherapy may be considered when specific allergens are present and cannot be avoided. Allergens such as grass or trees can pose as a major irritant for asthma (NHLBI, 2010).

Cost of Asthma Treatment

The cost of management varies by the severity and extent of the exacerbation and whether hospitalization is needed or if self-management can be used to control episodes of the disease. Some episodes require emergency room visits, but they are successfully treated and hospitalization is not required. More severe exacerbations may require hospitalization and costs are correspondingly higher. Through the use of the peak flow meter, which is a lower-cost alternative to pulmonary function tests, individuals in low-income countries could be provided with a measure of evaluation to offer early intervention preventing serious exacerbations. A group of lower-priced generic drugs, by oral and inhalation routes of administration, can keep the cost to the government-provided health services to a minimum. With lower-cost asthma medications, a greater benefit could be realized for the population who suffer with asthma.

The Global Initiative for Asthma (2010) recommends that countries identify low-cost drugs that can be made available for those who suffer from asthma. Otherwise, the cost of treatment for countries where the health of the population falls on the government will be far greater than can be supported. The report found that as much as 30% of the entire expenditure for health in a country would have to be spent on asthma medication alone if only 5% of the population had asthma and the cost of asthma treatment was in the range of US$30 (GINA, 2010). Guidelines for medications should include what is available as well as what is affordable for treatment of asthma.

Study Questions

1. Why is diabetes a growing major health issue for both developed and developing countries today?
2. What are the most important types of education for diabetics who live in developing countries with limited financial resources?
3. How do global environmental issues affect respiratory health in developed as well as developing countries? Give three specific examples.
4. What are the greatest challenges of chronic orthopedic diseases for people living in both developed and developing countries?

CONCLUSION

The World Health Organization has endorsed a global strategy to address NCDs and the common preventable risk factors related to lifestyle. While such a global strategy may seem ambitious, a global campaign will be necessary to reduce the burden of chronic NCDs on all regions of the world. One recommendation of the World Health Organization is for countries to develop activities that focus on (1) advocacy, (2) policy, (3) health promotion, (4) prevention, and (5) management of chronic conditions such as diabetes, chronic respiratory diseases, cardiovascular disease, blindness and visual impairment, and musculoskeletal diseases (WHO, 2010). This chapter has offered suggestions for addressing chronic NCDs globally; however, for a comprehensive public health approach, the strategies for interventions must include a broad-brush approach guided by the five major categories listed above.

Efforts designed to improve the world's health and reduce the incidence and prevalence of NCDs must address improvements in several areas:

1. Monitoring and surveillance of chronic health conditions and their cost and impact.
2. Health system changes to address the services needed for patients with NCDs, including addressing the need for cost-effective recommended pharmaceutical agents.
3. Policies to support health system changes that are needed and for public health safety.
4. Education for healthcare providers on screening diagnosis and management of NCDs.
5. Public health campaigns to educate the public on NCD recognition and prevention.
6. Health promotion and disease prevention programs such as worksite, faith-based, and other alternate site programs.
7. Funding of grassroots programs that offer innovative practices in the reduction of NCDs.
8. Increased research and strategies for applying evidenced-based findings to practice.

Through such a coordinated approach to NCD prevention and treatment, a significant impact may be achieved in reducing the incidence and prevalence of NCDs.

Case Study

C. Jones is a 63-year-old female with a five-year history of type 2 diabetes and worsening symptoms of chronic asthma with dyspnea and cough. She smoked two packs of cigarettes per day for 30 years, although she has not smoked since she was diagnosed with asthma two years ago. She lives alone on a farm in rural Georgia where she has an ample supply of oak, elm, and fruit trees as well as a large wooded area of mixed firs and other foliage nearby. She maintains several farm animals, including cattle, which provide milk and meat. She raises chickens, sheep, and goats for food and milk, and to sell at the market in town. She has two dogs, both of which live in the house with her. For heat in the winter, she uses a wood-burning stove and also loves to use it for cooking as often as possible. Her husband died two years ago, so she is responsible for the upkeep and maintenance of the farm although she has a farmhand, Mr. Ramirez, who works for her two to three days per week during nonharvest seasons. During harvest seasons, he works full time planting and maintaining the fields where she grows cotton, corn, and an assortment of vegetables. Mr. Ramirez arranges for migrant workers to supply labor to harvest the vegetables that she raises on the substantial farmland.

For control and management of her asthma symptoms, Jones has been on inhalers since she was diagnosed, but today she is having increased wheezing and is struggling to breathe. She is overweight at 5'6" in height and 180 pounds. She has managed her type 2 diabetes with diet and exercise but more recently has seen her blood sugars in the 200 range. Her most recent glycosylated hemoglobin test last week was 7.0% (normal is 4–6%).

On physical exam, she is anxious. Her blood pressure is 136/90 mmHg, pulse 120, and respiratory rate at 28. Her lungs wheeze bilaterally. No accessory muscles are being used and she is not cyanotic. Her lab values reveal: ABG 7.48; pO2: 58; pCO2: 40; O2 sat: 90%. Chest X-ray: diaphragms hyperinflated and no infiltrates are seen.

She is treated with albuterol and atrovent nebulizer and is started on a course of prednisone at 40 mg/day for three days, to be tapered down over two weeks. On day two of her prednisone, she calls to say that her blood sugar is 350 mg/dl.

Case Study Questions

1. What are Ms. Jones's risk factors for diabetes?
2. What are the triggers for asthma in Ms. Jones's environment?
3. What actions could be taken to treat her emergently?
4. What actions could be taken for long-term effect?

References

ADA. (2004). Gestational diabetes mellitus. *Diabetes Care Supplement*, 1, 88–90.

Arnaiz, N. O., Kaufman, J. D., Daroowalla, F. M., Quigley, S., Farin, F., & Checkoway, H. (2003). Genetic factors and asthma in aluminum smelter workers. *Archives of Environmental Health*, 58(4), 197–200.

Arshad, S., Bateman, B., & Matthews, S. (2003). Primary prevention of asthma and atopy during childhood by allergen avoidance in infancy: A randomized controlled study. *Thorax*, 58, 489–493.

Atkinson, M. A., & Eisenbarth, G. S. (2001). Type 1 diabetes: New perspectives on disease pathogenesis and treatment. *Lancet, 358*, 221–229.

Barnes, D., Openshaw, K., Smith, K., & van der Plas, R. (2002). What makes people cook with improved biomass stoves? A comparative international review of stove programs, *World Bank Technical Paper No. 242*, Energy Series. Washington, DC: The World Bank.

Beaglehole, R., & Yach, D. (2003). Globalisation and the prevention and control of non-communicable disease: The neglected chronic disease of adults. *Lancet, 362*, 903–908.

Centers for Disease Control and Prevention. (2004). *Chronic disease prevention*. Retrieved from http://www.cdc.gov/programs/chronic.htm

Chen, B., Hong, C., & Kan, H. (2004). Exposures and health outcomes from outdoor air pollutants in China. *Toxicology, 198*(1–3), 291–300.

Chui, D., Lau, J. S. K., & Yau, I. T. Y. (2004). An outcome evaluation study of the Rheumatoid Arthritis Self-Management Programme in Hong Kong. *Psychology, Health & Medicine, 9*(3), 286–291.

De Broeck, V., & Verjans, M. (2010). Work-related musculoskeletal disorders: Facts and figures. National Report: Europe. Retrieved from http://osha.europa.eu/en/resources/tero09009enc-resources/europe.pdf

Erikssen, G. (2001). Physical fitness and changes in mortality: The survival of the fittest. *Sports Medicine, 31*(8), 571–576.

European Occupational Safety and Health. (2010). *Strategic Framework 2014–2020*. Retrieved from: http://ec.europa.eu/social/main.jsp?catId=151&langId=en

Ezzati, M. (2004). Indoor air pollution and health in developing countries. *Lancet, 366*, 104–106.

Felson, D. T. (2000). Epidemiology of the rheumatic diseases. In W. Koopman (Ed.), *Arthritis & Allied Conditions*. New York: Lippincott, Williams and Collens.

Funnell, M. M., Brown, T. L., Childs, B. P., Haas, L. B., Hosey, G. M., Jensen, B., . . . Weiss, M. A. (2011). National standards for diabetes self-management education. *Diabetes Care, 34*, S89–S96.

Garancini, M. P., Calori, G., Ruotolo, G., Manara, E., Izzo, A., Ebbli, E., et al. (1995). Prevalence of NIDDM and impaired glucose tolerance in Italy: An OGTT–based population study. *Diabetologia, 38*, 306–313.

Global Initiative for Asthma. (2010). *Global strategy for asthma management and prevention*. Retrieved from http://www.ginasthma.org/

Hafstrom, I., & Hallengren, M. (2003). Physiotherapy in subtropic climate improves functional capacity and health-related quality of life in Swedish patients with rheumatoid arthritis and spondylarthropathies still after 6 months. *Scandinavian Journal of Rheumatology, 32*, 108–113.

Health Safety Executive. (2010). *The Health and Safety Executive Statistics 2009/2010*. Retrieved from http://www.hse.gov.uk/statistics/overall/hssh0910.pdf

Hedley, A., Ogden, C., Johnson, C., Carroll, M., Curtin, L., & Flegal, K. (2004). Prevalence of overweight and obesity among U.S. children, adolescents, and adults (1999–2002). *Journal of the American Medical Association, 291*(23), 2847–2850.

Helmick, C. G., Felson, D. T., Lawrence, R. C., Gabriel, S., Hirsch, R., Kwoh, C. K., Liang, M. H. … Stone, J. H. (2008). Estimates of the prevalence of arthritis and other rheumatic conditions in the United States. *Arthritis & Rheumatism, 58*(1), 15–25. doi:10.1002/art.23177.

International Diabetes Federation. (2009). Diabetes atlas. *Executive Summary* (4th ed.). Retrieved from http://www.idf.org/diabetesatlas/executive-summary.

International Diabetes Federation Consensus Workshop. (2004). Type 2 diabetes in the young: The evolving epidemic. *Diabetes Care, 27*, 1798–1811.

Katz, D. (2004). The burden of chronic disease: The future is prevention [Electronic version]. *Public Health Research, Practice, and Policy, 1*(2), 1.

Koster, I., von Ferber, L., Ihle, P., Schubert, I., & Hauner, H. (2006). The cost burden of diabetes mellitus: The evidence from Germany—the CoDIM Study. *Diabetologia, 49*, 1498–1504.

Lau, X., (2004). Lazy lifestyle a weighty issue. *Beijing Review, 47*(6), 28–29.

Lewis, R. D., Meyer, M. C., Lehman, S. C., Trowbridge, F. L., Bason, J. J., Yurman, K. H., et al. (2006). Prevalence and degree of childhood and adolescent overweight in rural, urban, and suburban Georgia. *Journal of School Health, 76*(4), 126.

Liebl, A., Mata, M., & Eschwege, E. (2002). Evaluation of risk factors for development of complications in type II diabetes in Europe. *Diabetología, 45*, S23–S28.

Liebl, A., Neiß, A., Spannheimer, A., Reitberger, U., Wagner, T., & Gortz, A. (2001). Costs of type 2 diabetes in Germany. Results of the Code-2 study. *Dutsch Medical Wochenschr, 126,* 585–589.

Magnusson, R. (2010). Global health governance and the challenge of chronic, non-communicable disease. *Journal of Law, Medicine and Ethics, 38*(3), 490–507.

Marmont, M., & Wilkinson, R. G. (Eds.). (2002). *Social Determinants of Health.* London: Oxford Press.

Masharani, U., Karam, J. H., & German, M. S. (2004). Pancreatic hormones and diabetes. In F. S. Greenspan, & D. G. Garner (Eds.), *Basic and Clinical Endocrinology* (7th ed., pp. 658–746). New York: Lange Medical Books/McGraw-Hill.

Masoli, M., Fabian, D., Holt, S., & Beasley, R. (2004). The global burden of asthma. Developed for the global initiative for asthma. *Allergy, 59*(5),469–478.

Michalsen, A., Klotz, S., Ludtke, R., Moebus, S., Spahn, G., & Dobos, G. (2003). Effectiveness of leech therapy in osteoarthritis of the knee. *Annals of Internal Medicine, 139,* 724–730.

Mohan, V., Deepa, M., Deepa, R., Shanthirani, C. S., Farooq, S., Ganesan, A., et al. (2006). Secular trends in the prevalence of diabetes and impaired glucose tolerance in urban South India—the Chennai Urban Rural Epidemiology Study. (CURES-17). *Diabetologia, 49,* 1175–1178.

Morgan, C. L., Currie, C. J., Stott, N. C. H., Smithers, M., Butler, C. C., & Peters, J. R. (2000). Estimating the prevalence of diagnosed diabetes in a health district of Wales: The importance of using primary and secondary care sources of ascertainment with adjustment for death and migration. *Diabetic Medicine, 17,* 141–145.

Nathan, D. M., Buse, J. B., Davidson, M. B., Heine, R. J., Holman, R. R., Sherwin, R., et al. (2006). Management of hyperglycaemia in type 2 diabetes: A consensus algorithm for the initiation and adjustment of therapy. *Diabetologia, 49,* 1711–1721.

National Health Interview Survey Data. (2007). *Lifetime asthma population estimates.* Retrieved online from: http://www.cdc.gov/asthma/nhis/05/table1-1.htm.

National Heart, Lung, and Blood Institute. (2010). Global initiative for asthma (GINA). Global strategy for asthma management and prevention, *NHLBI/WHO Workshop Report No. 02-3659.* Bethesda, MD: NLBHI.

National Institute of Diabetes, and Digestive and Kidney Disorders. (2011). *Diabetes overview.* Retrieved from http://diabetes.niddk.nih.gov/dm/pubs/overview/

National Institute of Neurological Disorders and Stroke. (2011). *Low back pain fact sheet.* Retrieved from http://www.ninds.nih.gov/disorders/backpain/detail_backpain.htm

Nikolic, I. A., Stanciole, A. E., & Zaydman, M. (2011). Chronic emergency: Why NCDs matter. *Health Nutrition and Population Discussion Paper.* Washington, DC: The World Bank.

Ogden, C. L., Carroll, M. D., Curtin, L. R., Lamb, M. M., & Flegal, K. M. (2010). Prevalence of high body mass index in U.S. children and adolescents, 2007–2008. *Journal of the American Medical Association, 303,* 242–249.

Ohmura, T., Ueda, K., Kiyohara, Y., Kato, I., Iwanoto, H., Nakayama, K., et al. (1993). Prevalence of type 2 (non-insulin dependent) diabetes mellitus and impaired glucose tolerance in the Japanese general population: The Hisayama study. *Diabetologia, 36,* 1198–1203.

Park, H. S., Kim, S. Y., Kim, S. R., & Lee, Y. C. (2010). Targeting abnormal airway vascularity as a therapeutical strategy in asthma. *Journal of the Asian Pacific Society of Respirology, 15,* 459–471. doi:10.1111/j.1440-1843 .2010.01723.x

Porth, C. M. (2009). *Essentials of pathophysiology: Concepts of altered health states.* Philadelphia: Lippincott Williams & Wilkins.

Reynolds, D. L., Chambers, L. W., Badley, E. M., Bennett, K. J., Goldsmith, C. H., Jamieson, E., Torrance, G. W, Tugwell, P. (1992). Physical disability among Canadians reporting musculoskeletal diseases. *Journal of Rheumatology, 19,* 1020–1030.

Rudd Center. (2011). *Fast food f.a.c.t.s. Food advertising to children and teens score.* Retrieved from http://fastfoodmarketing.org/

Ruta, L. M., Magliano, D. J., LeMesurier, R., Taylor, H. R., Zimmet, P. Z., & Shaw, J. E. (2013). Prevalence of diabetic retinopathy in type 2 diabetes in developing and developed countries. *Diabetic Medicine, 30*(4), 387–398. doi:10.1111/dme.12119.

Schneider Shafey, O., Dolwick, S., & Guindon, G. (2003). *Tobacco control country.* Retrieved from http://www .wpro.who.int/NR/rdonlyres/437C3114-24FE-45CA-9A62-8E119BC66CC6/0/TCCP2.pdf.

Schoenborn, C. A., Adams, P. F., & Barnes, P. M. (2002). Body weight status of adults: United States, 1997–98. *Advance Data from Vital and Health Statistics 330.* Hyattsville, MD: National Center for Health Statistics.

Smith, K. R., Mehta, S., & Maeusezahl-Feuz, M. (2004). Indoor air-pollution from household solid fuel use. In M. Eszzati, A. D. Lopez, A. Rodgers, & C. J. L. Murray (Eds.), *Comparative Quantification of Health Risks: Global and Regional Burden of Disease Attributable to Selected Major Risk Factors* (pp. 1435–1493). Geneva, Switzerland: World Health Organization.

Stewart, A. W., Mitchell, E. A., Pearce, N., Strachan, D. P., & Weilandon, S. K. (2001). The relationship of per capita gross national product to the prevalence of symptoms of asthma and other atopic disease in children. *International Journal of Epidemiology, 30,* 173–179.

Stratton, I. M., Cull, C. A., Adler, A. I., Matthews, D. R., Neil, H. A. W., & Holman, R. R. (2006). Additive effects of glycaemia and blood pressure exposure on risk of complications in type 2 diabetes: A prospective obser-vational study (UKPDS 75). *Diabetologia, 49,* 1761–1769.

Taiwo, O. A., Sircar, K. D., Slade, M. D., Cantley, L. F., Vegso, S. J. L, Rabinowitz, P. M., et al. (2006). Incidence of asthma among aluminum workers. *Journal of Occupational and Environmental Medicine, 48*(3), 275–282.

Tham, K. W., Zuraimi, M. S., Koh, D., Chew, F. T., Ooi, P. L. (2007). Associations between home dampness and presence of molds with asthma and allergic symptoms among young children in the tropics. *Pediatric Allergy Immunology, 18,* 418–424. doi:10.1111/j.139903038.2007.00544.x

Tseng, C. H., Tseng, C. P., Chong, C. K., Huang, T. P., Song, Y. M., Chou, C. W., et al. (2006). Increasing incidences of diagnosed type 2 diabetes in Taiwan: Analysis of data from a national cohort. *Diabetologia, 49,* 1755–1760.

Woolf, A., & Pfleger, B. (2003). Burden of major musculoskeletal conditions. *Bulletin of the World Health Organization, 81*(9), 646–656.

World Health Organization. (2001). *WHO and the bone and joint decade. The global economic and healthcare burden of musculoskeletal disease.* Retrieved from www.boneandjointdecade.org

World Health Organization. (2004). *Global strategy on diet, physical activity and health.* France: WHO Organiza-tion Press.

World Health Organization. (2006). *Tobacco: Deadly in any form or disguise.* Retrieved from http://www.who .int/tobacco/communications/events/wntd/2006/Report_v8_4May06.pdf

World Health Organization. (2008, April 18). Action plan for the global strategy for the prevention and control of noncommunicable diseases. *World Health Assembly Document A61/8.*

World Health Organization. (2010). *Global Recommendations on Physical Activity for Health.* Switzerland: WHO Organization Press.

World Health Organization. (2011). *Global Status Report on Noncommunicable Diseases 2010.* Retrieved from http://www.who.int/nmh/publications/ncd_report2010/en/

Wu, Y. (2006). Overweight and obesity in China. *British Medical Journal, 333,* 362. doi:10.1136/bmj.333.7564.362

Zan-bar, T, Aron, A., & Shoenfeld, Y. (2004). Acupuncture therapy for rheumatoid arthritis, *APLar Journal of Rheumatology, 7,* 207–214.

Zhao, Z., Zhang, Z., Wang, Z., Ferm, M., Liang, Y., & Norbäck, D.(2008). Asthmatic symptoms among pupils in relation to winter indoor and outdoor air pollution in schools in Taiyuan, China. *Environmental Health Perspectives.116*(1), 90–97. doi:10.1289/ehp.10576.

13

Global Perspectives on Violence, Injury, and Occupational Health

Carol Holtz

Objectives

After completing this chapter, the reader will be able to:

1. Compare and contrast types of violence, including physical, sexual, psychological, and neglect.
2. Discuss differences in global and U.S. violence statistics.
3. Explain causes of violence against women including intimate partner violence and violence during pregnancy.
4. Discuss culture and honor killings.
5. Examine issues of school violence including bullying and cyberbullying.
6. Characterize violence in war and related issues of post-traumatic stress disorder.
7. Compare and contrast U.S. and global statistics regarding injuries.
8. Discuss passenger and pedestrian road traffic injuries and fatalities in developed versus developing countries.
9. Discuss issues regarding injuries and fatalities related to drugs, alcohol, poisoning, and drowning worldwide.
10. Explain the need for protection from injury for populations worldwide within the workplace.
11. Discuss how public policy can promote occupational health both in the United States and globally.
12. Explain the special needs for health protection of healthcare workers.
13. Examine the issues of job stress and its relationship to an individual's general health.
14. Discuss special health issues of agricultural workers worldwide.
15. Discuss suicide in women in China.

INTRODUCTION: VIOLENCE AND INJURIES

Injuries and violence are a major global health issue. More than nine people die every minute of either an injury or as a result of violence. This amounts to 5.8 million people dying annually from either violence or an injury. Worldwide, road traffic accidents annually kill 1.3 million; suicides kill 844,000; and homicides kill 600,000. Many more people get treatment and survive injuries and violence (Centers for Disease Control and Prevention [CDC], 2014a).

Violence is the intentional use of physical force or power, threatened or actual, against oneself, another person, or a group or community that results in or has a high likelihood of injury, death, psychological harm, maldevelopment, or deprivation, and erodes the safety and security of families and communities (CDC, 2014a).

Worldwide, there are many different opinions regarding the definition of violence. Whether it involves children, youth, intimate partners, or is sexual in nature, violence is a significant worldwide health issue. Violence includes child abuse and neglect by caregivers, violence by youth (ages 10 to 29 years), intimate partner violence, sexual violence, elder abuse, self-inflicted violence, school violence, and collective violence, such as war or terrorism (Mahendra, Roehler, & Degutis, 2012).

Worldwide, injuries kill 5.8 million people yearly, which accounts for 9% of all global deaths. More than 40 million disability adjusted life years (DALYs) are lost as a result of violence. Up to 70% of women in some countries have experienced some form of intimate partner violence, and many have experienced sexual violence in their lifetime. Millions of children are victims of nonfatal abuse and neglect. Nearly 90% of deaths due to injuries (intentional and unintentional) occur in low- to middle-income countries. In many countries people who use bicycles, motorcycles, or are pedestrians account for up to 80% of all road traffic deaths (Mahendra, Roehler, & Degutis, 2012).

VIOLENCE AND INJURIES IN THE UNITED STATES

In 2011 the United States had injuries and unintentional violence which accounted for 51.3% of all deaths among people 1 to 44 years old, which is more than all the deaths from noncommunicable and infectious diseases combined. Within the United States, more than 187,000 people die from injuries each year (one person every three minutes). Approximately 32.4 million people are treated in emergency departments for injuries each year. Homicides disproportionately affect young adults, particularly those ages 15 to 24. It remains the second-leading cause of death and is more responsible for deaths in this age group than cancer, heart disease, birth defects, influenza, diabetes, and HIV combined. In 2011 more than 120,000 people were treated in U.S. hospital emergency rooms for acts of violence (CDC, 2014b; Simon & Hurvitz, 2014).

The U.S. rate of intentional homicides is 5 per 100,000 (The World Bank, 2014). The World Bank and the Inter-American Development Bank consider violence and insecurity to be major health obstacles. The United States has high rates of homicide and deaths related to firearms as compared to other developed countries, but when considering all countries of the world, the United States has lower rates of such fatalities than many other countries, including developing countries. Homicide rates for Africa, Central America, and South America are three times the U.S. rate.

Healthy People 2020 lists the objectives for reducing violence in the United States. These objectives include

1. Reducing homicides
2. Reducing firearm-related deaths
3. Reducing nonfatal firearm injuries
4. Reducing physical assaults
5. Reducing physical fighting among adolescents
6. Reducing bullying among adolescents
7. Reducing weapon-carrying adolescents on school property
8. Reducing child maltreatment deaths
9. Reducing nonfatal child maltreatment
10. Reducing nonfatal intentional self-harm injuries
11. Reducing children's exposure to violence
12. Increasing number of states and District of Columbia that link data on violent deaths (Modified from Simon & Hurvitz, 2014, Healthy People 2020 Violence Prevention Objectives).

Young people under age 18 are especially vulnerable to both injury and violence. Deaths are frequently due to road traffic injuries, suicides, homicides, wars, drownings, poisonings, and fires. The U.S. National Center for Injury Prevention and Control is primarily responsible for U.S. domestic issues; it also has established violence and injury prevention programs globally, which include:

1. Increased global awareness of injury and violence as preventable public health problems.
2. Partnering with others to promote global research on injury and violence.
3. Establishing standards and providing guidance for injuries and violence surveillance.
4. Training, mentoring, and providing guidance for injuries and violence and promoting guidance documents.
5. Supporting and promoting evidence-based strategies to prevent injuries and violence (Mahendra, Roehler, & Degutis, 2012).

Violence statistics in the United States are as follows:

Victims
- One in four women will experience domestic violence during her lifetime.
- Women experience more than 4 million physical assaults and rapes because of their partners, and men are victims of nearly 3 million physical assaults.
- Women are more likely to be killed by an intimate partner than men.
- Women ages 20 to 24 are at greatest risk of becoming victims of domestic violence.
- Every year, one in three women who is a victim of homicide is murdered by her current or former partner (Safe Horizon, 2014).

Facts about Violence
- Every year, more than 3 million children witness domestic violence in their homes.
- Children who live in homes where there is domestic violence also suffer abuse or neglect at high rates (30 to 60%).

- Children exposed to domestic violence at home are more likely to have health problems, including becoming sick more often, having frequent headaches or stomachaches, and feeling more tired and lethargic.
- Children are more likely to intervene when they witness severe violence against a parent, a situation that can place a child at great risk for injury or even death.
- Domestic violence is most likely to occur between 6 p.m. and 6 a.m.
- More than 60% of domestic violence incidents happen at home.
- Survivors of domestic violence face high rates of depression, sleep disturbances, anxiety, flashbacks, and other emotional distress.
- Domestic violence contributes to poor health for many survivors. For example, chronic conditions such as heart disease or gastrointestinal disorders can become more serious due to domestic violence.
- Among women brought to emergency rooms due to domestic violence, most were socially isolated and had fewer social and financial resources than other women not injured because of domestic violence.
- Without help, girls who witness domestic violence are more vulnerable to abuse as teens and adults.
- Without help, boys who witness domestic violence are far more likely to become abusers of their partners and/or children as adults, thus continuing the cycle of violence in the next generation (Safe Horizon, 2014).

A GLOBAL PERSPECTIVE OF VIOLENCE

What is acceptable in one geographic region of the world and in one specific culture may vary greatly from what is acceptable in another geographic region and culture. This includes what is acceptable behavior, what is unacceptable behavior, and what constitutes harm. For example, beating a child's arm, leg, or buttock in public school was a regular part of discipline generations ago, but today would be considered a crime in the United States or Great Britain, and a teacher who committed such an act could be considered for criminal prosecution (Krug, Dahlberg, Mercy, Zwi, & Lozano, 2002).

Categories of violence include physical, sexual, or psychological harm, or deprivation or neglect. These categories can be broken down further into the subcategories listed in Table 13-1.

To decrease world violence, a political commitment within nations must be made, and it must be recognized that change is possible. Recommendations to decrease violence in a nation from the *World Report on Violence and Health* (Krug, Dahlberg, Mercy, Zwi, & Lozano, 2002) include the following:

1. Create, implement, and monitor a national action plan for violence prevention.
2. Enhance the capacity for collecting data on violence. Many acts are hidden and unreported.
3. Define priorities and support research on causes, consequences, costs, and prevention of violence.
4. Promote primary prevention responses. Make improvements in parental training, family functioning, and measures to reduce firearms and firearm safety, and implement media campaigns to change attitudes, behaviors, and social norms.

TABLE 13-1 Types of Violence

Physical	Self Abuse Suicide	Interpersonal Family/Partner Child/Partner/Spouse Elder	Community Acquaintance Stranger	Collective Social Political Economic
Sexual		✓	✓	✓
Psychological	✓	✓	✓	✓
Deprivation and neglect	✓	✓	✓	✓

Data from Krug, E. G., Dahlberg, L. L., Mercy, J. A., Zwi, A. B., & Lozano, R. (2002). Summary. In *World Report on Violence and Health* (pp. 1–37). Geneva, Switzerland: World Health Organization.

5. Strengthen responses to victims of violence. Improve emergency responses, recognition of signs of violence situations, and referral of victims to agencies; support prevention programs; and increase reporting mechanisms and legal processes for victims.
6. Promote and monitor adherence to international treaties, laws, and other mechanisms to protect human rights.
7. Seek practical internationally agreed-upon responses to the global drug trade and global arms trade.

According to the United Nations (UN, 2012), the most dangerous places in the world for intentional homicides per 100,000 are as follows:

1. Honduras   90.4
2. Venezuela   53.7
3. U.S. Virgin Islands   52.6
4. Guatemala   39.9
5. Jamaica   39.3
6. Lesotho   38
7. Swaziland   33.8
8. St. Kitts and Nevis   33.6
9. South Africa   31
10. Colombia   30.8
11. Bahamas   29.8
12. Democratic Republic of the Congo   28.3
13. Rwanda   23.1

The highest world homicide rates by region or subregion per 100,000 population (UN, 2012) are as follows:

1. South Africa   31
2. Central America   26.5
3. South America   22.6
4. West and Central Africa   21.6

5. East Africa	20.8
6. Middle Africa	18.5

Suicide

More than 800,000 people each year worldwide commit suicide. Many use poisoning, hanging, or shooting to end their own lives. About 75% of suicides occur among people from poor or middle-income countries, although high suicide rates also persist in more developed nations. The World Health Organization [WHO] (2014a) states that the U.S. suicide rate is about average compared with worldwide rates; the nations of Guyana, North and South Korea have the highest rates. South Korea has the world's third highest rate with 28.9 out of every 100,000 people committing suicide. The United States is grouped among countries such as Australia, Spain, and much of Europe, with rates of between 10 and 14.9 per 100,000. Globally, suicide rates are highest in people aged 70 and over, but in some countries, the highest rates are found among the young. In the 15- to 29-year age group, suicide is the second-leading cause of death globally. Pesticide poisoning, hanging, and firearms use are among the most common methods of suicide globally, and evidence from Australia, Canada, Japan, New Zealand, the United States, and Europe shows that restricting access to these means can help to stop people from committing suicide (WHO, 2014a).

Some communities in India have a unique preventive method for curtailing domestic violence. A dharna is a public shaming and protest done in front of the home or workplace of abusive men. (Wolf, Gray, & Fazel, 2014). In the United States, a variety of violence prevention programs are promoted by the CDC and many U.S. state and city health departments. The U.S. public health approach recommends the following four steps to prevent violence:

1. Define the violence problem through systematic data collection.
2. Conduct research to find out why it occurs and who it affects.
3. Find out what works to prevent violence by designing, implementing, and evaluating interventions.
4. Promote effective and promising interventions in a wide range of settings and evaluate their impact and cost-effectiveness.

How children are raised affects their vulnerability and likelihood of becoming either a victim or a perpetrator as an adult. Examples of factors that play a role include alcohol abuse, being a victim of child maltreatment, or a psychological or personality disorder. Close relationships with others also affect one's possibility of becoming a victim or perpetrator when faced with the following issues:

- Poor parenting practices
- Marital discord and having friends who engage in violence
- Social, economic, and gender inequalities
- Weak economic safety nets

- Poor law enforcement
- Cultural norms about toleration of violence

One cause of violence is believed to be inequality in income and social status within countries. In countries where there are huge differences in incomes, such that some people are vastly wealthy in comparison to others living in extreme poverty, rates of violence are much higher. Violent crime and other forms of rebellion are seen as an expression of frustration for those who cannot their goals (Wolf, Gray, & Fazel, 2014).

CHILD MALTREATMENT (ABUSE) AND NEGLECT

Child maltreatment (abuse) and neglect is a serious problem that can have long-term harmful effects. The main goal of public health efforts is prevention by supporting families with skills and resources. One method of prevention is by teaching and supporting parental nurturing skills (CDC, 2014c). Child maltreatment includes all types of abuse and neglect of a child under the age of 18 by a parent, caregiver, or another person in a custodial role (e.g., clergy, coach, teacher). There are four common types of child maltreatment (abuse) and neglect:

- Physical abuse
- Sexual abuse
- Emotional abuse
- Neglect

Shaken baby syndrome is a form of child abuse that affects 1,200 to 1,600 children per year, and is an act that may result in serious permanent damage or even death. Twenty-five to 30% of shaken babies die from their injuries. Effects of child maltreatment may result in brain maldevelopment, sleep disturbances, panic disorder, and attention-deficit/hyperactivity disorder (ADHD). Long-term consequences of child maltreatment may also result in problematic behavior as adults, including smoking, alcoholism, drug abuse, eating disorders, severe obesity, depression, suicide, and sexual promiscuity. Victims of child maltreatment are twice as likely to be physically assaulted as adults. As many as one-third of parents who are maltreated as children are likely to mistreat their own children. The children who are most likely to suffer severe injury or death from such maltreatment are those younger than 4. Table 13-2 lists risk factors that can contribute to the need for protective factors for the child.

SEXUAL VIOLENCE

Sexual violence is defined as any act or attempt to obtain a sexual act, unwanted sexual comments or advances, or acts to traffic by any person regardless of the relationship to the victim, in any setting, including but not limited to home or work. Coercion may involve physical force or psychological intimidation, blackmail, or other forms of physical threats. It may also occur when the victim is unable to give consent, such as while drunk, asleep, or mentally incapable of understanding the situation. In addition, sexual violence may include denial of the right to use contraception or to use other protection against sexually transmitted diseases, or forced

TABLE 13-2 Risk Factors that Can Contribute to the Need for Protective Factors for the Child

Risk Factors	Protective Factors Needed for the Child
Disabilities or mental retardation, increasing caregiver burden	Supportive family environment
Social isolation of families	Nurturing parental skills
Parents' lack of knowledge of child development and needs	Stable family relationships
Poverty and unemployment	
Family disorganization and/or violence	
Substance abuse in family members	
Young and single parents	
Poor parent–child relationships	
Parental thoughts and emotions that support child maltreatment	
Parental stress and/or mental health issues	
Community violence	

abortion. It includes coerced sex in marriage and dating relationships, rape by strangers, rape during armed conflict, sexual harassment (including demands for sexual favors in return for jobs or school grades), sexual abuse of children, forced prostitution and sexual trafficking, child marriage, and violent acts against the sexual integrity of women, including female genital mutilation and obligatory inspections for virginity (CDC, 2010c).

Sexual trafficking involves physical coercion, deception, and bondage incurred by forced debt. Trafficked women and children are often promised work in domestic or service industries, but then are instead taken to brothels. Sexual violence has a tremendous impact on physical and mental health. As well as causing physical injury, it leads to a variety of short- and long-term reproductive health problems. The impact on mental health can be as serious as the physical impact and equally long-lasting. Deaths following sexual violence may come as a result of suicide, HIV infection, or murder. Murder can occur either during a sexual assault or later, as in "honor killings" from family members. People who have been sexually assaulted may be stigmatized and ostracized by their family or other community members. Coerced sex may result in sexual gratification of the perpetrator, although it is generally the result of the need for power and control over the person assaulted. Rape of either men or women is often used as a weapon of war as a form of attack on the enemy (CDC, 2010d).

Violence Against Women

An interview-based study of women and violence conducted in 10 countries by WHO (2005b), known as the Multi-country Study on Women's Health and Domestic Violence Against Women, revealed the prevalence, outcomes, and women's responses to such violence. In this study women older than the age of 15 located throughout the world reported experiences with violence both by partners and by nonpartners. The incidence of such violence ranged from 5% in Ethiopia to 65% in Samoa. Women reported higher levels of violence in urban settings than in rural settings, with the exception of Peru. When respondents were asked about forced sex by nonpartners after the age of 15, rates were highest (10 to 12%) in Peru, Samoa, and urban United Republic of Tanzania and lowest (1%) in Bangladesh and Ethiopia. Perpetrators included strangers, boyfriends, and male family members (not fathers) or male friends of the family. The WHO data revealed that women are more likely to experience acts of violence from people they know than from strangers. In 34 to 59% of all cases of physical violence against women, women who reported the act of violence had no one respond to help them.

To prevent and respond to such violence against women, WHO (2005b) made the following recommendations:

1. Promote gender equality and women's human rights. Violence against women is an extreme result of gender inequality. Improving women's legal and socioeconomic status is a key intervention in reducing women's vulnerability to violence.
2. Establish, implement, and monitor action plans to address violence against women. Governments need to publicly acknowledge that a problem exists, make a commitment to act on it, and plan and implement programs to address the violence against women.
3. Elicit social, political, religious, and other leaders in speaking out against violence against women. Men in positions of authority and influence can raise awareness of the problem of violence against women and challenge misconceptions and norms within a society.
4. Establish systems for data collection to monitor violence against women.
5. Develop, implement, and evaluate primary prevention programs against violence.
6. Prioritize the prevention of child sexual abuse.
7. Integrate programs to prevent violence into existing programs, such as those treating women for HIV/AIDS.
8. Make environments safer for women; for example, improve lighting and increase police vigilance.
9. Make schools safe for girls. Eradicate physical and sexual violence against girls in schools.
10. Include referral services for violence in established reproductive health services.
11. Strengthen formal and informal support systems with social workers and shelters for women living with violence.
12. Encourage the legal and justice systems to protect women from violence.
13. Support research on causes, consequences, and costs of violence against women.

Honor Killings

An honor killing is the murder of a family member or member of a social group by other members, due to a belief of the perpetrators and possibly other members of the community that the victim has brought dishonor to the family or the community. Dishonorable behavior is often identified as the manner of dressing, wanting to terminate an arranged marriage, wanting to marry someone of the individual's own choice, engaging in homosexual acts, engaging in heterosexual acts outside of marriage, or engaging in a nonsexual act that is considered inappropriate. Women who are targeted for honor killings may also be the victim of rape, or they may be seeking a divorce from an abusive husband. Honor crimes are acts of violence, usually murder, committed by male family members against female family members, whom the perpetrators perceive as having brought "dishonor" to their family. Sometimes people will commit suicide if they perceive themselves as dishonoring their family.

Honor killings have been reported in Egypt, Syria, Jordan, Turkey, Lebanon, Morocco, Pakistan, Syria, and Yemen, as well as in immigrant communities in France, Germany, and the United Kingdom. Some countries, such as Jordan, Syria, and Morocco, have laws stating that men are allowed to kill female relatives who commit illegitimate sexual acts. Countries where such acts are not legal but honor killings continue to occur include Turkey and Pakistan. According to the *New York Times* ("A Killing Sets Honor Above Love," 2010), in Dokan, Iraq, more than 12,000 women were victims of honor killings from 1991 to 2007. Although Kurdish law has stated since 2008 that honor killings are to be treated like any other murder, the practice continues and the crime is often staged to look like a suicide.

Intimate Partner Violence

Domestic or intimate partner violence comprises a range of sexually, psychologically, and physically coercive acts used against adult and adolescent women or men by current or former intimate partners. A CDC report on intimate partner violence indicated that 5.3 million intimate partners are victims of violence each year (CDC, 2014f). Such violence results in more than two million injuries and 1,300 deaths per year. Intimate partner violence occurs in all populations regardless of culture, socioeconomic status, or geographic location. Young women and those living at federal poverty levels are disproportionately more likely to be victims. As many as 324,000 women each year in the United States experience intimate partner violence during their pregnancy. According to the CDC data, 44% of women murdered by their intimate partners had visited an emergency room within the last two years of the homicide, and 93% had at least one injury visit. Firearms were the most common type of weapon used in such murders. In the United States, approximately 40 to 70% of female murder victims were killed by their husbands or boyfriends and had a history of being in an abusive relationship (CDC, 2014b; Stockman, Lucea, & Campbell, 2013).

The consequences of intimate partner violence include a 60% higher rate of health problems among these women as compared to women who have not been subject to abuse. Examples of these health issues include chronic pain, gastrointestinal disorders, and irritable bowel syndrome. Reproductive health problems may include unwanted pregnancy, premature labor and birth, sexually transmitted diseases, and HIV/AIDS. In addition, women often experience mental health problems such as anxiety and low self-esteem. They are also more likely to abuse alcohol and make suicide attempts. Women subjected to abuse are also more likely to be unemployed and to be recipients of public assistance (CDC, 2010d). Coerced or forced sexual initiation and sexual intimate partner violence contributes significantly to women's risk for HIV infection in countries where there is a high rate of HIV in the population (Stockman, Lucea, & Campbell, 2013).

Both men and women experience intimate partner violence, but women are two to three times more likely to report their situations. Hispanic women and women of American Indian/ Native Alaskan descent have a lower rate of reporting their victimization than non-Hispanic white women.

According to the CDC (2010d), characteristics of perpetrators of intimate partner violence include the following:

- Young age
- Heavy drinking
- Depression
- Personality disorders
- Low academic achievement
- Low income/poverty
- Witnessing or experiencing violence as a child
- Marital conflict or instability
- Male dominance in the family
- Economic stress
- Poor family functioning
- Weak community sanctions against domestic violence
- Traditional gender norms
- Social norms supportive of violence

The relationships of the perpetrators and the victims often featured the following characteristics (CDC, 2014a):

- Marital conflict
- Marital instability
- Male dominance in the family
- Poor family functioning
- Emotional dependence and insecurity
- Belief in strict gender roles
- Desire for power and control of a relationship, and exhibiting anger and hostility toward the partner

Low socioeconomic status and poverty are often linked to the causes of violence. Although domestic violence cuts across race, socioeconomic status, education, and income, African Americans experience a disproportionate amount of domestic violence compared with non-Hispanic white Americans. In recognition of this fact, the National Black Women's Health Project has identified domestic violence as the health issue of highest priority for African American women. African American women also are at a greater risk than non-Hispanic white women for contracting HIV as a result of domestic violence, and the number of deaths and serious injuries from such violence is greater in African American communities. African American women are more likely to kill a partner and are twice as likely to be killed because of domestic violence than are white women. Possible explanations for this imbalance in the rates of intimate partner violence are that African American women do not always see themselves as being in danger and are less likely to seek assistance as a result of violence. Moreover, African Americans are more likely to live in poverty and to have less access to transportation to geographically convenient shelters. In addition, a lack of culturally competent healthcare providers has resulted in the hesitancy of African American women to seek counseling and assistance for domestic violence (CDC, 2014a).

Intimate Partner Violence and Pregnancy

Domestic violence against women who are pregnant is a special case of intimate partner violence. The true incidence of physical abuse in pregnancy is not known but is suspected to range from 0.9 to 26% in developing countries. Most victims are reluctant to report such abuse. The effects of violence during pregnancy, which can be a blow to the abdomen, can include preterm labor and delivery, chorioamnionitis (infection of the amniotic fluid), premature rupture of membranes, low-birth-weight babies, intrauterine growth retardation, hemorrhage, fetal injury, and death of the mother and/or fetus. Indirectly, psychological stress and lack of access to prenatal care can also cause poor outcomes. Related responses to domestic violence include polysubstance (alcohol, drugs, and tobacco) abuse, which can harm the developing fetus (CDC, 2010d). Pregnancy can be a time of particular vulnerability because of changes in physical, emotional, social, and economic demands and needs. The time period has been known to extend beyond actual pregnancy and can start as early as one-year before conception until one year after childbirth. Prevalence rates in Africa and Latin America are higher than in Europe and Asia. Studies indicate a range of 3.9 to 8.7% incidence (Van Parys, Verhamme, Temmerman, & Verstraelen, 2014).

Sexual Violence Against Men and Boys

Sexual violence against men and boys is a significant problem that takes place in a variety of settings, including in the home, in the workplace, in schools, on the streets, in the military, during war, in prisons, and in police custody. Studies conducted mainly in developed countries indicate that men report a 5 to 10% rate of sexual abuse experienced while they were children. In developing countries, rates of child sexual abuse in boys have been reported as ranging from 3.6% in Namibia, to 13.4% in the United Republic of Tanzania, to 20% in Peru. Official statistics usually greatly underestimate the actual number of male rape victims (CDC, 2010d).

SCHOOL VIOLENCE

Violence is taking an increasing toll on American society. School violence is now a major problem that inhibits learning and causes physical and psychological harm to students. In the United States, an estimated 50 million students are enrolled in pre-kindergarten through 12th grade. Another 15 million students attend colleges and universities across the country. Although U.S. schools remain relatively safe, any amount of violence is unacceptable. Parents, teachers, and administrators expect schools to be safe havens of learning. Acts of violence can disrupt the learning process and have a negative effect on students, the school itself, and the broader community.

The potential for being threatened or injured by a weapon on school property has increased in recent years (CDC, 2014d). In addition, children may be bullied both at home and in their school environments. Victimized children often experience symptoms of withdrawal, anxiety, or depression, and many remain unhappy within their school environment. Prevention and intervention programs have been proven to reduce mental health problems during childhood.

As listed by the CDC (2014d) risk factors for perpetrators and victims for school violence include the following:

1. Substance abuse
2. Experiencing or witnessing violence and/or abuse within the home—physical, mental, and/sexual abuse/neglect
3. Depression
4. Low IQ and higher levels of aggression
5. Living in high-crime neighborhoods with gangs and exposure to community violence
6. School achievement problems such as ADHD, poor reading, and poor motor skills.

Approximately 30% of U.S. schoolchildren are exposed to bullying at school in grades 6 through 10. School bullying and cyberbullying are increasingly viewed as significant contributors to youth violence, including homicides and suicides. Studies of shootings at Columbine High School in Colorado and other U.S. schools indicate that bullying was a factor in these situations. Each day 160 U.S. children miss school because of the fear of being bullied. An estimated 100,000 children carry guns to schools each year. Of those who carry weapons to school, 285 have witnessed violence at home. Playground statistics reveal that every seven minutes a child is bullied and that responses from bystanders include adult intervention (4%), peer intervention (11%), and no intervention (85%). School bullying statistics reveal that 87% of school shootings are motivated by a desire to get back at those who have hurt them ("Bullying Statistics/Cyberbullying Statistics/School Bullying," n.d.).

In the United States, 11.1% of youths (15.1% of males and 6.7% of females) in grades 9 through 12 reported in a 2009 survey by the CDC that, within the past 12 months, they had been in a physical fight on school property. Five percent of students did not go to school on one or more days in the past 30 days because they felt unsafe at school or on their way to school. Also in 2009, in a national survey of youths in grades 9 through 12, 19.9% reported that they had experienced bullying on school property within the past 12 months (CDC, 2010c). Youth violence harms not only its victims but also their families, their friends, and entire communities.

Violent young people are also associated with other problems such as truancy, dropping out of school, substance abuse, reckless driving, and high rates of sexually transmitted diseases. Youth who witness physical or sexual abuse of other individuals in their homes or neighborhoods often get the idea that violence is an acceptable means of resolving problems (CDC, 2014d).

ELDER ABUSE

Elder abuse includes violence against individuals who are 60 and older, usually committed by a caregiver or a person whom the victim trusts. It may continue to occur because the older person is afraid to tell others or the police. Types of elder abuse include the following:

1. *Physical*: Hitting, kicking, pushing, slapping, burning or other means of force.
2. *Sexual*: Forcing an elder to have sex without consent.
3. *Emotional*: Behaviors that hurt the elder's self-worth or emotional well-being such as name calling, embarrassing the person, or not letting him or her see friends or family.
4. *Neglect*: Failure to meet the person's basic needs, including food, housing, clothing, and medical care.
5. *Abandonment*: Leaving the elder alone and withholding care.
6. *Financial*: Misusing the person's money, property, or assets.

Prevention strategies for elder abuse include these recommendations:

- Listening to the elders and their caregivers.
- Reporting abuse to Adult Protective Services.
- Educating about signs of elder abuse.
- Getting help from adult day care programs and caregivers who need help seeking counseling and treatment for psychological problems (CDC, 2010b).

VIOLENCE AND WAR

War is an organized and often prolonged conflict that is carried out by different groups of people. It is generally characterized by extreme violence, social disruption, and economic destruction. Violence related to war may result in increased health services costs, reduction in productivity, and decreased property values. Violence may cross international borders, especially when it is associated with illegal drug trade, small arms trade, sexual slavery, or terrorism. Sometimes violence is contained within cultural practices, such as violence against women and female genital mutilation. Today, people in many parts of the world face the prospect of violence as a result of war and terrorism. These situations affect large groups of civilians who are confronted with civil strife, food shortages, and population displacements. In the 20th century, 72 million deaths (nearly half of whom were civilians) occurred in 25 conflicts worldwide. From 1987 through 1997, 2 million children were killed and 4 to 5 million children were seriously injured during armed conflict.

Each year in Afghanistan 2,000 to 3,000 people are killed or injured by landmines and unexploded ordnance (UXO); about two people per 1,000 are permanently disabled. In recent years, frequency of rape and sexual violence has increased during and after conflicts. During the conflict in Bosnia in the early 1990s, estimates of the number of women raped ranged from 10,000 to 25,000 (CDC, 2014e).

As outlined by the CDC (2014e), efforts to address the high rates of violent deaths and the need to promote human security should include the following measures:

- Protect people in violent conflict.
- Protect people from the proliferation of arms.
- Support migrants, refugees, and internally displaced persons.
- Establish funds for postconflict situations.
- Encourage fair trade to benefit the poor.
- Provide minimum living standards everywhere.
- Give high priority to universal access to basic health care.
- Develop an equitable global system for patient rights.
- Provide basic education.

Within nations, efforts to reduce violence can also be directed toward religious and political leaders, who can work toward developing systems of openness and opportunity for their own constituents. Political violence is another threat to the health of many populations throughout the globe. Sousa (2013) studied the influence of lifetime and the influence of the past 30 days of political violence on the mental and physical health of adult Palestinian women from the West Bank. Political violence is the deliberate use of power and physical force (psychological, physical, and sexual) to achieve political goals. Findings revealed that religious support often was a force to strengthen survival of physical and mental health.

Bioterrorism also relates to war and poses a major threat to world health. Safeguarding the public's health, safety, and security became a high priority after the terrorist attacks on New York's World Trade Center and Washington, D.C.'s Pentagon on September 11, 2001. A few weeks later, on October 4, 2001, a Florida man was diagnosed with inhalation anthrax. His illness was traced to an anthrax agent that was dispersed throughout the U.S. postal system in New York, Washington, D.C., and other locations. This act of bioterrorism resulted in five deaths, thousands more people being tested, and many hundreds being treated for this illness.

As part of the U.S. response to these events, the Model State Emergency Health Powers Act, or Model Act, was developed. The Model Act provides states with power to detect and contain bioterrorism or a naturally occurring disease outbreak. Included are the following elements (Gostin et al., 2002):

- *Preparedness*: Preparing for a public health emergency
- *Surveillance*: Measures to detect and track public health emergencies
- *Management of property*: Ensuring adequate availability of vaccines, pharmaceuticals, and hospitals
- *Protection of persons*: Powers to compel vaccination, testing, treatment, isolation, and quarantine when clearly necessary
- *Communication*: Providing clear and authoritative information to the public

POSTTRAUMATIC STRESS DISORDER

Posttraumatic stress disorder (PTSD) is a chronic anxiety disorder triggered by traumatic events either by experiencing or witnessing it. As part of their symptoms, victims may reexperience the event through flashbacks, bad dreams, or frightening thoughts. They may engage in avoidance behaviors such as staying away from places or objects that serve as reminders of the bad experiences, may feel numb and lose interest in things that they normally enjoy, or may have trouble remembering the event. They may also be hyperaroused and easily startled, feel tense, have difficulty sleeping, or have angry outbursts. Signs and symptoms usually begin around three months after an event, but in some cases, may not occur until a year after the event. Triggering events may include rape, war, natural disasters, traumatic accidents or illnesses, or abandonment. Treatments include medication and psychological therapy. Unresolved problems can lead to permanent mental health disability or suicide (Mayo Clinic, 2014).

In a study conducted by the U.S. Department of Veteran Affairs, National Center for PTSD, between 2001 and 2003, the lifetime prevalence of PTSD among men was 3.6% and among women was 9.7%. Lifetime global prevalence of PTSD ranges from 0.3% in China to 6.1% in New Zealand (Gradus, 2007).

INJURY

Injuries cause approximately 10% of all deaths worldwide, with traffic accidents, self-inflicted injuries, violence, and war being the most common causes of traumatic deaths. All types of injuries are predicted to increase by the year 2020. Historically, global health-related problems tended to derive from infectious disease, pollution, and malnutrition; today, however, injury is attracting more attention as a major global health problem. A study comparing mortality from serious blunt trauma showed that the rates of these fatalities decreased as income increased; in this study, the examples cited to prove this point included a low-income country, Ghana; a middle-income country, Mexico; and a high-income country, the United States. *The higher rates of death in poorer countries were due to the increased time necessary to transport patients to a hospital emergency room setting and the less advanced care given in transit to the hospital.* Worldwide, an estimated 1.2 million people are killed in road crashes each year and as many as 50 million are injured. Projections indicate that these figures will increase by about 65% over the next 20 years unless there is new commitment to prevention (WHO, 2014b). Road traffic crashes in China kill more than 250,000 people annually, which is a higher number than in any other country in the world. Road accidents are the fourth leading cause of premature deaths in China, with drunk driving and speeding the major causes of the fatalities. The death rate of 21.3 per 100,000 population is more than twice the rate in Western Europe. Traffic accidents are also a major contributor to injuries. Almost 1.5 million people in China are living with permanent injuries due to road traffic accidents (Bhalla, Li, Duan, Wang, Bishai, & Hyder, 2013).

WHO reports that almost 12 million people die in traffic accidents each year, and this number is predicted to increase by 65% over the next 20 years. Most of this increase will be attributable to deaths in developing countries. In the United States, the estimated cost of serious trauma care for a single person is far greater than the cost of care for cancer and cardiovascular diseases. Thus, reducing the number of deaths and injuries from trauma could have a major worldwide positive economic impact. Significant advances in prehospital care in the form of advanced life support (ALS) and basic life support (BLS) have improved the mortality rates for serious injuries. Likewise, advances in technology in hospital emergency rooms and operative care, as well as intensive care unit (ICU) hospital care, have significantly improved patients' chances of survival in these scenarios. Unfortunately, many seriously injured patients who live in developing countries may not have the benefit of such care, owing to a lack of technology, lack of funds, or lack of transportation to healthcare facilities. Injuries traditionally have been considered to be random and unavoidable accidents, yet today intentional and unintentional injuries are considered to be preventable events. Injuries are among the world's leading causes of death, disability, or disease and affect people of all races, ages, and socioeconomic status. Worldwide, road traffic accidents and self-inflicted injuries are the leading causes of injury deaths (WHO, 2014b).

There is a significant gap in the burden imposed by trauma and injury in low- and middle-income countries of the world as compared to high-income countries. Fifteen percent of the world's population resides in high-income countries, with 60% of this high-income population having life spans exceeding 70 years. In contrast, the remaining 85% of the world's population lives in middle- and low-income countries, where only 25% of the population lives past 70 years. The newly independent countries of Eastern Europe, which are classified as middle-income countries, have the highest overall injury mortality rates. Countries in North America, Western Europe, Australia, and New Zealand, have the lowest injury rates. The main reasons for the higher rates of trauma and injury in low- and middle-income countries are inadequate systems of hospital and community-based emergency care. Roads used to transport trauma patients to hospitals are often unpaved and have few safety regulations. In addition, there is often little recognition of the need for road safety and public education on these issues in middle- and low-income countries. To bridge this significant gap, it is essential that trauma care services, research in trauma and injury, and comprehensive training programs for preventing injuries and violence that are unique to the specific demographic and environmental influences be developed (Hofman, Primack, Keusch, & Hrynkow, 2005; Zhang, Norton, Tang, Lo, Zhuo, & Wenkui, 2004).

Injuries and violence are also a great problem for U.S. older adults. To protect older Americans, many programs are being developed that address the following issues (CDC, 2010b, 2014f).

- Elder abuse and maltreatment
- Falls
- Traffic accidents with injuries
- Residential fire injuries
- Sexual abuse
- Suicide
- Traumatic brain injury

Road Traffic Injuries and Fatalities

A road traffic injury is a fatal or nonfatal injury that occurred as a result of a road traffic crash. A road traffic crash is a collision or incident that may or may not lead to injury, which occurs on a public road and involves at least one moving vehicle. In 1990, road accidents were the ninth leading cause of death in the world, and by 2020, they are expected to be the third leading cause of death if nothing is done to stop the trend. Every year, more than 1.3 million people around the world are killed in traffic accidents. Ninety percent of these deaths occur in poorer countries. These injuries are the single largest cause of death among persons 15 to 19 years of age. For each death from road traffic crashes, there are another 50 people who are injured or disabled from this cause. The majority of these deaths and injuries occur in developing countries where more people are now using cars, trucks, motorcycles, and mopeds, and where more pedestrians are vulnerable to injury and death from motor vehicles. The Southeast Asia and the Western Pacific regions of the world account for two thirds of global deaths due to road traffic accidents. The global losses related to injuries and deaths are estimated to be $518 billion (Dalal, Lin, Gifford, & Svanström, 2013). The CDC, in partnership with the U.S. National Highway Traffic Safety Administration, is also working to reduce deaths caused by alcohol-related road traffic injuries.

Worldwide, an estimated 1.2 million people are killed in road crashes each year and as many as 50 million are injured. Projections indicate that these figures will increase by about 65% over the next 20 years unless there is new commitment to prevention. Nevertheless, the tragedy behind these figures attracts less mass media attention than other, less frequent types of tragedy.

Wealthier countries are making significant progress in decreasing the numbers of traffic-related deaths and injuries. In developed nations, most of the victims of road accidents are drivers or passengers in vehicles. In contrast, most of those who die or are injured in road traffic accidents in developing countries are pedestrians who are too poor to own a vehicle. The child pedestrian injury is highest in South Asia and Sub-Saharan Africa. In places such as India, far more health spending is devoted to HIV/AIDS than to road traffic injuries, yet more people die from road traffic accidents than from HIV/AIDS. In addition to the losses due to injuries and deaths, many families lose the value of that person's earning potential, dramatically cutting essential household income. Moreover, road traffic injuries place a huge strain on healthcare budgets. For example, in Kenya, road traffic injuries account for 45 to 60% of all hospital admissions to surgical units (Watkins & Sridhar, 2009; WHO, 2009a). In the United States, every day, thousands of Americans are involved in motor vehicle crashes that result in injury or death: a teen driver killed just months after getting his license; an older driver disabled in a crash; a parent injured while driving intoxicated.

According to the CDC (2014a), the following occurred in the year 2011:

- More than 32,000 people in the United States died in a motor vehicle crash.
- Almost 10,000 people died at the hands of alcohol-impaired drivers.
- More than 2.6 million drivers and passengers were treated in emergency departments after being in a motor vehicle crash.

In the United States, teen drivers are especially vulnerable to traffic deaths. Forty percent of all teen deaths are attributable to motor vehicle accidents. Teens aged 16 to 19 are four times more likely than older drivers to have traffic accidents. Specifically, teenagers represent 10% of the U.S. population but account for 14% of all motor vehicle accidents. Moreover, the presence of other teen passengers increases the risk of accidents for teen drivers. Male teens have double the number of deaths from car accidents as female teens. The risk of such accidents is particularly high during the first years that teenagers are eligible to drive. Teens are more likely than older drivers to do the following:

- Underestimate the dangers in hazardous situations
- Have less experience coping with difficult driving situations
- Speed
- Run red lights
- Make illegal turns
- Ride with an intoxicated driver
- Drive while using alcohol and drugs
- Not use using a seat belt
- Texting and cell phone use

Male teens are less likely to use a seat belt than female teens. U.S. drivers older than 65 have higher rates of traffic accidents than all other drivers except teen drivers. The majority of fatal traffic accidents of older drivers occur during daytime and on weekdays. Although older drivers are more likely than younger drivers to use a seat belt, drivers 65 and older are more likely to die from injuries than younger drivers. Injury rates are twice as high among older men as they are among older women. Factors related to injury and deaths for older drivers include problems with vision, hearing, cognitive functions, and physical impairments (CDC, 2014a).

Child Passenger Safety

Motor vehicle injuries are the leading cause of death among children in the United States. In 2008, 968 children, 14 years and younger, died as occupants in motor vehicle accidents and another 168,000 were injured; many of these fatalities and injuries could have been prevented.

Of the children's deaths attributable to road crashes, 15% were a result of a drinking driver, and more than two-thirds of the children who died were in a vehicle with a drinking driver. In addition to children who are in vehicles with drinking drivers, many children are not restrained properly in the vehicles. Child restraint use is dependent on the driver's use of restraints; that is, nearly 40% of children riding with unbelted drivers were also unrestrained in the vehicles. Moreover, nearly 75% of car and booster seats are not used properly, increasing a child's risk of dying in a car accident (CDC, 2010a).

Injuries to children in motor vehicles can be prevented by the following measures:

1. Children should be put into a child safety seat, which reduces deaths in cars by 71%.
2. Adult drivers should not use alcohol when driving.
3. Booster seats should be used for all children younger than 8 years or less than 4 ft. 9 in. tall.
4. Children 12 and younger should ride in the back seat of a vehicle, which reduces injury by 40% (CDC, 2010a).

POISONING

Poisoning is a significant global public health problem. According to WHO data, an estimated 346,000 people die annually worldwide from unintentional poisoning. Of these deaths, 91%

occurred in low- and middle-income countries. In the same year, unintentional poisoning caused the loss of over 7.4 million years of healthy life (i.e., DALYs) (WHO, 2014c).

Lead is a toxic metal, the widespread use of which has caused extensive environmental contamination and health problems in many parts of the world. It is a cumulative toxicant that affects multiple body systems, including the neurologic, hematologic, gastrointestinal, cardiovascular, and renal systems. Children are particularly vulnerable to the neurotoxic effects of lead, and even relatively low levels of exposure can cause serious, and in some cases, irreversible, neurological damage. Globally, lead exposure is estimated to account for 0.6% of disease, with the highest burden in developing regions. Childhood lead exposure is estimated to contribute to about 600,000 new cases of intellectual disabilities every year. Reductions in the use of lead in gasoline, paint, plumbing, and solder have resulted in substantial reductions in blood lead levels. However, significant sources of exposure still remain, particularly in developing countries. Interventions to reduce lead poisoning include eliminating nonessential uses of lead, such as in paint, ensuring the safe recycling of lead-containing waste, educating the public about the importance of safe disposal of lead-acid batteries and computers, and monitoring of blood lead levels in children, women of child-bearing age, and workers (WHO, 2014c).

ALCOHOL-RELATED INJURIES

In the United States, excessive alcohol consumption causes more than 10,000 deaths per year, and between 20 and 30% of the patients seen in all emergency rooms have alcohol-related problems. Half of all alcohol-related deaths are the result of injuries from motor vehicle accidents, falls, fires, drowning, homicides, and suicides. Thirty percent of Americans will at some stage in their lives be involved in an alcohol-related crash (CDC, 2014g).

As outlined by the CDC (2014g), preventable actions and programs can be developed, such as the following:

- Suspend driver's licenses of those who drive intoxicated.
- Lower the illegal blood alcohol concentration level for U.S. adult drivers to 0.08% in all states.
- Establish a zero tolerance policy for drivers younger than age 21 who consume alcohol.
- Establish sobriety checkpoints and have community education about drinking and driving.
- Raise state and federal alcohol excise taxes.
- Have compulsory blood alcohol testing after all traffic accidents with injuries.

FIRES AND BURNS

Burns are injuries of the skin and sometimes of the underlying tissue, muscle, nerves, and organs. They can be caused by hot liquids, flames, hot surfaces, sunlight or radiation, electricity, or chemicals. Primary prevention is the most effective means of combating burns (CDC, 2014f). Prevention methods suggested by the CDC (2014f) include

- Enclose open fires, and limit the height of fires in homes, especially in developing countries.
- Promote use of safe stoves and fuels.

- Have housing fire safety regulations and inspections.
- Educate the public.
- Establish and comply with industrial safety regulations.
- Promote the use of smoke detectors, fire alarms, and escape systems for fires.
- Refrain from smoking in bed.
- Promote the use of nonflammable children's pajamas.
- Lower the temperature of hot water taps in homes.

In the United States, four of every five fires occur in the home; cooking is the main cause of residential fires and smoking is the second leading cause of fires. Most fire-related deaths are attributable to smoke or toxic gas inhalation. Those persons at greatest risk from fires are children younger than 5, adults older than 65, African Americans and Native Americans, persons living in poverty, residents of rural areas, and inhabitants of substandard housing (CDC, 2014f).

Fires occur more in the winter season, and more deaths occur among those persons without home smoke detectors. However, homes in developing nations do not tend to have smoke detectors, and more residents of these countries tend to cook by fire within their homes (CDC, 2014f).

DROWNING

Drowning is the process of experiencing respiratory impairment from submersion/immersion in liquid; outcomes are classified as death, morbidity, and no morbidity. WHO (2014d) outlines key global factors, including the following:

- Drowning is the third-leading cause of unintentional injury death worldwide, accounting for 7% of all injury-related deaths.
- There are an estimated 372,000 annual drowning deaths worldwide.
- Global estimates may significantly underestimate the actual public health problem related to drowning.
- Children, males, and individuals with increased access to water are most at risk of drowning.

The global burden and death from drowning is found in all economies and regions, however (WHO, 2014d).

- Low- and middle-income countries account for 95% of unintentional drowning deaths.
- Over half of the world's drowning occurs in the WHO Western Pacific region and WHO Southeast Asia region.
- Drowning death rates are highest in the WHO African region, and are 10 to 13 times higher than those in the United Kingdom or Germany respectively.

Despite limited data, several studies reveal information on the cost impact of drowning. In the United States, 45% of drowning deaths are among the most economically active segment of the population. Coastal drowning in the United States alone accounts for US$273 million each year in direct and indirect costs. In Australia and Canada, the total annual cost of drowning injury is US$85.5 million and US$173 million respectively (WHO, 2014d).

There is a wide range of uncertainty around the estimate of global drowning deaths. Nonfatal drowning statistics in many countries are not easily available or are unreliable. Age is one of the major risk factors for drowning. This relationship is often associated with a lapse in supervision. In general, children under five have the highest drowning mortality rates worldwide. Canada and New Zealand are the only exceptions, where adult males drown at higher rates (WHO, 2014d).

Examples of global drowning statistics compiled by WHO (2014d) include the following:

- Australia: drowning is the leading cause of unintentional injury death in children aged one to three.
- Bangladesh: drowning accounts for 43% of all deaths in children aged one to four.
- China: drowning is the leading cause of injury death in children aged one to fourteen.
- United States: drowning is the second-leading cause of unintentional injury death in children aged one to fourteen.

Males are especially at risk of drowning, with twice the overall mortality rate of females. They are more likely to be hospitalized than females for nonfatal drowning. Studies suggest that the higher drowning rates among males are due to increased exposure to water and riskier behavior such as swimming alone, drinking alcohol before swimming alone, and boating. Increased access to water is another risk factor for drowning. Individuals with occupations such as commercial fishing or fishing for subsistence, and using small boats in low-income countries are more prone to drowning. Children who live near open water sources, such as ditches, ponds, irrigation channels, or pools are especially at risk (WHO, 2014d).

Other factors associated with an increased risk of drowning, such as:

- Being a member of an ethnic minority, those with lower socioeconomic status, lack of higher education, and members of rural populations all tend to be associated with an increased risk, although this association can vary across countries.
- Infants left unsupervised or alone with another child around water.
- Unsafe or overcrowded transportation vessels lacking flotation devices.
- Alcohol use, near or in the water.
- Medical conditions, such as epilepsy.
- Tourists unfamiliar with local water risks and features.
- Floods and other cataclysmic events such as tsunamis.

Drowning prevention strategies should be comprehensive and include engineering methods which help to remove the hazard, legislation to enforce prevention and assure decreased exposure, education for individuals and communities to build awareness of risk and to aid in response if a drowning occurs, and prioritization of research and public health initiatives to further define the burden of drowning worldwide and explore prevention interventions. Eliminating exposure to water hazards is the most effective strategy for drowning prevention. Measures included in this strategy focus on draining unnecessary accumulations of water or altering the environment to create barriers to open water sources (WHO, 2014d).

Examples of specific strategies should include:

- Development and implementation of safe water systems, such as drainage systems, piped water systems, and flood control embankments in flood prone areas.
- Building four-sided pool fences or barriers preventing access to standing water.
- Creating and maintaining safe water zones for recreation.
- Covering of wells or open cisterns.
- Emptying buckets and baths, and storing them upside-down (WHO, 2014d).

OCCUPATIONAL HEALTH

There are no true global surveillance systems for occupational illness and injury. The International Labour Organization (ILO) collects data from member countries and periodically publishes global and regional estimates. The World Health Organization has an ongoing effort to estimate the global burden of disease. Both organizations state that their statistics greatly underestimate the true burden of global injury due to work.

Global Injuries and Fatalities

Work-related injuries and illnesses are events or exposures in the work environment that cause or contribute to a health condition or significantly aggravate a preexisting condition. These illnesses or injuries may result in death, loss of consciousness, time away from work, restricted work activity, or medical treatment beyond first aid. Significant work-related injuries or illnesses may be diagnosed by a physician or other healthcare professional (CDC, 2014h).

Occupational illnesses may consist of any of the following:

- Skin diseases or disorders caused by exposure to chemicals, plants, or other substances. The worker may get problems such as contact dermatitis, eczema, rash, ulcers, chemical burns, or inflammations.
- Respiratory problems associated with breathing hazardous biological products, chemicals, dust, gases, vapors, or fumes. Examples include pneumonitis, pharyngitis, rhinitis, tuberculosis (TB), occupational asthma, toxic inhalation injury, and chronic bronchitis.
- Poisoning, which can occur from exposure to lead, mercury, arsenic, carbon monoxide, hydrogen sulfide, or other gases.
- Other occupational illnesses, such as heatstroke, sunstroke, heat exhaustion, freezing, frostbite, decompression sickness, anthrax, HIV, and hepatitis B.

Occupational injuries could include broken bones, cuts, or fractured eardrums. Injuries can result in sick days away from work, a transfer to another location or assignment, or permanent job loss. Workplace injuries, illnesses, and fatalities continue to occur at very high rates worldwide, contributing to the worldwide burden of health (CDC, 2014h).

The ILO (2013) estimates that more than 2.3 million women and men globally die from work-related accidents or diseases every year; this corresponds to over 6,000 deaths every day. Worldwide, there are approximately 340 million occupational accidents and 160 million victims of work-related illnesses annually. The ILO updates these estimates at intervals, and the updates indicate an increase of accidents and ill health. Some of the major findings in the ILO's latest statistical data on occupational accidents and diseases and work-related deaths on a worldwide level include the following:

- Diseases related to work cause the most deaths among workers. Hazardous substances alone are estimated to cause 651,279 deaths a year.
- The construction industry has a disproportionately high rate of recorded accidents.
- Younger and older workers are particularly vulnerable. The aging population in developed countries means that an increasing number of older persons are working and need special consideration.

Noise-induced hearing loss is a significant problem among workers in a variety of settings. This hearing loss is irreversible. Workers in heavy industry, factories, coal and iron mining, construction, and airports are among the many employees who can become partially or completely deaf from occupational hazards of noise production at the workplace. In addition, exposure to excessive noise at the workplace may produce hearing problems in the newborns of pregnant women. Workers need to use hearing protection devices at work whenever they are exposed to harmful noise (Azizi, 2010).

In the Japanese workplace, employers are required to provide annual health checkups for workers. A national law mandates that an occupational physician be assigned to companies employing at least 50 workers. This law has effectively lowered the incidence of coronary heart disease among the workers. About 60% of women and 70% of men over the age of 20 receive some type of medical exam once a year. The primary aim is to reveal general health problems within the workers. These requirements are prescribed by the Industrial Safety and Health Law, established in 1972 (Okamura, Sugiyama, Tanaka, & Dohi, 2014). As in Japan, the European Union workers also have the Agency for Safety and Health at Work which identifies health issues among workers. Cardiovascular diseases and stroke are the most common identifiable health issues found (Guazzi, Faggiano, Mureddu, Faden, Niegauer, & Temporelli, 2014).

The U.S. Occupational Safety and Health Administration (OSHA) is an agency of the Department of Labor. Congress established the agency under the Occupational Safety and Health Act, which President Nixon signed into law on December 29, 1970. OSHA's mission is to "assure safe and healthful working conditions for working men and women by setting and enforcing standards and by providing training, outreach, education and assistance United States Department of Labor." OSHA calculates that 6,000 employees die each year in the United States from injuries in the workplace, and another 50,000 die from illnesses caused by exposure to workplace hazards. This burden costs U.S. businesses more than $125 billion annually. Federal criteria as per OSHA standards used to address worker safety consist of the following requirements (OSHA, 2014):

- Provide well-maintained tools and equipment.
- Provide medical examinations.
- Provide training to OSHA standards.

- Report accidents or fatalities within eight hours.
- Keep records of work-related accidents, injuries, or illnesses.
- Post prominently employee rights and responsibilities.
- Provide employees with access to their medical and exposure records.
- Do not discriminate against employees who exercise their rights under the OSHA Act.
- Post citations and violations at or near the worksite.
- Respond to survey requests.

Acute trauma at work is a leading cause of death and disability among workers in the United States; it can occur with a sudden application of force or violence that causes injury or death. In 2000, there were 5,915 workplace deaths in the United States from acute traumatic injury. The National Institute for Occupational Safety and Health (NIOSH) is currently conducting research to identify and prioritize the problems with injury surveillance studies, to quantify and prioritize risk factors with analytic injury research, to identify existing or new strategies to prevent occupational injuries through prevention and control research, and to implement the most effective injury control measures with communication and dissemination of recent information and technology (CDC, 2014a).

Occupational health is often neglected in developing countries because of competing social, economic, and political issues. Indeed, the majority of developing countries lack the ability to establish new occupational health policies and regulations. In recent decades, however, many U.S. manufacturing jobs have moved to developing countries where labor and taxes are much more economical. Thus, much of U.S. manufacturing has made a dramatic shift from well-regulated, high-wage, often unionized plants to low-wage, unregulated, and nonunion plants in the developing world. In turn, workers in developing countries have often been subjected to high noise and temperature levels, unguarded machinery, and other safety hazards. In countries such as Indonesia and Guatemala, limited or no safety regulations exist within occupational settings. Other countries, such as China or Mexico, may have safety regulations, but they may not be fully enforced. One problem in Mexico and some other countries is the nation's level of international indebtedness to private banks, the World Bank, and the International Monetary Fund. This results in a level of national dependency on foreign investment, which discourages the host country from pushing for occupational health policies.

Hashim and Bofetta (2014) report from research studies that there is a decline in cancers attributable to environmental and occupational carcinogens such as asbestos, arsenic, and indoor and outdoor air pollution in most developed countries, but for those living in developing countries, the pollution is likely to grow and thereby cause an increase in some cancers due to pollution. These individuals are at greater risk for asbestos exposure due to a lapse in industrial cleanliness, effective protective legislation, and lack of education about asbestos handling. Countries accounting for the world's greatest asbestos consumption include Russia, China, India, Kazakhstan, Ukraine, Thailand, Brazil, and Iran.

All forms of asbestos are now banned in 52 countries, including all of the European Union. Despite all that is known about the health dangers of asbestos, the annual world production continues. More than 2 million tons are still produced annually. Russia is the world's leading producer, followed by China, Kazakhstan, Brazil, Canada, Zimbabwe, and Colombia. International agencies such as WHO have called for a worldwide ban (LaBour et al., 2010).

Municipal solid waste handling and disposal has become a great public health concern for workers employed in this area as well as for the general environment of a community. Because these workers are exposed to many pathogens and toxic substances from the waste itself and from its decomposition, they suffer significant rates of occupational diseases. A study conducted in Athens, Greece, concluded that respiratory diseases are significantly increased in these workers (Athanasiou, Makrynos, & Dounias, 2010).

Occupational healthcare reform in the Russian Federation is urgently needed and occupational diseases of Russian workers are 10 to 100 times higher than reported by official statistics. Annually, 190,000 workers who are employed in dangerous and hazardous industries die from occupational environmental problems and injuries. Russian employers are not legally held accountable for neglecting safety rules and for underreporting of occupational diseases (ODs). Almost 80% of all Russian industrial enterprises are considered dangerous or hazardous for health. Hygienic control of working conditions is minimal or totally excluded in the working environments. (Dudarev & Odland, 2013).

Safety of Healthcare Providers

Healthcare facilities around the world employ over 59 million workers who are exposed to a complex variety of health and safety hazards everyday including:

- Biological hazards, such as TB, hepatitis, HIV/AIDS, SARS.
- Chemical hazards, such as glutaraldehyde, ethylene oxide.
- Physical hazards, such as noise, radiation, slips, trips, and falls.
- Ergonomic hazards, such as heavy lifting.
- Psychosocial hazards, such as shiftwork, violence, and stress.
- Fire and explosion hazards, such as using oxygen, alcohol sanitizing gels.
- Electrical hazards, such as frayed electrical cords.

Healthcare workers (HCWs) need protection from these workplace hazards just as much as mining or construction workers do. Yet, because their job is to care for the sick and injured, HCWs are often viewed as "immune" to injury or illness. Their patients come first. They are often expected to sacrifice their own well-being for the sake of their patients. Indeed, protecting HCWs has the added benefit of contributing to quality patient care and health system strengthening. Some of the same measures used to protect patients from infections, such as adequate staffing, can protect HCWs from injury (WHO, 2014e).

In the United States, needlestick injuries have decreased from 1 million exposures in 1996 to 385,000 exposures in 2000. This decline has resulted from the development and application of OSHA's blood-borne pathogens standard. The success in decreasing needlesticks may largely be attributed to the elimination of needle recapping and the use of safer needle devices, sharps collection boxes, gloves and personal protective gear, as well as other universal precautions. Increased risk for HIV from needlesticks can result from deep injury, visible blood on the device, high viral titer status of the patient (especially a newly infected patient), a patient in the terminal state, and the device being used to access an artery or vein. The U.S. surveillance for healthcare workers identified the following devices as being responsible for most needle-stick injuries:

- Hypodermic needles (32%)
- Suture needles (19%)
- Winged steel needles (butterflies) (12%)
- Scalpel blades (7%)
- IV and catheter needles (6%)
- Phlebotomy needles (3%)

The most common circumstances that cause injuries involve hollow-bore needles, which can be filled with blood (OSHA, 2014).

The 2014 Ebola virus disease outbreak poses serious health risks for workers in various occupations and has had a significant occupational mortality, especially among HCWs. These casualties add to the global shortage of health workers, which particularly affects the countries experiencing this outbreak. Within its mandate, ILO is collaborating with the WHO in specific activities to address important occupational safety and health and other issues arising out of this outbreak in relation to the world of work (CDC, 2014i).

Job Stress

In the American workplace, 25% of employees view their jobs as the number one stressor in their lives. Job stress can be defined as the harmful physical and emotional responses that happen when the requirements of the job do not match the capabilities, resources, or needs of the worker, leading to poor health or injury.

Job stress is not the same as job challenge, which often energizes workers. Possible causes of job stress include differences in the individual personality and coping styles as well as certain working conditions of the job itself. Certain jobs may be more likely to lead to stress than other jobs. Factors that lead to stress on the job include the following:

- Heavy workloads
- Infrequent rest breaks
- Long working hours
- Shift work
- Routine tasks that have little inherent meaning
- Having little or no participation in decision making
- Poor communication in the organization
- Insensitivity to family needs
- Conflicting or uncertain job expectations
- Too much responsibility
- Job insecurity
- Unpleasant or dangerous physical conditions such as crowding, noise, or air pollution

Healthcare expenses are 50% greater for workers who report high levels of job stress. An increase in job stress may result in an increase in risk for any or several of the following conditions (CDC, 2014h):

- Cardiovascular disease
- Musculoskeletal disorders
- Psychological disorders
- Workplace injuries
- Suicide
- Cancer
- Ulcers
- Impaired immune function

Some employers assume that stressful working conditions are expected and that companies must constantly increase the pressure on workers so that they will remain productive and profitable. In reality, stress in the workplace is often associated with greater absenteeism, tardiness, and job quitting. Low morale, health and job complaints, and employee turnover often are the first signs of job stress. Remedies for job stress include stress management and employee assistant programs to help employees cope with difficult work, personal stressors, and organizational change. Employers also need to work with their employees to solve problems early before they become too large, causing greater damage to workers or the company (CDC, 2014h).

Reproductive Health

Job stress and workplace hazards can cause problems related to reproductive health in employees. Such reproductive disorders may include developmental disorders, spontaneous abortion, low birth weight, preterm birth, and congenital anomalies. Other potential disorders include reduced fertility, infertility, impotence, and menstrual disorders.

Occupational Lung Disease

Many occupational lung diseases are related to a specific occupation or exposure to hazardous materials, such as asbestosis, coal workers' pneumoconiosis (black lung), silicosis (exposure to fine sand as in ceramic workers), berylliosis, byssinosis (brown lung, exposure to raw cotton), and farmer's lung. Workplace exposures can cause or worsen adult-onset asthma, chronic obstructive pulmonary disease (COPD), which encompasses emphysema and chronic bronchitis, and lung cancer (CDC, 2014j).

Occupational lung cancer is the most frequent occupational cancer and is caused by exposure to substances such as asbestos, arsenic, chloroethers, chromates, ionizing radiation, nickel, and polynuclear aromatic hydrocarbons. NIOSH estimates that millions of workers are exposed to substances that have been tested and found to be cancer-causing, although only 2% of all chemicals in commerce have undergone such testing. These occupational exposures account for about 10.3% of lung cancer cases worldwide. An estimated 14% of COPD is due to occupational exposure (CDC, 2014j).

Occupational or work-related asthma is the most common form of occupational lung disease. An estimated 15 to 23% of new adult asthma cases in the United States are due to occupational exposures. These exposures in the workplace also can worsen preexisting asthma. Symptoms usually occur while the worker is exposed at work but, in some cases, they develop several hours after the person leaves work and then subside before the worker returns to the job. In later stages of the disease, symptoms can occur away from work after exposure to common lung irritants such as air pollution or dust (CDC, 2014j).

Other occupational lung diseases that threaten workers include:

- *Asbestosis*: This progressive disease, which causes scarring on lung tissue, is caused by exposure to asbestos. In the United States, 1.3 million employees in construction and industry have had exposures to asbestos on the job, and in 2002 there were 6,343 deaths from asbestosis.
- *Black lung disease (pneumoconiosis)*: This chronic occupational lung disease is caused by the prolonged breathing of coal mine dust, which contains silica and carbon. Approximately 1 of every 20 U.S. miners studied has X-ray evidence of black lung disease. For some miners, the disease evolves into a more severe form, called progressive massive fibrosis. Black lung disease is not reversible, and there is no specific treatment for it (CDC, 2014j).
- *Brown lung disease (byssinosis)*: This is a chronic obstruction of the small airways in the lungs, causing impaired lung function. It occurs when a worker breathes dust from hemp, flax, and cotton processing. In the United States, more than 30,000 textile workers have been affected by this problem.
- *Silicosis*: This disease results from exposure to free crystalline silica in mines, in blasting operations, and in stone, clay, and glass manufacturing. The silica causes scar tissue in the lungs and increases the risk of TB.
- *Hypersensitivity pneumonitis*: This disease results from exposure to fungus spores from moldy hay, bird droppings, or other organic dust. These contaminants inflame the lung sacs, create scar tissue, and decrease lung functioning (CDC, 2014j).

All forms of asbestos are now banned in 52 countries worldwide, having been replaced with safer products. Nonetheless, a significant number of countries continue to use, import, and export asbestos. All forms of asbestos cause asbestosis, a fibrotic lung disease, as well as malignant mesothelioma, lung and laryngeal cancers, and potentially ovarian, gastrointestinal, and other cancers. Approximately 125 million people globally are exposed to asbestos in their working environments today, and many more have had such exposures in previous years. NIOSH estimates that current rates of exposure to asbestos will lead to five deaths from lung cancer and two deaths from asbestosis for every 1,000 workers who are exposed to asbestos during their lifetime. In the United Kingdom, at least 3,500 people die each year from this exposure, and this number may increase to 5,000 deaths per year in the future (CDC, 2014j).

In Asian countries such as China and India, there is ongoing use of asbestos despite substantial evidence of the link, even at low-level exposure, between this substance and the development of pulmonary fibrosis and lung cancer in humans. The continued use of this toxic material is allowed by these countries' poor occupational health and safety systems (CDC, 2014j).

Agricultural Safety

Agriculture is one of the most hazardous of all economic sectors, and many agricultural workers suffer occupational accidents and ill health each year. It is also the largest sector for female employment in many countries, especially in Africa and Asia. Agriculture employs approximately 1 billion workers worldwide, or more than one-third of the world's labor force, and accounts for approximately 70% of child labor worldwide (ILO, 2014).

Farmers are at high risk for both fatal and nonfatal injuries. Leading causes of agricultural machinery injuries include entanglements, being pinned or stuck by machinery, falls, and runovers. Nonmachinery injuries include falls from heights, animal-related trauma, and being stuck against objects. Frequently encountered injuries include limb fractures, open wounds, intracranial (head) injuries, and spinal cord injuries. Workers in agriculture have double the mortality rates because of inadequate training and safety systems. In the United States, agriculture workers make up only 3% of the workforce but account for almost 8% of all work-related accidents. In Italy, 9% of the workforce is farm workers, but they account for 28.9% of work-related injuries. In this setting, the greatest dangers are posed by cutting tools and machinery such as tractors and harvesters, and exposure to pesticides and other chemicals.

Facts related to safety in U.S. farming, as provided by the NIOSH (2014), include the following:

- Approximately 1,854,000 full-time workers were employed in production agriculture in 2012.
- An estimated 955,000 youth under 20 years of age resided on farms in 2012, with about 472,000 youth performing farm work. In addition to the youth who live on farms, an estimated 259,000 youth were hired to work on U.S. farms in 2012.
- In 2012, 374 farmers and farm workers died from a work-related injury, resulting in a fatality rate of 20.2 deaths per 100,000 workers. Tractor overturns were the leading cause of death for these farmers and farm workers.
- The most effective way to prevent tractor overturn deaths is the use of a Roll Over Protective Structure (ROPS). In 2012, 59% of tractors used on U.S. farms were equipped with ROPS. If ROPS were placed on all the tractors manufactured since the mid-1960s that are used on these farms, the prevalence of ROPS-equipped tractors could be increased to over 80%.
- On average, 113 youth under 20 years of age die annually from farm-related injuries (1995–2002), with most of these deaths occurring to youth 16 to 19 (34%).
- Of the leading sources of fatal injuries to youth, 23% involved machinery (including tractors), 19% involved motor vehicles (including ATVs), and 16% were due to drowning.
- Every day, about 167 agricultural workers suffer a lost-work-time injury. Five percent of these injuries result in permanent impairment.
- In 2012, an estimated 14,000 youth were injured on farms; 2,700 of these injuries were due to farm work.

Study Questions

1. How do culture, politics, geography, and economics play roles in violence within a community?

2. Why do populations in developing countries as compared to developed countries have higher death rates from road traffic accidents?
3. What is the relationship between domestic violence and school violence for an individual child?
4. What are some occupational health hazards related to mining and manufacturing?
5. Explain why farming can be hazardous to a person's health.
6. How do "honor killings" and female genital mutilation relate to culture and health for women?

Case Study 1: Alliance Ntakwinja (Democratic Republic of Congo)

A 22 year old married woman with two children, living in the Democratic Republic of Congo revealed that she was raped by four men who came to her house. Her husband was home and they took him outside and tied him to a tree. Later she was taken to a local hospital where she spent three weeks recovering from her injuries. Other women who were on the same hospital ward were also raped with subsequent injuries. An organization called Women to Women funded by Soroptimist International, later contacted her and she was able to get job training making soap, which financially helps her entire family. This organization helps women survivors rebuild their lives and is committed to end violence to women and girls by raising awareness about violence against women and advocating for governments to be accountable and responsible for protecting women and girls. This organization gives refuge, protection and rehabilitation for women who have experienced violence, which includes safe housing and mental health care.

Case Study 1 Questions

1. Within the context of culture, what are the implications of rape for this woman, her family, and her community?
2. What could be done to prevent this situation from happening? What are the barriers to overcome?

Data from Harvey, M. (2013). ENOUGH IS ENOUGH: End Violence Against Women. Initial results on prevalence, health outcomes and women's responses. Global Day of Action on International Women's Day. *Soroptimist International. This case study appears with kind permission of Women for Women International, who help women survivors of war rebuild their lives. To find out more about their work and sponsorship, visit www.womenforwomen.org. Interview by Nicola York.*

Case Study 2: Women and Suicide in China

Background

China accounts for 26% of all suicides worldwide. Suicide is the fifth-leading cause of death in the country overall and is the leading cause of death for young women in the country. Suicide is four to five times more frequent in rural settings than in urban ones. Suicide rates are higher among women than among men in China (WHO, 2009b).

Situation

Zhang Xihuan, a 45-year-old woman with hepatitis B, was building a new home and needed to borrow extra money for the project. Her debt from her out-of-pocket health expenditures, as well as from her house loan, gave her great anxiety and depression. The shame of not being able to pay her bills and owing money caused her to make a quick decision to end her life by drinking a bottled pesticide. The cultural shame of owing money and the overwhelming burden of her disease both contributed to her decision to end her life.

Case Study 2 Questions

1. Explain the contributing factors in Mrs. Zhang's behavior.
2. Which types of political, social, economic, and cultural-based interventions are needed to decrease this sort of violence in China?
3. Why are rural women more prone to suicide than urban men?
4. Why is China a higher risk area for suicide than other areas of the world?

Data from World Health Organization. (2009b). Women and suicide in rural China. *Bulletin of the WHO*, *87*(12), 885–964.

References

A killing sets honor above love. (2010, November 21). *New York Times*, p. 9.

American Lung Association. (2005). *Occupational lung disease fact sheet*. Retrieved from http://www.lungusa
.org/site/pp.as[?c=dv:IL9O0E&b=35334

Athanasiou, M., Makrynos, G., & Dounias, G. (2010). Respiratory health of municipal solid waste workers. *Occupational Medicine* [Advance access publication on September 5, 2010]. doi:10.1093/occmed/Kqq127

Azizi, M. H. (2010). Occupational noise-induced hearing loss. *International Journal of Occupational and Environmental Medicine 1*(3), 118–123.

Bhalla, K., Li, Q., Duan, L., Wang, Y., Bishai, D., & Hyder, A. (2013). The prevalence of speeding and drunk driving in two cities in China: A mid-project evaluation of ongoing road safety interventions. *Injury, 44*. Supp. 4. S49–56.

Bullying statistics/cyberbullying statistics/school bullying (n.d.). Retrieved from http://www.how-to-stop-bullying.com/bullyingstatistics.html

Centers for Disease Control and Prevention. (2010a). *Child passenger safety: Fact sheet*. Retrieved from http://www.cdc.gov/MotorVehicleSfety/Child_Passenger_Safety/CPS-Factsheet.html

Centers for Disease Control and Prevention. (2010b). *Elder maltreatment fact sheet*. Retrieved from http://www.cdc.gov/violenceprevention

Centers for Disease Control and Prevention. (2010c). *Understanding school violence: Fact sheet*. Retrieved from http://www.cdc.gov/ViolencePrevention/pdf/SchoolViolence_FactSheet-a.pdf

Centers for Disease Control and Prevention. (2010d). *World report on violence and health*. Retrieved from http://www.cdc.gov/violenceprevention

Centers for Disease Control and Prevention. (2014a). *Worldwide injuries and violence*. Retrieved from http://www.cdc.gov/injury/global/

Centers for Disease Control and Prevention. (2014b). *Intimate partner violence*. Retrieved from http://www.cdc.gov/violenceprevention/intimatepartnerviolence/

Centers for Disease Control and Prevention. (2014c). *Child maltreatment: Data sources*. Retrieved from http://www.cdc.gov/violenceprevention/childmaltreatment/datasources.html

Centers for Disease Control and Prevention. (2014d). *About school violence*. Retrieved from http://www.cdc.gov/violenceprevention/youthviolence/schoolviolence/

Centers for Disease Control and Prevention. (2014e). *War-related injury prevention*. Retrieved from http://www.cdc.gov/nceh/publications/factsheets/War-relatedInjuryPrevention.pdf

Centers for Disease Control and Prevention. (2014f). *Injury prevention and control*. Retrieved from http://www.cdc.gov/injury/

Centers for Disease Control and Prevention. (2014g). *Alcohol and public health: Alcohol-related disease impact (ARDI)*. Retrieved from http://apps.nccd.cdc.gov/DACH_ARDI/Default/Default.aspx

Centers for Disease Control and Prevention. (2014h). *Occupational safety and health risks*. Retrieved from http://www.cdc.gov/niosh/programs/global/risks.html

Centers for Disease Control and Prevention. (2014i). *Ebola*. Retrieved from http://www.cdc.gov/vhf/ebola/hcp/safety-training-course/

Centers for Disease Control and Prevention. (2014j). *Occupational respiratory disease surveillance*. Retrieved from http://www.cdc.gov/niosh/topics/surveillance/ords/

Dalal, K., Lin, Z., Gifford, M., & Svanström, L. (2013). Economics of global burden of road traffic injuries and their relationship with health system variables. *International Journal of Preventative Medicine* (12), 1442–1450.

Dudarev, A., & Odland, J. (2013). Occupational health and health care in Russia and Russian Arctic: 1980–2010. *International Journal of Circumpolar Health, 72*. Retrieved from http://www.circumpolarhealthjournal.net/index.php/ijch/article/view/20456

Gostin, L., Sapssin, J., Teret, S., Burris, S., Mair, J., Hodge, J., & Vernick, J. (2002). The model state emergency health powers act: Planning for and response to bioterrorism and naturally occurring infectious diseases. *Journal of the American Medical Association, 288*(5), 622–628.

Gradus, J. (2007). *Epidemiology of PTSD*. National Center for PTSD, U.S. Department of Veteran Affairs. Retrieved from http://www.ptsd.va.gov/professional/pages/epidemiological-facts-ptsd.asp

Guazzi, M., Faggiano, P., Mureddu, G., Faden, G., Niebauer, J., & Temporelli, P. (2014). Worksite health and wellness in the European Union. *Progress in cardiovascular diseases. 56*(5), 508–514. doi:10.1016/j.pcad.2013.11.003

Harvey, M. (2013). *ENOUGH IS ENOUGH: End violence against women. Initial results on prevalence, health outcomes and women's responses*. Global Day of Action on International Women's Day. Soroptimist International.

Hashim, S., & Boffetta, P. (2014). Occupational and environmental exposures and cancers in developing countries. *Annals of Global Health, 80*(5), 393–411.

Hofman, K., Primack, A., Keusch, G., & Hrynkow, S. (2005). Addressing the growing burden of trauma and injury in low- and middle-income countries. *American Journal of Public Health, 95*(1), 13–17.

International Labour Organization. (2013). *Global employment trends*. Retrieved from http://ilo.org/global/research/global-reports/global-employment-trends/2013/lang--en/index.htm

Krug, E. G., Dahlberg, L. L., Mercy, J. A., Zwi, A. B., & Lozano, R. (2002). Summary. In *World Report on Violence and Health* (pp. 1–37). Geneva, Switzerland: World Health Organization.

LaBour, J., Castleman, B., Frank, A., Gochfeld, M., Greenberg, M., Huff, J., . . . Watterson, A. (2010). The case for global ban on asbestos. *Environmental Health Perspectives, 118*(7), 897–901.

Mahendra, R., Roehler, D., & Degutis, L. (2012). CDC Injury center at 20 years: Celebrating the past, protecting the future. *Journal of Safety Research, 43*(4), 227–326.

Mayo Clinic. (2014). *Post-traumatic stress disorder*. Retrieved from http://www.mayoclinic.org/diseases-conditions/post-traumatic-stress-disorder/basics/definition/con-20022540

National Institute for Occupational Safety and Health. (2014). *Agricultural safety*. Retrieved from http://www.cdc.gov/niosh/topics/aginjury/default.html.

NationMaster. (2010). Crime statistics: Murders per capita most recent by country. Retrieved from http://www.nationmaster.com/graph/cri_mur;erca;-crime-murders-per-capita

Okamura, T., Sugiyama, D., Tanaka, T., & Dohi, S. (2014). Worksite Wellness for the Primary and Secondary Prevention of Cardiovascular Disease in Japan: The Current Delivery System and Future Directions. *Progress in Cardiovascular Diseases, 56*(5), 515–521. doi:10.1016/j.pcad.2013.09.011

Occupational Safety and Health Administration. (2014). *What is occupational safety and health administration (OSHA)?* Retrieved from http://searchcompliance.techtarget.com/definition/Occupational-Safety-and-Health-Administration-OSHA

Radim, R., Binkova, B., Dejmek, J., & Bobak, M. (2005). Ambient air pollution and pregnancy outcomes: A review of the literature. *Environmental Health Perspectives, 113*(4), 375–382.

Safe Horizon. (2014). *Domestic violence: Statistics and facts.* Retrieved from http://www.safehorizon.org/page/domestic-violence-statistics--facts-52.html

Simon, T., & Hurvitz, K. (2014). Healthy people 2020 objectives for violence prevention and the role of nursing, *The Online Journal of Issues in Nursing, 19*(1). doi:10.3912/OJIN.Vol19No01Man01

Sousa, C. (2013). Political violence, health, and coping among Palestinian women in the West Bank. *American Journal of Orthopsychiatry, 83*(4), 505–519.

Stockman, J., Lucea, M., & Campbell, J. (2013). Forced sexual initiation, sexual intimate partner violence and HIV risk in women: A global review of the literature. *AIDS Behavior. 17*(3), 832–847. doi:10.1007/s10461-012-0361-4.

United Nations. (2012). *UN Office of Drugs and Crime. World drug report.* Retrieved from http://www.unodc.org/unodc/data-and-analysis/WDR-2012.html

Van Parys, A., Verhamme, A., Temmerman, M., Verstraelen, H. (2014). Intimate partner violence and pregnancy: A systematic review of interventions. *PLOS One.* Retrieved from http://www.plosone.org/article/info%3Adoi%2F10.1371%2Fjournal.pone.0085084

Watkins, K., & Sridhar, D. (2009). *Road Traffic Injuries: The Hidden Development Crisis: Making Roads Safe.* First Ministerial Conference on Road Safety. Moscow.

Wolf, A., Gray, R., & Fazel, S. (2014). Violence as a public health problem: An ecological study of 169 countries. *Social Science & Medicine, 104,* 220–227. doi:10.1016/j.socscimed.2013.12.006

The World Bank. (2014). *Intentional homicides.* Retrieved from http://data.worldbank.org/indicator/VC.IHR.PSRC.P5

World Health Organization. (2005b). *Multi-Country Study on Women's Health and Domestic Violence Against Women* (pp. 1–28). Geneva, Switzerland: Author.

World Health Organization. (2009a). *Global Status Report on Road Safety* (pp. 1–43). Geneva, Switzerland: Author.

World Health Organization. (2009b). Women and suicide in rural China. *Bulletin of the WHO, 87*(12), 885–964.

World Health Organization. (2014a). *Preventing suicide: A global imperative.* Retrieved from http://www.who.int/mental_health/suicide-prevention/world_report_2014/en/

World Health Organization. (2014b). *Violence and injury protection.* Retrieved from http://www.who.int/violence_injury_prevention/en/

World Health Organization. (2014c). *Poisoning prevention and management.* Retrieved from http://www.who.int/ipcs/poisons/en

World Health Organization. (2014d). *Drowning.* Retrieved from http://www.who.int/mediacentre/factsheets/fs347/en/

World Health Organization. (2014e). *Occupational health.* Retrieved from http://www.who.int/occupational_health/en/

Zhang, J., Norton, R., Tang, K., Lo, S., Zhuo, J., & Wenkui, G. (2004). Motorcycle ownership and injury in China. *Injury Control and Safety Promotion, 11*(3), 159–163.

14

Global Perspectives on Nutrition

Carol Holtz
Marvin A. Friedman
Emily Peoples

Objectives

After completing this chapter, the reader will be able to:

1. Compare and contrast good and poor nutrition in developed and developing nations.
2. Discuss the "human right to food."
3. List the nutritional challenges for the 21st century.
4. Discuss types of nutritional deficiencies, including iron-deficiency anemia and niacin, vitamin A, vitamin B, iodine, and zinc micronutrient deficiencies.
5. Explain protein–energy malnutrition.
6. Discuss obesity in developing and developed countries.
7. Discuss the role of fiber in good nutrition.
8. Compare and contrast food safety and security worldwide in developed and developing countries.
9. Discuss the worldwide relationship between poverty and nutrition levels.
10. Define and discuss food emergencies.
11. Compare and contrast nutritional challenges among developed and developing countries.
12. Describe the worldwide nutritional challenges of childbearing women.
13. Discuss the worldwide challenges of nutrition in older adults.
14. Discuss the clinical examples regarding nutritional challenges.

INTRODUCTION

Good nutrition is the basis for health, for people of all developmental levels, and for infant and children's growth and development. In addition, it is correlated to a more effective immune system and reduction of a number of diseases. In considering nutritional status, two classes of nutrients are distinguished: macronutrients and micronutrients. Macronutrients make up the bulk of the diet and consist of fats, starches, and protein (amino acids); they primarily provide energy. Micronutrients are frequently enzyme cofactors or catalyze other reactions; they are required in much smaller amounts than macronutrients.

Despite the incentives to overcome malnutrition, it continues to be a worldwide problem for all countries, affecting about one third of the world's population. Some forms of malnutrition, such as stunting, are showing modest but uneven declines; other forms, such as anemia in women of reproductive age, are unchanged. Yet other problems, such as overweight and obesity, are increasing.

Traditionally the World Health Organization (WHO) focused on the issue of deficiencies induced by disease, but more recently the agenda for both developing and developed countries is the improvement of global nutrition related to overnutrition, especially obesity. Worldwide, obesity and malnutrition are leading causes of such chronic diseases as cardiovascular disease, cancer, hypertension, and diabetes. Deficiency diseases include scurvy, a vitamin C deficiency; blindness that results from vitamin A deficiency; kwashiorkor, a protein deficiency; goiter, an iodine deficiency; pellagra, a niacin deficiency; anemia that results from an iron deficiency; vitamin B_{12}, or folic acid, deficiency; and many more. Significant morbidity, mortality, and economic costs are associated with these kinds of nutritional imbalances (WHO, 2014).

Despite the incentives to overcome malnutrition, it remains a problem of staggering size worldwide. Malnutrition affects all countries. Almost one in three people on the planet experience it. For every country it represents a substantial drag on sustainable development. Efforts to combat it are gathering momentum and are beginning to deliver results, but turning the tide of decades of neglect will not be easy. While some forms of malnutrition, such as stunting, are showing modest but uneven declines, other forms, such as anemia in women of reproductive age, are stagnant. And still others, such as overweight and obesity, are increasing.

Malnutrition is considered to be the world's leading threat to life and health today. The following is a common scenario: An infant has marginal macronutrient intake, usually as a result of maternal milk supply drawing to an end. The infant then develops diarrhea from an intestinal parasite or other infectious agent. This disease is promoted by low immune response from macronutrient deficiency. Unable to stop the consequent water–sodium imbalance, the infant dies of dehydration. Even if the infant survives, the long-term consequences of this bout with disease can be catastrophic.

It is difficult to imagine living on less than $1 per day, yet 1.2 billion people in the world do so. With this limited amount of income, it is very difficult to maintain a healthy and adequate diet. Every day 24,000 people worldwide die from hunger and malnutrition, the majority of whom are young children as described in the preceding scenario. In addition to macronutrient deficiency, nearly 33% of the world suffers from micronutrient malnutrition, which results in the following problems:

- Decreased mental and physical development
- Poor pregnancy outcomes

- Decreased work capacity for adults
- Increased illness
- Premature death
- Diseases
- Deficiencies in zinc, leading to immune deficiency, growth retardation, and diarrhea
- Bone loss
- Blindness (WHO, 2014)

OBTAINING A NUTRITIONAL ASSESSMENT

Dietary habits, cooking methodology, and soil composition vary within the world's geographic locations and tend to result in different nutritional deficiencies (Tsang, Sullivan, Ruth, Williams, & Suchdeov, 2014). The ability to produce an accurate nutritional assessment continues to be a challenge. Nutritional excesses are frequently appearing globally with different outcomes, and it is difficult to differentiate between the influence of overnutrition resulting in obesity, as well as the relationship of excess iron intake and decreased intelligence (Senior, Charleston, Lihoreau, Buhl, Raubenheimer, & Simpson, 2015). The primary concerns for nutritionists are the nutritional deficiencies resulting in chronic health issues, which include the impact on behavior, immunology, birthweight and neonatal survival, and obesity, which are the subjects of current research. These topics are often difficult to quantify.

Many regulatory agencies publish what are called "market basket surveys," which enable researchers to identify and quantitate what people eat (Callan, Hinwood, & Devine, 2014). Once the nutrient content is determined, these market baskets yield knowledge regarding nutrient uptake. Another way to accomplish surveys on population eating is by diet recall, asking people to recall what they have eaten within one day, seven days, or 28 days (Cremaschini et al., 2015). The short one-day questionnaire is more accurate as compared to extended days recall. People can more accurately remember what they ate yesterday as compared to a week or longer period of time.

WHO indicates a need for improvement in the global nutrition of women and children and created the following goals:

Global Nutrition Targets for 2025 (WHO, 2014)
1. Reduce stunting by 40% in children under five
2. Reduce anemia by 50% in women of reproductive age
3. Decrease low-birth-weight babies by 30%
4. No increase in overweight children
5. Increase the rate of exclusive breastfeeding in the first six months up to at least 50%
6. Reduce and maintain childhood wasting to less than 5%

FREEDOM FROM HUNGER: A HUMAN RIGHT

In the International Covenant on Economic, Social and Cultural Rights (ICESCR), freedom from hunger is described as a human right. More specifically it was agreed, "The right to food is a human right inherent in all people, to have regular permanent and unrestricted access, either directly or by means of financial purchases, to have quantitatively and qualitatively adequate and sufficient food corresponding to the cultural traditions of people to which the consumer belongs, is one that ensures a physical and mental, individual and collective fulfilling and dignified life free of fear" (UN Committee on Economic, Social and Cultural Rights [CESCR], 1999, p. 3). The signatory parties to this agreement concluded that the right to adequate food is linked to the inherent dignity of the human person. Furthermore, "the right to adequate food is realized with every man, woman and child, alone or in community with others, having physical access at all times to adequate food or means for its procurement" (CESCR, 1999, p. 3).

In addition, a human rights framework was addressed by the Universal Declaration of Human Rights, which was adopted by the United Nations in 1948. According to this document, to fulfill the right to food is to not interfere with one's ability to acquire food. To protect the right to food is to make sure that others do not interfere with the right to food. The right to food and the right to be free from hunger are outlined in article 25 of the Universal Declaration of Human Rights, which describes a minimum standard of living that includes the right to housing, clothing, health care, and social services. To fulfill the right to food, it is necessary to facilitate social and economic environments that foster human development and to provide food to people in an emergency or in circumstances when they are unable to provide for food by themselves (CESCR, 1999).

Today, not only are there problems from lack of quantity and quality of food to satisfy the dietary needs of individuals, that is, food that is both free from adverse substances and acceptable—but there are also worldwide issues with overnutrition (obesity). Overweight or obesity are prevalent global problems, and increasing numbers from emerging or transition economy nations are now facing health challenges related to these issues similar to the problems encountered by the developed world. Overweight and obesity in both developed and developing nations are creating chronic health problems and costing these countries' economies hundreds of millions of dollars (WHO, 2015a). This is an even more extreme problem among individuals migrating from global areas where food is not available, to developed countries where overeating is easy.

WHO's Nutrition for Health Development established major goals at the World Summit for Children in 1990 and the International Conference on Nutrition in 1992, which with some modification in 2003, were still relevant in 2015. They include the elimination of the following:

- Famine and related deaths
- Starvation and nutritional deficiency diseases caused by natural and human-made disasters
- Iodine and vitamin A deficiency

In addition, these goals called for reduction of the following:

- Starvation and widespread hunger
- Undernutrition, especially in women, children, and the aged
- Other micronutrient deficiencies, such as iron deficiency

- Diet-related communicable and noncommunicable diseases
- Barriers to breastfeeding
- Poor sanitation, hygiene, and unclean drinking water

Strategies for implementing these goals include the following measures:

- Developing new nutritional health policies and programs
- Improving household food security
- Improving food quality and safety
- Preventing and treating infectious diseases
- Promoting breastfeeding
- Promoting diets with micronutrient supplements
- Assessing and monitoring nutritional programs

Stunting and low-body-weight problems are due to persistent undernutrition. The combination of food distribution imbalance, rising fuel costs, and the global financial crisis beginning in 2007 has had negative impacts on global nutrition. The question is how long these crises will last and how they will affect food availability. Of particular interest is the U.S. Environmental Protection Agency's (USEPA's) and Brazilian government's requirement that a percentage of corn production be allocated for ethanol production, which will likely result in a substantial increase in food and livestock costs (USEPA, 2010).

TYPES OF NUTRITIONAL CHALLENGES

Micronutrient Deficiencies

Micronutrient deficiencies are widespread among 2 billion people worldwide. These are silent epidemics of vitamin and mineral deficiencies affecting people globally of all genders, races, and geographic locations. Not only do they cause specific diseases, but they also exacerbate infectious and chronic diseases, thereby affecting morbidity, mortality, and quality of life. Deficiencies related to chronic diseases include osteoporosis, osteomalacia, thyroid deficiency, colorectal cancer, and cardiovascular disease. Consumption of folic acid and fortified foods by pregnant women is well known to prevent many congenital malformations and cognitive impairments. Deficiencies in micronutrients increase the severity of illnesses such as HIV/AIDS and tuberculosis (Tulchinsky, 2010).

Micronutrient deficiencies include deficiencies of iron, iodine, and vitamin A as well as zinc, folate, and other B vitamins. In many settings, more than one micronutrient deficiency exists, which necessitates interventions that address multiple micronutrient deficiencies. Areas of prevalence are especially extensive in Southeast Asia and Sub-Saharan Africa. These deficiencies are mainly caused by inadequate food intake, poor quality of foods, poor bioavailability because of inhibitors, types of preparation, and presence of infections, especially as a result of poor water quality (WHO, 2015b).

Iodine Deficiency Disorders

Iodine deficiency is the world's most prevalent, yet easily preventable, cause of brain damage. Today we are on the verge of eliminating it—an achievement that will be hailed as a major public health triumph that ranks with getting rid of smallpox and poliomyelitis. Iodine deficiency disorders (IDD), which can start before birth, jeopardize children's mental health and often their very survival. Serious iodine deficiency during pregnancy can result in stillbirth, spontaneous abortion, and congenital abnormalities such as cretinism, a grave, irreversible form of mental retardation that affects people living in iodine-deficient areas of Africa and Asia. However, of far greater significance is IDD's less visible, yet pervasive, mental impairment that reduces intellectual capacity at home, in school, and at work. A simple solution is to add iodized salt to the diet (WHO, 2015b). Iodizing table salt is one of the best and least expensive methods of preventing IDD. The target is the elimination of IDD through universal salt iodization. Progress has been dramatic since the primary intervention strategy for IDD control with the universal salt iodization, adopted in 1993. Salt was chosen because it is widely available and consumed in regular amounts throughout the year, and because the cost of iodizing it is extremely low for about US$0.05 per person per year. This solution has been implemented in most countries where iodine deficiency is a public health problem. Globally, UNICEF estimates that 66% of households now have access to iodized salt (WHO, 2015b).

Iron-Deficiency Anemia

Iron deficiency is the most widespread nutrient deficiency in the world, affecting more than two billion people. It is best known for causing anemia, a condition in which the body manufactures an inadequate number of red blood cells. Although iron deficiency is the main cause of anemia, other causes may be related to nutrient deficiencies such as vitamin B_{12} and folic acid, as well as nonnutritional causes such as malaria, genetic abnormalities (thalassemia), and chronic disease. Iron deficiency, which is diagnosed based on low hemoglobin or hematocrit levels, develops over time. Populations especially vulnerable to iron-deficiency anemia are young children and women of childbearing age.

When a person experiences decreased numbers of red blood cells, which normally carry oxygen throughout the body, the individual has a decreased oxygen level and develops symptoms of weakness and fatigue. This problem has profound effects on infants and children by limiting learning capacity and impairing the immune system.

Within the region of Southeast Asia, millions of people are affected by this problem, mainly adolescent girls and childbearing-age women (due to menstruation) and young children. Pregnant women with iron-deficiency anemia are more likely to die in childbirth as a result of postpartum hemorrhage, or to have their fetus or newborn die as a result of decreased oxygen levels in the tissues. Research indicates that children who have this problem have a five- to seven-point reduction in IQ score. The main contributing factors to iron-deficiency anemia include inadequate intake of iron, poor iron availability from cereal-based diets, and high intestinal worm infections. According to WHO, iron-deficiency anemia is second only to tuberculosis as the world's most prevalent and costly health problem. In India and parts of Africa, more than 80% of the population has this condition (Healthline, 2015). Iron supplementation improves iron status during pregnancy and the postpartum period, and infants born to mothers who take iron during pregnancy benefit by being protected from iron-deficiency anemia. Iron-deficiency disorders in pregnant women cause fetal and infant thyroid function alterations. Countries such as China, Pakistan, India, Indonesia, and Ethiopia continue to have insufficient dietary iron intake (Boy et al., 2009).

Signs and symptoms of iron-deficiency anemia include pallor, fatigue, and weakness. Adaptation occurs such that the disease may go unrecognized for a long period of time. In severe cases, patients may have difficulty in breathing. In addition, unusual obsessive cravings, known as pica, may be evident; dirt, white clay, or ice may be consumed. Also, patients may experience hair loss and lightheadedness. Other symptoms may include mouth ulcers, sleepiness, constipation, tinnitus (ringing in the ears), fainting, depression, missed menstrual cycle, heavy menstrual cycle, itching, or poor appetite (National Institutes of Health [NIH], 2012).

Adding micronutrients to such products such as table salt has been practiced for many years to replenish deficient levels of iodine; a form of table salt with iron fortification has also been manufactured to help combat iron-related anemia may also sometimes have a rusty taste.

Niacin Deficiency (Pellagra)

Pellagra, also known as "black tongue," is found among populations who consume corn as the main staple of their diet, a practice often seen in Mexico, northern Italy, and South America. Because corn is deficient in the amino acid tryptophan, and because tryptophan is required for biosynthesis of niacin, these populations are particularly sensitive to niacin deficiency. Signs of niacin deficiency include photosensitivity, red skin lesions, and dementia, and the condition can lead to mortality. Pellagra is easily treated with niacin supplements. Genetically engineered maize that has a high tryptophan content and does not cause pellagra is also available; a Nobel Prize was awarded for the development of this bioagricultural product (WHO, 2015b).

Vitamin A Deficiency

Vitamin A deficiency (VAD) occurs because of inadequate storage of vitamin A, caused either by inadequate intake of food rich in vitamin A or by severe and repeated illnesses. Approximately two billion people in the world are at risk for vitamin A deficiency, along with iodine or iron deficiencies. This problem is especially prevalent in Southeast Asia and Sub-Saharan Africa, and pregnant women and young children are at greatest risk. In many of these areas, more than one micronutrient deficiency exists, so that interventions must address multiple micronutrient deficiencies. Severe vitamin A deficiency is usually associated with signs of night blindness and decreased levels of vitamin A (less than 0.35/dL). Serum retinol is the biochemical indicator of vitamin A status. VAD is the leading cause of preventable blindness in children and increases the risk of disease and death from severe infections. In pregnant women, VAD causes night blindness and may increase the risk of maternal mortality. Vitamin A deficiency is a public health problem in more than 50% of all countries, especially in Africa and Southeast Asia, hitting hardest young children and pregnant women in low-income countries (WHO, 2015b).

Crucial for maternal and child survival, supplying adequate vitamin A in high-risk areas can significantly reduce mortality. Conversely, its absence causes a needlessly high risk of disease and death.

- For children, lack of vitamin A causes severe visual impairment and blindness, and significantly increases the risk of severe illness, and even death, from such common childhood infections as diarrheal disease and measles.
- For pregnant women in high-risk areas, vitamin A deficiency occurs especially during the last trimester when demand by both the unborn child and the mother is highest. The mother's deficiency is demonstrated by the high prevalence of night blindness during this period. The impact of VAD on mother-to-child HIV transmission needs further investigation.
- WHO's goal is the worldwide elimination of vitamin A deficiency and its tragic consequences, including blindness, disease, and premature death. To successfully combat VAD, short-term interventions and proper infant feeding must be backed up by long-term sustainable solutions. The arsenal of nutritional "well-being weapons" includes a combination of breastfeeding and vitamin A supplementation, coupled with enduring solutions, such as promotion of vitamin A-rich diets and food fortification. Food fortification takes over where supplementation leaves off. Food fortification, for example, sugar in Guatemala, maintains vitamin A status, especially for high-risk groups and needy families. For vulnerable rural families, for instance in Africa and Southeast Asia, growing fruits and vegetables in home gardens complements dietary diversification and fortification and contributes to better lifelong health. Vitamin A is available from raw, colored foods such as carrots or tomatoes (WHO, 2015b).

Vitamin D Deficiency

This nutritional deficiency is unique among vitamin deficiencies. Vitamin D is required for the absorption of calcium and translocation to bones and teeth. Deficiency of this micronutrient in children results in rickets, which is a failure of the long bones to mature. In adults, it causes osteoporosis (fragile bones) and osteomalacia (bone thinning). Chronic vitamin D deficiency eventually also causes dermal lesions. What makes this vitamin unique is that the body easily produces a large amount of vitamin D from the reaction of sunlight and sterol (a cholesterol derivative). In the absence of sunlight, the body cannot get enough vitamin D from diet alone. This disease was first seen among nuns in Europe who were always completely covered by their habits and generally worked inside. Now, vitamin D is added to milk, which is the major source of dietary calcium (Pettifor, 2008).

Rickets is a disease widely recognized in many developing countries today. Its origin was identified only in the early part of the 20th century with the discovery of vitamin D, and the advent of ultraviolet light irradiation therapy meant that rickets could be eradicated. Today rickets is still found in some breastfed African American infants, and in Europe it is often found in children of recent immigrants from India, Pakistan and Bangladesh, North Africa, and the Middle East. In the Middle East, vitamin D deficiency and rickets continue to be problems despite abundant all-year sunshine. Infants, adolescent females, and pregnant women are particularly at risk, especially in areas where social and religious customs prevent adequate sunlight exposure of pregnant women and their adolescent daughters (Pettifor, 2008).

Iodine-Deficiency Disorder

Iodine deficiency is the leading cause of preventable brain damage in childhood. Iodine deficiency is found in populations with no access to saltwater fish (seawater is high in iodine) or as a result of consuming vegetables such as broccoli that bind with iodine and make iodine unavailable for absorption. During the last decade, worldwide improvement in the prevalence of this micronutrient deficiency has been realized through low-cost prevention measures such as the iodization of salt (WHO, 2015b).

Under normal conditions the body has small amounts of iodine, housed mainly in the thyroid gland and used for the synthesis of thyroid hormones. Iodine deficiency causes hypothyroidism (goiter), which can lead to the syndrome called iodine-deficiency disorder (IDD). In developed countries, iodine intake correlates with obesity and basal metabolic rate because the hormone requiring iodine—thyroxin—regulates basal metabolism rate.

Worldwide data on urinary iodine levels and goiter are monitored via the WHO's Global Database on Iodine Deficiency Disorders. These disorders comprise deficiencies resulting from decreased intake of the element iodine, which is essential in minute amounts for normal growth and development. Thyroid failure causing irreversible brain damage can occur if the iodine deficiency occurs in the period ranging from fetal life to three months after birth. Iodine deficiency causes a decreased mean IQ loss of 13.5 points in children (WHO, 2015b). During the past century, iodine fortification has been implemented into foods such as bread, milk, water, and salt. Salt has been the most commonly fortified product because it is widely used and available. WHO recommends the addition of 20 to 40 milligrams of iodine per kilogram of salt to meet daily iodine requirements, assuming that the average consumption is 10 grams per day. It is necessary that the iodine content of iodine-fortified foods be monitored during manufacturing to ensure that the prescribed levels are maintained. Iodine fortification is safe, but excessive intake may produce hyperthyroidism. Problems caused by iodine deficiency include goiter, psychomotor defects, impaired mental function, and slow cognitive development. The universal iodization of salt has been very successful in bringing the prevalence of these conditions down in many countries (WHO, 2015b).

Nuclear events, such as the one that occurred in Chernobyl, in the former Soviet Union, cause the production of I^{131}, the radioactive form of iodine. Consumption of this isotope results in thyroid cancer. Similarly, irradiation of the head and neck, as was common in acne therapy in the 1950s, also caused conversion of iodine to I^{131} and a consequent epidemic of thyroid cancer (WHO, 2015b).

Zinc Deficiency

Dietary zinc deficiency is unlikely in healthy persons. Secondary zinc deficiency can develop in the following individuals:

- Patients with hepatic insufficiency (because the ability to retain zinc is lost)
- Patients taking diuretics

- Patients with diabetes mellitus, sickle cell disease, chronic renal failure, or malabsorption problems
- Patients with stressful conditions (e.g., sepsis, burns, head injury)
- Elderly institutionalized and homebound patients (common)

Maternal zinc deficiency can cause fetal malformations and low birth weight. Zinc deficiency in children causes impaired growth and impaired taste (hypogeusia). Other symptoms and signs in children include delayed sexual maturation and hypogonadism. In children or adults, symptoms include alopecia, impaired immunity, anorexia, dermatitis, night blindness, anemia, lethargy, and impaired wound healing. Zinc deficiency should be suspected in undernourished people with typical symptoms or signs. However, because many of these symptoms and signs are non-specific, low albumin levels, which are also common in zinc deficiency, make serum zinc levels difficult to interpret. Diagnosis usually requires the combination of low levels of zinc in serum and increased urinary zinc excretion. If available, isotope studies can measure zinc status more accurately. Treatment consists of elemental zinc 15 to 120 mg/day, given orally, until symptoms and signs resolve (Boy et al., 2009; Johnson, 2008).

Hypozincemia is usually a nutritional deficiency but can also be associated with malabsorption, diarrhea, chronic liver disease, chronic renal disease, sickle cell disease, diabetes, and malignancies. Zinc deficiency, however, is typically the result of inadequate dietary intake of zinc. Decreased vision, smell, and memory are also connected with zinc deficiency. Moreover, a deficiency in zinc can cause malfunctions of organs and their related functions. One sign that may be caused by zinc deficiency is white spots, bands, or lines on the fingernails (Boy et al., 2009; Johnson, 2008).

One third of the world population is at risk of zinc deficiency, with the percentage of the population at risk ranging from 4 to 73% depending on the country. Zinc deficiency is the fifth-leading risk factor for disease in the developing world. Providing micronutrients, including zinc, has been identified as one of the four quick positive solutions to major global problems. Zinc food fortification and supplementation to children in developing countries have been proven to decrease diarrhea, pneumonia, and childhood mortality (Boy et al., 2009; Johnson, 2008).

Protein–Energy Malnutrition

Protein–energy malnutrition (kwashiorkor) is a global health problem and is potentially fatal, often causing death in children, mainly in developing countries where the environment is characterized by unsafe water, reductions in macronutrients, and deficiencies in many micronutrients. Kwashiorkor is an example of various levels of inadequate protein or energy intake. Although it mainly occurs in infants and children, it can be found in persons of any age in the life cycle. In the United States, secondary protein–energy malnutrition is seen in elderly people who live in nursing homes and in children in poverty. Such malnutrition may result from AIDS, cancer, kidney failure, inflammatory bowel disease, and other disorders. It usually appears in people who have chronic disease or chronic semistarvation, and takes three forms:

- *Dry (thin, desiccated)*. Marasmus results from near-starvation with a deficiency of protein and calories. The marasmic child consumes little food, usually because the mother is unable to breastfeed, and appears very thin as a result of loss of body muscle and fat. This is the predominant form of protein–energy malnutrition in most developing countries. It occurs when energy intake is insufficient for the body's requirements and the body uses up its own reserves. Marasmic infants have hunger, weight loss, growth retardation, and wasting of fat and muscle. The chronic phase of this disease is made acute when an incident of diarrhea takes place. This diarrhea usually takes on fatal consequences.

- *Wet (edematous, swollen)*. Kwashiorkor is an African word meaning "first child–second child"; it refers to the fact that a first child may develop protein–energy malnutrition when a second child is born and replaces the first child at the breast. In many poor areas of the world, the weaned child is then fed a thin gruel of poor nutritional quality and has organic failure to thrive. Edema results because the protein deficiency is greater than the energy deficiency. Increased carbohydrate intake is accompanied with decreased protein intake, and a decrease in albumin causes the edema. Those affected get thinning and discoloration of the hair and have an increased vulnerability to infections. The body weight increases due to edema.
- *Combined form (between the two extremes)*. In marasmic kwashiorkor, children have some edema and more body fat than marasmus.

Treatment of these conditions includes the following measures:

- Correcting fluid and electrolyte imbalances.
- Treating infections (causing diarrhea) with antibiotics.
- Supplying macronutrients (primarily milk-based formulas) by diet therapy and malnutrition ranges from 5 to 49% (WHO, 2015b).

OBESITY

Worldwide, at least 2.8 million people die each year as a result of being overweight or obese, and an estimated 35.8 million (2.3%) of global DALYs are caused by overweight or obesity. Overweight and obesity lead to adverse metabolic effects on blood pressure, cholesterol, triglycerides, and insulin resistance. Risks of coronary heart disease, ischemic stroke, and type 2 diabetes mellitus increase steadily with increasing body mass index (BMI), a measure of weight relative to height. Raised body mass index also increases the risk of cancer of the breast, colon, prostate, endometrium, kidney, and gall bladder. Mortality rates increase with increasing degrees of overweight, as measured by BMI. To achieve optimum health, the median BMI for an adult population should be in the range of 21 to 23 kg/m2, while the goal for individuals should be to maintain BMI in the range 18.5 to 24.9 kg/m2. There is increased risk of comorbidities for BMI 25.0 to 29.9, and moderate to severe risk of comorbidities for BMI greater than 30.

The BMI metric correlates the amount of body fat with height but does not directly measure body fat. Other modes of measuring body fat include skinfold thickness and waist circumference, calculation of waist-to-hip circumference ratios, and other diagnostic measurements such as ultrasound, computed tomography (CT), and magnetic resonance imaging (MRI). For children and adolescents, the BMI ranges are defined by taking into account normal male and female variations of body fat for specific ages (WHO, 2015c).

Childhood Obesity in the United States

About one in eight preschoolers is obese in the United States. Obesity among low-income preschoolers declined from 2008 through 2011, in 19 of the 43 states and territories studied. Children who are overweight or obese as preschoolers are five times as likely as normal-weight children to be overweight or obese as adults. Obese children are more likely to become obese adults and suffer lifelong physical and mental health problems. Obesity rates in low-income preschoolers, after decades of rising, began to level off from 2003 through 2008 and now are showing small declines in many states. However, too many preschoolers are obese. State and local officials can play a big part in reducing obesity among preschoolers (WHO, 2015c) by taking any of the following steps.

- Create partnerships with community members such as civic leaders and child care providers to make community changes that promote healthy eating and active living.
- Make it easier for families with children to buy healthy, affordable foods and beverages in their neighborhood.
- Help provide access to safe, free drinking water in places such as community parks, recreation areas, child care centers, and schools.
- Help local schools open up gyms, playgrounds, and sports fields during nonschool hours so more children can safely play.
- Help child care providers use best practices for improving nutrition, increasing physical activity, and decreasing computer and television time.

About one in five (19%) black children and one in six (16%) Hispanic children between the ages of two and five are obese. Obese children are more likely to be obese later in childhood and adolescence. In these older children and adolescents, obesity is associated with high cholesterol, high blood sugar, asthma, and mental health problems. Children who are overweight or obese as preschoolers are five times as likely as normal-weight children to be overweight or obese as adults (WHO, 2015c).

Adult Obesity

Some key facts about adult obesity as provided by WHO (2015c) are as follows:

- Worldwide obesity has more than doubled since 1980.
- In 2014, more than 1.9 billion adults, 18 years and older, were overweight. Of these over 600 million were obese.
- 39% of adults aged 18 years and over were overweight in 2014, and 13% were obese.
- Most of the world's population live in countries where overweight and obesity kills more people than underweight.
- Obesity is preventable.

Overweight and obesity are defined as abnormal or excessive fat accumulation that may impair health. The BMI is a simple index of weight-for-height that is commonly used to classify overweight and obesity in adults. It is defined as a person's weight in kilograms divided by the square of his height in meters (kg/m^2).

The World Health Organization provides the following definitions of overweight and obesity (2015c):

- A BMI greater than or equal to 25 is overweight.
- A BMI greater than or equal to 30 is obesity.

Causes of Obesity and Overweight

Obesity and overweight are caused by an energy imbalance between calories consumed and calories expended. Globally, there has been an increased intake of energy-dense foods that are high in fat and a decrease in physical activity due to the increasingly sedentary nature of many forms of work, changing modes of transportation, and increasing urbanization.

Changes in dietary and physical activity patterns are often the result of environmental and societal changes associated with development and lack of supportive policies in sectors such as health, agriculture, transport, urban planning, environment, food processing, distribution, marketing, and education (WHO, 2015c).

Consequences of Overweight and Obesity

Raised BMI is a major risk factor for noncommunicable diseases such as:

- Cardiovascular diseases (mainly heart disease and stroke), which were the leading cause of death in 2012.
- Diabetes.
- Musculoskeletal disorders (especially osteoarthritis—a highly disabling degenerative disease of the joints).
- Some cancers (endometrial, breast, and colon).

The risk for these noncommunicable diseases increases with an increase in BMI. Childhood obesity is associated with a higher chance of obesity, premature death, and disability in adulthood. But in addition to increased future risks, obese children experience breathing difficulties, increased risk of fractures, hypertension, early markers of cardiovascular disease, insulin resistance, and psychological effects.

The "Double Burden" of Disease

Many low- and middle-income countries are now facing a "double burden" of disease. They continue to deal with the problems of infectious disease and undernutrition; they are also experiencing a rapid upsurge in noncommunicable disease risk factors such as obesity and overweight, particularly in urban settings. Often undernutrition and obesity exist side by side within the same country, the same community, and even the same household.

Children in low- and middle-income countries are more vulnerable to inadequate prenatal, infant, and young child nutrition. At the same time, they are exposed to high-fat, high-sugar, high-salt, energy-dense, micronutrient-poor foods, which tend to be lower in cost but also lower in nutrient quality. These dietary patterns in conjunction with lower levels of physical activity result in sharp increases in childhood obesity while undernutrition issues remain un-solved (WHO, 2015c).

Prevention and Reduction of Overweight and Obesity

Individuals can

- limit energy intake from total fats and sugars.
- increase consumption of fruit and vegetables, as well as legumes, whole grains, and nuts.
- engage in regular physical activity (60 minutes a day for children and 150 minutes per week for adults).

The food industry can play a significant role in promoting healthy diets by

- reducing the fat, sugar, and salt content of processed foods.
- ensuring that healthy and nutritious choices are available and affordable to all consumers.
- practicing responsible marketing especially those aimed at children and teenagers.
- ensuring the availability of healthy food choices and supporting regular physical activity practice in the workplace (WHO, 2015c).

Obesity in China

Tsung Chen (2004), in his article on obesity in Chinese children, states that China used to be known for her slender people. Now China is fighting obesity, especially childhood obesity, simi-lar to other parts of the world. The proportion of obesity among children under the age of 15 increased from 15% in 1982 to 27% in 2003. Predisposing factors for the increasing prevalence of childhood obesity in China includes fast food and physical inactivity. Effective advertise-ments of fast-food giants in the United States such as McDonald's and Kentucky Fried Chicken plus physical inactivity are important risk factors for obesity in Chinese children. Television viewing is also a problem. Each hourly increment of television viewing is associated with a 1 to 2% increase in the prevalence of obesity in urban china. Childhood obesity is more prevalent in urban areas than in rural areas, not only because children in rural China are physically more active, but also because urban boys consume more fat than rural boys: 23 to 30% versus 16 to 20%. In addition, urban children in China are engaged in more homework because they are un-der pressure to achieve scholastically, whereas rural Chinese children are engaged more in field work because of economic necessity.

Fiber Consumption

Dietary fiber, also known as food roughage or bulk, is found mainly in fruits, vegetables, whole grains, and legumes. It is best known for its ability to relieve constipation, but is also known to lower the risk of type 2 diabetes, heart disease, and diverticular disease. There are two types of fiber:

- *Insoluble fiber* promotes movement of material through the gastrointestinal system, in-creasing bulk in stool. Examples include whole wheat flour, wheat bran, and numerous vegetables.

- *Soluble fiber* dissolves in water, making a gellike material, which aids in lowering blood cholesterol and glucose levels. It is found in oats, beans, peas, apples, citrus fruits, carrots, and barley.

Low-fiber foods include refined or processed foods such as canned fruits and vegetables, pulp-free juice, white breads and pastas, and non-whole-grain foods. Since the low-carbohydrate fad has passed, whole grains have made a comeback as part of the mainstream diet in the developed world. Eating a diet rich in whole grains has been associated with significant benefits, such as reduction in the rates of certain types of cancers, heart disease, type 2 diabetes, and weight management. The 2005 International Food Information Council (IFIC) Foundation guideline calls for at least three servings of whole grains per day, and particularly for young children, the servings need to be gradually increased (IFIC Foundation, 2005).

The fiber content of different whole-grain foods varies between 0.5 and 4 grams of fiber per serving, depending on the food category and serving size. Whole grains are the entire seed of plants, which contains all of the parts—the bran, germ, and endosperm—found in the original grain seed. They can take the form of a single food such as oatmeal, brown rice, barley, or popcorn, or can be an ingredient in another food such as bread or cereal. Examples include whole wheat, whole oats, whole-grain corn, popcorn, brown rice, whole rye, whole-grain barley, wild rice, buckwheat, bulgur (cracked wheat), millet, quinoa, and sorghum (IFIC Foundation, 2005). Oats are a good source of dietary fiber and are particularly helpful in the treatment of diabetes and cardiovascular disorders. Oat bran, in particular, is a good source of B-complex vitamins, protein, fat, and minerals, as well as soluble fiber (Butt, Tahir-Nadeem, Kashif Iqbal Khan, Shabir, & Butt, 2008).

When grain is refined, most of the bran and some of the germ is removed, which results in loss of fiber, B vitamins, vitamin E, trace minerals, unsaturated fat, and other nutrients. In the United States, by law, enriched fortified grains must also contain folic acid (IFIC Foundation, 2005).

In a study of 5,686 American preschoolers, Kranz (2006) noted that children are not likely to be consuming fiber at the recommended level, and are even less likely to do so as their age increases. The reason is that the children have increased independence in food selection as they age. Medium-income non-Hispanic white children were less likely to have adequate daily fiber intake than low-income non-Hispanic white children. Although low-income families were more likely to consume fewer processed and refined foods because of financial restrictions, higher-income families bought and consumed more fresh fruits, vegetables, and whole-grain products than middle-income families.

FOOD SAFETY AND SECURITY

Food prevents illness and maintains normal growth and development. Food security may be defined as steady access to sufficient nutritious foods to maintain an active healthy life. Those who have food security have access to clean, safe, and nutritious food at all times. They are able to acquire necessary foods without having to scavenge or steal. In contrast, food insecurity exists when there is limited or uncertain availability of safe and nutritious food. In this situation, food may not be easily acquired in safe and socially acceptable ways. The long-term effects of food insecurity are ill health, reduction in physical and cognitive growth and development, disease vulnerability, and, if untreated, eventually death (Hall & Brown, 2005).

Food insecurity is a state in which there is a nonsustainable food supply that interferes with optimal self-reliance and social justice. People who lack nutritionally adequate and safe food in their diet must often use severe coping strategies to obtain food, such as scavenging, stealing, and going to food banks. Those most susceptible to food insecurity are single heads of households, older adults, children without parents or guardians, landless people, those living in war zones, migrants, and immigrants. Persons with food insecurity are living with unhealthy diets and poor health status.

"Hunger," "famine," and "starvation" are commonly used terms when addressing people with food insecurity. These terms are defined as follows:

- *Hunger*: lethal, recurrent, and involuntary experiences of uneasy or painful sensations caused by lack of food. Hidden hunger is associated with deficiencies in micronutrients, may be less recognized and reported, and can be deadly. Hunger related to food insecurity leads to malnutrition.
- *Famine*: a sudden decrease in the level of food consumption for a large number of people. Lack of nutrients over at least several days can lead to starvation.
- *Starvation*: a severe lack of food that can occur without famine. For example, starvation may result from an inequitable social system, poverty, landlessness, civil disturbance, political injustice, government greed, or incompetency. Starvation is a severe reduction in vitamin, nutrient, and energy intake. It is the most extreme form of malnutrition (Kregg-Byers & Schlenk, 2010).

Food insecurity in the United States affected 11.7% of married couple households in 2003, and was present in 32.3% of families with a female head of the household and no spouse. Today in the United States, women are more likely to live in poverty than men, which greatly increases their risk of experiencing food insecurity. In households with food insecurity, often the first foods to be eliminated are fruits and vegetables, causing the family members to lack essential vitamins and minerals. This population is more likely to become overweight or obese from diets that include more energy-dense foods than fruits and vegetables, and that contain more refined grain, sugars, and fats, which cost less per calorie. Food-insecure women and children are ultimately at greater risk for chronic illnesses, including cancers and cardiovascular diseases (Olson, 2005).

In 2008, more than 14% of all U.S. households—49 million people—were food insecure. Most adults living in food-insecure households are not able to afford balanced meals, and worry about the adequacy of their food supply, running out of food, cutting the size of their meals, or skipping meals. Common responses to food insecurity include food budget adjustments, reduced food intake, and consumption of energy-dense foods (including refined grains, foods with added saturated trans-fats, and foods with added sugar), which are of poor nutritional quality and less expensive calorie-for-calorie than alternatives. In addition, U.S. adults living in food-insecure homes tend to eat fewer weekly servings of fruits, vegetables, and dairy, and lower levels of micronutrients, including B-complex vitamins, magnesium, iron, zinc, and calcium. These diet patterns are linked to the development of chronic diseases such as diabetes, hypertension, and hyperlipidemia. Nutritional problems, which may also occur in children within these households, include iron-deficiency anemia, acute infection, chronic illness, and developmental and mental health problems. In addition, overweight and obesity are found in both adults and children who experience food insecurity (Seligman, Laraia, & Kushel, 2010).

In addition to the aforementioned concerns about food security, the term "food security" now has a new meaning that may differ from its traditional definition—that is, it may be defined in terms of food safety. Put simply, food has become a weapon of bioterrorism. Besides having terrorism-related concerns about disease threats such as anthrax and smallpox, the world population now has major concerns relating to the safety of food and water supplies, which could be a source of the intentional spread of illness. Toxic substances might be put into the food and water supply that could include radioactive particles, microorganisms (e.g., *E. coli* 0517:H7, *Salmonella, Shigella*), or botulism toxin (a very deadly substance) (WHO, 2014).

The International Food Safety Authorities Network (INFOSAN) was developed by WHO in cooperation with the Food and Agriculture Organization (FAO) of the United Nations to promote the exchange of food safety information and to improve collaboration among international food authorities. Its goal is preventing the international spread of contaminated food. This organization has 143 members representing most countries of the world (WHO, 2014).

One example of a global concern related to the world food supply is bird flu, a disease that infected chickens in Southeast Asia as a result of failure to segregate these animals from wild birds. Once the chickens entered the food chain, they had the potential to transmit the disease.

Following natural disasters, food in affected areas may become contaminated and be at risk for outbreaks of food-borne illnesses such as diarrhea, dysentery, cholera, and typhoid fever. Poor sanitation and lack of clean drinking water have caused massive epidemics of food-borne diseases. Contaminated water may be considered to be an unclean food and should be boiled or given additives (biocides) to be made safe before it is consumed or added to foods. Some examples of food and water issues after a major flood include the following (WHO, 2014):

- Agriculture harvested from an area that has been flooded may be contaminated with microorganisms from raw sewage or microorganisms and chemicals in the flood water.
- Produce that was stored in the affected areas may be contaminated by flood waters.
- Foods that have not been contaminated need to be protected against sources of contamination.
- All foods distributed with mass feeding programs should be fit for human consumption and be nutritionally and culturally appropriate.
- Consumers need education in food preparation in more primitive conditions to promote food safety.

NUTRITION AND POVERTY

The significance of poverty relates not only to low income. Perhaps more significant components of poverty include limited or no access to health services, safe water, literacy, and education. There is a two-way association between poverty and health—that is, poverty is one of the main factors related to poor health, and poor health can lead to poverty. Poverty causes people to be exposed to environmental risks such as poor sanitation, unhealthy food, violence, and natural disasters. Those in poverty are less prepared to cope with their problems, putting them at greater risk for illness and disability.

Nutritional status depends on both food and nonfood factors. The nonfood factors include education and hygiene. As of 2010, 925 million people in the world experienced significant hunger. This includes 19 million in developed countries, 37 million in the Near East and North Africa, 53 million in Latin America and the Caribbean, and 239 million in Sub-Saharan Africa (World Hunger Education Service, 2012).

Poverty affects nutrition throughout the life span, causing both infectious and noncommunicable diseases and leading to a reduced learning capacity. Beginning in pregnancy, the fetus, when compromised with malnutrition, has slower intrauterine growth and as a result is small for gestational age. After being born, these low-birth-weight children do not respond to environmental stresses as well as their larger counterparts. Lifetime challenges from malnutrition affect the normal cognitive, psychomotor, and affective behavior in children, and later as they become adults, they have less resistance to infection (a weaker immune system) throughout the life span. Pregnant teens in poverty are more likely to have malnutrition and again expose the fetus and newborn to even greater risks. Low height for age (stunting) is the most frequently seen manifestation of malnutrition worldwide, with more than 30% of the world's children manifesting stunting. Poor quality and quantity of milk during the first two years of life results in shorter and more disease-prone individuals. Adults in poverty often use their money to buy more high-energy (calories) foods of low nutritional quality, which may not resolve nutritional deficiencies in vitamins or protein, but contribute to overweight and obesity. Older adults affected by poverty often suffer a long history of poor nutrition and frequent illnesses (both infectious and noncommunicable). Many have to continue working to help their adult children and grandchildren. The most common scenario of food-related disease among poverty-stricken populations in developing countries is one in which children, aged two to five, obtain bacterial infections from unsafe drinking water. This results in diarrhea, which, without antibiotics, is virtually impossible to cure. The child with diarrhea develops an electrolyte imbalance and protein and calorie deficits. Because poor children are not equipped with any reserve to fight this infection, the consequences of this diarrhea are more often fatal. Antibiotic treatment along with oral rehydration therapy (ORT) early in the disease will save numerous lives on a global basis.

Many poor women lack folic acid during pregnancy by not getting supplements from a prenatal care clinic, which can result in neural tube defects (NTDs). An NTD is a type of birth defect affecting the brain and spinal cord. The neural tube forms within 28 days after conception and develops into the brain and spine. NTDs occur when the neural tube fails to close properly, which can result in neural tissue being exposed and susceptible to damage. Adequate folic acid consumption has been shown to decrease the risk of neural tube defects. The neural tube closes before a woman usually knows she is pregnant. To prevent NTDs for all pregnancies, planned and unplanned, the World Health Organization recommends that women capable of becoming pregnant consume 400 micrograms of folic acid each day. It is often difficult to consume the equivalent of 400 micrograms of folic acid daily through an unfortified diet so increasing levels of folic acid in staple foods through fortification increases the likelihood that the target population will receive adequate amounts of folic acid needed to prevent NTDs (Centers for Disease Control and Prevention [CDC], 2015a).

NUTRITIONAL EMERGENCIES

WHO assists with worldwide nutritional emergencies through numerous projects developed to provide assistance as needed. Some of its projects include the development of the following (WHO, 2014):

- A manual that provides an explanation or how-to guide for managing nutritional needs of a community in an emergency, including the estimation of energy, protein, and nutrient requirements for a specific population.
- A field guide to determine nutritional requirements, current nutritional status, and methods for prevention and treatment of protein–energy malnutrition and micronutrient deficiency diseases.
- Specific guides for prevention and control of scurvy, pellagra, and thiamine deficiency.
- Guides for feeding infants and young children.
- Training modules for humanitarian aid workers.
- Guides for caring for the nutritionally vulnerable people of a population.
- Training modules for management of severe malnutrition.

Burundi, a Sub-Saharan African nation, has a significant problem with acute malnutrition in the general population, which is especially acute in children younger than five. This outcome is a consequence of armed conflicts resulting in displacement of people, the inability of people to work their land, and changes in weather patterns that have caused severe agricultural problems. To combat this situation, International Medical Corp (IMC), an emergency nongovernmental organization (NGO), has implemented a comprehensive program for treatment and prevention of malnutrition in three Burundian provinces (Muyinga, Rutana, and Kirundo) since 1998. The program consists of three therapeutic feeding centers, one in each province, and 38 supplementary feeding centers, 12 to 14 in each province. The therapeutic feeding centers provide inpatient, high-intensity treatment to the severely malnourished, and the supplementary feeding centers provide rations and treatment in an ambulatory (outpatient) center. UNICEF, USAID, and other NGOs have partnered with IMC to make a more dramatic impact in combating the acute malnutrition (Mach, n.d.).

In September 2006, the Global Alliance for Improved Nutrition (GAIN) signed an agreement with the United Nations International Children's Emergency Fund (UNICEF) to support flour fortification in Central and Eastern Europe in an effort to improve maternal, infant, and child health. GAIN is an organization that was created to fight vitamin and mineral deficiency. This type of malnutrition affects more than two billion people globally, and produces major health problems such as limited cognitive and psychomotor function, blindness, and death (GAIN, 2006).

NUTRITIONAL CHALLENGES IN VULNERABLE POPULATIONS

Infants and Children

The vast majority of children who die of hunger will not die in a high-profile emergency, but rather will die unnoticed by anyone other than their families and neighbors. There are approximately 400 million hungry children in the world, including an estimated 146 million who are younger than five. These children will most likely die or have long-term disabilities unless the following occurs (Gerberding, 2006):

- The children are identified and support from local organizations can reach them in their local communities.
- Local organizations are able to initiate interventions.
- Water purification and transport systems are established.
- Antibiotics can be made available.
- Complementary interventions such as childhood immunizations, education, and food security are also given.

Each year undernutrition contributes to the deaths of approximately 5.6 million children younger than five. In the least developed countries of the world, 42% of children are stunted in growth and 36% are underweight. Insufficient folic acid among childbearing-age women contributes to 200,000 babies being born with birth defects worldwide. Iron deficiency contributes to 60,000 deaths among women in pregnancy and childbirth and decreases cognitive development in 40 to 60% of the children of the developing world. Food fortification, supplementation, and dietary improvements have been successful in eliminating most of these problems in the developed world and could result in similar improvements in the developing world (Gerberding, 2006; WHO, 2014).

As we have said, children younger than five are generally much more vulnerable to nutritional challenges and have higher mortality rates during major emergencies such as earthquakes or tidal waves because of increased rates of communicable diseases and diarrhea as well as very high rates of undernutrition. During major emergencies, donations of infant formula and other powdered milk products can actually do more harm than good for these children. Infants and small children do better if they are breastfed only. Mothers and infants need to be kept together during such crises, and mothers should continue breastfeeding. In addition, maternal nutrition cannot be ignored and must be addressed. Any breastmilk substitutes for feeding infants and young children should be given only after the children's needs are carefully assessed and under strict medical supervision and hygienic conditions; there should be no general distribution of such products. Children older than six months should also be given fortified foods or micronutrient supplements under supervised programs (WHO, 2014).

Safe water is also essential for nutrition. In settings with poor access to safe water and hygiene, children experience diarrhea and malnutrition. Diarrheal infections kill almost 2 million children younger than five annually, and cause short- and long-term morbidity among millions more. Children with diarrhea frequently lose their appetites and do not absorb food, leading to nutritional deficiencies. In addition, malnourished children are at higher risk for diarrheal diseases. These children commonly have poor height and weight gains. Foods prepared with unsafe water or unclean hands expose children to diarrhea, causing illnesses and further promoting malnutrition (Gerberding, 2006). A significant percentage of infants anywhere from four to six months can be given complementary feedings, which usually consist of cereals or gruels.

Undernutrition and infectious diseases, both individually and in combination, have drastic effects on children worldwide, with more than 50% of all deaths of children due to the infectious diseases of pneumonia, diarrhea, malaria, measles, and AIDS. Undernutrition is a very important cause of these deaths—as many as 35% of all child deaths worldwide are a result of undernutrition. Undernutrition is a form of malnutrition that encompasses stunting (low height for age), wasting (low weight for age), and micronutrient deficiencies. As noted earlier, micronutrient deficiencies are common in children worldwide. A variety of interventions for undernutrition are available, including fortifications of condiments and other foods (Peterson, 2009).

As stated in "Global Childhood Malnutrition" (2006), in the developing world there are 146 million children younger than five who are underweight. Undernutrition is the cause of 5.6 million deaths per year. In countries such as India, Bangladesh, and Pakistan, many children also have iron-deficiency anemia and iodine deficiency. From 1990 to 2002, China reduced its number of underweight children from 19 to 8% ("Global Childhood Malnutrition," 2006). Low birth weight (LBW) correlates with nutrition-related early childhood mortality. Thirty million newborns each year in developing countries (24% of the 126 million births per year) suffer from intrauterine growth retardation (IUGR). The world prevalence for of IUGR/LBW is 11% of all newborns in developing countries (13.7 million babies annually). Incidence in Asia (excluding Japan) is highest in the world with 28.3% (accounting for 80% of all newborns worldwide); next are middle and Western Africa with incidence of 14.9% and 11.4%, respectively. Almost 30% of South Asian women are moderately or severely underweight and do not gain a sufficient amount of weight during pregnancy to allow for fetal growth (Underwood, 2002). In rural areas of Southeast Asia, breastfeeding is common for infants and young children, but this practice is decreasing in urban areas. A very interesting social structure has evolved in which the poor and the wealthy perform breastfeeding, while the middle class, due to problems with the mothers having to work, use bottle feeding.

South African children younger than five have a relatively high mortality rate and high prevalence of stunting. HIV and diarrheal disease are the leading causes of childhood morbidity and death in this country. One way to reduce the high rates of diarrhea and mortality is by micronutrient supplementation. A study conducted by Chagan et al. (2009) of the effect of micronutrient supplementation on children with diarrheal disease, some of whom had HIV, demonstrated the efficacy of zinc combined with multiple micronutrients in reducing diarrhea morbidity in rural South African children.

Childbearing Women

Pregnancy itself contributes to nutritional challenges even among the most nutritionally stable women in developed countries, but for pregnant women who are poor in developed and developing countries, the challenge of adequate nutrition is by far much greater. One specific nutritional issue specific to childbearing-age women is folic acid deficiency. Folic acid is readily available from green leafy vegetables, but many populations' diets are marginally deficient in these components. Folic acid is necessary for nucleic acid production (i.e., DNA and RNA synthesis). A population marginally deficient in folic acid will appear normal at first glance. However, this deficiency results in numerous birth defects, particularly cleft lip and palate, and spina bifida. Because most populations are marginally deficient in this vitamin, it is logical that folic acid supplements should be taken during pregnancy. This may be a problem, as most developmental anomalies are induced in the first three months of pregnancy, and for at least half of that time most women do not know they are pregnant. Folic acid is an essential water-soluble B vitamin that is used in the prevention of folate-deficiency anemia. In 1998, the United States mandated that all enriched flour be fortified with folic acid. Canada and Chile enacted similar laws for fortification of folic acid in wheat flour. At present, such fortification is mandatory in more than 50 countries. Where folic acid is fortified in flour, it has been shown to decrease neural tube defects in newborns.

Vitamin B_{12} deficiency is also widespread and the supplement (a safe additive) can also be added to flour to prevent pernicious anemia (Oakley & Tulchinsky, 2010).

Older Adults

National estimates reveal that there are more than 36 million older adults in the United States, 58% of whom are female. Among this group, the rate of food insecurity ranges from 6 to 16%. Good nutrition is particularly important for older adults because inadequate diets may contribute to or exacerbate diseases, or delay recovery from illnesses. This group consistently has lower intakes of nutrients such as protein, iron, zinc, vitamins B_6 and B_{12}, riboflavin, and niacin. Of particular note is the incidence of scurvy in elderly men. Many of these individuals eat primarily canned food, and the heat processing used during the canning process destroys ascorbic acid (vitamin C).

Poverty in older adults frequently causes them to do the following:

- Consume fewer than three meals per day.
- Have a lower intake of energy, vitamin C, iron, zinc, and calcium.
- Have iron-deficiency anemia.
- Have reduced bone density or osteoporosis.
- Have oral health problems (tooth decay and gum disease).

Strategies to assist older U.S. adults by enhancing their food security include an increase in dietitians and health professionals and federal nutrition programs for elders such as the Older Americans Act Nutrition Program (meals-on-wheels program) and the Food Stamp Program (SNAP) (CDC, 2015a).

The elderly population is a swiftly expanding age group. In 2009, individuals over the age of 60 represented 11% of the total population and that number is expected to grow to 15% by the year 2025 and 22% by 2050. This elderly age bracket is more susceptible to illnesses or becoming chronically debilitated, requiring more healthcare resources (Chwang, 2012). As the number of individuals defined as elderly increases, the strain on the healthcare system and the economy will continue to grow as well. Prevention of illness and disability is vital to keeping people healthy and keeping them healthy for longer. Prevention becomes increasingly important with its multitude of benefits including improving quality of life for these older adults in addition to reducing strain on the healthcare system. Eating healthy diets and maintaining a good nutritional status is an important part of healthy aging and acts as a preventative measure for many health conditions (Chang, Nayga, & Chan, 2011). Many studies have been performed to examine the nutritional status of the elderly and the results of these studies show significant incidence of undernutrition. López-Contreras, Torralba, Zamora, and Pérez-Llamas (2012) reported the rates of undernutrition to be 5 to 20% in community-dwelling older adults and 20 to 30% in institutionalized older adults. Institutionalized older adults are more likely to suffer from undernutrition with some studies showing as many as 42% of elderly individuals in nursing homes receiving less than the recommended dietary intake for their age (Jain, Purnima, Jain, & Gupta, 2013; López-Contreras, Torralba, Zamora, & Pérez-Llamas, 2012). Clearly there is a need for enhanced nutrition in the elderly age group and nurses are in a prime position to enact positive changes in the nutritional status of older adults.

Aspects of Aging That Impact Nutrition

Many aspects of aging can impact the nutritional status of elderly individuals. Physiological factors include both normal, age-related changes as well as pathological changes that are common in this age group. Some normal parts of aging that can impact nutritional status include reductions in taste and smell, decreased motility in the esophagus, slowed gastric emptying, changes in the digestive tract that impair absorption of nutrients, and dental problems such as weakened enamel and increased sensitivity (Chwang, 2012; López-Contreras, Torralba, Zamora, & Pérez-Llamas, 2012).

Certain pathological conditions common to this age group can significantly impact the diet of an elderly person. Xerostomia, dry mouth, frequently affects older adults with studies reporting the incidence at anywhere from 10 to 46% (Hopcraft & Tan, 2010). A lack of saliva dissuades many xerostomia sufferers from eating or eating the variety of foods they need. Xerostomia can be caused by radiation treatments to the head and neck, dehydration, diabetes, and many medications (Visvanathan & Nix, 2010).

Dysphagia, difficulty swallowing, is another pathological condition affecting older adults that can interfere with nutrition (Chwang, 2012). Loss of teeth is a major issue for elderly individuals that can severely impair nutritional status (Chwang, 2012). About 50% of older Americans have lost at least some of their teeth. Loss of teeth leads to avoidance of fruits and vegetables in the diet and the addition of foods that are soft and tend to be more refined. These foods are typically lacking in vitamins, minerals, and fiber while being high in cholesterol and sodium. Diets high in these foods can lead to becoming overweight in addition to lacking necessary nutrients (American Geriatrics Society, 2012). Loss of functionality, such as mobility impairments or visual impairments, causes problems for older adults in the area of nutrition as well (Chwang, 2012). These impairments make it difficult for elderly individuals to perform tasks such as grocery shopping and food preparation (U.S. Department of Health and Human Services, 2012).

With all of these factors that put older adults at greater risk for malnutrition, it is easy to see how such large percentages of this population do suffer from undernutrition and the importance of intervening to improve the nutritional status of elderly individuals. Understanding the importance of good nutrition, specifically as it applies to this elderly age group, is another vital component of being prepared to enact positive changes.

Importance of Good Nutrition to Healthy Aging

A good diet is essential to maintaining good health across the life span and is even more relevant to the elderly of all global areas because it promotes healthy aging. Healthy aging and a good diet in particular have been shown to reduce morbidity (Jain, Purnima, Jain, & Gupta, 2013). A healthy diet reduces the risk of developing many conditions such as heart disease, hypertension, high cholesterol, diabetes mellitus, cancer, anemia, bone loss, and stroke (National Institute on Aging, 2012). Some elderly individuals may already have some of these chronic conditions, but that does not make a healthy diet any less important. A healthy diet can help reduce the severity and better manage the effects of some conditions, such as hypertension and diabetes (National Institute on Aging, 2012). A poor diet can lead to undernutrition, which is correlated with an overall lower quality of life, chronic disability, increased comorbidities, increased cases of hospital admissions and readmissions, impaired cognitive function, depression, an increased mortality rate, impaired skin integrity, constipation, and sleeping problems (American Geriatrics Society, 2012; Lara-Pulido & Guevara-Cruz, 2012; López-Contreras, Torralba, Zamora, & Pérez-Llamas, 2012; National Institute on Aging, 2012).

Imbalances of specific nutrients in the diet can cause or increase the older adult's risk for many conditions. Lack of B vitamins can cause nerve damage or anemia (American Geriatrics Society, 2012). Deficient iron intake can also cause anemia (Chang, Nayga, & Chan, 2011). Calcium is an important nutrient for bone health and inadequate intake of calcium increases the risk for fractures and osteoporosis in older adults (American Geriatrics Society, 2012; Chang, Nayga, & Chan, 2011). Excess sodium in the diet can raise blood pressure, which can be problematic especially for those elderly individuals already diagnosed with hypertension. Cholesterol is another nutrient that can have negative impacts when taken in excess of the recommended levels. Hypercholesterolemia, an increase of lipids in the blood, is a risk factor for many cardiovascular and peripheral vascular diseases (Chang, Nayga, & Chan, 2011).

Protein is a major nutrient of high importance to nutritional status. Protein is necessary to build muscle and prevent the breakdown of muscle (Tieland, Borgonjen-Van den Berg, Loon, & Groot, 2012). Sarcopenia, a decrease in skeletal muscle mass, occurs as a normal part of aging in about 15 to 50% of the elderly population (Chwang, 2012). Sarcopenia leads to many problems when performing the activities of daily living, such as preparation of food and personal hygiene, and is associated with increased mortality rates (Chwang, 2012). Adequate protein intake can help to delay or prevent the onset of sarcopenia or slow its progression in an individual already affected (Tieland, Borgonjen-Van den Berg, Loon, & Groot, 2012). A study by Tieland, Borgonjen-Van den Berg, Loon, and Groot (2012) established that 10% of the community-dwelling elderly has protein intake levels below the recommended amount and 35% of the institutionalized elderly persons had protein intake levels below the recommended amount.

Hydration

Any discussion of nutrition for any age group would be incomplete without briefly covering water intake. Water is also an essential nutrient, and older adults require at least 1,500 milliliter of fluid intake per day, more if they are more active (McCarthy & Manning, 2012). Many older adults intake just enough fluid to prevent outright, acute dehydration, but the fluid intake is still low enough that it does have negative health effects such as constipation, urinary tract infections, impaired cognitive function, and an increased risk for falls (McCarthy & Manning, 2012). A normal part of aging is a diminished sense of thirst, which can reduce the amount of fluid an older adult takes in (U.S. Department of Health and Human Services, 2012). It is recommended that elderly individuals be encouraged to drink water throughout the day, even if they do not feel thirsty, as well as before and after any activity (McCarthy & Manning, 2012; U.S. Department of Health and Human Services, 2012). Older adults suffering from urinary incontinence frequently limit their fluid intake in an attempt to assist in managing their incontinence (McCarthy & Manning, 2012). It is important to intervene with these patients and educate them on the negative effects of limiting fluid intake as well as better methods for managing incontinence, such as pelvic floor exercises.

Evaluation and Assessment

Evaluation of nutritional status is not as simple as measuring body mass index, which has been proven to be only moderately accurate as an indicator of nutritional status (Kozakova, Jarosova, & Zelenikova, 2012). Kozakova, Jarosova, and Zelenikova (2012) conducted a study comparing three of the most widely used assessment tools for evaluation of nutritional status: the Mini Nutritional Assessment (MNA), the Subjective Global Assessment (SGA), and the Malnutrition Universal Screening Tool (MUST). The Mini Nutritional Assessment is designed for use with individuals over the age of 65 and consists of six questions intended to identify persons who are malnourished or at risk for becoming malnourished (Nestle Nutrition Institute, n.d.). The Subjective Global Assessment involves several questions evaluating medical history and physical examination values with the final overall score reflecting malnutrition or risk for malnutrition. Finally, the Malnutrition Universal Screening Tool scores points in three areas: BMI, recent weight loss, and current disease state (Kozakova, Jarosova, & Zelenikova, 2012).

The Kozakova, Jarosova, and Zelenikova study (2012) compared these three assessment tools and found the Mini Nutritional Assessment to be the most accurate. The MNA is the only tool specifically geared for older adults and proved to be the most reliable and more accurate indicator of current malnutrition as well as the best indicator of risk for malnutrition (Kozakova, Jarosova, & Zelenikova, 2012). Other studies have also identified the MNA as the best tool for assessing nutritional status in elderly individuals (Chwang, 2012). When comparing the Mini Nutritional Assessment to evaluations of nutritional status based on BMI, the MNA was found to be much more sensitive to malnutrition than a simple body mass index (Kozakova, Jarosova, &

Zelenikova, 2012). The MNA is a very good indicator of risk for malnutrition even when there is no evidence of malnutrition. This is important because early diagnosis of malnutrition and risk for malnutrition is vital to preserving the individual's health and correcting the problem before it progresses further (Lara-Pulido & Guevara-Cruz, 2012). Although the MNA includes questions on levels of physical functionality and mental health status, these are two areas that are worth delving into more deeply if the elderly individual in question has any impairments, as physical functionality and mental health status both significantly impact the older adult's ability to achieve adequate levels of nutrition (Chang, Nayga, & Chan, 2011).

Nutritional Education

For positive changes in diet to be enacted, elderly individuals and their caretakers both need to be knowledgeable regarding nutrient requirements and how to ensure those requirements are met in the diet. Jain, Purnima, Jain, and Gupta (2013) reported the results of a study on the knowledge bases of older adults regarding nutrition. The study was conducted on adults both in nursing homes and dwelling in the community. The results of the study showed that the majority of elderly individuals were consistently scoring unsatisfactorily on nutrition knowledge tests (Jain, Purnima, Jain, & Gupta, 2013). The first step in improving nutritional status in our elderly population is to teach these older adults what nutrients they require on a daily basis, how to get those nutrients, and how to manage some of the difficulties their age group faces in regard to nutrition.

The U.S. Department of Health and Human Services (2012) has extensive literature on recommended daily intake for older adults. There are many valid sources on the Web detailing appropriate nutrient intake for this group, and most sites offer geriatric-friendly, printable versions as well. For adults over the age of 50, the recommended daily serving of protein is 5 to 7 ounces, keeping in mind that 3 ounces of meat, poultry, or fish is about the size of a deck of playing cards. However, meat, poultry, and fish are not the only sources of protein. Also equivalent to an ounce of meat, poultry, or fish is a single egg, a tablespoon of peanut butter, one-fourth of a cup of beans, or an ounce of nuts (U.S. Department of Health and Human Services, 2012). The recommended daily serving of grain is 5 to 10 ounces, an ounce of grain being equivalent to such items as a muffin, a slice of bread, or a cup of cereal (U.S. Department of Health and Human Services, 2012). Dairy intake is recommended at 3 cups per day (U.S. Department of Health and Human Services, 2012). Good sources of dairy include fat-free or low-fat milk, cheese, or yogurt. The recommendations for fruit are 1.5 to 2.5 cups per day, and the recommended amount of vegetables is 2 to 3.5 cups (U.S. Department of Health and Human Services, 2012). Intake of oils should be limited to about 5 to 8 teaspoons per day and should be taken from healthier options such as nuts, olives, or avocados (U.S. Department of Health and Human Services, 2012). It is important to encourage fiber intake as well. Eating fruits and vegetables with the skins on and consuming whole grains are good ways to increase fiber intake. Adequate fiber intake can prevent constipation, as long as plenty of water is taken in as well. To assist in estimating amounts without having to painstakingly measure everything, the U.S. Department of Health and Human Services guidelines provide some handy references as well. A fist represents about a cup, the tip of a finger represents a teaspoon, half of a baseball is about half a cup, and a ping pong ball represents 2 tablespoons (U.S. Department of Health and Human Services, 2012).

Required daily caloric intake varies from individual to individual based on variables such as gender and activity level. For older adults, daily required calories range anywhere from 1,600 to 2,800 based on gender and activity level (U.S. Department of Health and Human Services, 2012).

Elderly individuals experience metabolic changes as a normal part of aging leading to increases in body fat percentages, decreases in lean muscle mass, and loss of appetite (Chwang, 2012; U.S. Department of Health and Human Services, 2012). A decrease in activity level may accompany aging for many older adults as well, further reducing their caloric need (National Institute on Aging, 2012). Although they may experience a loss of appetite and require fewer calories overall, it is important to remember that older adults still require many nutrients. Nutrient-dense foods are foods with high concentrations of nutrients in them and are an important part of the elderly individuals' diet (National Institute on Aging, 2012). Examples of nutrient-dense foods include Greek yogurt, beans, sweet potatoes, nuts and seeds, strawberries, and pineapple (Fries, n.d.).

There are many recommendations to improve nutritional status in the elderly. Encouraging healthy snacks between meals, nutritional supplement drinks such as Boost, a brightly lit and positive eating environment, socialization with meals, and healthy flavor enhancers such as spices, herbs, and lemon juice are all recommended to encourage a good diet in the elderly population (Chwang, 2012; U.S. Department of Health and Human Services, 2012). Some older adults struggle with affording food, shopping for food, and preparing food. An important part of nutritional education for these individuals is assistance learning how to eat on a budget. Recommendations include buying store labeled items and items on sale as well as buying only as much as the individual is sure to use and freezing leftovers to avoid waste (U.S. Department of Health and Human Services, 2012). Additionally, there are government programs to assist elderly individuals in affording food, shopping for food, and having meals delivered to their homes if needed. One excellent resource is www.eldercare.gov, which puts older adults and their caretakers in touch with community resources including meal services and transportation aid. The website has an easy-to-use locator to help elderly individuals identify a myriad of community resources available to them.

Study Questions

1. Discuss the causes and possible remedies of childhood, and adult hunger and malnutrition in both developed and developing countries.
2. Explain the human right "freedom from hunger." Do you believe that all people living in the world should have this right? Why?
3. Why is having good nutrition during pregnancy especially important for women throughout the world?
4. Compare and contrast nutritional deficiencies, such as iron-deficiency anemia, niacin, vitamin A, vitamin B, iodine, and zinc micronutrient deficiencies.

5. Describe some nutritional challenges and relate potential solutions for children, middle-age, and older adults worldwide.
6. Explain why obesity is a major health problem in both developed and developing nations.

Case Study 1: Micronutrient: Iodine Deficiency

Prior to the initiation of a nationwide program in China to eliminate iodine deficiency in 1995, more than 20% of Chinese children between the ages of 8 and 10 years were found to have enlarged thyroid glands. In addition, there were approximately 400 million people living in China at risk for developing a disorder associated with iodine deficiency.

The National Iodine Deficiency Disorders Elimination Program was introduced by the Chinese government in an effort to combat this national health problem. The focus of the program was to produce, package, and distribute iodized salt nationwide. One challenge that had to be overcome for the program to be successful was that many people lived in salt-producing areas and on salt hills and consumed only raw salt; thus they were reluctant to pay for commercially produced salt.

The efforts of the program were primarily supported by the World Bank, UNICEF, and WHO. At its beginning, a nationwide health campaign was initiated to inform the public of the ill effects of iodine deficiency and to explain how essential it was to purchase only the fortified salt. Ensuring that the people across the nation would have access to the iodized salt, salt-producing factories were instructed to improve and increase their technology for production. New centers were also built for iodation and packaging. Licensing regulations, including quality control, were put into place by the government in an attempt to ban the sale of noniodized salt (Center for Global Development, 2006).

Five years after the initiation of the program, 94% of the country was receiving iodized salt as compared to only 80% at the start of the program. The quality of the product had also dramatically improved. The health of schoolchildren has shown a significant improvement. Total goiter rates declined to 6.5% in 2002 (Center for Global Development, 2006).

An Essential Micronutrient: Iodine

Iodine is a trace element that participates in the synthesis of thyroxine, a hormone secreted by the thyroid gland. Thyroxine stimulates cell oxidation and regulates the basal metabolic rate. It also helps regulate protein synthesis in the brain and other organs. The majority of iodine found in the body is contained in the thyroid gland. The recommended daily intake of iodine is 90 micrograms (mcg) for preschool children, 120 mcg for school children, 150 mcg for adults, and 200 mcg for pregnant and lactating women. Iodine is naturally found in seafood and in soil and water around the world.

Iodine deficiency results when intake falls below the recommended levels. The principal disorder associated with deficient levels is enlargement of the thyroid gland, or goiter. Gland enlargement occurs as a result of continuous secretion of thyroid-stimulating hormone (TSH) despite low blood levels of thyroid hormone and the increase in the amount of thyroglobulin that accumulates in thyroid follicles. The gland thereby increases in size; in some cases, it may weigh up to 700 grams or more. Iodine deficiency can also cause profound damage to the developing brain in utero and during the growing years of infancy and childhood. Stillbirths and miscarriages can result during pregnancy (Williams & Schlenker, 2003).

Case Study 1 Questions

1. What were the challenges for supplying commercially produced fortified salt to the people of China?
2. Why is commercially produced fortified salt needed in the diet to maintain health?
3. How did the iodine deficiency challenge get resolved?

Case Study 2: Micronutrient: Vitamin A

To reduce vitamin A deficiency in Sub-Saharan Africa, the International Potato Center, supported by the Department for International Development, has developed a sweet potato variety that is enhanced with the provitamin A form known as beta-carotene. This orange-fleshed sweet potato is being promoted to alleviate vitamin A deficiency among children and pregnant and lactating women. In a project led by South African scientists, schoolchildren between the ages of 5 and 10 were given a portion of boiled, mashed orange-fleshed sweet potato, weighing 125 grams, each day over 53 school days. A similar group of children received the same portion of white-fleshed sweet potato. Blood tests showed that the orange-fleshed sweet potato provided 2.5 times the recommended dietary allowance of vitamin A for that age group. The vitamin A stored in the liver in this group of children increased by 10% as compared to a 5% decline in vitamin A liver stores in those children consuming the white variety of sweet potatoes (South African Medical Research Council, 2004).

An Essential Nutrient: Vitamin A

Vitamin A is a fat-soluble vitamin that has many physiological functions:

- It helps with visual adaptation to light and darkness and prevention of night blindness.
- It is essential for optimal growth of soft tissues and bones.
- It maintains the integrity of epithelial cells such as the mucous membranes.
- It maintains normal skin.
- It supports the immune system in the formation of T lymphocytes.

The recommended daily allowance for vitamin A is 300 mcg for children 1 to 3 years of age, 400 mcg for children 4 to 8 years of age, 600 mcg for children 9 to 13 years of age, and 700 mcg for women and 900 mcg for men ages 14 and older. Two dietary sources of vitamin A exist. Retinol, or preformed vitamin A, is the natural form that can be found in animal food sources and is associated with fats. Beta-carotene is the provitamin A form and is found in orange-yellow and dark green leafy vegetables. The clinical signs of vitamin A deficiency include conditions such as xerophthalmia, an abnormally dry and thickened surface of the cornea and conjunctiva; night blindness; and keratinization, where epithelial cells become dry, flat, and hard (National Institutes of Health, 2006b).

Case Study 2 Questions

1. What role did the sweet potato have in providing vitamin A to the people of Sub-Saharan Africa?
2. What are the health problems occurring with vitamin A deficiency?

Case Study 3: Micronutrient: Iron

Iron-deficiency anemia has been a major health problem for more than four decades in Sri Lanka. Women of childbearing age and those who are pregnant are at highest risk, as are preschool children and children in primary school. The rate of anemia is especially high among groups of low socioeconomic status living in crowded environmental conditions and those prone to recurrent infections. A national survey found that 58% of children in primary school were identified as anemic (International Nutrition Foundation, n.d.).

A research study was conducted in Colombo, Sri Lanka, using 453 school children between the ages of 5 and 10, who presented with and without infection. The study examined the effects of iron supplementation on both iron status and morbidity and was designed as a longitudinal, randomized, controlled, double-blind supplementation trial. Baseline information was collected on each child that consisted of a detailed medical history, height and weight, venous blood sample, socioeconomic status, and morbidity from respiratory and gastrointestinal illness (deSilva, Atukorala, Weerasinghe, & Ahluwalia, 2003).

The intervention consisted of iron supplementation for eight weeks. The children were given 60 mg of elemental iron (ferrous sulfate) every day. The control group received placebo capsules of lactose. Field investigators followed up with each of the children at their homes every two weeks to ensure high compliance. After supplementation was completed, all children were reassessed according to the preintervention parameters (deSilva, Atukorala, Weerasinghe, & Ahluwalia, 2003).

Of the 363 children who completed the eight-week iron supplementation, 52.6% of the children had anemia. After the children took iron supplements, there was a significant improvement in iron status as indicated by the serum hemoglobin and ferritin concentrations in both groups of children with and without infections. In addition, those children who received the iron had a lower number of upper respiratory tract infections and total number of sick days (deSilva, Atukorala, Weerasinghe, & Ahluwalia, 2003).

An Essential Nutrient: Iron

Iron is found in the body bound to protein; it is present in blood as the heme portion of hemoglobin and in muscle as myoglobin, bound to a transport protein as transferrin, and stored as a protein–iron compound as ferritin. It has many functions, such as the following:

- Participates in the transportation of oxygen from the lungs to the tissues as a component of hemoglobin.
- Acts as a catalyst of oxidative enzyme systems for energy production.

- Converts beta-carotene to vitamin A.
- Synthesizes collagen.
- Removes lipids from the bloodstream.
- Detoxifies drugs in the liver.
- Helps in the production of antibodies.

The recommended daily allowance for iron for the following age groups is as follows:

- Infants 7 to 12 months: 11 mg per day
- Children 4 to 8 years: 10 mg per day
- Children 9 to 13 years: 8 mg per day
- Children 14 to 18 years: 11 mg per day for males; 15 mg per day for females
- Women aged 19 to 50 years: 18 mg per day
- Men aged 19 to 50 years: 8 mg per day
- Women aged 51 and older: 8 mg per day
- Men aged 51 and older: 8 mg per day

Iron can be found in organ meats such as liver, dark green vegetables, and grains. The principal disorder associated with iron deficiency is anemia. Anemia can lead to various symptoms such as fatigue, pale skin, difficulty maintaining body temperature, glossitis, slow cognitive and social development, and decreased immune function. Common causes of iron-deficiency anemia are increased iron losses, inadequate dietary intake, and inadequate absorption of iron usually secondary to diarrhea (National Institutes of Health, 2006a).

Case Study 3 Questions

1. Explain why iron is important for health of both children and adults.
2. Discuss the effects of iron-deficiency on both children and adults.
3. What types of foods are high sources of iron?

Case Study 4: Protein–Energy

Mr. Williams, a 70-year-old man with long-standing insulin-dependent diabetes mellitus, renal insufficiency, and heart failure, was admitted to the hospital with fatigue, weakness, and weight loss. The nursing staff discovered a 4-inch-diameter decubitus ulcer located over his sacrum. His caretaker gave a detailed history of his eating patterns over the previous three months, indicating a progressive decline in his food intake. Mr. Williams is 5 feet 11 inches tall (180 cm) and his present weight is 125 pounds (56 kg). His calculated BMI is 17.2.

Causes of Unintentional Weight Loss in the Elderly

Unintentional weight loss often occurs in the elderly. There are many causes and situations that can signal and alert one to malnutrition, especially in the elderly population. Many chronic disorders of the cardiovascular, endocrine, gastrointestinal, and neurological systems can play a role in weight loss, along with infections and malignancy. Psychiatric and eating disorders such as anorexia nervosa and bulimia also predispose an individual to weight loss. As a person ages, grief and depression can result from separation from family or loss of a spouse, which may leave a person living and eating alone. The side effects of many medications can also cause an individual to be anorexic and interfere with the utilization of food nutrients. Variables that actually interfere with the ability to eat include ill-fitting dentures, loss of teeth, problems with swallowing, and decreased sensation of taste and smell. All of these factors play a role in nutritional intake. Economic factors may also place the elderly at risk for malnutrition, including low socioeconomic status, insufficient income to purchase food, and inadequate living conditions such as the lack of heating or cooling and the lack of appliances to prepare meals (Jensen, Friedmann, Coleman, & Smiciklas-Wright, 2001; Williams & Schlenker, 2003).

Physical features of protein–energy malnutrition include the following:

- Reduction in body weight
- Muscle wasting with loss of strength
- Reduction in cardiac and respiratory muscular capacity
- Thinning of skin
- Decreased basal metabolic rate
- Hypothermia
- Edema
- Immunodeficiency
- Apathy

Treatment for Protein–Energy Malnutrition

Nutritional therapy for Mr. Williams is aimed at improving tissue integrity, muscle function, and immune function by providing enhanced amounts of protein and energy intake. Optimal dietary protein should be supplemented to the patient to ensure that an adequate supply of necessary amino acids is obtained for tissue synthesis. Calories need to be provided in amounts that will meet his energy output demands (Akner & Cederholm, 2001). Mr. Williams will also benefit from enhanced oral supplements to aid in healing of his pressure sore (European Pressure Ulcer Advisory Panel, n.d.). In addition, supplementation of arginine, vitamin C, vitamin A, and zinc has been shown to be beneficial for the treatment of pressure sores (Langer, Schloemer, Knerr, Kuss, & Behrens, 2003; Schmidt, n.d.).

Essential Nutrition: Protein

Proteins are made up of amino acids that are necessary for the body to function properly, for growth, and for maintenance of body tissue. Proteins are the principal source of nitrogen and are essential for many body functions, including the following:

- Building new body tissues and repairing old ones
- Supplying amino acids for making enzymes and hormones
- Regulating fluid and acid–base balance

- Providing resistance from disease
- Providing transport mechanisms
- Providing energy

Protein requirements are influenced by the rate of growth, body size, rate of protein synthesis, quality of the protein, and dietary intake of fats and carbohydrates. The recommended dietary allowance (RDA) for both men and women is 0.80 gram per kilogram of body weight per day (Institute of Medicine, 2005). Additional protein is needed during illness and disease, trauma, prolonged immobilization, pregnancy, and lactation. Protein needs of infants and children vary according to their age and patterns of growth.

Sources of proteins can be described as either complete proteins or incomplete proteins. A food that supplies a sufficient amount of the nine indispensable (essential) amino acids is called a complete protein. All proteins from animal sources are considered to be complete proteins. Foods from this group include chicken, beef, pork, fish, shellfish, eggs, and the milk food groups. Incomplete proteins are foods that lack one or more essential amino acids; they include foods such as some fruits, grains, and vegetables (National Library of Medicine, 2006). The following are the nine indispensable (essential) amino acids (Institute of Medicine, 2005):

- Histidine
- Isoleucine
- Leucine
- Lysine
- Methionine
- Phenylalanine
- Threonine
- Tryptophan
- Valine

Case Study 4 Questions

1. Explain why protein is needed for the health of children and adults.
2. Which food sources supply protein in the diet?
3. What problems occur with limited protein intake in both children and adults?

Case Study 5: Obesity

Dorothy is a 36-year-old female who has been diagnosed with hypertension by her family doctor. Her other significant medical history includes insulin-dependent diabetes mellitus. She reports that she has always had a sedentary job and lifestyle. Dorothy's weight is 204 pounds, her height is 66 inches, and she has a waist circumference of 38 inches. Her blood pressure is 170/95 mm Hg and her heart rate is 86. She has acknowledged that she has been taking her blood pressure at home and it has been at least 156/95 mm Hg on several occasions.

According to the USDA's Dietary Guidelines for Americans (2005b), Dorothy's BMI is 33, indicating that she is considered obese. Another index that can be useful to identify obesity is the measurement of waist and waist/hips circumference.

Case Study 5 Questions

1. Discuss the relationship of obesity with chronic health diseases such as diabetes, cardiovascular disease, and hypertension.
2. What can be done to decrease obesity in populations in developed as well as developing countries?

References

Akner, G., & Cederholm, T. (2001). Treatment of protein–energy malnutrition in chronic nonmalignant disorders [Electronic version]. *American Journal of Clinical Nutrition, 74*, 6–24.

American Geriatrics Society. (2012). *Nutrition: Unique to older adults.* Retrieved from http://www .healthinaging.org/aging-and-health-a-to-z/topic:nutrition/info:unique-to-older-adults/

Boy, E., Mannar, V., Pandav, C., de Benoist, B. Viteri, F., Fontaine, O., & Hotz, C. (2009). Achievements, challenges, and promising new approaches in vitamin and mineral deficiency control. *Nutrition Reviews, 67*(suppl 1), S24–S30.

Butt, M., Tahir-Nadeem, M., Kashif Iqbal Khan, M., Shabir, R., & Butt, M. (2008). Oat: Unique among the cereals. *European Journal of Nutrition, 4*, 68–69.

Callan, A., Hinwood, A., & Devine, A. (2014). Metals in commonly eaten groceries in Western Australia: A market basket survey and dietary assessment. *Food Additives, Part A Chemical Analysis Control Exposure Risk Analysis, 31*(12), 1968–1981.

Centers for Disease Control and Prevention. (2015a). *Food Fortification Network.* Retrieved from http://www.ffinetwork.org/

Centers for Disease Control and Prevention. (2015b). *Childhood obesity.* Retrieve from http://www.cdc.gov/ vitalsigns/childhoodobesity/index.html

Centers for Disease Control and Prevention. (2003). *Food safety and nutrition.* Retrieved from http://www.cdc .gov/nceh/globalhealth/priorities/foodnutrition.htm

Center for Global Development. (2006). *Case 14: Preventing iodine deficiency disease in China.* Retrieved from http://www.cgdev.org

Chagan, M. K., Van den Broeck, J., Luabeya, K., Mpontshane, N., Tucker, K. L., & Bennish, M. L. (2009). Effect of micronutrient supplementation on diarrhoeal disease among stunted children in rural South Africa. *European Journal of Clinical Nutrition, 63*, 850–857.

Chang, H., Nayga, R., & Chan, K. (2011). Gendered analyses of nutrient deficiencies among the elderly. *Journal of Family and Economic Issues, 32*(2), 268–279.

Chen, T. (2004). Obesity in Chinese children. *Journal of the Royal Society of Medicine, 97*(5), 254.

Chwang, L. (2012). Nutrition and dietetics in aged care. *Nutrition & Dietetics, 69*(3), 203–207.

Costarelli, V., & Manios, Y. (2009). The influence of socioeconomic status and ethnicity on children's excess body weight. *Nutrition and food Science, 39*(6), 676.

Cremaschini, M., Moretti, R., Brembilla, G., Valoti, M., Sarnataro, F., Spada, P., Mologni, G., Franchin, D., Antonioli, L., Parodi, D., Barbaglio, G., Masanotti, G., & Fiandri, R. (2015). Assessment of the impact over one year of a workplace health promotion programme in the province of Bergamo. *Medicina del Lavoro (Industrial Medicine), 106*(3), 159–171.

deSilva, A., Atukorala, S., Weerasinghe, I., & Ahluwalia, N. (2003). Iron supplementation improves iron status and reduces morbidity in children with or without upper respiratory tract infections: A randomized controlled study in Colombo, Sri Lanka [Electronic version]. *American Journal of Clinical Nutrition, 77,* 234–241.

European Pressure Ulcer Advisory Panel. (n.d.). *Nutritional guidelines for pressure ulcer prevention and treatment.* Retrieved from http://www.epuap.org

Fries, W. (n.d.). *10 nutrient rich foods for a healthy diet.* Retrieved from http://www.webmd.com/vitamins-and-supplements/lifestyle-guide-11/healthy foods?page=1

Global Alliance for Improved Nutrition. (2006). *Gain signs grant agreement with UNICEF to support flour fortification in the CEE/CIS region.* Retrieved from http://www.gainhealth.org/ch/FN/index.cfm?contentid=fp5C67729.1143.F7CC.3

Gerberding, J. (2006). *Initiative to combat child hunger.* FDCH Congressional Testimony: 9/26/2006. Committee name: Senate Foreign Relations. Accession number: 32Y1742177555. Retrieved from http://wf2la7.webfeat.org/WSvZG1118/url=http://web.ebscohost.com/ehost/delivery?vid

Global childhood malnutrition. (2006). *Lancet, 367*(9521), 1459.

Hall, B., & Brown, L. (2005). Food security among older adults in the United States. *Topics in Clinical Nutrition, 20*(4), 329–338.

Harder, B. (2004). Double credit. *Science News, 166*(18), 276–277.

Healthline (2015). Retrieved from https://www.google.com/search?q=healthline+(2015)&sourceid=ie7&rls=com.microsoft:en-US:IE-Address&ie=&oe=&gws_rd=ssl

Hopcraft, M., & Tan, C. (2010). Xerostomia: An update for clinicians. *Australian Dental Journal, 55*(3), 238–244.

IFIC Foundation. (2005, March/April). Whole grains on the rise. *Food Insight,* 4–6.

Institute of Medicine. (2005). Protein and amino acids. In *Dietary Reference Intakes for Energy, Carbohydrates, Fiber, Fat, Fatty Acids, Cholesterol, Protein, and Amino Acids (Macronutrients).* Retrieved from http://www.nap.edu/catalog/10490.html

International Food Policy Research Institute. 2015. *Global Nutrition Report 2015: Actions and Accountability to Advance Nutrition and Sustainable Development.* Washington, DC.

International Nutrition Foundation. (n.d.). *Case studies on successful micronutrient programs: The Sri Lankan experience.* Retrieved from http://www.inffoundation.org

James, W. P. T., Simitasiri, S., Hag, U., Tagwirery, J., Norum, K., Uauy, R., & Swaminathan, M. S. (2000). Ending malnutrition by 2020: An agenda for change in the millennium. *WHO Food and Nutrition Bulletin, 21S,* 1S–76S.

Jain, M., Purnima, Jain, P., & Gupta, K. (2013). Appraisal of nutrition and health related knowledge, attitude and practices of rural and urban elderly using a gender lens. *Indian Journal of Gerontology, 27*(3), 519–529. Retrieved from http://www.gerontologyindia.com/

James, W. P. T., Simitasiri, S., Hag, U., Tagwirery, J., Norum, K., Uauy, R., & Swaminathan, M. S. (2000). Ending malnutrition by 20120: An agenda for change in the millennium. *WHO Food and Nutrition Bulletin, 21S*–76S.

Jensen, G. L., Friedmann, J. M., Coleman, C. D., & Smiciklas-Wright, H. (2001). Screening for hospitalization and nutritional risks among community-dwelling older persons [Electronic version]. *American Journal of Clinical Nutrition, 74,* 201–205.

Johnson, L. (2008). Zinc deficiency. In *Merck Manual.* Whitehouse State, NJ: Merck and Company.

Kozakova, R., Jarosova, D., & Zelenikova, R. (2012). Comparison of three screening tools for nutritional status assessment of the elderly in their homes. *Biomedical Papers of the Medical Faculty of the University Palacký, Olomouc, Czechoslovakia, 156*(4), 371–376. doi:10.5507/bp.2011.057

Kranz, S. (2006). Meeting the dietary reference for fiber: Sociodemographic characteristics of preschoolers with high fiber intakes. *American Journal of Public Health, 96*(9), 1538–1541.

Kregg-Byers, C., & Schlenk, E. (2010). Implications of food insecurity on global health policy and nursing practice. *Journal of Nursing Scholarship, 42*(3), 278–285.

Labbok, M., Clark, D., & Goldman, A. (2004). Breast-feeding: Maintaining an irreplaceable immunological resource. *Nature Reviews, 4,* 565–572.

Langer, G., Schloemer, G., Knerr, A., Kuss, O., & Behrens, J. (2003). Nutritional interventions for preventing and treating pressure ulcers. *Cochrane Database of Systematic Review, 4,* CD003216.

Lara-Pulido, A., & Guevara-Cruz, M. (2012). Malnutrition and associated factors in elderly hospitalized. *Nutricion Hospitalaria, 27*(2), 652–655

López-Contreras, M., Torralba, C., Zamora, S., & Pérez-Llamas, F. (2012). Nutrition and prevalence of undernutrition assessed by different diagnostic criteria in nursing homes for elderly people. *Journal of Human Nutrition & Dietetics, 25*(3), 239–246.

Mach, O. (n.d.). *Improving nutrition in Burundi.* Global Health Council, International Medical Corp. Retrieved from http://www.globalhealth.org/reports/printview-report.php3?id=53

Marvin, S., & Medd, W. (2004). Fat city. *World Watch, 18*(5), 10–14.

McCarthy, S. & Manning, D. (2012). Water for well-being: Promoting oral hydration in the elderly. *Australia & New Zealand Continence Journal, 18*(2), 52–56.

Monteiro, C. A., Moura, E. C., Conde, W. L., & Popkin, B. M. (2004). Socioeconomic status and obesity in adult populations of developing countries: A review. *Bulletin of the World Health Organization, 82*(12), 940–946.

Morris, J. (2006, September 26). World Food Programme. Statement by James T. Morris, Executive Director World Food Program to the United States Senate, Foreign Relations Committee. Hearing: Ending Child Hunger and Undernutritional Initiative.

Nash, M. (2003). Obesity goes global. *Time, 162*(8), 53–54.

National Institute on Aging. (2012). *Eating well as you get older.* Retrieved from http://nihseniorhealth.gov/eatingwellasyougetolder/benefitsofeatingwell/01.html

National Institutes of Health. (2006a). *Dietary supplement fact sheet: Vitamin A and carotenoids.* Retrieved from http://ods.od.nih.gov

National Institutes of Health. (2006b). *Dietary supplement fact sheet: Iron.* Retrieved from http://ods.od.nih.gov

National Institutes of Health. (2010). *Dietary supplement fact sheet: Iron.* Retrieved from http://www.ncbi.nlm.nih.gov/pubmedhealth/PMH0001610

National Library of Medicine. (2006). Medline Plus. *Medical encyclopedia: Protein in diet.* Retrieved from http://www.nlm.nih.gov

Nead, K., Halterman, J., Kaczorowski, Auinger, P., & Weitzman, M. (2004). Overweight children and adolescents: A risk for iron deficiency. *Pediatrics, 114*(1), 104–108.

Nestle Nutrition Institute. (n.d.). *MNA: Mini-nutritional assessment.* Retrieved from http://www.mna-elderly.com/

Oakley, G., & Tulchinsky, T. (2010). Folic acid and vitamin B_{12} fortification of flour: A global basic food security requirement. *Public Health Reviews, 32*(1), 284–296.

Olson, C. (2005). Food insecurity in women. *Topics in Clinical Nutrition, 20*(4), 321–328.

Pena, M., & Bacallao, J. (2002). Malnutrition and poverty. *Annual Reviews of Nutrition, 22,* 241–253.

Peterson, K. (2009). Childhood undernutrition: A failing global priority. *Journal of Public Health Policy, 30*(4), 455–464.

Pettifor, J. (2008). Vitamin D &/or calcium deficiency rickets in infants & children: A global perspective. *Indian Journal of Medical Research, 127,* 245–249.

Ramakrishnan, U. (2002). Prevalence of micronutrient malnutrition. *Nutrition Review, 60*(5), S46–S52.

Schmidt, T. R. (n.d.). *What's new in nutrition: Wound care in long-term care.* Retrieved from http://www.novartisnutrition.com

Seligman, H., Laraia, B., & Kushel, M. (2010). Food insecurity is associated with chronic disease among low-income NHANES participants 1,2. *Journal of Nutrition, 140*(2), 304–311.

Senior, A. M., Charleston, M. A., Lihoreau, M., Buhl, J., Raubenheimer, D., & Simpson, S. J. (2015). Evolving nutritional strategies in the presence of competition: A geometric agent-based model. *Computational Biology, 11*(3). E1004111.

Shah, S., Selwyn, B., Luby, S., Merchant, A., & Bano, R. (2003). Prevalence and correlates of stunting among children in rural Pakistan. *Pediatrics International, 45,* 49–53.

Shahar, S., Adznam, S., Rahman, S., Yusoff, N., Yassin, Z., Arshad, F., Sakian, N., Salleh, M., & Samah, A. (2012). Development and analysis of acceptance of a nutrition education package among a rural elderly population: an action research study. *BMC Geriatrics, 12,* 24. doi:10.1186/1471-2318-12-24.

South African Medical Research Council. (2004). *Not an ordinary sweet potato.* Retrieved from http://www.mrc.ac.za/mrcnews/sep2004/sweetpotato.htm

Stallings, S., Wolman, P., & Goodner, C. (2001). Contribution of food intake patterns and number of daily food encounters to obesity in low-income women. *Topics in Clinical Nutrition, 16*(4), 51–60.

Stettler, N. (2004). Comment: The global epidemic of childhood obesity: Is there a role for the paediatrician? *Obesity Reviews, 5*(suppl 1), 1–3.

Tieland, M., Borgonjen-Van den Berg, K., Loon, L., & Groot, L. (2012). Dietary protein intake in community-dwelling, frail, and institutionalized elderly people: scope for improvement. *European Journal of Nutrition, 51*(2), 173–179.

Tsang, B., Sullivan, K., Ruth, L., Williams, T., Suchdev, P. (2014). Nutritional status of young children with inherited blood disorders in western Kenya. *African Journal of Tropical Medical Hygiene, 90*(5), 955–962. Doe: 10.4269/ajtmh.13-0496.Epub

Tulchinsky, T. (2010). Micronutrient deficiency conditions: Global health issues. *Public Health Reviews, 32*(1), 243–256.

Ulrich, C. (2005). Iron plays a major role in nutrition. *Human Ecology, 32*(3), 7–11.

Underwood, B. (2002). Health and nutrition in women, infants, and children: Overview of the global situation and the Asia enigma. *Nutrition Reviews, 60*(5), S7–S13.

UN Committee on Economic, Social and Cultural Rights. (1999). *General Comment No. 12: The Right to Adequate Food (Art. 11 of the Covenant),* 12 May 1999. Retrieved from http://www.refworld.org/docid/4538838c11.html.

USAID. (2005). *USAID announces contribution to global nutrition.* Retrieved from http://www.usaid.gov/our_work/global_health/home/News/nutrition_program.html

U.S. Department of Agriculture. (2005a). *About WIC.* Retrieved from http://www.fns.usda.gov/wic/aboutwic/mission.htm

U.S. Department of Agriculture. (2005b). *Dietary guidelines for Americans.* Weight management (Ch. 3). Retrieved from http://www.health.gov/dietaryguidelines/dga2005/document/html/chapter3.htm

U.S. Environmental Protection Agency. (2010). *EPA finalizes regulations for national renewable fuel standard program for 2010 and beyond.* Retrieved from http://www.epa.gov/otaq/renewablefuels/420f10007.pdf

U.S. Department of Health and Human Services. (2012). *Healthy eating after 50.* Retrieved from http://www.nia.nih.gov/health/publication/healthy-eating-after-50

Visvanathan, V., & Nix, P. (2010). Managing the patient presenting with xerostomia: A review. *International Journal of Clinical Practice, 64*(3), 404–407.

Williams, S. R., & Schlenker, E. D. (2003). *Essentials of nutrition & diet therapy* (8th ed.). St. Louis, MO: Mosby.

World Health Organization. (2014). *Global Nutrition Report.* Retrieved from http://www.who.int/nutrition/global-target-2025/en/

World Health Organization. (2015a). *Obesity and overweight.* Retrieved from http://www.who.int/mediacentre/factsheets/fs311/en/

World Health Organization. (2015b). *Micronutrient deficiencies.* Retrieved from http://www.who.int/nutrition/topics/ida/en/

World Health Organization. (2015c). *Global Health Observatory (GHO) data. Overweight and obesity.* Retrieved from http://www.who.int/gho/ncd/risk_factors/obesity_text/en/

World Hunger Education Service. (2012). *World Hunger and Poverty Facts and Statistics.* Retrieved from http://www.worldhunger.org/articles/Learn/world%20hunger%20facts%202002.htm

15

Global Perspectives on Environmental Health

Marvin A. Friedman

Objectives

Upon completing this chapter, the reader will be able to:

1. Discuss the basic principles of the science of toxicology.
2. Relate the sources, pathways, receptors, and controls of toxicants.
3. Explain processes and endpoints in the human body associated with exposure to toxic agents.
4. Relate various responses associated with different routes of toxic exposure, metabolic pathways, mechanisms of distribution within the body, and elimination processes as they relate to potential pharmacological responses.
5. Describe risk assessment and risk management as they are applied to toxic agents in the environment.
6. Explain the relationship of major aspects of environmental toxicology and chemistry.
7. Discuss the significance of the dose and response to noxious substances.
8. Describe the occurrence and significance of major classes of environmental toxicants.
9. Compare and contrast different populations at risk for environmental health problems based on past history, age, geography, and occupational and environmental exposures.
10. Discuss environmental quality, public health, sustainability, regulatory science, and public communication related to environmental pollution and contamination.

INTRODUCTION

Environmentally induced diseases can result from lack of knowledge about the adverse effects of electromagnetic, ionizing, and nonionizing radiation and environmental chemicals, or from intentional or ethical decisions that weigh the pros and cons of competing alternatives resulting in population exposure to toxic chemicals. This chapter relates examples of how epidemics have resulted from a failure to know and understand environmental risks from both human-made stimuli and natural contaminants as well as environmental risks that resulted from societal, economic, or ethical decisions. In addition, a moral or ethical framework to assess environmental decisions based on risk is described. The regulatory framework under which many governments implement these decisions will be explained as well. Upon completion of this chapter, the reader will have a broader and deeper understanding of how humans interact with their environment.

GLOBAL ISSUES: LESSONS IN ENVIRONMENTAL HEALTH

Much has been written and speculated on the issue of global health and sustainable development. Explanations will be provided regarding how to evaluate eco-disasters such as tsunamis, reactor melt-downs, and air contamination. This chapter is not a compendium of possibilities, however, but rather a development of how to think about and evaluate new scenarios. Speculation about problems for which there are no hard data is difficult and unreliable. However, environmental problems can be solved through application of diligent scientific procedures.

What Happened to the Mink?

In the early 1980s, reproductive complications were observed in mink (Aulerich & Ringer, 1977). Several dietary components were evaluated to determine whether they were the cause of this failure for mink to reproduce. Neither the Coho salmon, which made up the major component of their diet, nor other species of Great Lakes fish appeared to cause this response in experimental mink. Diets and carcasses were evaluated for mercury and chlorinated pesticides, and there was no correlation. Analysis of the pathological signs suggested that polychlorinated biphenyl (PCB) might be the causative agent. However, no other species was presenting with these signs. With feeding of groups of mink on 30 ppm PCB diets or salmon from the Great Lakes, the signs were identical to those of wild mink. It turns out that mink are extremely sensitive to the reproductive effects of PCBs and there were enough PCBs in Great Lakes Coho salmon to induce the detrimental reproductive effects.

The next issue was to determine the source of the PCBs. It was determined that the major use of PCBs was as a heat transfer agent in electrical transformers (International Agency for Research on Cancer [IARC], 1978). At first glance, this use would not suggest an etiology for the high levels of PCBs that were observed in the mink and Coho salmon. However, PCBs are not metabolized to any large extent and, therefore, were stable in the environment. Because they were fat soluble and only marginally water soluble, the PCBs accumulated in the fat of the fish, which then accumulated in the fat of the mink. During the winter, as the mink lost their fat, their blood levels of PCBs would increase sharply. The PCBs caused increased drug metabolism that was reflected in alteration of circulating sex hormone levels that then adversely affected mink reproduction.

The science did not end here. It turned out that PCBs were contaminated with another chlorinated, environmentally stable hydrocarbon, tetrachlorodibenzodioxin (TCDD, more simply known as dioxin), which was three orders of magnitude more toxic than PCBs (Mandal, 2005). This substance was even more widely distributed and was found not only associated with PCBs but also in landfills associated with paper mills that chlorinated their waste at elevated temperatures. This discovery led to a change in the paper-making process in which chlorine dioxide—rather than chlorine—is used. Chlorine replacement due to environmental contamination will be a continuing theme in this chapter; it is a costly step that does not necessarily translate to developing countries.

Parenthetically, the PCB toxic response was replicated in humans when a Japanese family used PCBs for cooking instead of cooking oil; the signs of toxicity were the same. This chapter evaluates what makes one species more sensitive than another, how we characterize the toxicity of materials, and how we can extrapolate risk to environmental exposures. Although there was no human reproductive toxicity observed in these studies, the studies did cause a careful evaluation by regulatory agencies of the safety of Great Lakes fish, particularly to the Canadian aboriginal population, who consume large quantities of these animals.

Considering the prolonged exposure to very low, subclinical exposures to PCBs, the subsequent health effects are not obvious; the issue being whether there are any health consequences of the contamination. Extrapolation from the mode of action to possible sequelae is the most logical way to approach this problem. PCBs act through interaction with a cytoplasmic and nuclear receptor that changes the pattern of metabolism of many substances, including hormones and neurotransmitters (Nikolerisa & Hanssonb, 2015). As a result, there are two obvious target pathways which deserve evaluation, namely reproduction and developmental behavior. In animals models, effects are seen in these systems (Bell, 2014). However, reproduction and developmental behavior are notoriously poor predictors of human effects so the final impact on human health is still an open issue.

What About the Cats in Japan?

In the 1950s, the domestic house cat population in Japan demonstrated a highly unusual central neurotoxicity characterized by a staggered gait and other signs—a condition referred to as Minimata disease, named after the Japanese seaside town where the phenomenon was observed (Takeuchi, D'Itri, Fischer, Annett, & Okabe, 1977). A chemical plant had initiated the manufacture of acetaldehyde and dumped waste methyl mercury in Minimata Bay. Methyl mercury, being fat soluble and not metabolized by fish, accumulated in fish in the bay. The cats ate these fish exclusively in their diet. Subsequently, people living in Minimata began to show the same neurological signs, which also included tunnel vision and learning deficits.

Methyl mercury is a well-known neurotoxin that causes neuropathies in experimental animals and has been studied as a pesticide. In the 1960s, grain was shipped to Iraq for planting that was treated with methyl mercury as a pesticide (Rustam & Hamdi, 1994). This pesticide was purple in color, and it was not expected that people would eat the grain; rather, they were instructed to plant it. They prepared it as bread, however, and a clear dose-response was noted between bread consumption and tunnel vision, peripheral neuropathies, terata, and other forms of methyl mercury toxicity.

Methyl mercury is a component of sea water and accumulates in pelagic (oceangoing) fish. Considerable debate has arisen about the safety of pelagic fish due to methyl mercury contamination. Island populations consuming diets consisting almost exclusively of fish have been studied, but to date these results are inconclusive (Board on Environmental Science and Toxicology, 2000). When methyl mercury is used as an herbicide, such as on golf courses, where the water is not free flowing like the ocean, its concentration can become excessive and the fish in the local waters can represent a source of toxicity.

As we have described, modes for animal developmental behavior are not good predictors of human toxicity. More relevant would be epidemiological data. In order to have epidemiological data that can discern an effect, a population with relatively large exposure to methyl mercury and one with no exposure must be available. Large exposure would be expected from a population consuming large amounts of fish. As a corollary, a behavioral or IQ test must be relevant to these populations and not beyond their sphere of experience. The population of the Seychelles Island consumed a diet extremely rich in fish (Davidson et al., 2011). This same population appeared on the surface to have developmental issues, as might be predicted by the animal models (Newland, Reed, & Rasmussen, 2015; Watson et al., 2013). At issue then is whether the behavioral models are relevant for this population.

Why Do We Discuss Selenium?

The biological effects of selenium represent the best example of environmental health and toxicology. Selenium is a metal that is found in abundance in many parts of the world and concentrates in some plants. Most selenium is consumed as the sulfur amino acids methionine and cysteine, as the selenium can replace the sulfur in these compounds. There is a nutritional requirement for selenium in several biochemical pathways. In New Zealand, China, and Finland, for example, selenium deficiency has been a major public health problem; in these countries, selenium intake is less than 50 mcg/day. Selenium deficiency is characterized by cardiomyopathy and muscle pain (Dodig & Cepelak, 2004; Rederstorff, Krol, & Lescure, 2006). In contrast, in other areas of the world, selenium is present in excess (Dodig & Cepelak, 2004). In these areas, a characteristic neurotoxicity is observed when levels exceed 250 mcg/day. Consideration of selenium deficiency or excess in the absence of knowledge of the other biological properties might lead to other toxic effects.

Vitamin A

Vitamin A, α-tocopherol, is a necessary component of the human diet. Vitamin A, which is needed for vision, is a fat-soluble vitamin that becomes concentrated in the liver (Fishman, 2002; Russell, 1967). Vitamin A, like selenium, also has toxic properties when consumed in excess. This toxicity has been documented among Arctic explorers and Eskimos who consume polar bear. Polar bears live on a diet rich in fish, which in turn are rich in vitamin A. When Arctic explorers consumed polar bear liver, their dose of vitamin A was enormous. As this example demonstrates, a nutrient that receives little attention in the Western diet can be a serious toxin in other conditions. A deficiency of vitamin A is characterized by night blindness, which is then followed by the development of connective tissue disorders. Chronic toxicity affects the skin, the mucous membranes, and the musculoskeletal and neurological systems. Vitamin A toxicity is not necessarily restricted to polar bear consumption, however, as megadose vitamins are becoming popular.

Lessons to Be Learned

All materials have toxicity when their exposure reaches high enough doses. In the case of methyl mercury and PCBs, those animals with the highest consumption of these materials were harbingers of human exposure. With selenium and vitamin A, toxicities arise from both deficiencies and excesses. As they demonstrate, just because a material is required as part of the human diet does not mean it has no toxicity.

PRINCIPLES OF ENVIRONMENTAL HEALTH

Definitions

For the purposes of this chapter, infectious agents are excluded from the discussion to the extent possible. Very frequently, there is a trade-off between infectious agents and chemicals: Examples include food preservatives and water purification, not to mention antibiotics and other pharmaceuticals and antiseptics. Due to the ability of microorganisms to reproduce, infectious disease almost always represents a greater public health concern than chemical contamination.

Assessment of environmental health is couched in technical terms that have clear definitions. Sometimes these definitions have connotations that public health professionals must ignore. For example, workplace exposure to toxic substances is different from environmental exposure. However, contamination of rivers with pharmaceutical agents is an environmental event. The use of estrogens as birth control agents in women, for example, would not be considered environmental. These hormones are excreted in urine and may end up in river water (Shore, Gurevitz, & Semesh, 1993). In one case, this phenomenon resulted in developmental and reproductive problems in striped bass that almost killed the species. Prior to delineating the impact of environmental chemicals on public health, it is important to clarify these terms.

Environment

The environment is defined as the air we breathe, the water we drink, and the food we eat. None of these environmental components is pure in the chemical sense. That is, there is no chemical definition of air, water, or food, as each is a mixture and has both major and minor components contributed by natural sources. For example, the air in the forest contains chemical substances (e.g., terpenes) that volatilize from trees in the forest. Although these substances are natural components of the forest air, they are intentional additives in cleaning products, and in some cases have pesticidal and biocidal activity. The same caveat applies to food. Although a synthetic diet can be constructed from purified starches, proteins, and fatty acids, no one consumes this diet. Therefore, a qualifier is usually appropriate with an environmental component, such as "forest air" or "Great Lakes water."

Environmental Agent

An environmental agent is the chemical or infectious agent or radiation source that is alleged to induce an environmental health incident. Such an agent is associated with two critical characteristics.

First, the quality of data linking the agent with the effect is important. Although Koch's postulates can be applied to infectious agents, it is more difficult to apply them directly to environmental health. Koch's postulates are as follows:

1. The pathogen must be present in all hosts diagnosed with the disease.
2. The pathogen must be isolatable from the diseased host.
3. The pathogen must be purifiable.
4. The purified pathogen must cause the specific disease.
5. The pathogen must be isolated from the host used in step 4.
6. The pathogen in step 5 must be shown to be the same pathogen purified in step 3.

To do this, one would have to demonstrate that the environmental agent was present in the affected population, that the agent could cause the environmental outcome, and that it was present in sufficient quantities to account for the effects.

Second, there must be an analytical technique for the agent in question. Of course, that requires a detailed definition of the environmental agent. For example, it is not sufficient to suggest that the neurological behavior observed in the cats at Minimata Bay was caused by methyl mercury. Instead, the neurological signs must be demonstrated in experimental animals following methyl mercury treatment. Methyl mercury had to be isolated from the cats at doses that would cause the disease. The first step in any environmental evaluation is always the development of an analytical method.

Adverse Health Effect

An adverse health effect is usually defined in preclinical toxicology as any significant deviation from the norm. In the human environment, applying this definition is not always easy. The best example of such difficulty in defining adverse health effects lies in the manufacture of hypnotics. These substances are safe and effective in people even when used in large doses. Sleep induction is a therapeutic response. However, in the manufacturing environment, they may cause workers to fall asleep on the job; this is an adverse outcome. As this example demonstrates, the definition of adverse health effect is subjective: It is the induction of an effect that the exposed population does not intend or want. This has already been demonstrated with environmental exposure to estrogens that can also inhibit reproduction in the environment.

Risk

Risk is the probability that an adverse outcome will occur. Individual risk is the probability that an individual will suffer from an adverse outcome. The opposite of individual risk is population risk—the expected number or percentage of adversely affected individuals in a population who will suffer an adverse outcome. Obviously, exposure of three people to a material that will cause one adverse event in a million is different from exposing 300 million people to that risk.

Risk has three components: exposure, causation, and dose-response. The calculation and interpretation of risk will be dealt with in great detail later.

Ecology

Receptors for adverse events are not restricted to humans but are also present in wildlife, including fish. Due to the varied spectrum of species and their different physiologies, a substantial difference in sensitivity has been observed. Subtle questions can be asked with regard to protection of the environment. For example, are environmental evaluations performed by protecting most of the species exposed or by protecting the total population?

Toxicology

Toxicology is the study of the adverse effects of materials, chemicals, or radiation on living organisms. Although not explicit in the definition, what makes a toxicologist different from other scientists is that a toxicologist relates dose and response rather than just studying response. The terms "adverse effects" and "toxicological effects" are used interchangeably in this chapter.

Physiologically or Toxicologically Significant Adverse Health Effects

Although the issue of what qualifies as a significant adverse effect might seem easily resolved, it is actually very difficult to state with clarity. For example, an environmental substance that only causes weight loss at a specific dose is not considered to be inducing an adverse effect. However, when that same substance is evaluated as a pharmaceutical for that purpose, it is considered therapeutic. Looking at the same situation in reverse, one can look at a material that can be used safely and effectively as a hypnotic. The dose at which it manifests the hypnotic response is not a toxic dose but rather a dose that produces a pharmacologically beneficial event. However, when this material is manufactured in the workplace and exposure takes place at a level sufficient to induce a hypnotic dose, the workers fall asleep, and there are substantial problems thereafter.

To put matters in perspective, one can consider how to evaluate additives for food that decrease calorie availability or promote weight loss. When a manufacturer evaluates an inert ingredient such as a nonmetabolizable starch for use in breads, cookies, and cakes, the U.S. Food and Drug Administration (FDA) requires at least a 100-fold safety margin be maintained. Of course, adding 100 times the amount to be used in breads, cakes, and cookies will result in body weight loss, as the test animals do not eat enough food to compensate for the starch. It then appears that there is a toxic response characterized by weight loss. Because such components are food additives and not drugs, a margin of safety is required before they can be included in foods for the general public. Thus the definition of "adverse effect" is not always obvious.

Similarly, with large sample sizes or sensitive assays, small effects that have no physiological significance can be detected even while the response has no toxicological significance. The terms "statistical significance" and "toxicological significance" relate to different levels of findings: The former is dependent on characteristics of the assay and the sample size, while the latter deals with hazards. It is necessary to have statistical significance before toxicological significance becomes an issue. It is important to evaluate whether effects observed in populations around the world are real adverse health effects or just statistical anomalies caused by large sample sizes or sensitive assays.

Global Catastrophic Risk

There are a few risks whose consequences can be so significant that normal considerations of cost, benefit, weight of the evidence, and concentration dependency are not considered. The most obvious of these is climate change, which results from destruction of the ozone layer of the atmosphere and consequent warming of the surface of the Earth by a few degrees Celsius. The postulate underlying the theory of global warming is that release of carbon dioxide or fully halogenated hydrocarbons (to be discussed later in this chapter) into the atmosphere can decrease the density and effectiveness of the stratospheric filter for radiation. Although the data are poor and the effects immeasurable, if true, this outcome would mean a global catastrophe. Of course, the causation must be human-made so that it becomes actionable. Global warming from volcanoes is an entirely different environmental scenario as there is not much that can be done to affect volcanoes. Therefore, the threat must be dealt with as if it were absolutely true. Such mega-events are not common, but when present require an entirely different way of thinking about risk. Treatment of drinking water, safety of vaccines, and contamination of foodstuffs all fit into this global catastrophic risk.

PRINCIPLES OF TOXICOLOGY

A detailed and comprehensive treatise on toxicology is beyond the scope of this chapter. However, there are some very critical concepts that can be covered here.

Intrinsic Activity

Intrinsic activity can be defined as the maximum response that can be induced by a toxicant. It can be seen in Figure 15-1, which is an idealized schematic. Of the four curves, two have the same intrinsic activity and two have the same potency. For intrinsic activity, the maximum response is 40 at both high and low potency, whereas the maximum at the low dose is 8. Intrinsic activity is a biological property of a substance. For example, the diuretic properties of a substance such as melamine and the porphyrin-modifying properties of lead and iron are intrinsic activities; they may be considered as a physical property of the substance. Such activities are generally determined in animal experiments or in vitro studies, but sometimes are identified in humans first as anecdotal observations, such as the observation that vinyl chloride was a human carcinogen. In the European Union, a classification system for intrinsic activity has been developed, where category 1 is an activity known to occur in humans, category 2 is an activity that will probably occur in humans, and category 3 is an activity that has been identified only in animals.

Intrinsic activity does have degrees of effectiveness associated with it. That is, the maximum effect of a substance can differ between two substances. For example, one substance may induce more chromosomal anomalies than another at the maximum dose tested.

One can compare the bladder cancer–inducing activity of chemicals as an example. Several materials such as melamine or saccharine will precipitate in the bladder. This precipitate can irritate the walls of the bladder and cause tumors to be produced. Very seldom does the incidence of tumors produced by this mechanism exceed 15% even at doses such as 6,000 ppm in the diet (Heck & Tyl, 1985; Melnick, Boorman, Haseman, Montali, & Huff, 1984). In contrast, some aromatic amines cause bladder cancer in rats in 50% of the animals.

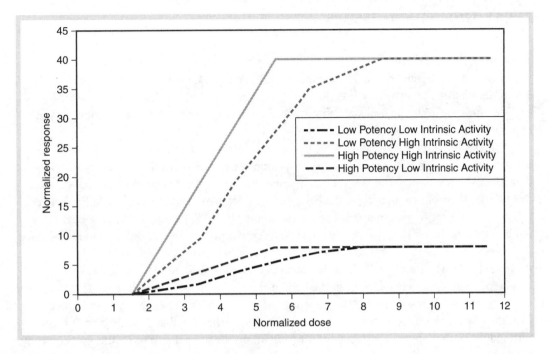

FIGURE 15-1 Comparison of Potency and Intrinsic Activity

Potency

Potency relates to the dose at which an effect is observed. The units of expression of potency are either expressions of doses where no responses occur or expressions of doses where a 50% response occurs. In the case of the doses with no response, the "no observed adverse effect" level (NOAEL) is used; it depends on the dose spacing and sensitivity of the assay to detect responses. The NOAEL is the experimental dose at which no adverse effect has been observed, but this experimental point is highly dependent on the protocol, quality of data, experimental design, and sample size. The poorer the design, the lower the quality of the data, or the smaller the sample size, the higher the NOAEL.

In the case of measuring a 50% response, the ED_{50} (effective dose in 50% of the population), LD_{50} (lethal dose in 50% of the population), or benchmark dose (BMD; a curve-fitting exercise) is used. These metrics are the most reproducible experimental observations. Finally, a mathematical curve fitting can be used that will generate the best-fitting curve—that is, the curve that takes into account all of the data points. This mathematical expression can then be used to generate a theoretical 10% dose-response, which is the BMD. Because this is a mathematical curve fitting, virtually any dose can be used or the statistical bounds could also be used. In Figure 15-1, the ED_{50} for the higher-potency material is 4; for the lower-potency material, it is 6.

The concepts of potency and intrinsic activity underscore the inability to compare the adverse effects of substances. Either potency or intrinsic activity can be a variable.

LEGAL AND ETHICAL ISSUES

Laws and Regulations

Governing of democratic nations is accomplished in two ways. First, laws are passed by an elected legislature that provides direction for governance. Second, within these laws is the delegation of responsibility to, or establishment of, an executive agency for implementation and enforcement of these laws.

The executive agencies deal with the details of implementation and interpretation of the legislation. As an example, the U.S. Congress passed the Federal Insecticide, Pesticide and Rodenticide Act, which gave the U.S. Environmental Protection Agency (EPA), a part of the executive branch, control over the sale and labeling of biocides. This separation of authority between legislative and executive branches is not unique to the United States, but rather is global in nature. Serious abuses in this system occur when there is no legislative branch to write the laws, such that the executive branch writes the laws, establishes the regulations, and performs the enforcement. This system typically leads to corruption and environmental deterioration.

Legal challenges to regulations in the United States, for example, which make for interesting news, deal with whether the regulatory agency has the authority to perform a specific task as identified by legislation, or whether the regulatory agency has acted as described by law. Citizens may then challenge the regulatory enforcement on the basis that it was either not correctly carried out by law or that the law did not authorize the agency to act the way it did.

Perhaps the best example of the difference between regulation and legislation can be seen in the failed attempts of the FDA to regulate cigarette smoking. Clearly, the FDA is responsible for a major component of public health, and clearly cigarette smoking is detrimental to public health. However, there was no authorization in the Food, Drug, and Cosmetic Act that would allow the FDA to regulate smoking. Cigarette smoke is neither a food nor a food additive, and Congress chose not to change the legislation to authorize FDA regulation of tobacco products. Tobacco is also not considered a drug, as manufacturers do not make any health-related claims for cigarette smoke. It was only recently that the FDA embarked on regulating cigarette smoke by declaring cigarettes to be a drug delivery system, delivering nicotine as a drug (Centers for Disease Control and Prevention [CDC], 2007; FDA, 1995). This allegation brought cigarettes under the Food, Drug, and Cosmetics Act and, therefore, made them subject to FDA regulation. Otherwise, independent of the adverse health effects of cigarettes, the FDA was powerless to regulate tobacco smoke.

Regulation Versus Ethics

Ethics becomes an issue when there are no laws or regulations available to support regulatory enforcement. The critical issue associated with ethical decisions lies in the values involved. Values have many varied definitions, and can be parsed into moral values, ethical values, family values, religious values, and so on. Based on the soft and personal nature of values, interpreting them for environmental (economic) decision making is virtually impossible. Ethical considerations must either be converted to some form of regulation or cannot be major decision criteria for environmental issues.

An example of an ethical decision is Proposition 6 in California, a regulation to ban consumption of horse meat (Alpen, Powers-Risius, Curtis, & DeGuzman, 1998; CDC, 2007). There was no public health issue involved in this proposition and no laws under which to regulate horse meat. Thus the state made a decision that it was unethical to slaughter horses for the purpose of human consumption.

WHAT IS THE ENVIRONMENT?

As noted earlier, the environment consists of the air we breathe, the water we drink, and the food we eat. Public health concerns about each of these aspects of the environment are very different.

Air Pollution

There are four major classes of air-polluting gases: irritating chemicals, asphyxiating chemicals, air toxics, and atmospheric reactants.

Irritants

Irritants damage the surface of the respiratory tract. Highly water-soluble irritants such as formaldehyde cause irritation of the upper respiratory tract, whereas less water-soluble irritants such as nitrogen oxides cause lower respiratory tract irritation.

Hydrogen chloride is very water soluble and is an upper respiratory tract irritant. Its inhalation causes effects in the nose, for example. As a response to contact with upper respiratory tract irritants, individuals will hold their breath or breathe more shallowly. The major chronic effect of upper respiratory tract irritants is loss of the sense of smell through toxicity to the olfactory epithelium. Sulfur dioxide is another example of an upper respiratory tract irritant.

Oxides of nitrogen such as nitrogen dioxide are lower respiratory tract irritants; exposure to these substances is accompanied by chest pains. The other major environmental irritant gases are ozone and chlorine, which oxidize in the lower respiratory tract. In each case, the result is fibrotic/scarring lesions in the irritated portion of the lung with an accompanying loss of function. Lower respiratory tract irritants can also cause emphysema and other typical pulmonary lesions.

It is extremely import to differentiate irritants from foul-smelling materials. Odor is not necessarily a characteristic of toxic vapors. Foul smells are designed to elicit an avoidance response.

Asphyxiates

Asphyxiates cause suffocation or lack of oxygen transport to the body. The major asphyxiate is carbon monoxide; overexposure to this gas leads to a chemical asphyxiation. Carbon dioxide induces a similar response but at markedly higher concentrations.

Toxics

The third class of pollutant gases comprises toxins—gases that are absorbed through the lungs and have adverse systemic effects. For example, hydrogen cyanide has direct effects on the blood, but not on the lungs. A wide variety of other materials, when inhaled, produce systemic toxicity. Anesthetic and neurotoxic gases, such as ether and toluene, are in this class. Virtually any material when inhaled can be absorbed into the lung to some extent.

High-molecular-weight polymers and water-insoluble chemicals are not absorbed into the bloodstream, but rather are deposited into the lungs and remain there. These materials may be removed by a system that moves them up the trachea for excretion or to be swallowed. The body defenses against these materials may have a side effect of irritating the adjacent lung tissue. Macrophages are designed to kill bacteria in the lungs by producing peroxide. An effect of some particulates is to kill the macrophages, thereby causing peroxide buildup in the lungs, which eventually proves toxic. Finally, exercise can accentuate lung toxicity through increase in the respiratory rate. With increased respiration, the dosage increases.

Atmospheric Reactants

Chemical reaction of pollutants with atmospheric constituents can induce serious environmental degradation. The two major classes of these air pollutants are smog and greenhouse gases.

Smog. Photochemical smog is a concern in most major urban centers. Smog is caused by a reaction between sunlight and emissions, mainly from human activity such as automobile exhaust and fireplaces. Photochemical smog is the chemical reaction of sunlight, nitrogen oxides (NOx), and volatile organic compounds (VOCs) in the atmosphere, which leaves behind airborne particles (called particulate matter) and ground-level ozone. Nitrogen oxides are released in the exhaust of fossil fuel–burning engines in cars, trucks, coal power plants, and industrial manufacturing factories. VOCs are vapors released from gasoline, paints, solvents, pesticides, and other chemicals.

Greenhouse Gases. Some organic substances—the most notable and avoidable being fully halogenated substances such as chlorofluorocarbons (CFCs)—decrease the atmospheric filter for sunshine. The greenhouse gases may interact with ozone, which filters sunlight and provides a stable temperature on Earth. Perhaps the most significant of these gases is carbon dioxide, which is produced by burning fossil fuels and by the setting of concrete. Methane is produced by livestock farming and rice paddies. Sunlight and other radiation turn methane and carbon dioxide into free radicals, which then interact with ozone.

Water Pollution

Pollution of drinking water can take the form of either chemical or microbial contamination. Microbial contamination is beyond the context of this chapter, except to note that it necessitates chemical treatment of water. In the absence of chemical treatment, epidemics of cholera and typhus can occur, as well as *E. coli* infection. On a global basis water contamination is a leading cause of death as an inducer of diarrhea.

Treatment of microbial contamination is not difficult, but it is costly. It generally involves killing the organisms with chlorine, chlorine dioxide, or ozone. The costly part is not only the treatment phase, but also the transport of the water to the site of use. In developing countries without water purification plants, boiling water is effective as a microbial decontamination measure. In general, chemical oxidants are added to the water to sterilize it. Historically the most popular of these compounds has been chlorine. Chlorine is an inexpensive and effective agent for this purpose. The downside of chlorine use is twofold: It is difficult and risky to transport, and the chemical reaction between chlorine and the biological agents in water results in the production of chloroform and other trihalomethanes that are carcinogens at high doses in experimental animals. Chemical reaction rate constants show that the bromine analogues—bromoforms—are also produced from this process. For this reason, newer water treatment facilities tend to use either peroxide or chloramine. Peroxide is very effective at eliminating other chlorination by-products such as TCDD, which is among the most toxic of all organic chemicals and is highly persistent in the environment. Paper mills, which may have a very high organic content waste, use the more costly peroxide process to avoid TCDD production. Chloramine is not without its disadvantages, however, as it appears to increase the level of nitrosamines in the water. Nitrosamines are highly carcinogenic chemicals more commonly found in nitrite-preserved meats.

The issues involved in the evaluation and trade-off of these treatment methods are closely analogous to the ethical decisions discussed previously. Possibly the worst alternative is microbiological contamination, but only peroxide is without a potentially toxic sequelae. Yet the concentrations of halogenated contaminants are very low following water treatment, and the nitrosamine concentration resulting from this process amounts to less than 0.5% of dietary intake of these compounds. Regulatory risk assessment methods assume that there is no risk-free dose.

Radiation

Radiation represents an electromagnetic spectrum that covers many facets from visible light, to ultraviolet light, to infrared to radio waves, to microwaves, and so forth. From a health viewpoint, radiation can be condensed into three facets: ionizing, nonionizing, and thermal radiation.

Ionizing Radiation

Ionizing radiation consists of high-energy radiation such as gamma rays, X-rays, and other high-energy particles. These forms of radiation penetrate the skin and are not stopped by most boundaries. Biologically, they ionize chemicals in the body, which has two effects. First, the ionization mutates DNA. Dividing cells with damaged DNA either will be repaired, will die, or will be transformed into cancer cells. Approximately one million DNA lesions per cell per day are produced as a result of background radiation. In the case of other cellular components, contact with ionizing radiation causes them to become oxidized. The resulting oxidative stress has many sequelae such as aging and many diseases. The most significant lesion entails chromosome breakage, a nonrepairable phenomenon. However, it appears to be at least a second-order reaction; thus, at low levels of radiation, the risk of chromosome breakage is exponentially less than at high doses.

Nonionizing Radiation

Nonionizing radiation (UV radiation) is responsible for suntans and other dermal responses (Elnazar, Ghazy, Ghoneim, Taja, & Abouelella, 2015). It does not penetrate the skin to any great depth. While the chemical reaction resulting in tanning is not deleterious, nonionizing radiation can cross-link dermal DNA, thereby inducing mutagenic reactions. This results in severe dermatological responses such sunburns and melanomas.

Thermal Radiation

Long-wave radiation such as microwave or radar causes water molecules to heat up and produce a thermal effect. This effect is usually not a concern to the environment.

PERSISTENT ORGANICS

Water contamination results in exposure from two sources. First and most obvious is drinking the water. Second, and not as obvious, is consumption of fish and seafood harvested from the water. The ability of materials to accumulate and persist in wildlife is a measurable characteristic of organic and inorganic chemicals. Some of the most recognizable of these persistent chemicals are DDT, PCBs, and TCDD. The environmental concern is not that these compounds are toxic at ambient concentrations, but rather that they can accumulate in biota to reach toxic levels as discussed earlier with methyl mercury. On a global basis, these persistent organic pollutants are being banned with the same aggressiveness as those that cause global warming.

Clearly, low-cost chlorination will continue to predominate in countries where the social costs of its elimination cannot be borne by the economy. In the Western world, one of the other water treatment methods will be selected.

Toxics

In the same way that there are toxic substances in the air, so there can also be toxic substances in water. Toxicants are defined as materials in water that exert toxic effects through systemic absorption. Establishing an acceptable dose for materials in water over a lifetime is difficult. In addition, estimating consumption of water toxics is complicated. In the United States, individuals move frequently and their exposure to any particular drinking water source is, on average, limited to 10 years. Most individuals have an average consumption of 3 liters of water per day.

Toxics in drinking water may include pesticides, heavy metals, nitrosamines, halogenated materials from chlorination, and other pollutants, depending on the area, groundwater source, purification methods, and so on. There is currently no economically sound way to remove metals from drinking water, so these components represent a special problem. Symptomatology in a population exposed to chemically contaminated drinking water will not be restricted to a single individual, but rather will appear in large numbers of the overall population. For example, contamination of water with large amounts of iron salts will result in liver and blood problems in many people. If only a single individual is found to have a problem, the causative agent is not likely present in the community's drinking water.

A special subset within the general population when it comes to water pollution is people who have wells. Because the well can be contaminated in its construction, use, or the water supply it accesses, a family deriving its water from that source can have toxic symptoms separate from the overall population. For example, one family in Japan lined its well with an acrylamide polymer that had not sufficiently polymerized to remove the acrylamide (Igisu, Goto Kawamura, Koto, & Izumi, 1975). The entire family then came down with acrylamide neurotoxicity, while the rest of the population remained healthy.

Biological Oxygen Demand

When microorganisms in water metabolize pollutants to nontoxic carbon dioxide, they utilize oxygen in this process. As a side note, the degradability of an organic chemical is measured in terms of the demand it presents on oxygen. Such oxygen depletion can be disastrous to animals in the water that require oxygen, such as fish. Fish kills can be caused by adding to water various nutrients that microorganisms metabolize, thereby depleting the available oxygen. Another way to stimulate growth of oxygen-depleting organisms is to add a cofactor to the water that had previously been growth limiting. Runoff of phosphate used in fertilizer from agricultural and suburban land, for example, provides much needed phosphate to algae, which then grow and deplete the oxygen in the water in which they live. This reaction is ruinous to many lakes and estuaries such as the Everglades. Globally, this problem has become more extensive as the equation for the value of conservation versus agricultural production has shifted to favor agricultural production in the developing world.

FOOD

The inclusion of food in this chapter is not meant to imply that food is toxic. However, food can serve as a source of pharmacologically active substances that must be considered in disease causation. These substances can arise through food storage, manufacture, or cooking, or they can be integral parts of the food being consumed. For example, some Guam inhabitants chew on cycad nuts ("The Cycad Story Extended," 1970). As a result, these individuals may develop a disease similar to amyotrophic lateral sclerosis (ALS, also known as Lou Gehrig's disease).

There are two ways of looking at food contamination. Historically, epidemiologists have been primarily concerned with low levels of very potent contaminants. In reality, there may be an even higher risk associated with high levels of low-potency substances.

For example, the presence of nitrosamines in nitrite-preserved foodstuffs has been the subject of extensive research. These substances cause cancer at low doses in virtually every species tested, including humans. Nevertheless, their presence in foodstuffs appears so low that they do not represent a public health risk. Nitrosamines are generally the result of food preservation using nitrites or are produced by the conversion of nitrate to nitrite in the stomachs of neonates and subsequent in vivo nitrosation. They are found in low levels in drinking water as a result of chloramine purification as well.

In contrast, polyunsaturated fatty acids are another cancer risk, albeit one with very little animal data to support their carcinogenic role. These chemicals are present in very high levels in many foods, delivering very significant doses to people who consume these foodstuffs. Even though they appear to have low potency, they may represent a much greater risk than the much more potent nitrosamines, simply because of the volumes in which they are consumed.

The argument about "risk versus potency" of components in foods approaches absurdity when nitrosamines are compared with the use of salt. Salt represents a real public health problem, even though it is a naturally occurring substance (Hussein & Brasel, 2001).

Food Storage

Contamination of food during storage can be a major source of toxic substances. Peanuts provide a perfect example of this problem. Peanuts, being approximately 50% fat, are an excellent substrate for mold growth. The mold *Aspergillus flavus* has been particularly well studied (Hussein & Brasel, 2001). This mold produces a unique metabolite, aflatoxin, which is among the most highly carcinogenic substances known. In many areas of the world, such as central Africa, this mold growth results in a substantial increase in liver cancer cases. Some areas of China also exhibit the same increased cancer incidence from aflatoxin consumption. Peanuts are not the only aflatoxin substrate, however; *Aspergillus* can also grow on corn, wheat, and so on. The FDA monitors aflatoxin contamination very closely, and foodstuffs are carefully assayed for aflatoxin content.

Many storage molds produce very potent toxins (Howlett, 1996). A laundry list will not be provided here, as this list grows continually with the discovery of new molds.

Food Manufacture

The contamination of food and beverages by chemicals during manufacture is a heavily regulated issue in the developed world. Many developing nations follow FDA or European Union (EU) regulations for their internal food manufacture industries. The United States and the EU have different approaches to this issue, however ("Evaluation of Certain Food Contaminants," 2006; Hattan & Kahl, 2002).

In the United States, industry must supply FDA not only with safety information that is correlated with expected exposure, but also with efficacy data in the case of direct food additives. Chemicals are evaluated on a single-use basis; that is, if a chemical is used in more than one process, each process is evaluated independently. Each chemical is also evaluated independent of the foodstuff. For example, the fortification of breakfast cereals does not consider the presence of these nutrients in the milk added to the cereal.

In contrast, the EU has developed a list of substances that are considered acceptable for food use. In addition, the EU has created a list of chemicals that are not allowed for use in foods. Efficacy is not an issue in the EU when it comes to food additives.

Consider the example of the addition of calcium to breakfast cereal. The FDA would consider the nutrient properties of calcium and set a standard for addition of calcium in breakfast cereal. It would not consider the calcium level in milk added to the breakfast cereal, arguing that cereal can be consumed without milk. In the EU, calcium salts are approved for use in foodstuffs, so calcium may be added to cereal or even milk by any food manufacturer.

Cooking

Production of toxicants by cooking is a completely unregulated activity. The most readily apparent cooking contaminants are associated with grilling food at high temperatures. The charred surfaces of meats and other grilled foodstuffs are rich in polynucleated aromatic hydrocarbons (PAHs). These materials are carcinogenic and mutagenic, and they induce reproductive disorders when present at elevated concentrations. The chemistry that produces PAHs occurs at elevated temperatures from all organics. For example, smoke from fires or automobile exhaust may contain high levels of these materials. Once highly significant air pollutants, PAHs are now tightly regulated in the developed world.

In contrast, amino acids reaction with creatine—found in muscle tissue—causes the production of heterocyclic amines (HCAs). The major source of these chemicals is cooking of muscle meat from animals and fish. Epidemiologists have linked this cooking process with cancer of the stomach. Frying, broiling, and barbequing cause much more HCA production than baking or microwaving, as they induce higher temperatures in the foodstuff.

In the same fashion as HCAs are produced by heating muscle meat at high temperatures, acrylamide is produced by heating starchy foods in excess of 230°F. Acrylamide has long been established as a human neurotoxin due to its mishandling in industry, particularly grouting. An industrial intermediate, it is used in the manufacture of polymers for water treatment, mining, paper manufacture, and sludge dewatering. Excessive heating of the amino acid asparagine in the presence of reducing sugars also produces acrylamide. In the mid-1980s, acrylamide was found to cause cancer in laboratory rats and to influence chromosomal segregation in male reproductive tissue (Maronpot, 2015). It is found in greatest quantities in those starchy foods cooked at the highest temperatures, such as potato chips. This elevated cooking process is used to drive out the water in the food product so that the temperature can exceed the boiling point of water. For example, acrylamide has been found in the crust of bread but not in the middle.

Saturated fatty acids have been found in low levels in meats. To increase their shelf life, some foodstuffs are treated with antioxidants to keep the unsaturated fatty acids from going rancid, which in turn elevates the saturated fatty acid content. Saturated fatty acids have been associated with many maladies, including memory loss and cancer.

Intrinsic Pharmacologically Active Chemicals

There is no end of naturally occurring chemicals in food that have pharmacological activity. For example, the puffer fish—considered a delicacy in Japan—is rich in tetrodotoxin, an extremely potent neurotoxin. Consequently, preparation of puffer fish must be done by a licensed individual who can remove the poisonous gland. Some mushrooms contain α-amanitin, which was developed into the anticancer drug amantadine. The existence of such potent agents has spawned an effort by the pharmaceutical industry to seek biological substances that occur naturally and develop them into commercial medications.

The presence of these substances in foodstuffs does not have a large impact on the Western world, where diets are relatively standard. In the developing world, however, it is a different story. As noted earlier, consumption of cycad nuts in Guam (and the Philippines) has resulted in amyotrophic lateral sclerosis. In the Western world, concern about foodstuffs focuses on those materials that are present in large amounts and have low potency, such as cholesterol. In the developing world, the more potent contaminants become more important. That is not to say that there is not also toxicity from low-potency chemicals. For example, iron toxicity is rampant in some areas of China and Africa as a result of cooking in rusty pots.

Food allergies are another area where intrinsic properties of food represent serious medical hazards. To some individuals, peanuts are extremely toxic. The incidence of this allergy is low, perhaps one person per million population. However, with 300 million inhabitants in America, it is questionable whether this risk can be economically regulated (Schoessler, 2005).

SUSTAINABLE DEVELOPMENT

According to the United Nations, sustainable development is the process of developing land, cities, business, communities, and so on, so that the result "meets the needs of the present without compromising the ability of future generations to meet their own needs" ("The Environment Becomes a Political Issue," 1988). One of the factors that sustainable development must overcome is environmental degradation, but it must do so without foregoing the needs related to economic development, social equality, and justice. To accomplish this goal, a balance must be struck between industrial development, pollution control with an absence of environmental degradation, and attention to the needs for the future. We have discussed air pollution with its toxics and oxidants, water pollution with its toxics and persistent organic chemicals, and the protection of our food supply. An unsustainable situation occurs when natural capital (the sum total of nature's resources) is used up faster than it can be replenished. Sustainability requires that human activity, at a minimum, use nature's resources only at a rate at which they can be replenished naturally. Implicit in this concept is the idea that pollution prevention is as important or more important than pollution development.

Study Questions

1. Explain, with examples, why it is important to human health to pay attention to environmental incidents caused by chemicals, infectious agents, or radiations. How do these agents cause global environmental health incidents?
2. Relate the problems of selenium deficiency and excess. What are some contributing factors in the environment that can cause these abnormalities? What solutions can correct these abnormal conditions? What other substances also have potential problems with excess and deficiency?
3. What is meant by dose and potency?
4. Explain how food can be contaminated during storage. What are the health implications? What are the important factors to consider while protecting our food supply?
5. Discuss how some methods of cooking food can cause harm to the body.
6. Explain, compare, and contrast examples of sustainable and unsustainable developments.

Case Study 1: Micronutrient: Aflatoxin B1

In 1960, more than 100,000 young turkeys on poultry farms in England died from an apparently new liver disease that was termed "Turkey X disease." It was soon found that ducklings and young pheasants were also affected, and heavy mortality among these fowl populations was experienced. This disease became associated with feed, particularly peanut meal from Brazil. Subsequently it was found that a potent toxin, aflatoxin B1, was present in the feed. Aflatoxin B1 was produced by a storage mold that grew on the peanuts because of the relative humidity on the surface of the peanuts. Visual selection of peanuts for human consumption could eliminate the aflatoxin contamination.

Chronic toxicology studies in rats revealed that aflatoxin B1 is among the most potent carcinogens known, causing liver cancer in rats (Figure 15-2). However, there are some geographic areas in the world where aflatoxin exposure causes no increase in liver cancer. Confounding environmental factors involved in aflatoxin-related liver cancer based on the global distribution of liver cancer and aflatoxin exposure can be present in some world locations, such as central Africa. Within central Africa, hemosiderosis, produced by iron toxicity from using rusty cooking utensils, causes liver cancer (Mandishona et al., 1998).

In China, there is a high rate of hepatitis B virus, which acts synergistically with aflatoxicosis. Knowledge of this phenomenon is enormously significant in preventing liver cancer.

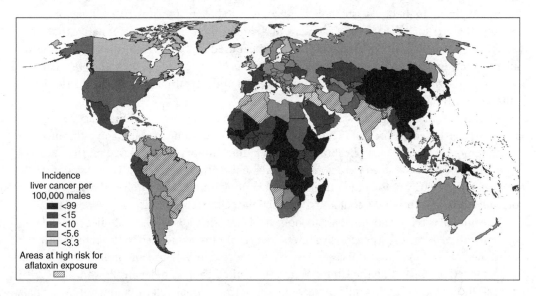

FIGURE 15-2 Correlation Between Populations with High Liver Cancer Rates and High Risk of Chronic Exposure to Aflatoxin Contamination
Reproduced from National Institute of Environmental Health Sciences. *Liver cancer data from the GLOBOCAN 2002 database.* Retrieved from http://www-dep.iarc.fr/GLOBOCAN_frame.htm. Aflatoxin data from Williams et al. (2004). Human aflatoxicosis in developing countries. *American Journal of Clinical Nutrition, 80,* 1106–1122.

Specifically, the same techniques that are useful in Africa will not have utility in China. In both cases, hygienic food storage will be effective. In Africa, upgrading the cooking utensils will produce a sharp drop in liver cancer; in China, an upgrade in cooking utensils could prevent hepatitis B (Chen & Zhang, 2011; Yu & Yuan, 2004). An important lesson to be learned here is the same one that was presented with methyl mercury—namely, that domestic or wild animals can be a sentinel of human disease.

Case Study 1 Questions

1. Earlier in this chapter, the presence of aflatoxin in peanuts was discussed. Are there any other foods that might be contaminated by aflatoxin?
2. As there may have been two factors required for the appearance of human cancer, is the risk from aflatoxin overestimated?

Case Study 2: Balkan Nephropathy

Balkan nephropathy is an interstitial nephropathy first identified in the 1920s in people living along the Danube River (Cosyns, 2003). It was not a typical nephropathy, from a morphological standpoint, and was restricted to adults—that is, no children presented with the disease. Chronic exposure to dietary aristocholic acid appears to be a major causative risk factor for this nephropathy. Aristocholic acid may come from *Aristolochia clematitis,* a plant native to the endemic region, and its seeds may comingle with wheat used for bread. According to the International Agency for Research on Cancer, several *Aristolochia* species have been used in traditional Chinese medicine as antirheumatics, as diuretics, and in the treatment of edema. Aristolochic acids are constituents of these plant species.

After the recognition of these acids' role of Balkan nephropathy, the American Public Health Service tested aristocholic acid in rats and mice for chronic toxicity. This substance caused tumors at the site of application as well as kidney tumors in rats. Based on these toxicology studies, follow-up studies were done on individuals with nephropathy. High rates of urethral cancer, primarily of the upper urinary tract, among individuals with renal disease who had consumed botanical products containing aristocholic acids were found.

The human carcinogenicity of aristocholic acids was first identified in studies of Belgian patients with nephropathy (progressive interstitial renal fibrosis) related to the consumption of herbal medicines. More than 100 cases have been reported in Belgium and more than 170 cases in other locations, including the United States, the United Kingdom, Japan, Taiwan, and China. Clinical studies found significantly increased risks of transitional-cell carcinoma of the urinary bladder and upper urinary tract among Chinese renal-transplant or dialysis patients who had consumed Chinese herbs or drugs containing aristocholic acids, using nonexposed patients as the reference population. This is the first "known human carcinogen" that was first discovered in animals.

Case Study 2 Questions

1. Should the FDA regulate the import and use of herbal medicines? If so, how should the FDA do so?
2. How would you compare the risk and hazards from aristocholic acid and aflatoxin?

References

Alpen, E. L., Powers-Risius, P., Curtis, S. B., DeGuzman, R. (1998). *California Proposition 6. Prohibition on Slaughter of Horses for Human Consumption.* Retrieved from https://ballotpedia.org/California_Proposition_6,_Prohibition_on_Slaughter_of_Horses_for_Human_Consumption_(1998)

Aulerich, R. J., & Ringer, R. K. (1977). Current status of PCB toxicity to mink, and effect on their reproduction. *Archives of Environmental Contamination and Toxicology, 6*(2–3), 279–292.

Bell, M. R. (2014). Endocrine disrupting actions of PCB's on brain development and social and reproductive behaviors. *Current Opinions in Pharmacology, 19*, 134–144.

Board on Environmental Science and Toxicology. (2000). *Toxicological effects of methylmercury.* Washington, DC: National Research Council.

Centers for Disease Control and Prevention. (2007). *Selected Actions of the U.S. Government Regarding the Regulation of Tobacco Sales, Marketing, and Use.* Atlanta, GA: Author.

Chen, J. G., & Zhang, S. W. (2011). Liver cancer epidemic in China: Past, present and future. *Seminars in Cancer Biology, 21*(1), 59–69.

Cosyns, J. (2003). Aristolochic acid and "Chinese herbs nephropathy": A review of the evidence to date. *Drug Safety, 26*(1), 33–48.

The cycad story extended. (1970). *Food, Cosmetics, and Toxicology, 8*(2), 217–218.

Davidson, P. W., Cory-Slechta, D. A., Thurston, S. W., Huang, L. S., Shamlaye, C. F., Gunzler D., Watson, G., van Wijngaarden, E., Zareba, G., Klein, J. D., Clarkson, T. W., Strain, J. J., & Myers, G. J. (2011). Fish consumption and prenatal methylmercury exposure: Cognitive and behavioral outcomes in the main cohort at 17 years from the Seychelles child development study. *Neurotoxicology. 32*(6), 711–717. doi:10.1016

Dodig, S., & Cepelak, I. (2004). The facts and controversies about selenium. *Acta Pharmacopeia, 54*(4), 261–276.

The environment becomes a political issue. Highlights of the Brundtland Commission Report. (1988). *UN Chronicles, 25*(1), 38–39.

Elnazar, S., Ghazy, A., Ghoneim, H., Taja, A., & Abouelella, A. (2015). Effect of ultra violet irradiation on the interplay between Th1 and Th2 lymphocytes. *Frontier Pharmacology, 6*, 56. doi:10.3389/fphar.2015.00056

Evaluation of certain food contaminants. (2006). *World Health Organization Technical Reporting Service, 930.*

Fishman, R. A. (2002). Polar bear liver, vitamin A, aquaporins, and pseudotumor cerebri. *Annals of Neurology, 52*(5), 531–533.

Food and Drug Administration (FDA). (1995). Regulations restricting the sale and distribution of cigarettes and smokeless tobacco products to protect children and adolescents: Proposed rule regarding FDA's jurisdiction over nicotine-containing cigarettes and smokeless tobacco products: Notice. *Federal Register,* pp. 41314–41787.

Hattan, D. G., & Kahl, L. S. (2002). Current developments in food additive toxicology in the USA. *Toxicology, 181–182*, 417–420.

Heck, H. D., & Tyl, R. W. (1985). The induction of bladder stones by terephthalic acid, dimethyl terephthalate, and melamine (2,4,6-triamino-S-triazine) and its relevance to risk assessment. *Regulatory Toxicology and Pharmacology, 5*(3), 294–313.

Howlett, J. (1996). ILSI Europe Workshop on Food Additive Intake: Scientific assessment of the regulatory requirements in Europe, 1995. Brussels summary report. *Food Additives and Contaminants, 13*(4), 385–395.

Hussein, H. S., & Brasel, J. M. (2001). Toxicity, metabolism, and impact of mycotoxins on humans and animals. *Toxicology, 167*(2), 101–134.

Igisu, H., Goto, I., Kawamura, Y., Koto, M., & Izumi, K. (1975). Acrylamide encephaloneuropathy due to well water pollution. *Journal of Neurology, Neurosurgery, and Psychiatry, 38*(6), 581–584.

International Agency for Research on Cancer (IARC). (1978). IARC monographs on the evaluation of the carcinogenic risk of chemicals to humans. Polychlorinated biphenyls and polybrominated biphenyls. *IARC Monograph Programme on the Evaluation of the Carcinogenic Risk of Chemicals to Humans, 18.*

Mandal, P. K. (2005). Dioxin: A review of its environmental effects and its aryl hydrocarbon receptor biology. *Journal of Comparative Physiology, 175*(4), 221–230.

Mandishona, E., MacPhail, A. P., Gordeuk, V. R., Kedda, M. A., Paterson, A. C., Rouault, T. A., & Kew, M. C. (1998). Dietary iron overload as a risk factor for hepatocellular carcinoma in black Africans. *Hepatology, 27*(6), 1563–1566.

Maronpot, R. R., Thoolen, R. J., & Hansen, B. (2015). Two year carcinogenosity study of acrylamide in Wistar Han rats with utero exposure. *Exploratory Toxicological Pathology., 67*(2), 189–195.

Melnick, R. L., Boorman, G. A., Haseman, J. K., Montali, R. J., & Huff, J. (1984). Urolithiasis and bladder carcinogenicity of melamine in rodents. *Toxicology and Applied Pharmacology, 72*(2), 292–303.

Newland, M. C., Reed, M. N. & Rasmussen, E. (2015). A hypothesis about how early developmental methylmercury exposure disrupts behavior in adulthood. *Behavioral Processes, 114*, 41–51. doi:10.1016/j.beproc.2015.03.007.

Nikolerisa, L., & Hanssonb, M. (2015). Unraveling the estrogen receptor(er) genes in Atlantic salmon (Salmo salar) reveals expression differences between the two adult life stages but little impact from polychlorinated biphenyl (PCB) load. *Molecular and Cellular Endocrinology, 400*, 10–20.

Paracelsus. (1567). *Theiohratus ex Hohenheim Eremita: Von de Besucht.* Dilogen.

Prohibition of Horse Slaughter and Sale of Horse Meat for Human Consumption Act of 1998. (1998). California Proposition 6.

Rederstorff, M., Krol, A., & Lescure, A. (2006). Understanding the importance of selenium and selenoproteins in muscle function. *Cellular and Molecular Life Sciences, 63*(1), 52–59.

Russell, F. E. (1967). Vitamin A content of polar bear liver. *Toxicon, 5*(1), 61–62.

Rustam, H., & Hamdi, T. (1994). Methyl mercury poisoning in Iraq: A neurological study. *Brain, 97*(3), 500–510.

Schoessler, S. Z. (2005). The perils of peanuts. *School Nurse News, 22*(4), 22–26.

Shore, L. S., Gurevitz, M., & Semesh, M. (1993). Estrogen as an environmental pollutant. *Bulletin of Environmental Contamination and Toxicology, 51*(3), 361–366.

Society of Toxicology. (2011). *Toxicology definition.* Retrieved from http://toxicology.org

Takeuchi, T., D'Itri, F. M., Fischer, P. V., Annett, C. S., & Okabe, M. (1977). The outbreak of Minamata disease (methyl mercury poisoning) in cats on Northwestern Ontario reserves. *Environmental Research, 13*(2), 215–228.

USFDA. (1995). Regulations restricting the sale and distribution of CigFish consumption and prenatal methylmercury exposure: cognitive and behavioral outcomes in the main cohort at 17 years from the Seychelles child development study.

Watson, G. E., van Wijngaarden, E., Love, T. M., McSorley, E. M., Bonham, M. P., Mulhern, M. S., Yeates, A. J., Davidson, P. W, Shamlaye, C. F, Strain, J. J., Thurston, S. W., Harrington, D., Zareba, G., Wallace, J. M., & Myers G. J. (2013). Neurodevelopmental outcomes at 5 years in children exposed prenatally to maternal dental amalgam: The Seychelles Child Development Nutrition Study. *Neurotoxicology Teratology, 39*, 57–62. doi:10.1016/j.ntt.2013.07.003

Yu, M. C., & Yuan, J. M. (2004). Environmental factors and risk for hepatocellular carcinoma. *Gastroenterology, 127*(5 suppl 1), S72–S78.

16

International Social Work Practice in Health Care

Monica Nandan

Objectives

After completing this chapter, the reader will be able to:

1. Understand the role of social workers in a global health context.
2. Analyze the role of international social workers as they promote human rights.
3. Evaluate how social workers address the social determinants of health.
4. Explain how social workers intervene in addressing health challenges caused by:
   a. Discrimination
   b. Elderly and aging
   c. Disasters, wars, and violence
   d. Substance abuse
   e. Spirituality, grief, caregiving, dementia
   f. Adherence to healthcare regime
5. Understand how social workers operate as culturally competent health workers and interdisciplinary health team members.
6. Distinguish social work roles in four countries.

INTRODUCTION

Globalization and economic policies instituted by the World Health Organization (WHO) and the International Monetary Fund (IMF) are unfortunately widening the income disparities across the globe, creating health inequities within and between countries (International Federation of Social Workers [IFSW], 2012). Unequal distribution of health care is not a natural phenomenon but is the result of a combination of poor social and health policies and programs, cultural values, research inequalities, and unfair economic distribution (Fish, 2009). For instance, although life expectancy and access to high-quality health care is excellent in countries such as Japan and Canada, these characteristics are low and poor in several Sub-Saharan African countries (Bywaters, McLeod, & Napier, 2009).

Access to health care is moving from a voluntary social utility to a commercialized industry across the globe, resulting in dismantling of universal health care in several countries. Other challenges in the global healthcare arena include limited funding for healthcare research, escalating healthcare costs, lack of access to quality care, and draining medical skills across borders of countries where stark healthcare disparities exist. These contextual elements are creating different types of challenges for healthcare service recipients and providers (IFSW, 2012; Rosenberg, 2006). More specifically, health challenges created by the aforementioned reasons are creating "social, legal, and ethical dilemmas for individual, families, and healthcare providers. These psychosocial implications of health care are what social workers are trained to address" (National Association of Social Workers [NASW], 2005, p. 5). Through collaborative efforts with other healthcare professionals, social workers focus on enhancing individual, family, and community well-being (Martone & Munoz, 2009).

Tackling inequalities in health care is a major focus of social work (Auslander, 2014. Social workers do not accept status quo and challenge the constraints and injustices of the world. They promote social change while implementing the principles of human rights and social justice (Davis, 2009). Often, structural determinants of health are largely responsible for major health inequalities across the globe. For instance, debt repayments, unfair trade practices, gender inequalities, poor policies of pharmaceutical companies, and lack of public health infrastructure exist in Zimbabwe and South Africa. Conversely, in Sri Lanka and Kerala (India)—where commitment for promoting health as a social goal exists, there also exists a social welfare orientation towards development, community participation in healthcare decisions, universal coverage for all and intersectorial collaboration to promote population health (Bywaters, McLeod, & Napier, 2009).

Health inequalities affect every facet of an individual's life. "Health inequalities are differences in health which are not only unnecessary and avoidable but, in addition, are considered unfair and unjust" (Hudson, 2012, p. 108). Hence, social workers cannot ever disconnect from being involved in correcting health inequalities because they are always focusing on the social determinants—that often create the inequalities—and on promoting social justice (Bywaters, McLeod, & Napier, 2009). Social workers focus on providing resources, information, and opportunities to individuals in a manner that these individuals feel empowered to make changes in their lives (Davis, 2009). "Remedial, prevention and developmental functions are not mutually exclusive and, as social workers in many developing countries are now demonstrating, it is possible to integrate these different functions within the same practice setting" (Midgley, 2001, p. 22). Involving governmental entities and policy makers is as important in addressing chronic health inequalities as providing direct services, and social workers are best suited for both these approaches (Raniga & Zelnick, 2014).

Often, social workers across the globe focus on risk factors that result in childhood deaths, HIV and AIDS, hypertension, overweight and obesity, respiratory illnesses caused by pollution, deaths due to infection from unsafe water and sanitation, and death due to alcohol consumption. Through multisystemic, culturally sensitive interventions, social workers across the globe attempt to create change to reduce the potency of the risk factors (Rosenberg, 2006). Furthermore, they conduct comprehensive person-in-environment assessments and provide multidimensional interventions across the entire spectrum of healthcare services from primary care, community health, rehabilitation, and acute care to long-term and mental health care (Yellowless & Hardy, 2014). Social work practice settings and intervention techniques (at various system levels) vary greatly across the globe, from social workers playing instrumental roles in developed countries such as the United Kingdom, Australia, Canada, and the United States, emerging roles in countries such as China and Saudi Arabia (Albrithen & Yalli, 2012; Heinonen, Jiao, Deane, & Cheung, 2009; Qiuling & Chapman, 2014; Yalli & Cooper, 2008), and negligible roles in Sub-Saharan countries (Estes, 2010). Globally, within the healthcare arena, social workers hold positions of therapists, advocates for policy change, community organizers and developers, program developers, case managers, just to name a few (Bywaters, McLeod, & Napier, 2009).

Healthcare social workers have struggled to reach a healthy balance between prevention and curative interventions, managing relationships on interdisciplinary healthcare teams, and accountability for what they do in health care (Auslander, 1997). The rapidly changing sociopolitical and economic context of health services is requiring social workers to constantly adapt; the social worker's focus is moving away from inpatient care to more community-based health care, and health promotion with a public health philosophy. These changes are also necessitating that social workers develop novel and innovative practice models because the models are not cross-culturally relevant. Social workers are being required to provide more information to clients and patients for them to make appropriate choices regarding their care presently and in the future (Auslander, 2014).

Social workers are committed to "maximizing the well-being of individuals and society . . . [by] emphasizing principles of social justice and respect for human dignity and human rights. . . . [M]inimum standards of human rights include also the right to adequate housing, income, employment, education and health care (Australian Association of Social Workers, 2013). Generally, the health of individuals is embedded in the larger living and working conditions in which they find themselves (Williams, Costa, Odunlami, & Mohammed, 2008). More specifically, the health of women in rural China is impacted not only by the physical environment, but also by their social and economic contexts (Heinonen, Jiao, Deane, & Cheung, 2009). Ida Cannon, a pioneer healthcare social worker, wrote that the complexities of social problems often necessitate medical and social interventions; consequently, social workers are integral in all healthcare settings (Judd & Sheffield, 2010). Social workers' ability to assess a broad range of factors (e.g., physical, social, emotional, environmental) that can influence a person's health and well-being makes them a valuable member of any health team (Yellowless & Hardy, 2014). "Through their unique and multi-layered perspective social work professionals intervene with the person in the context of their social environments and relationships, recognizing the impact of the social, cultural, economic, psychological and emotional, political, legal and environmental determinants on health and overall well-being" (Yellowless & Hardy, 2014, p. 5).

Throughout this book, reference is made to increasing rates of disabling, acute, and chronic conditions across the lifespan of populations. This chapter provides an overview of (1) international social work and human rights, (2) select challenges in global health and the role of social work, (3) social work practice in a global context, and (4) illustrations of healthcare social work practice in four countries.

INTERNATIONAL SOCIAL WORK AND HUMAN RIGHTS

In July 2001, the International Association of Schools of Social Work (IASSW) and the International Federation of Social Workers (IFSW) adopted the following definition of international social work:

> The social work profession promotes social change, problem solving in human relationships and the empowerment and liberation of people to enhance well-being. Utilizing theories of human behavior and social systems, social work intervenes at the points where people interact with their environments. Principles of human rights and social justice are fundamental to social work. (IFSW, 2012)

International social workers play a momentous role in promoting human rights and social justice, providing humanitarian assistance and supporting rebuilding communities after disasters (Estes, 2010). Health is a social justice and a human rights issue in a global context. International social workers possess a unique knowledge and skill set for positively facilitating sustainable solutions for recurrent local, regional, and national health challenges. In developing countries, these professionals attempt to eliminate barriers to development that have historically oppressed disenfranchised populations, for example, elderly women, persons with mental illness, and political and economic refugees (Estes, 2010). Social workers are problem solvers who create empowering environments for their clients and are social change agents when institutions are the cause of problems. For example, when institutions create barriers to accessing affordable health care, social workers become agents of change (Fleming et al., 2011).

INTERNATIONALIZATION OF SOCIAL WORK

Although social work as a profession began in Europe (Amsterdam) and only recently spread to the United States, it has evolved internationally to address global issues of famine, poverty, disaster, war, and immigration. In the 1920s, the profession found its way to South America, the Caribbean, India, and South Africa (Kendall, 1990). The IASSW and the IFSW assisted with spreading the profession across the globe and with organizing practitioners and educators. Today, renewed emphasis is being placed by social work programs to sensitize students to the international dimension of practice in their own countries (Estes, 2010).

In developed countries, the term "social work" is in common use whereas in developing countries the terms "social development" and "developmental social welfare" seem to be used (Estes, 2010). Development-focused social workers often function as caseworkers, community organizers, social planners, and educators. Within these roles, they promote individual and community empowerment, institution building, and community and region building. They also challenge existing policies (e.g., healthcare policies) that detrimentally impact vulnerable populations. Their primary goal is to promote human rights and social justice in all arenas through advocacy and social development (Estes, 2010). Essentially, social workers—with a long history of strengths-based, person-in-environment and systems approach—are well positioned to deal with prevention, intervention, and "post-vention" strategies in a global health context (IFSW, 2012). Healthcare social workers are employed in thousands of nongovernmental and quasi-governmental organizations that contribute to developmental work (including health care) across the world. Globally, social workers use three types of practice models that are relevant to health care: (1) services delivered at the individual level to restore their functioning; (2) services delivered through a social welfare model that is instituted through universal social welfare policies, which also covers health issues; and (3) services delivered through community organizing and community development in which residents are involved in designing their future that promotes population health through affordable and accessible care (Estes, 2010).

SOCIAL DETERMINANTS OF HEALTH AND SOCIAL WORK

Article 25 of the United Nations (UN) Declaration of Human Rights states that individuals have the right to:

> a standard of living adequate for health and well-being of self and of family, including food, clothing, housing and medical care and necessary social services, and the right to security in the event of unemployment, sickness, disability, widowhood, old age or other lack of livelihood in circumstances beyond [their] control. (UN, 1948)

According to the UN and IFSW, all individuals have the right to social conditions that promote health and well-being, and they also have the right to access services that promote health and assist with dealing with illnesses (IFSW, 2012). Health not only has physical and medical genesis, but also has several social determinants (Aho, Kauppila, & Haanpaa, 2010; Bywaters, McLeod, & Napier, 2009; Drenth, Herbst, & Strydom, 2013). Social factors play an important role in how individuals maintain or change their health behaviors. Social constructs, such as finances, employment, education, information, access to services and networks, all impact the extent to which an individual or family can access health care and participate in self-care. It is difficult to systematically address health inequalities unless these social constructs are addressed (Bywaters, McLeod, & Napier, 2009).

Social workers often address these social factors. For instance, social workers interact with a child who is living in extreme poverty, an adolescent interacting with the criminal justice system, and individuals subjected to human trafficking or interpersonal violence. Most likely, these individuals will have compromised physical and emotional health, which social workers can play an instrumental role in restoring. Social workers address these constructs at micro (individual and family), mezzo (organizational and community), and macro (policy) levels to impact physical and emotional health (Bywaters, McLeod, & Napier, 2009).

Healthcare social workers assist patients and clients to adapt and adjust to their health conditions, which enable them to improve their social functioning (Malinga & Miupedziswa, 2009).

They also view their patients or clients as partners and coproducers of change, wherein the latter participates with social workers to create sustainable change in the health of communities. Social workers also attempt to address the social determinants of health through cross-sector alliances (Estes, 2010).

SELECT CHALLENGES IN GLOBAL HEALTH AND THE ROLE OF SOCIAL WORK

Population health is impacted by societal discrimination, normal aging process, disasters, wars and violence, mental health and substance abuse, grief, and nonadherence to health regimes. In this section the reader will understand some of the implications of these elements across the globe and the roles played by social workers to improve population health and well-being.

Discrimination

Unfortunately, the ostracizing of same-sex couples and discriminatory actions towards them has been shown to result in mental health problems among those self-identifying as lesbian, gay, bisexual (LGB). These mental health challenge are manifested in substance misuse, higher rates of suicide, and deliberate self-harm (Fish, 2009). Attitudes of healthcare professionals toward this population, or limited understanding about their needs, further compromises their health. Although the United Nations (UN) has considered sexual orientation as a status protected from discrimination since 1979, the human rights of this population segment is still at risk. Laws, which often reflect a culture's value, have been discriminatory toward LGB populations across the globe. Because the LGB population does not have a legally protected status in most societies, they are vulnerable to discrimination and, many times, to violence (Faria, 1997).

This issue is even more challenging for individuals seeking asylum. The LGB population fears that their families will become targets in the country of origin, especially if they have "come out." Challenges are similar for homeless youth who self-identify as LGB as they are bullied and subjected to violence (Fish, 2009). Globally, with growing risks of health and safety of those identifying with this population, social workers are best equipped to promote change through activism and policy advocacy (Fish, 2009). In any of the aforementioned situations, social workers can do case advocacy, consumer advocacy, and legislative advocacy for creating social changes, in addition to building individual self-esteem, worth, and dignity (Faria, 1997).

During the joint meeting of the IFSW and the IASSW in 2000, social work practitioners, educators, and researchers realized the necessity for cultural competency, especially in responding to HIV and AIDS across the globe. Understanding the sociocultural dynamics surrounding the epidemic's progression necessitates that social workers and other healthcare practitioners design prevention programs that are culturally sensitive (Rowe, 2007).

Similarly, discrimination against indigenous Australians has made them susceptible to health problems. Even today, this group suffers from an unusually high rate of incarceration, experiences of violence and abuse, as well as lower rates of employment and education. Consequently, substance abuse is higher in this population segment. Further, not only do they experience barriers to accessing health care, they themselves distrust the healthcare system and its professionals (Whiteside, Tsey, & Cadet-James, 2009).

Empowerment plays a significant role in health promotion particularly because individuals can have a sense of control over their lives by participating in decision making that impacts them. The Family Wellbeing Empowerment (FWE) program has assisted with increasing the self-worth of indigenous Australians, including their ability to cope with stress and their ability to help others with the same. The community empowerment that ensued resulted in effectively addressing endemic issues of mental health, substance abuse, high rates of chronic conditions, and family violence (Whiteside, Tsey, & Cadet-James, 2009). These authors emphasize that personal and community empowerment is important to address socioeconomic inequalities whether at local or international levels. Feeling empowered creates a sense of health and well-being. Social workers are often integral members of such organizations and programs.

Individuals living with disabilities are also subjected to discrimination across the world; almost 25% of the world's population is living with some form of disability. This population has been marginalized, segregated, and stigmatized not only in developing countries but also within industrialized nations. Wars, famine, and disasters contribute to injuries that often result in disability. In the 1980s, the UN identified the human rights of individuals living with disability as a priority. Social workers work with individuals living with disabilities as well as with their family members and other caregivers. They provide direct casework, individual counseling, group work, policy advocacy, and community development on behalf of individuals living with disabilities. They have advocated for policies to provide more affordable and accessible health care and rehabilitation to these individuals across the globe, and they have fought for policies that are antidiscriminatory (IFSW, 2012).

Mental Health and Substance Abuse

Discrimination and stigma due to religion, ethnicity, and cultural differences has caused a rise in mental health problems in Scotland, especially among immigrant populations. Discrimination against people suffering from mental illness continues to exist. Immigrants—from India, Pakistan, and China living in Scotland—who suffer from mental illness fear shame, feel concern about their family's reputation, and worry about prospective marriages. Immigrants from such cultural backgrounds continue to believe that there is no cure for mental illness, and hence, they do not seek assistance.

One intervention does not fit all situations, nor do individuals deal with mental illness in the same fashion. Communities and society vary in how they respond to mental illness. During assessment and in designing interventions, social workers incorporate cultural contexts of individuals suffering from mental illness. In these instances, social workers hold workshops within ethnic communities to apprise them about mental health and the types of interventions that are culturally appropriate. Often, ethnic "insiders" facilitate these workshops so that the message is heard. The community organizing and community development approaches employed by social workers and other professionals toward addressing the mental health of immigrant populations in Scotland has been successful. The social isolation of and the shame experienced by immigrants suffering from mental illness has been reduced through seminars on mental health and partnerships created with community members for designing culturally appropriate interventions (Quinn & Knifton, 2009).

> One of the most interesting aspects of my work is discovering those amazing individuals in rural parts of Kerry who may have been living with chronic mental illnesses . . . I am not restricted by the structures within the Mental Health Services or the limitations of the hospital based social workers or the statutory obligations of our Child Protection Colleagues. (Mike Mansfield, as cited in Fleming et al., 2011)

The incidence and course of mental health conditions such as schizophrenia varies between developed and developing countries. International research consistently demonstrates that schizophrenia has a more favorable outcome in developing countries. This condition has elevated levels in urban versus rural settings. Mental health is not an equal opportunity condition. Several risk factors such as "geography, SES, race, and other personal characteristics and community conditions have now been systematically documented in hundreds of studies" (Hudson, 2012, p. 117).

Social workers are concerned with the influence of social and economic factors (e.g., class, ethnicity, gender) on an individual's experience of their mental illness. They are concerned with restoring individual, family, and community well-being; promoting an individual's control over their lives; and with promoting the principles of social justice. Often, creating change in a health situation requires both change at the individual level and the social level (Harvey, 2009). Social workers' person-in-environment perspective allows them to consider the impact of social and physical environment on individuals. They can assess the role of place in generating and perpetuating mental illness. Social workers partner with clients for determining what is best for their situation, in mobilizing natural support systems, and advocating for enhancing the resources available in a community to address mental illness (Hudson, 2012).

With economic growth, globalization, and improving standards of living in developing countries, substance abuse is on the rise (Fewell et al., 2011). Though the disease process for substance abuse is similar across countries, consequences of substance abuse are different across borders as are the available resources for healing. In traditional countries such as Ghana, substance abuse is frowned upon. In these societies, working with individuals suffering from addiction, social workers are integrating indigenous healers and traditional health practitioners with traditional Western medicine. They also use more family-based approaches in dealing with addiction patients.

Internationally, harm reduction models for dealing with substance abuse is more common than the disease model which dominates in the West. As mentioned earlier, cultures vary in how they view individuals suffering from addiction. Intercultural competence among mental health workers and caseworkers is very important in order to understand the worldview of individuals from different cultural and sociopolitical environments. International social workers have to be incredibly self-aware and non-judgmental in their acceptance of other cultures when they work with addiction patients across the globe (Fewell et al., 2011).

Elder Care and Aging

With improvement in hygiene and medical technology, people across the globe are living longer and there is a gradual shift in "concern for human health from physical to psychological" (Chong, 2007, p. 92). According to WHO (2015), by 2020, the number of people over the age of 60 can add to more than a billion. Additionally, of the 10 countries with the highest proportion of aging population, half are in developing countries (e.g., China, India, Indonesia, Brazil, and Pakistan). Psychological disorders among the elderly population is growing and the common conditions include Alzheimer's, depression, anxiety, alcohol addiction, suicide, schizophrenia, paranoia, autism, as well as fears and phobias (Turner, 1992). Alzheimer's disease takes a toll on the elderly person and on caregivers, who are predominantly family members (Pinson, Register, & Roberts-Lewis, 2010).

Supporting the caregivers, especially of elderly suffering from Alzheimer's disease, is a significant focus among social workers. The emotional and physical strain placed on caregivers, such that it impacts their health, is not unusual and is well documented. With their clinical and organizational skills, social workers can mobilize religious communities across the globe to assist caregivers, especially to provide respite to the primary caregiver. Additionally, they have developed and coordinated caregiver support groups, and conducted psycho-educational workshops as well as stress management seminars for caregivers. Social workers have also organized massage therapy for caregivers, and assisted caregivers with preparing for medical appointments of their loved ones (Pinson, Register, & Roberts-Lewis, 2010).

The physical and mental health of the elderly population is closely related (Drewnowski et al., 2003). Health promotion is a significant element in elder care. Social workers are advocating for transferring some of the medical and health service expenditures toward promoting the health of the elderly population (Chong, 2007). Social workers intervene at individual, family, social network, and community levels on behalf of the aging population, by focusing on providing empowering environments for this population and moving from remedy to prevention services (Chong, 2007). To address the emotional needs of the population, social workers focus on enhancing their problem-solving abilities to reduce their dependence on family, friends, and service providers.

To what extent are medical communities and families continuing to provide the physical and emotional care required by the aging population? Given the gradual dismantling of the joint families and geographic social networks across the world, maintaining a positive mental health of the aging population is clearly a challenge. The number of elderly people who are single due to divorce, separation, widowhood, or never marrying is growing, reducing the number that can turn to nuclear families for support, assistance, or advise (Chong, 2007). To address the health-related needs of a Chinese aging population that is living alone without any pension, social workers and community service planers need to focus more attention on designing community-based health services in areas with a high concentration of isolated elderly population (Liu & Bern-Klug, 2011).

In general, social workers play an instrumental role in assessing the mental and emotional health of this population, involving them in the decision-making process to promote their health and independence, developing or strengthening existing social networks, and advocating for policies that promote independence and emotional well-being. More specifically, social workers assist isolated elderly individuals to build or rebuild their social network, after performing a thorough network analysis of existing support systems (Drewnowski et al., 2003).

High suicide rates, depression, and social isolation are common occurrences among the elderly population worldwide (Hooyman & Kiyak, 2002; Kahn, Hessling, & Russell, 2003). Unfortunately, in Asian countries, societal attitude toward elderly suicide is more lenient. "Timely action is seldom undertaken to save lives, possibly because it is considered natural that elderly people would want to die or to end their lives because they will die very soon anyway" (Chong, 2007, p. 98).

Another challenge experienced by the elderly is the generation of grandparents who are raising grandchildren, particularly in African nations where AIDS/HIV has taken a heavy death toll on parents. A majority of the AIDS orphans reside in Africa and are being raised by grandparents. Such caregiving not only takes a physical, social, material, and psychological toll on grandparents, but has also made them more vulnerable to violence from the community (Angwe, 2012). Social development workers cannot only provide emotional support to the grandparents, but also through community organizing, mobilize other grandparents to support each other to preempt vulnerability to violence.

Mourning rights for widows are rather cruel in several African nations, where they are subjected to physical torment (e.g., head shaving; expulsion from home). Particularly in Nigeria, childless widows are at a higher risk for abuse, robbery, and violence, and are accused of witchcraft for unexplained phenomenon in local communities. Sadly, in a province in Nigeria, elderly women are subjected to gang-rape for ritualistic purposes. Essentially, elderly women are seriously threatened by poverty, physical and financial abuse, loneliness, and emotional suffering. Ironically, even though most African nations are highly religious and care for the elderly is part of a moral fabric of society, dwindling family structures are leaving many elderly populations vulnerable to violence (Angwe, 2012).

The role of social workers as policy advocates and community organizers is very important for creating social change in these communities. They can collaborate with the UN and Human Rights Commissions to enact new, and enforce existing, policies particularly protecting rights of women and childless widows. With high levels of illiteracy among women in African countries, social workers can organize forums to provide individuals an opportunity to consult with them, and to share their concerns with other women in the community. Communal living in several African nations enables these forums to serve as informal mediums to resolve conflicts, reduce isolation, and offer social and emotional support to aging population. Essentially, ending elderly abuse requires both social and legal approaches for which social workers can mobilize community members and advocate with policy makers for change (Angwe, 2012). Additionally, in the absence of universal health care for elderly citizens—who often have to rely on their meager pensions or savings for accessing healthcare services—social workers can advocate for low-cost health screenings in communities which can greatly prevent abuse and violence against vulnerable aging populations.

Disasters, Wars, and Violence

According to the UN Commission on Human Rights, at least 50 countries have some form of conflict in place across the world and over 25 million individuals are displaced each year (UN Commission on Human Rights, 1994). This number grows exponentially when we take into account human-made and natural disasters (IFSW, 2012). Internal armed conflicts in countries, ethnic and religious fights, mass violation of human rights, general violence in communities and natural disasters create injuries, traumas, deaths, disablement and displacement, or forced migration of people which has detrimental impact on population health (IFSW, 2012).

In disasters, wars, and violence, not only physical health care but emotional and mental health care is required to mend bodies and broken hearts. Psychosocial well-being is as important as physical well-being in disaster situations. Individuals displaced in such a fashion are vulnerable populations, often subjected to discrimination; they are distraught with emotional trauma and grief related to loss of family members, limbs, and possessions due to war or disasters. Women, children, and the elderly populations are the most severely impacted in these situations (IFSW, 2012). International social workers and social development workers need to focus on the emotional and material needs of these populations, providing them with crisis intervention, grief counseling, and case management to ensure they can access needed services after a disaster or war.

In post-war Libya, the mental health status of several citizens was negatively impacted. Those with pre-existing mental health conditions experienced worsening of their mental health and well-being during the war. Professionals within the limited number of mental health facilities were unable to cope with burgeoning urgent needs. Since the war, more educational programs for psychologists, nurses, and social workers have emerged in this country. To reduce the stigma attached to mental illness, these professionals are raising awareness about mental health (WHO, 2013).

Several American states have Disaster Medical Assistance Teams (DMATs), including several highly trained medical professionals who not only triage patients during disaster situations but also provide the necessary interventions and medical care. Social workers are active members on such teams (Malamud, 2010). According to the manager of the DMATs of the National American Red Cross in Washington, over 50% of the 4,000 disaster mental health volunteers across the United States are social workers (Dale, 2011). Nonetheless, there is always a need for dedicated case managers and mental health professionals who can provide a range of services "across the disaster continuum from preparedness, response and recovery" (National Voluntary Organizations Active in Disaster, 2015). Not only are social workers well trained to provide these services, they are adequately equipped to coordinate and manage volunteer efforts in such situations. The strengths-based approaches and systems' focus employed by social workers helps increase the resilience of individuals and communities after disasters. A high level of need exists for social workers in disaster management, and a tremendous shortage of qualified workers is the reality in the international arena (Dale, 2011).

Social workers in New Zealand have experienced a variety of disaster situations (e.g., earthquakes, mining accidents, car accidents), where they have responded with exceptional crisis management skills. Not only do they comfort the relatives and friends of clients, they set up a relatives' center that will provide information about community resources after a disaster. They will call the next of kin for those clients who must be evacuated; they collect data concerning those who are missing, ensure all social workers are accounted for, and assist medical personnel as needed. They do this often with compromised telephone service, little computer access, and light accessibility (Maher & Maidment, 2013).

Healthcare social workers in Australia are integrated into hospital disaster response teams. They play an instrumental role in providing emotional support to victims and their families, referring them to community-based assistance, and in grief and bereavement counseling. After a disaster, they are also vital professionals for victim identification and in the department of forensic medicine (Pockett, 2006).

Domestic and Family Violence

Domestic and family violence is now considered a health issue. Hospitals and healthcare settings are ideal settings in which to screen for domestic and family violence. Early identification and intervention by health professionals can greatly reduce health complications resulting from such violence (Power, Bahnisch, & McCarthy, 2011). Social workers play an instrumental role in screening patients in the emergency departments in Australian hospitals. Using an ecological framework for screening and interventions, social workers address the issue at the individual and family levels (micro), at organizational and service delivery levels (mezzo), and at legal and policy levels (macro). Within this framework, social workers are prepared to address contextual and structural determinants of domestic and family violence and accordingly design programs (Power, Bahnisch, & McCarthy, 2011).

Spirituality plays a major role in working with immigrant South Asian individuals (e.g., Punjabi Sikh men) who have mental health and substance abuse issues, and who have participated in domestic violence (Thandi, 2011). Spirituality can play a major role in the prevention and intervention with such patients. Services provided in Punjabi by social workers are culturally appropriate and sensitive to the nature of the therapeutic relationship. These very issues influence the victim's ability to seek services in domestic violence situations. Incorporating spirituality into the therapeutic relationship with Punjabi men is very helpful, as is providing educational workshops on substance abuse and mental illness to community members from South Asian countries (Thandi, 2011). Religious leaders and community members, along with social workers, can help sustain the change that Punjabi men may like to create in their lives.

Spirituality, Grief, Caregiving, and Dementia

The rate of growth of dementia, particularly Alzheimer's disease, continues to increase worldwide and the concomitant burden on caregivers continues to rise (Pinson, Register, & Roberts-Lewis, 2010). Spiritual care, spiritual needs, spiritual pain, and spiritual well-being are important concepts in the areas of grief, dementia, and health care (Callahan, 2015). Although spirituality is called by different names across cultures and communities, people served by social workers often draw upon their spiritual strength (Canda & Furman, 2010). Spirituality assists humans with gaining meaning and purpose within their culture (Hall, Livingston, Brown, & Mohabir, 2011). Spirituality is equally important when dealing with mental health issues particularly of refugees and asylum seekers (Zoma, 2014).

Faith and spirituality play a major role in assisting caregivers and patients suffering from cognitive and physical impairments. With the help of social workers, faith-based organizations and local congregations have been providing support—emotional, physical, financial, and spiritual—to individuals living with impairments, and to their caregivers. Additionally, social workers are continuing to become more competent in spiritual practice, especially in the realm of death and hospice care.

Death and grief both signify the vulnerability of individuals, and hence, need the attention of social workers (Drenth, Herbst, & Strydom, 2013). In South Africa, bereavements caused by HIV/AIDS epidemic, tuberculosis, fatal motor accidents, and crime is on the rise. Though grief is a normal response in such situations, about 10 to 20% of bereaved individuals experience complicated grief. Complicated grief often arises during the coexistence of several situations—individuals experiencing multiple losses, a difficult manner of death, or the death of a child (Drenth, Herbst, & Strydom, 2013).

Social workers focus on the loss experiences of individuals and the impact on their psychological and social functioning. They are well equipped to assist individuals and families in the following grief-invoking situations: complicated grief situations, families with members diagnosed with HIV/AIDS, children engaging in delinquent behaviors after the death of a parent, individuals engaging in substance abuse after loss of a close family member or friend, individuals who have attempted suicide, and families that have experienced a death normally stigmatized by society (Drenth, Herbst, & Strydom, 2013, p. 367).

Unfortunately, gender inequalities exist in accessing grief-related services in some African nations. In addition to providing clinical services during grief, social workers advocate for accessing comprehensive palliative care, which in Africa has become a human rights issue. These professionals also challenge the status quo in the health care of African society, which often continues to disenfranchise vulnerable and oppressed population groups (Drenth, Herbst, & Strydom, 2013).

Mourning the death of a lesbian or gay partner may be impaired due to societal issues, which, in turn, may give rise to an atypical manifestation of grief. In such situations, social workers assist the surviving partner with first describing the nature of their relationship and subsequently assessing the cause of impaired resolution of grief. The social worker can assist the client to affirm his or her relationship and then assist the client, where appropriate, with alternative rituals to bring closure to the relationship and begin a therapeutic grieving process (Faria, 1997).

Finally, Islam is the fastest-growing religion in the world and the second largest faith. Spirituality is important for social work interventions with Muslim populations from South Asian countries. Social workers need to acknowledge, and when appropriate, apply their values and belief systems during assessment and intervention. Faith is a critical aspect of the lives of

Muslim families, and social workers need to incorporate it into building a positive relationship with Muslim individuals and families. Social workers must maintain a working relationship with Islamic clergy while working therapeutically with individuals and families (Hall, Livingston, Brown, & Mohabir, 2011).

Adherence in Healthcare Regime

Adherence to a healthcare regime is impacted by social and economic factors such as poverty, minority status in society, access to health systems, health condition–related factors, therapy or treatment factors. Other patient-related factors include their attitudes toward, and beliefs about, health conditions and care, knowledge about the health conditions, resources, communication about health services, and larger cultural factors that influence each of the above elements (Vourlekis & Ell, 2008). Health behaviors and outcomes are the result of a patient's predispositions (e.g., knowledge, coping skills, attitude), reinforcements (e.g., social support systems), and enabling factors (e.g., resource acquisition, system responsiveness).

Social work case managers play an active role in teaching patients health-related self-management skills for maintaining their well-being, and through counseling reducing the psychological stresses caused by ill-health. Similarly, they also facilitate communication between healthcare providers and patients to enhance the quality of understanding of patients and family members. They also make referrals to community resources as needed for patients. These three illustrations indicate how social workers influence patients' predispositions, reinforcements, and enabling factors that influence patients' adherence to medical regime. Culturally competent social work care managers integrate individualized services for patients with services from multiple systems as needed (Vourlekis & Ell, 2008).

SOCIAL WORK PRACTICES IN A GLOBAL CONTEXT

International healthcare social workers not only have to be culturally competent practitioners, but they also serve as significant members on interdisciplinary healthcare teams in different settings.

Cultural Competency of Healthcare Social Workers

In an international context, the more vulnerable the population being served in healthcare settings, the more relevant it is for social workers and other healthcare providers to be culturally competent (Ng, Popova, Yau, & Sulman, 2007). Delivering culturally competent care is one way to reduce the gaps in health status across diverse populations (Anderson et al., 2003). Ng and coauthors have written, "Social workers often bridge the gap between patients' cultural and linguistic needs and the understanding of multidisciplinary staff" (Ng, Popova, Yau, & Sulman, 2007, p. 139). Qualified and well-trained social workers in health settings often understand the history, culture, health beliefs, and practices of different native and immigrant groups and take leadership roles in designing appropriate health-related services to enhance access and health outcomes (Ng, Popova, Yau, & Sulman, 2007).

Interdisciplinary Teams

Interdisciplinary care is becoming more common in acute care setting, in mental health and in public health clinics, as professionals are beginning to recognize that patient care is neither one discipline's sole responsibility nor prerogative. Social workers can—and they need to—take more active roles in building and supporting collaborative team, which often have positive outcomes on patient health, especially pertaining to chronic conditions such as diabetes, mental health, HIV, and the like (Emmer, 2003).

One of the main goals of interdisciplinary primary care health teams is to enable individuals in their self-care by empowering them and subsequently toward illness prevention (Department of Health and Children, 2001). Another goal of such teams is to reduce health inequalities. People's health is not affected only by the level of health care in a country, but also by its accessibility. Social workers, through advocacy, promote affordable and accessible health care and create individualized care plans that support human dignity, respect, and choices; all these factors, in turn, enhance individual health status (Fleming et al., 2011).

Social workers play a vital role in interdisciplinary healthcare teams, particularly those serving dying patients, or patients who are managing chronic pain (Aho, Kauppila, & Haanpaa, 2010). These patients need medical, psychological, and social supports, and social workers can particularly assist in alleviating some of the psychological and social distresses that can aggravate situations of dying patients or those in chronic pain. Patients suffering from acute and chronic pain are often susceptible to depression and substance abuse. Consequently, the role of social workers in such situations cannot be underestimated. Social workers in Finland are very knowledgeable about community resources that can help dying patients and those in chronic pain. In addition to providing individual and family counseling, social workers can make referrals easily and also coordinate case management (Aho, Kauppila, & Haanpaa, 2010).

Similarly, in Ireland, social workers serve a key role in primary care teams, along with general practitioners, nurses, healthcare assistants, physiotherapists, occupational therapists, administrators, and clerical staff. Social workers operate as social change agents within these teams, conducting holistic assessments, consulting with other health and social service providers, educating in health and social care, and capacity building in communities, in addition to the traditional role of providing therapeutic counseling (Fildes & Cooper, 2003). These teams employ an interdisciplinary approach to primary care in Ireland (Fleming et al., 2011) by focusing on social determinants of health while managing population health.

Social workers focus on the "social" elements of population health (IFSW, 2012). Using Dahlgran's health framework (1995, c.f., Fleming et al., 2011), social workers primarily link people's physical, emotional, social, and economic well-being. Engaging community members to identify and address social determinants of health is a key role played by social workers in Ireland (Fleming et al., 2011). As primary team members, social workers promote health by conducting group work on anxiety management, self-esteem, healthy eating, and by promoting health fairs, particularly in rural communities. Essentially, social workers operate in a preventive health capacity and assist individuals avoid further deterioration of life circumstances that can have detrimental effects on their physical and emotional health.

In Saudi Arabia as well, social workers—though limited in number—collaborate with physicians and other healthcare professionals on these teams to ensure that optimum services are provided to patients. On such teams they serve as a link between the team and patients (Albrithen & Yalli, 2012). Unlike healthcare social workers in developed countries, these workers wear many additional hats in Saudi Arabia—fundraisers, community organizers, capacity builders, and patient advocates for monitoring and reporting family complaints in hospitals. For the most part, Saudi Arabia is a hierarchical patriarchal society, with limited resources, autonomy, and support afforded to hospital social workers. Social workers need to share the same gender with their clients in order to serve them; this limits the number of cases seen by a single social worker (Albrithen & Yalli, 2012).

ILLUSTRATIONS OF HEALTHCARE SOCIAL WORK PRACTICES IN FOUR COUNTRIES

Tremendous variability exists in how social work is practiced across the globe. Some illustrations of variability were evident in the preceding sections of the chapter. Additional overview of healthcare social work practice across the globe is provided below.

Botswana

Culture and stigma attached to health conditions influence the nature of care sought by Botswana residents. Traditional or folk care is common in Botswana, and many times patients wish to leave the hospital setting to seek such care instead. In instances where families are unable or unwilling to take the primary responsibility (e.g., feeding, bathing, etc.) for caring for their loved ones in hospitals, social workers shoulder the burden of deciding how to address this caregiving gap within the hospital. Weakened traditional social networks make discharge planning very difficult for social workers. Botswana hospitals also receive a fair volume of undocumented individuals. Once these individuals die, social workers are responsible for ensuring the body is disposed (Malinga & Miupedziswa, 2009).

In Botswana, healthcare social workers focus on enabling clients and patients to adapt and adjust to their health condition and with improving their social functioning (Malinga & Miupedziswa, 2009). They are hired to provide counseling services to patients and families in hospitals. Generic practice social workers in Botswana do not have the credentials to practice as counselors. Some, however, are receiving additional certification for working with AIDS/HIV, in palliative care, and in bereavement and grief counseling. Their impact is particularly felt in their work with individuals, families, and communities affected by AIDS/HIV. The stigma attached to this condition in particular results in patients not receiving treatment, or in being abandoned in hospitals because families decline to provide food and other amenities. Such situations are very challenging for social workers since they have to make some difficult decisions about the care of individuals suffering from AIDS/HIV.

Undocumented immigration into Botswana creates additional burdens on the healthcare system and hospitals, especially when patients die in the hospital and social workers are responsible for the last rites. Finally, with only 66 trained social workers nationally, burnout rate in

Botswana is high among the social workers who have very limited resources at their disposal to address endemic epidemics (Malinga & Miupedziswa, 2009). Clearly, this country can benefit from more trained social workers who have the necessary resources to address such complex health issues.

South Africa

South African healthcare experience incorporates both developed and developing nation's characteristics. High rates of poverty, violence, and an influx of refugees strain the health and healthcare system of South Africa. Consequently, healthcare social workers in South Africa incorporate the understanding of both developed and developing countries with regard to health care and illness. They use Western and indigenous treatments paradigms, while being sensitive to the diverse cultures and religion practiced in South Africa. Social workers understand the significance of dreams, evil spirits, and ancestors in causing illness; use of medicine to harm others; the responsibility of indigenous healers for diagnosis, healing and protection of individuals; and different roles of different types of healers such as diviners, herbalists, faith healers, and prophets (Carbonatto, 2009, p. 256). Social workers play a crucial role in providing resources such as food, safe drinking water and sanitation, education, essential medicines, and services to mothers and children, as well as providing resources for controlling local endemic diseases. Their primary focus is on HIV/AIDS and other sexually transmitted diseases, maternal, child and women's health, nutrition, spread of communicable diseases, chronic health conditions, and mental health and substance abuse (Carbonatto, 2009).

Lack of adequate hospitals and clinics inhibits health across South Africa. About 80% of the population is served by public health services and 20% by private, state-of-the-art hospitals. Being team players and working collaboratively with other healthcare professionals, families, and the community is key for social work practice in South Africa.

New Zealand

Hospital social workers in New Zealand are an essential part of the emergency department, available 24 hours a day, and seven days a week. They are an important member of the trauma response team—which responds to postdisaster emergency situations. Particularly, when the Canterbury region experienced several earthquakes between 2007 and 2012, social workers played an instrumental role in comforting and assisting relatives and friends of clients. Other illustrations of their assistance were provided under the section on "disaster, war and violence" (Maher & Maidment, 2013).

Unfortunately, with the Health and Disability Act of 1993 passed in New Zealand, the role of social workers in medical healthcare settings is continuing to dwindle. They are involved with the elderly population and their families primarily around episodic crises in hospitals. They are not actively involved in the prevention and primary care arena yet. Healthcare social work in primary care is still in its infancy in this country. Working with the elderly population is relationship-oriented work that can realize better results if approached from a primary care framework. Unfortunately, in a context that emphasizes targets, cost efficiencies, and reduction of risk, social work with the elderly can become challenging. "One of the essential components of creating a healthy society means moving resources from secondary care to primary health care" (Foster & Beddoe, 2012, p. 41). Regrettably, this is not occurring with regard to social work services.

Australia

The state of Queensland, Australia, is practicing the devolution of centralized health services, and is radically shifting responsibilities to local and community health centers. This government is attempting to reduce hospital demand and improve the transition of patients from hospital to home by focusing on services in the communities (Queensland Government, 2013). Social workers in Queensland conduct comprehensive health assessments and provide interventions for the entire continuum of health—physical, cognitive, emotional, social, and spiritual—in diverse settings (e.g., rural, urban, acute care, mental health, primary care, and academic healthcare settings). They are hired in positions that are available to other healthcare providers in allied healthcare fields, such as case management, drug and alcohol counseling, clinical therapy, generic mental health care, and the like (Yellowless & Hardy, 2014).

Conclusion

Healthcare social workers practice in a wide range of settings across the globe and the nature of practice varies from direct clinical work with patients in hospitals to public health and prevention work in community settings. "Social workers who have learned from the strengths, creativity and survival skills of service users have much to offer to national and global initiatives on health inequalities" (Davis, 2009, p. 272). They are strong advocates for eliminating health inequity through policy change and community development and for creating empowering environments for vulnerable populations—vulnerable because of their physical, emotional, or situational difficulties (Yellowless & Hardy, 2014). The interdependent nature of the world today—especially as it pertains to health and health care—is necessitating international collaborations and cultural competency among social workers, particularly with vulnerable populations crossing borders as refugees and undocumented immigrants (Estes, 2010). For effective health care and international social work practice, it is imperative for partnerships among healthcare providers—traditional and indigenous—family and community members and religious organizations.

Study Questions

1. Describe the various types of social work services provided to patients and clients experiencing discrimination, disasters, wars, and violence.
2. What is the role of healthcare social workers in addressing health inequalities across the globe and what are some of the strategies employed by them?
3. How do you perceive the role of social workers in interdisciplinary teams?
4. Compare and contrast the roles of healthcare social workers in the four countries with those in the United States (or your home country).

5. How can you collaborate with social workers to enhance the quality of care provided to patients in inpatient and outpatient settings? More specifically, what knowledge and skills do they possess that complements yours?
6. Globally, what are some common challenges experienced by social workers in health care, and are they similar to the challenges experienced by your profession?

Case Study

Mrs. Xing migrated with her son and daughter-in-law 12 years ago to New Zealand, but has not adapted to the culture. She has limited English skills and spends most of her time at home with the school-aged grandchildren. She is living with anxiety and in fear, limiting her interactions with neighbors. She is predominantly dependent on her son for financial support. During her annual checkup, the general practitioner (GP) refers Mrs. Xing to a social worker in the community.

Case Study Questions

1. What types of psychological assessments can a social worker perform on Mrs. Xing?
2. What types of interventions can the social worker employ?
3. How can she engage Chinese community members?
4. If Mrs. Xing is admitted to the hospital, what can a nurse do to learn about her background? What types of questions can a nurse ask in this situation?

Data from Foster, S., & Beddoe, L. (2012). Social work with older adults in primary health—Is it time to move our focus? *Aotearoa New Zealand Social Work Review, 24*(2), 37–48.

References

Aho, H., Kauppila, T., & Haanpaa, M. (2010). Patients referred from a multidisciplinary pain clinic to the social worker, their general health, pain condition, treatment, and outcome. *Scandinavian Journal of Pain, 1*(4), 220–226. doi:10.1016/j.sjpain.2010.09.009

Albrithen, A., & Yalli, N. (2012). The perception of organizational issues of social work practitioners in Saudi hospitals. *Journal of Social Service Research, 38*(3), 273–291.

Anderson, L. M., Scrimshaw, S. C., Fullilove, M. T., Fielding, J. E., Normand, J., & the Task Force on Community Prevention Services. (2003). Culturally competent healthcare systems a systematic review. *American Journal of Preventive Medicine, 24*(3S), 68–79.

Angwe, B. (2012, August 21–24). *Open-Ended Working Group on Ageing for the Purpose of Strengthening the Protection of the Human Rights of Older Persons.* (Third working session.) In United Nations, General Assembly, 7–8(65), 182 (2012). Retrieved from http://social.un.org/ageing-working group/documents/Chairssummary3rdsessionOEWGfinal.pdf

Auslander, G. K., Rosenberg, G., & Weissman, A. (2014). *International Perspectives on Social Work in Health Care: Past, Present, and Future.* New York: Haworth Press.

Australian Association of Social Workers. (2013). Practice Standards. Australia, Canberra.

Bywaters, P., McLeod, E., & Napier, L. (2009). *Social Work and Global and Health Inequalities: Practice and Policy Developments.* Bristol: Policy Press.

Callahan, A. M. (2015). Key concepts in spiritual care for hospice social workers: How an interdisciplinary perspective can inform spiritual competence. *Social Work & Christianity, 42*(1), 43–62.

Canda, E. R., & Furman, L. D. (2010). *Spiritual Diversity in Social Work Practice the Heart of Helping* (2nd ed.). New York: Oxford University Press.

Carbonatto, C. L. (2009). The challenge of training social workers for healthcare in South Africa. In P. Bywaters, E. McLeod, & L. Napier (Eds.), *Social Work and Global Health Inequalities and Policy Developments* (pp. 250–264). Great Britain: Policy Press.

Chong, A. M. (2007). Promoting the psychosocial health of the elderly—The role of social workers. *Social Work in Health Care, 44*(1–2), 91–109.

Dale, M. (2011). Building resilience after disaster volunteering experiences called "wonderfully rich and professionally rewarding." *NASW NEWS, 56*(8).

Davis, A. (2009). Addressing health inequalities: The role of service user and people's health movements. In P. Bywaters, E. McLeod, & L. Napier (Eds.), *Social Work and Global Health Inequalities Practice and Policy Developments* (pp. 265–274). Great Britain: Policy Press.

Department of Health and Children. (2001). *Primary Care: A New Direction: Quality and Fairness-A Health Systems for Your Health Strategy.* Dublin: Hawkins House.

Drenth, C. M., Herbst, A. G., & Strydom, H. (2013). Complicated grief in South African context: A social work perspective. *British Journal of Social Work, 43*(2), 355–372.

Drewnowski, A., Monsen, E., Birkett, D., Gunther, S. V., Su, J., & Marshall, G. (2003). Health screening and health promotion programs for the elderly. *Disease Management & Health Outcomes, 11*(5), 29–309.

Emmer, L. (2003). The social worker as part of an interdisciplinary team. *Adolescent Health, 3*(1), 1–3.

Estes, R. (2010). *United States-Based Conceptualization of International Social Work Education.* (Paper). Retrieved from http://www.cswe.org/File.aspx?id=31429

Faria, G. (1997). The challenge of health care social work with gay men and lesbians. In G. K. Auslander, G. Rosenberg, & A. Weissman (Eds.). *International Perspectives on Social Work in Health Care: Past, Present and Future* (pp. 65–72). New York: Haworth Press.

Fewell, C., Gilbert, D. J., MacMaster, S., Maison, T., Holleran Steiker, L., & Straussner, S. L. (2011). International social work: Experiences and implications regarding substance abuse. *Journal of Social Work Practice in the Addictions, 11*(4), 398–407.

Fildes, R., & Cooper, B. (2003). *Preparing for Change: Social Work in Primary Health Care.* Canadian Association of Social Workers. (Paper). Retrieved from http://www.casw-acts.ca/sites/default/files/attachements/Preparing%20for%20Change.%20Social%20Work%20in%20Primary%20Health%20Care%20Report_0.pdf.

Fish, J. (2009). All thing equal? Social work and lesbian, gay, and bisexual (LGB) global health inequalities. In P. Bywaters, E. McLeod, & L. Napier (Eds.), *Social Work and Global Health Inequalities Practice and Policy Developments* (pp. 144–149). Great Britain: Policy Press.

Fleming, T., Flood, S., Gumulka, S., Jacob, D., Parkinson, R., & Reilly, P. (2011). *The Role of Social Work in Primary Care in Ireland Social Workers in Primary Care Special Interest Group of the IASW.* (Draft).

Foster, S., & Beddoe, L. (2012). Social work with older adults in primary health—Is it time to move our focus? *Aotearoa New Zealand Social Work Review, 24*(2), 37–48.

Gofin, J., & Gofin, R. (2011). *Essentials of Global Community Health.* Sudbury, MA: Jones & Bartlett Learning.

Hall, R. E., Livingston, J. N., Brown, C. J., & Mohabir, J. A. (2011). Islam and Asia Pacific Muslims: The implications of spirituality for social work practice. *Journal of Social Work Practice, 25*(2), 205–215.

Harvey, D. (2009). Conceptualizing the mental health of rural women: A social work and health promotion perspective. *Rural Society, 19*(4), 353–362.

Heinonen, T., Jiao, Y., Deane, L., & Cheung, M. (2009). Social work in rural China: Advancing women's health and well-being in the village. In P. Bywaters, E. McLeod, & L. Napier (Eds.), *Social Work and Global Health Inequalities Practice and Policy Developments* (pp. 172–177). Great Britain: Policy Press.

Hooyman, N. R., & Kiyak, H. A. (2002). *Social Gerontology: A Multidisciplinary Perspective* (6th ed.). Boston, MA: Pearson.

Hudson, C. G. (2012). Disparities in the geography of mental health: Implications for social work. *Social Work, 57*(2), 107–119.

International Federation of Social Workers. (2012). *Global Standards*. Retrieved from http://ifsw.org/policies/global-standards/.

Judd, R. G., & Sheffield, S. (2010). Hospital social work: Contemporary roles and professional activates. *Social Work in Health Care, 49*(9). doi:10.1080/00981389.2010.499825

Kahn, J. H., Hessling, R. M., & Russell, D. W. (2003). Social support, health, and well-being among the elderly: What is the role of negative affectivity? *Personality and Individual Differences, 35*(1), 5–17.

Kendall, K. A. (1990). *The International in American Education*. New York: Hunter College School of Social Work.

Liu, J., & Bern-Klug, M. (2011). Elder's expectations of community health services in China. *Indian Journal of Gerontology, 25*(4), 532–552.

Maher, P., & Maidment, J. (2013). Social work disaster emergency response within a hospital setting. *Aotearoa New Zealand Social Work Review, 25*(2), 69–77.

Malamud, M. (2010). Devastating earthquake in Haiti has many stepping up to help victims social workers "uniquely skilled" to respond. *NASW NEWS, 55*(3).

Malinga, T., & Miupedziswa, R. (2009). Hospital social work practice in Botswana: Yesterday, today and tomorrow. *Journal of Social Development in Africa, 24*(1), 91–117.

Martone, J., & Munoz, L. (2009). Lessons on migration, globalization, and social work: Two personal accounts on international field placements in Mexico. *Journal of Poverty, 13*(3), 359–364.

Midgley, J. (2001). Issues in international social work: Resolving critical debates in the profession. *Journal of Social Work, 1*(1), 21–35. doi:10.1177/146801730100100103

National Voluntary Organizations Active in Disaster. (2015, May). *Disaster Emotional Care Points of Consensus*. Ratified by full membership.

Ng, J., Popova, S., Yau, M., & Sulman, J. (2007). Do culturally sensitive services for Chinese in-patients make a difference? *Social Work Health Care, 44*(3), 129–143.

Pinson, S. M., Register, K., & Roberts-Lewis, A. (2010). Aging, memory loss, dementia, and Alzheimer's disease: The role of Christian social workers and the church. *Social Work & Christianity, 37*(2), 188–203.

Pockett, R. (2006). Learning from Each Other: The Social Work Role as an Integrated Part of the Hospital Disaster Response. *Social Work in Health Care, 43*(2), 131–149. Retrieved from "http://dx.doi.org/10.1300/J010v43n02_09

Power, C., Bahnisch, L., & McCarthy, D. (2011). Social work in the emergency department-implementation of a domestic and family violence screening program. *Australian Social Work, 64*(4), 537–554.

Qiuling, A., & Chapman, M. V. (2014). The early professional experience of a new social worker in China. *Journal of Social Work Education, 50*(2), 322–333. doi:10.1080/10437797.2014.885266

Queensland government. (2013). *Queensland health*. Retrieved from https://publications.qld.gov.au/storage/f/2014-06-03T23%3A46%3A13.459Z/blueprint-for-better-healthcare-screen.pdf

Quinn, N., & Knifton, L. (2009). Addressing mental health inequalities in Scotland through community conversation. In P. Bywaters, E. McLeod, & L. Napier (Eds.), *Social Work and Global Health Inequalities Practice and Policy Developments* (pp. 187–192). Great Britain: Policy Press.

Raniga, T., & Zelnik, J. (2014). Social policy education for change: South African student perspectives on the global agenda for social work and social development. *International Social Work, 57*(4), 386–397.

Rosenberg, G. (2006). Welcome to the ninth Doris Siegel memorial fund colloquium. In G. Rosenberg, & A. Weissman (Eds.), *International Social Health Care Policy, Programs, and Studies* (pp. 1–4). New York: Haworth Press.

Rowe, W. (2007). Cultural competence in HIV prevention and care: Different histories, shared future. In S. Dumont, & M. St-Onge (Eds.), *Social Work, Health, and International Development: Compassion in Social Policy and Practice* (pp. 45–54). Binghamton, NY: Haworth Press.

Thandi, G. (2011). Reducing substance abuse and intimate partner violence in Punjabi Sikh communities. *Sikh Formations: Religion, Culture, Theory, 7*(2), 177–193.

Turner, F. J. (1992). *Mental Health and the Elderly: A Social Work Perspective*. New York: Free Press.

United Nations. (1948). The universal declaration of human rights. *Claiming Human Rights Guide to International Procedures Available in Cases of Human Rights Violations in Africa*. Article 25. Retrieved from http://www.claiminghumanrights.org/udhr_article_25.html#at27

UN Commission on Human Rights. (1994). *UNHCR's Operational Experience with Internally Displaced Persons*, Geneva.

Vourlekis, B., & Ell, K. (2008). Best practice case management medical adherence. *Social Work in Health Care, 44*(3).

WHO. (2015). *Ageing and health*. Retrieved from http://www.who.int/mediacentre/factsheets/fs404/en/

WHO. (2013). *Libya. Mental health and psychosocial support programme in Libya "Building Back Better"*. Retrieved from http://www.who.int/features/2013/mental_health_libya/en/

Whiteside, M., Tsey, K., & Cadet-James, Y. (2009). Empowerment as a social detriment of Indigenous Australian health: the case of the Family Wellbeing Programme. In P. Bywaters, E. McLeod, & L. Napier (Eds.), *Social Work and Global Health Inequalities Practice and Policy Developments* (pp. 165–171). Great Britain: Policy Press.

Williams, D. R., Costa, M. V., Odunlami, A. O., & Mohammed, S. A. (2008). Moving upstream: How interventions that address the social determinants of health can improve health and reduce disparities. *Journal of Public Health Management and Practice, 14*, S8–17.

Yalli, N., & Cooper, N. (2008). The perceptions of hospital social workers in Saudi Arabia regarding the organisational factors that impact on their role. *International Journal of Social Welfare, 17*(3), 247–250. doi:10.1111/j.1468-2397.2008.00559.x

Yellowless, J., & Hardy, F. (2014). Queensland branch position paper on the role of social work in health care. *Australian Association of Social Workers*. Canberra, Australia.

Zoma, M. (2014). Respecting faiths, avoiding harm: psychosocial assistance in Jordan and the United States. *Forced Migration*. Retrieved from http://www.fmreview.org/faith/zoma

SECTION III

LIFE SPAN HEALTH ISSUES

17

Global Health in Reproduction and Infants

Carol Holtz

Objectives

After completing this chapter, the reader will be able to:

1. Define reproductive health and reproductive rights.
2. Discuss the international health issues related to male and female reproduction, including human rights and public policy, infertility, family planning (contraception), pregnancy, childbirth, and infant health.
3. Discuss the history and background related to global reproduction and infant health.
4. Compare and contrast adolescent and adult reproductive issues, challenges, and rights.
5. Compare and contrast global perspectives, laws, and practices of legal and illegal abortions and maternal mortality consequences.
6. Relate the global progress of development toward Millennium Development Goal 5: Reduce the maternal mortality ratio as defined by the number of maternal deaths per 100,000 live births by three quarters between 1990 and 2015.
7. Discuss HIV status and reproductive health consequences.

BACKGROUND

Maternal and infant mortality is the key indicator of international health development, and the challenge for reduction has long been a goal for developing countries. Maternal mortality and HIV/AIDS are the two leading causes of death among women of reproductive age worldwide. For the first time in the mid-2000s, women in every country gained a longer life expectancy at birth then men, and also during the last half of the 2000s women's risk of death from pregnancy-related complications was reduced by greater than 90% in many developed countries.

However, a huge disparity still exists in maternal mortality rates between developing and developed countries. The estimated maternal mortality for Sub-Saharan Africa remains at 500 deaths per 100,000 live births. Two countries in that region have the world's highest ratios. Chad has 1,100 deaths per 100,000 live births and Somalia has 1,000 deaths per 100,000 live births. More than 300,000 women die each year globally from pregnancy-related conditions with 99% occurring in developing countries (Canudas-Romo, Liu, Zimmerman, Ahmed, & Tsui, 2014).

Millennium Developmental Goal (MDG) number 5 calls for the reduction in maternal mortality (deaths per 100,000 live births) by three-quarters by 2015, and the establishment of universal access to high-quality reproductive health care. Evidence suggests that there is a relationship between maternal education and protection for maternal and infant mortality. Karlsen and colleagues (2011) collected data from 287,035 inpatients giving birth in 373 institutions in 24 countries in Africa, Asia, and Latin America, and found that women with no education are 2.7 times more likely to die from childbirth. Women with one to six years of education were twice as likely to die from childbirth-related causes than women with 12 years of education or more (Karlsen et al., 2011; Zureick-Brown et al., 2013).

Newborn survival (birth to 28 days) has improved slowly in most regions of the world. Globally, in 2012, 44% of all deaths of children under five occurred during the neonatal period, which was up from 37% in 1990. Each year, 6.6 million children under five years old die, including 2.9 million newborns. An additional 2.6 million babies are stillborn annually. Maternal deaths can have terrible consequences for the whole family, and child deaths are often linked to maternal health via perinatal causes, suboptimal care and poor nutrition in pregnancy, and preterm delivery. Newborns and mothers are at the highest risk for death at the time of childbirth, with about one-third of neonatal deaths occurring within the first 24 hours after birth. The risk of maternal death is highest within 48 hours after delivery (Darmstadt et al., 2013).

Important maternal health indicators include:

1. *Basic services* such as clean and reliable water, sanitation facilities, electricity, power generators, refrigerators, and sterilization of medical equipment.
2. *General medical services* such as a blood bank, safe blood, biochemical and clinical laboratories, adult intensive-care units, and neonatal intensive care units.
3. *Basic lab screening testing,* which includes tests for protein in the urine, HIV, syphilis, and urine cultures.
4. *Anesthesia,* which includes doctors, nurses, and paramedics in the hospital or on call.
5. *Emergency obstetric services,* which includes parenteral antibiotics, oxytocic drugs, anticonvulsants, blood transfusions, and neonatal resuscitation, maternal cardio-pulmonary resuscitation, hysterectomies, and staff skilled in performing and caring for a women needing a caesarian section.
6. *At least one OB/GYN resident* on call and a continuous educational program.

Reproductive health is important because it contributes to the general economic growth of a nation, equality in gender, and democratic governance. Poor or inadequate sexual and reproductive health contributes to one-third of the world's burden of disease for women of childbearing age and one-fifth of the total world population. The greatest need for reproductive health services is among the poorest people in the developing countries. Improved contraception in developing countries could prevent 52 million unintended birth (Karlsen et al., 2011; Zureick-Brown et al., 2013).

Although the estimated annual rate of decline in the maternal mortality rate fell short by about 2.3% of the MDG goal 5, the annual number of deaths worldwide has declined by 34% between 1990 and 2008 (from about 546,000 deaths to 358,000 deaths). The majority of maternal mortality has shifted from Asia to Sub-Saharan Africa. Differences in fertility, the HIV/AIDS epidemic, and access to reproductive care are related to these shifts. Countries with poor maternal and infant health generally have weak healthcare systems, are in a social crisis, or both. Sex discrimination and lack of healthcare services, lack of equal rights, and lack of power for women all contribute to this health problem. Violence against women, rape, and sexual coercion threaten women's human rights and reproduction. Contraceptive use has increased, but now an estimated 201 million women in developing countries have unmet needs for birth control, and 60 million unplanned pregnancies occur annually (Karlsen et al., 2011; Vanderkruik, Tunçalp, Chou, & Say, 2013: Zureick-Brown et al., 2013).

The countries with the highest numbers of maternal deaths in 2008 were India (63,000), Nigeria (50,000), the Democratic Republic of the Congo (19,000), and Afghanistan (18,000). The maternal mortality rate ranges from the developed countries such as Greece with 2 for every 1,000 live births, Denmark (5/100,000), Sweden (5/100,000), and Australia (8/100,000) to developing countries with high rates such as Kenya (530/100,000), Zimbabwe (790/100,000), Somalia (1,200/100,000), and Afghanistan (1400/100,000) (Karlsen et al., 2011; Vanderkruik, Tunçalp, Chou, & Say, 2013; Zureick-Brown et al., 2013).

DEFINITION OF REPRODUCTIVE HEALTH

The United Nations (UN) Conference on Population and Development defines reproductive health as "a state of complete physical, mental, and social well-being and not merely the absence of disease or infirmity, in all matters relating to the reproductive system and to its functions and processes. Reproductive health therefore implies that people are able to have a satisfying and safe sex life and that they have the capability to reproduce and the freedom to decide if, when, and how often to do so. Implicit in the last condition are the rights of men and women to be informed and to have access to safe, effective, affordable, and acceptable methods of family planning of their choice, as well as other methods of their choice for regulation of fertility that are not against the law, and the right of access to appropriate healthcare services that will enable women to go safely through pregnancy and childbirth and provide couples with the best chance of having a healthy infant" (United Nations Family Planning Association [UNFPA], 2011).

Gender inequality has a direct influence on reproductive health, which results in poor reproductive and mental health outcomes, including unwanted pregnancy, unsafe abortions, maternal mortality, sexually transmitted diseases (STDs), and depression. In poor countries with a strong male dominance, women usually have little control of their sex lives, are rarely able to choose whom to marry, when to have sex, how many children to have, or whether to use contraception or protection against STDs. Men are often permitted to have multiple sex partners, and women remain uninformed and passive about sexuality, which increases their risk of exposure to human immunodeficiency virus (HIV) and other STDs. Women often internalize the local cultural norm that says they are inferior to males, an attitude that may be reflected in the patterns of female feticide and infanticide in some countries. Women's greater rate of malnutrition contributes to maternal and infant mortality. Pregnant women who are also malnourished more frequently have low-birth-weight babies. During pregnancy, the women may have anemia, making them vulnerable to postpartum hemorrhage, leading to shock and death (UNFPA, 2011).

PRETERM BIRTHS

Approximately 15 million preterm births (before 37 weeks' gestation) occur every year and 1.1 million of those will die owing to preterm birth related complications. Preterm birth is the leading cause of death in the first month of life due to increased risk for respiratory, infectious, metabolic, and nervous system morbidities. These risks continue to be a major problem for children under five. Preterm children also have a greater risk of childhood and early adult illnesses, such as hypertension and diabetes. Greater than 60% of preterm births occur in low- and middle-income countries. Of these births, 45 to 50% are caused by spontaneous preterm labor, 30% by premature rupture of membranes, and 15 to 20% are initiated by the healthcare provider (Vogel, Lee, & Souza, 2014).

Factors that increase the risk for preterm deliveries are as follows:

- Young or advanced age
- Race
- Multiple pregnancy
- Shorter pregnancy intervals
- Infections
- Chronic or acute medical conditions
- Poor nutrition, lifestyle factors
- Psychological factors
- Genetic predisposition (Vogel, Lee, & Souza, 2014)

In Latin America and Asia diseases such as pyelonephritis, diabetes and preeclampsia positively affect the high rates of preterm births, and in Africa, malaria, and HIV/AIDS are additional causes to preterm births (Vogel, Lee, & Souza, 2014).

REPRODUCTIVE RIGHTS

According to the United Nations' Programme of Action of the International Conference on Population and Development, 1995, para. 7.3, as cited in *World Population Monitoring 2002* (UN, 2004; UNFPA, 2011):

> Reproductive rights embrace certain human rights that are already recognized in national laws, international human rights documents, and other consensus documents. These rights rest on the recognition of the basic right of all couples and individuals to decide freely and responsibly

the number, spacing, and timing of their children and to have the information and means to do so, and the right to attain the highest standard of sexual and reproductive health. It also includes their right to make decisions concerning reproduction free of discrimination, coercion, and violence, as expressed in human rights documents . . . The promotion of the responsible exercise of these rights for all people should be the fundamental basis for government and community-supported policies and programs in the area of reproductive health, including family planning. As part of their commitment, full attention should be given to the promotion of mutually respectful and equitable gender relations and particularly to meeting the educational and service needs of adolescents to enable them to deal in a positive and responsible way with their sexuality.

The key issues about reproductive human rights that stand out in this UN document are (1) family planning, (2) adolescent issues, (3) reproductive rights, (4) HIV/AIDS, and (5) violence against women (UN, 2004; UNFPA, 2011).

An example of the lack of personal reproductive rights in that country is evident in a law established in China. On June 1, 1995, the Chinese government passed the Maternal and Infant Health Care Law to decrease the number of congenital anomalies (birth defects) in the country. This law requires that couples obtain a premarital exam for serious genetic diseases and "relevant medical disorders," as well as prenatal testing. If a serious disorder is found, the law dictates that long-term contraception or sterilization must take place or the couple may not marry. People who have diseases or problems such as schizophrenia, psychoses, leprosy, HIV/AIDS, and STDs are subject to this law. Within this law also is a mandated right for all pregnant women to have the right to prenatal care, which includes education about pregnancy and general health care, and health care for the newborn. Encouragement is given to the couple to electively abort a pregnancy in which a fetus is known to have a serious genetic disorder or a serious defect, or a pregnancy in which the life of the mother may be jeopardized from the pregnancy (Law of the People's Republic of China on Maternal and Infant Care, 1995).

The one-child policy, known officially as the family planning policy, was the population control policy of the People's Republic of China. Many demographers considered the term "one-child" a misnomer, as the policy allowed many exceptions: for example, rural families were permitted to have a second child if the first child was a girl or was disabled, and ethnic minorities were exempt. Foreigners living in China and residents of the Hong Kong and Macau were also exempt from the policy. In 2007, approximately 35.9% of China's population was subject to the one-child restriction. This law, however, was modified. In November 2013, the Chinese government announced that it would further relax the policy by allowing families to have two children if one of the parents is an only child. Demographers estimate that the policy averted 200 million births between 1979 and 2009. The previous rules allowed two children for couples in which both parents were only children. The old policy also made exceptions for China's officially recognized ethnic minorities and rural couples whose first child was a girl or was disabled. The government estimates that the change will allow an additional 15 to 20 million couples to expand their families, helping to stem a plummeting birthrate that experts say has left China with a dangerous demographic imbalance in both age and gender. But only about half of those couples are willing to have two children, according to research by the National Health and Family Planning Commission cited in state news media (Levin, 2014).

As of January, 2016, China's Health and Family Planning Commission relates that 90 million couples now qualify for a second child under the new rules. The one-child policy was in place for more than three decades in China to control population growth. Abuses of forced abortions and sterilizations and led to more boys being born than girls. The two-child policy will increase the number of new babies born in China every year from 16 million to between 20 million and 24 million (Baculinao, 2016).

Reproductive human rights issues in the United States have also been challenged. Workplace barriers for breastfeeding contribute to low breastfeeding rates in the United States as well as in other global locations. The American Academy of Pediatrics recommends breastfeeding through the first six months of an infant's life, and continued breastfeeding until at least 12 months of life. Of the 50 states, only 23 states have adopted laws to encourage breastfeeding (if mothers wish to do so) in the workplace. Federal law did not provide any protection to working mothers until the 2010 enactment of the reasonable "break time" provision of the Patient Protection and Affordable Care Act, which required that new mothers be given time to pump breastmilk for (not feed) children younger than one year of age; the law exempts from this requirement employers who demonstrate hardship (Murtagh & Moulton, 2011).

INFECTIONS AND PREGNANCY/INFANT HEALTH

Pregnancy-related infections are a cause of maternal and fetal/newborn morbidity and mortality and are extremely important and often preventable, contributing to about 50,000 maternal deaths annually. The World Health Organization (WHO) defines "puerperal sepsis" as an infection of the genital tract occurring any time between the rupture of membranes in pregnancy and the 42nd day postpartum. The impact of infection includes deaths and disability from infections of the urinary tract, soft tissue, abortion-related infections, and intrauterine infections. Infection is the third leading cause of maternal mortality, causing 10 to 12% of all maternal deaths, disproportionately occurring in developing countries. The risk of death from puerperal sepsis is 2.7 times higher in Africa, 1.9 times higher in Asia, and 2.1 higher in Latin America than in developed countries (Gravett et al., 2012).

ADOLESCENT REPRODUCTIVE HEALTH

Across the globe, adolescents and young adults often face a transition into adulthood with insufficient knowledge and experience. It is important to educate them for effective health promotion and prevention of diseases and unwanted pregnancies. Menarche (the age at which reproduction is physically possible) varies greatly across societies. In a recent study of 67 countries, researchers concluded that menarche is reached earlier in developed societies as compared to developing societies. It is associated with socioeconomic class, literacy rates, and nutrition. The onset of sexual activity today typically takes place during adolescence, a period of growth, experimentation, and identity search. Lack of access to health information among adolescents may be due to social, cultural, and sometimes legal barriers. It results in adolescents who are often poorly informed and do not make responsible choices, which may lead to sexual and reproductive health problems (WHO, 2014a).

Globally, approximately 16 million adolescent girls give birth every year, the majority of whom live in low- and middle-income countries. Stillbirths and newborn deaths are 50% higher among infants of adolescent mothers as compared to women 20 to 29 years of age. Infants of adolescent mothers are more likely to have low birth weights as well. In addition, an estimated three million girls, ages 15 to 19, have unsafe abortions each year (WHO, 2014a).

Many factors converge to create environments in which teens are prone to giving birth. Some of these factors as compiled by WHO (2014a) can include:

1. Societies in which girls are under cultural pressure to marry and bear children quickly. In middle- and low-income countries 30% marry before the age of 18 and 14% marry before the age of 15.
2. Girls have limited education and employment prospects. Education is a major protective factor in decreasing teen pregnancies.
3. Many adolescents have no knowledge about preventing pregnancy or are unable to obtain contraceptives.
4. There is a lack of sex education in many countries.

Teen pregnancy and childbearing bring substantial social and economic costs through immediate and long-term impacts on teen parents and their children. In most developed countries of the world, the majority of teenagers become sexually active, and at least 75% have had sexual intercourse by the time they are 20 years old. Teenagers in the United States are becoming sexually active with more partners as compared to teenagers of other developed countries such as Canada, Sweden, France, and the United Kingdom. U.S. teenagers also have high rates of pregnancy, childbearing, and abortion as compared to their peers in other developed countries. A major factor to explain that last point is that U.S. teenagers use fewer types of contraception than teens of other developed countries. This decrease in use is due to negative attitudes toward teen sexual activity, restriction of access to reproductive health services, and lack of motivation to prevent pregnancy. The U.S. infant mortality rate ranks 27th among developing countries with wide disparities among race, socioeconomic status, and geography. In the southern region of the United States, as compared to other regions of the country, there is an excess of infant deaths per 1,000 live births. Some of this regional disparity is due to a greater proportion of African American births with preterm deliveries. Premature births, congenital anomalies, and sudden unexpected infant deaths (SUIDs) were the three leading causes of death of infants in the South.

Preterm births were about 20% higher in the U.S. South, highest in the states of Alabama, Mississippi, and Louisiana. Sexually transmitted diseases disproportionately affect teenagers as compared to older women of childbearing age. Syphilis, gonorrhea, and chlamydia are the most common STDs in teens. The United States has higher rates of STDs than other developed countries such as the United Kingdom, France, Canada, and Sweden, because of the lower use of condoms and higher numbers of sexual partners among U.S. teenagers (Hirai et al., 2014; WHO, 2014a, 2014b).

CULTURAL INFLUENCES ON REPRODUCTIVE HEALTH

Cultures directly affect programs and policies related to reproductive health. For example, Islamic law condemns prostitution, homosexuality, and premarital sex. Thus, the interpretation of the Koran presents challenges for establishing reproductive health programs for teenagers in many Muslim countries. For example, in Morocco—a mostly Muslim country in northern Africa—there is opposition to sex education and condom promotion for unmarried adolescent use, yet in other Muslim countries there are clear guidelines for sex education. In Iran in the late 1980s, fatwas declared that family planning methods were allowed. In Egypt since the 1960s, all major family planning and reproduction health programs were supported by religious leaders (Beamish & Abderrazik, 2003). Childbirth educators need to assess their own cultural competence, beginning with an understanding of their own background and how it affects interactions with families.

The following are examples of cultural influences on Latina/Hispanic women.

Prenatal

- Women are taught to avoid foods that are considered to be "hot" by their culture (e.g., chilies and coffee) because it is believed to cause the child to be born with spots and to be more susceptible to rashes.
- Foods such as shrimp, fish, oysters, and other shellfish are sometimes removed from the diet and the quantity of eggs are reduced to avoid giving birth to a child with bad body odors.
- Women are encouraged to eat foods that are high in iron such as beans.
- Women use plenty of cream as it is believed to aid in the production of better breast milk.
- Women are encouraged be stay active (especially by walking) as this is said to help develop a healthier baby with a better temperament.
- To avoid problems with the umbilical cord, women are discouraged from wearing anything around the neck and from clothing that contains elastic, and they are told to not reach upward for things, such as clothing on a clothesline.
- As the culture is very respectful of its elders, women will often look to mothers, aunts, and grandmothers for advice on all topics both during pregnancy and otherwise.
- Some traditional Hispanic beliefs say that if the woman's face stays nice and smooth, she will not gain much weight; if her stomach becomes pointed she will have a boy; and if the mother is more tired and gains more weight she will have a girl.
- Women are given medallions, a red ball, or a rosary that is secured with a large safety pin to the clothing to prevent malformations in the child.
- Intercourse may be halted during pregnancy as it is believed to be harmful to the baby. It can begin again one to three months after the birth.

Labor and Delivery

- Some Hispanic woman may believe that they should not take any pain medications as the medication may not be good for the baby.
- If the baby was in a malposition for birth, crawling on the hands and knees can help to bring the baby back into the correct position for birthing.
- Woman in rural areas often give birth to their children at home with only a midwife present; however, hospital birthing is considered to be safer.
- Screaming during the labor and delivery is considered to be harmful to the baby.
- Some traditional pain management techniques include controlled breathing, walking, counting forward and backward, or reciting letters of the alphabet.
- The family may want to take the umbilical cord, placenta, or both to their home with them after the birth. The placenta may be planted below a fruiting tree as it is believed the child will grow and bear fruit as the tree grows.
- The mother may want to have bright clothing as it is said to encourage a baby with a better attitude and intelligence. Makeup is also not worn during the labor and delivery.

Postpartum

- Mothers practice the *Quarentena*, which is a length of time (usually around 40 days after the birth) during which the mother and child are to remain in the home with limited visitors so that they can properly bond and are not exposed to infections from outside. During this time, some mothers may only take sponge baths.
- It is thought that fresh air is healthiest for the baby, and perfumes and scented cleaning agents should not be used in the home with the baby.
- The baby must be kept warmly wrapped and wear socks at all times to keep from becoming chilled.
- Cloth diapers may also be favored as the plastic on disposable diapers is believed to be bad for the baby's skin.
- After several months of breastfeeding, some mothers believe that the nutritional value of their breast milk declines and that drinking a small amount of beer daily can help produce *levadura*—a stronger more healthy milk.
- Women may give the baby certain herbal teas (made with fresh herbs, not from tea bags) to help calm a baby who may have colic. The mother may also rub a food item into the back of the knees as it is believed to help develop strong bones.
  (The above has been modified from Hispanic cultural views on pregnancy; prenatal through postpartum, Purnell & Paulanka, *Transcultural Health Care: A Culturally Competent Approach*, 2005, pp. 409–410.).

FERTILITY

The age of childbearing varies greatly among countries. In Africa, the ages of women who are bearing children are evenly distributed between younger and older women. In most other major areas of the world, however, the majority (two-thirds) of childbearing takes place before age 30. In many developed countries today, the age at which women have their first child has increased. Women are having children later in life and are having fewer children than previous generations, which has resulted in a below-replacement-level fertility rate in many developed countries. Lower fertility rates in developed countries are attributable to factors such as industrialization, urbanization, modernization of societies, improved access to education, improved survival of children, and increased use of contraception (UN, 2004).

Men are physiologically capable of reproducing longer than women and often marry later and become fathers at older ages than women. Women who have children closely spaced in age and who give birth when they are younger than 18 or older than 34 have higher risks of morbidity and mortality for both themselves and their babies (UN, 2004).

Cultural Influences on Reproduction

In the Arab culture, the bride's status in her husband's household is unstable until she gives birth to her first baby and proves that she is fertile; she is then obligated to have a second child because of the fear that an only child may die and leave the parents childless. After the second child is born, the pressure to continue having children exists if there are only female children. Women are expected to continue having children until at least one son is born. The need to have a male child is great, to preserve the family name. Muslims believe that their religion requires them "to be fruitful and multiply" (Kridli, 2002).

Infertility: Cultural and Religious Issues

Infertility is the biological failure to conceive by normal sexual activity without contraception or to carry a pregnancy to full term; it affects both men and women of reproductive age. This definition contrasts with intentional childlessness, which may be due to cultural, social, economic, or psychological factors. Infertility rates are especially high in Sub-Saharan Africa, where many individuals have reproductive tract infections caused by STDs, particularly gonorrhea and HIV infections. Unsafe abortions may also be responsible for infertility problems among residents of countries with transition economies. In developed countries, infertility rates are higher than might be expected in spite of available legal abortions and treatment of STDs, mainly due to significant delays in childbearing. In many cultures, infertility causes stress, social exclusion, and stigma. In some cultures, women who are infertile may be divorced, neglected, abused, and given lower social status. Universally, infertility usually results in serious psychological stress for the couple. Approximately 8 to 12% of couples worldwide experience infertility problems of some type (WHO, 2010b).

In a masters' thesis in Makeree University in Uganda, Komurembe (2010) described the challenges of fertility within the culture of Uganda. Fertility rates in Uganda at 6.7 are one of the highest in the world, which has been attributed to the cultural and gender practices amongst the communities. This research report was compiled basing on the findings of a field study carried out in two subcounties of Ntungamo and Itojo. The study set out to identify the cultural practices that influence fertility. The study's findings indicated that although the respondents were knowledgeable about family planning methods, the majority were not using them for a variety of reasons, which included the cultural beliefs in extending the family lineage, polygamy, early marriages, extramarital sex, and sexual rituals. Respondents believed that influences on fertility also included subordination of women, women's economic dependence on men, and women's lack of control over information sources.

In Mexico, problems of reproductive health are associated with pregnancy in adolescents, STDs, and genitourinary neoplasms. Infertility affects 10% of couples, usually as a result of asymptomatic infections. Education, poverty, nutrition, and pollution are problems that also must be solved (Centers for Disease Control and Prevention [CDC], 2014a).

In many cultures the inability to produce a child is considered a personal tragedy that often affects the whole family as well as the community. Womanhood is frequently defined through fertility. Infertility in many cultures is blamed on the woman, resulting in social stigma, social isolation, domestic violence, and polygamy. Researchers from Tehran, Iran, conducted a study that explored infertility from the perspective of infertile Iranian women. Themes that emerged included spousal abuse, marital instability, social isolation, and low self-esteem. In some cultures, the problem is solved by adopting a child, remarriage, or divorce. In Iran men can take a second wife, with or without a divorce, to satisfy the need for producing offspring. About 24.9% of women in Iran are infertile at some time in their lives, and many seek help at the various nongovernmental organization (NGO) reproductive health research centers (Behboodi-Moghadan, Salsali, Efterhar-Ardabily, Vaismoradi, & Ramezanzadeh, 2013).

Religion and culture are often major influences on fertility treatments. According to Jewish law, an infertile couple should undergo diagnosis and treatment. Most Jewish infertile couples may do almost anything to have a child, including the use of reproductive technology. In fact, Israel, a predominately Jewish country, is one of the leading countries of the world in the research and development of reproductive technology. Insemination of husband's sperm is permitted, and some groups of Jews permit insemination of another man's sperm if absolutely necessary. In vitro fertilization and embryo transfer are also permitted by most groups of Jewish people. Most Christian groups state that marriage does not confer upon spouses the duty to have a child, but the right to have intercourse. Sterility can be an occasion for other important services to humanity such as adoption, educational work, assistance to families, and assistance to disadvantaged children. Islam allows all treatments for infertility as long as they involve only the husband and the wife; adoption is not permitted. Polygamy is practiced today in many Islamic societies, which creates more opportunities for fertility within a family structure. In contrast, the Roman Catholic Church states that assisted reproduction—including artificial insemination, in vitro fertilization (IVF), and embryo transfer—is not allowed (Schenker, 2005).

Within Judaism, fetal reduction for multiple-gestation pregnancies is allowed by most Jews. Catholics, however, consider this practice to be an abortion, which is not permitted. In Islam, fetal reduction is allowed if the other fetuses or the mother's life is in jeopardy (Schenker, 2005).

The status of the human embryo is quite controversial in the United States. Not all embryos created in IVF clinics are used for pregnancy implantation. Clinics may put "extra" created embryos in cryopreservation, to be donated for reproductive use for couples, research, or disposal. Disposal of excess embryos creates many moral and ethical issues, which continue to be widely debated. Currently some 400,000 embryos are frozen in storage in the United States, and many others exist in other countries as well. Depending on the culture, religion, and geographic location, human embryos are regarded as anything from a cluster of cells to an actual human being (Gurmankin & Caplan, 2004).

FAMILY PLANNING AND CONTRACEPTION

Family planning allows people to decide the number, spacing, and timing of the births of their children. Research clearly links adequate spacing of the birth of children with decreased maternal and infant morbidity and mortality. At present, 60% of the world's individuals or couples use family planning as compared to 10% in the 1960s (Table 17-1). Contraception is the intentional prevention of a pregnancy by natural or artificial methods. Family planning and contraception use are closely correlated to a woman's or the couple's urbanization, education, socioeconomic status, and approval by culture.

According to a survey of women 15 to 44 years of age in the United States, the most common forms of contraception are as follows:

- Oral contraceptive pill
- Female sterilization
- Male condom
- Male sterilization
- Injectable Depo-Provera

Family planning services should be integrated within primary healthcare services, which should include education and counseling for informed contraception decision making for the couple. In addition, care for STDs, cervical cancer screening, and breast cancer screening need to be included as part of primary health care. Family planning serves the following purposes (WHO, 2010):

- It promotes gender equality and empowers women and families.
- It can reduce maternal deaths by 32% and deaths of newborns and children by 10%.

TABLE 17-1 Worldwide Contraceptive Use

Country	Percentage of Population Using Contraceptives (%)
Africa	<10
Eastern Europe	35
Russian Federation	70–74
Western Europe	71–77
Latin America	73
United States	82
China	83

Data from United Nations (UN). (2004). *World Population Monitoring 2002: Reproductive Rights and Reproductive Health.* New York: Author.

- It can potentially decrease unwanted pregnancies by 71%.
- It can decrease HIV transmission by as much as 80% with the promotion of consistent and correct condom use.
- It slows population growth, thereby significantly reducing poverty and hunger.

According to a UN report, in China, premarital sex is no longer taboo, and norms and behaviors are changing. Most sexually active people do not want a pregnancy, yet many lack knowledge of contraception. Many unmarried women are embarrassed about obtaining contraception and do not want their sexual activity to be revealed. Many believe that family planning centers are for married women only, yet the government has made these services available to all (WHO, 2010).

According to a Muslim jurist who uses the Koran, under a fatwa (ruling) related to family planning in Islam, family planning is permitted. There is a wide variation of opinion among Muslim authorities regarding family planning, however. Some Muslims do not believe in family planning and state that children are a great asset: The larger the number of Muslims, the greater the power. The higher courts in Jordan have stated that family planning is acceptable in Islam, but decisions on this issue are left to the couple (Hasna, 2003).

Mogilevkina and Odlind (2003) report that historically in Ukraine, as in other countries of the former Soviet Union (now known as the Commonwealth of Independent States), abortion was used as a method of birth control. This policy reflected negative attitudes toward contraception. Researchers' data from 1999 showed that the abortion rate was 121 abortions per 100 deliveries, and 36.7 abortions per 1,000 women of reproductive age. Today, contraception services are increasing in Ukraine, yet abortion remains common and 32.5% of women do not use any form of contraception.

Emergency Contraception

One example of a moral dilemma regarding emergency contraception was reported by Zwillich (2005). In the United States, a small group of conservative pharmacists have refused to fill prescriptions for the emergency contraception medication called levonorgestrel (Barr Pharmaceuticals), which prevents pregnancy when taken within 72 hours of unprotected sex. The drug works by inhibiting ovulation, interfering with fertilization, and blocking implantation in the wall of the uterus.

Abortion

Elective abortion is the voluntary termination of a pregnancy, which in most cases, is done prior to viability of the fetus. In 1973, the U.S. Supreme Court ruled that induced abortions must be legal in all states as long as the pregnancy is less than 12 weeks' gestation. Individual states can regulate abortion in a second-trimester pregnancy and prohibit abortion that is not life threatening after 12 weeks' gestation. Some states have established additional regulations regarding use of the procedure in the third trimester of pregnancy, such as requiring a 24-hour waiting period for counseling or requiring parental approval for minors (Boonstra & Nash, 2014).

Grimes and colleagues (2006) state that abortion is a persistent and preventable epidemic. According to WHO, an unsafe abortion, which represents a human rights issue, is a procedure for terminating an unintended and unwanted pregnancy either by people without necessary skills or in an environment that does not conform to minimum medical standards. It endangers women, the majority of whom live in developing countries, where abortion is highly restricted by law, or in countries where, although legally permitted, abortions are not easily accessible. In these settings women often obtain secret abortions from medical practitioners, paramedical workers, or traditional healers. Legal abortions by trained healthcare providers are a safe procedure with minimum morbidity and mortality.

According to WHO's (2010a) *Packages of Interventions for Family Planning, Safe Abortion Care, Maternal, Newborn, and Child Health,* women should be provided safe abortion services to the full extent of the local law within a specific geographic location. In addition, women need access to treatment for complications due to spontaneous or unsafe abortion, as well as information and counseling services. In some parts of the world, women are forbidden to have any information, counseling, or procedure related to an elective abortion.

History of Elective Abortion

According to the Childbirth by Choice Trust (1999), abortion has been practiced in almost all regions throughout the world since the earliest times. Women have been faced with unwanted pregnancies and have chosen to abort a fetus regardless of religious or legal sanction, often risking their lives in the process. In primitive societies, abortions were induced by poisons, herbs, sharp sticks, and pressure on the abdomen, causing vaginal bleeding. Ancient Chinese and Egyptians used surgical instruments, much like modern ones of today. Socrates, Plato, and Aristotle were known to suggest abortion, while Hippocrates recommended it on occasion. St. Augustine (354–430 AD) related that the animation and sensation of pregnancy occurred at 40 days after conception; prior to the first 40 days, abortion was not considered homicide. Pope Innocent III wrote that quickening—the time of perception of fetal movement—was the moment that abortion became homicide. In 1869, Pope Pius IX declared excommunication for those who had an abortion at any stage of fetal development. From the late 1800s until World War II, abortion was restricted almost everywhere in the world. Later, countries in Eastern and Central Europe relaxed some of the laws, followed by most of the developed countries during the 1960s and 1970s (Childbirth by Choice Trust, 1999).

In January 2012, WHO and the Guttmacher Institute released a study of global abortion trends indicating that women are not influenced by the nation or local law in which they reside when they make their decision to have an abortion. If it is illegal in their area of residence, women often seek abortions in unsafe conditions by untrained people. In 2008, the estimated annual number of deaths from unsafe abortion worldwide declined from 56,000 in 2003 to 47,000 in 2008. Complications from unsafe abortion accounted for an estimated 13% of all maternal deaths worldwide in both years. In countries where abortion is legal, researchers found that abortion was safe, whereas in countries where it is illegal, the procedure is dangerous. Globally, there are 28 abortions for every 1,000 women of childbearing age, and studies show that abortion accounts for 13% of women's deaths during pregnancy and childbirth. Data suggests that the best way to reduce abortion rates is to make contraception more available rather than banning the practice altogether. The study found that in Eastern Europe, where contraception has become more accessible, abortion rates have decreased by 50% (Infoplease, 2014).

Worldwide, nations have different ways of addressing the rules and regulations regarding abortion. Between 1995 and 2003, the abortion rate (the number of abortions per 1,000 women of childbearing age (15–44 years) for the world overall dropped from 35 to 29 and remained virtually unchanged, at a rate of 28 per 1,000, in 2008. Nearly half of all abortions worldwide are unsafe, and nearly all unsafe abortions (98%) occur in developing countries. In the developing world, 56% of all abortions are unsafe, compared with just 6% in the developed world. The proportion of abortions worldwide that take place in the developing world increased between 1995 and 2008 from 78 to 86%, in part because the proportion of all women who live in the developing world increased during this period. In 2008, six million abortions were performed in developed countries and 38 million in developing countries. In 2008, there were 29 abortions per 1,000 women aged 15 to 44 in developing countries, compared with 24 in the developed world (Alan Guttmacher Institute, 2014).

In the Sub-Saharan region, mainly South Africa, abortion was legalized in 1997, an area of the world that has the lowest abortion rate for all countries of this region, which is 15 per 1,000 women (2008). East Africa has the highest rate, at 38 per 1,000 women of childbearing age, followed by Middle Africa at 36 per 1,000 women, West Africa at 28 per 1,000 women, and North Africa at 18 per 1,000 women. In Europe, abortion is generally legal. In Western Europe, the rate is 12 per 1,000 women, while in Eastern Europe it is 43 per 1,000 women. The significant difference in rates between the two regions reflects the relatively low contraceptive use in Eastern Europe, as well as a high degree of reliance on condoms, withdrawal, and the rhythm method, all which have higher failure rates. In Europe, 30% of pregnancies end in abortion; there is a higher proportion in Eastern Europe with a rate of 43 per 1,000 women. Western Europe, Southern Africa, and Northern Europe have the lowest abortion rates in the world. The abortion rate fell in Latin America from 37 to 32 per 1,000 women in 2008. In Latin America, abortion rates range from 29 to 39 per 1,000 women. In Cuba, abortions are generally safe; the country has the lowest proportion of abortions in the region that are unsafe (46%), compared with nearly 100% in Central and South America. In Asia, abortion rates between 2003 and 2008 ranged from 26 per 1,000 in South Central Asia and Western Asia to 36 per 1,000 in Southeastern Asia. Abortion incidence appears to have risen in China since 2003, after an extended period of decline. Evidence shows that this is due to an increase in premarital sexual activity and disruptions in access to contraceptive services because of increased urbanization (Alan Guttmacher Institute, 2014).

Abortion is legal in many areas of the world, yet the criteria for permitting it vary. Some countries permit abortions only to save the woman's life. The laws are generally more restrictive in the developing world than in the developed nations. In countries where abortion is strictly illegal or very restrictive, unsafe abortions are performed against the law and can cause unnecessary morbidity and mortality. Globally, one in eight maternal deaths is due to an unsafe abortion. The highest rates of maternal death by unsafe abortion are found in Africa, with a rate of seven deaths per 1,000 unsafe abortions, followed by Asia, with four deaths per 1,000 unsafe abortions. The most frequent complications from unsafe abortions are sepsis, incomplete abortion, hemorrhage, and abdominal cavity injury. The regions that have highly restrictive abortion laws are not associated with lower abortion rates. For example, the abortion rate in African countries is 29 per 1,000 women of childbearing age and 32 per 1,000 in Latin America where abortion is illegal under most circumstances in the majority of countries. These rates can be compared to 12 per 1,000 in Western Europe, where abortion is generally legal.

An estimated 19 to 20 million elective abortions take place every year, with 97% of these procedures occurring in developing countries. These procedures are among the most neglected of global health challenges. An estimated 68,000 women die each year worldwide from unsafe abortions, and many millions more are permanently injured. The leading causes of death in such cases are hemorrhage, infection, and poisoning. Legal abortions, by contrast, have a mortality rate of one per 100,000 procedures (Grimes et al., 2006).

Maternal deaths from abortions are very difficult to report with any accuracy because many of the procedures are illegal and secret, and there are powerful disincentives for reporting such data. Approximately half of such deaths occur in Asia, and most of the remainder occurs in Africa. Examples of unsafe elective abortion methods used worldwide include the following toxic solutions:

- Toxic solutions
  - Turpentine
  - Laundry bleach
  - Detergent solutions
  - Acid
  - Laundry bluing
  - Cottonseed oil
  - Arak (strong liquor)
  - Teas and herbal drinks
  - Boiled avocado or basil leaves
  - Drugs such as Pitocin
- Objects placed through the cervix:
  - Sticks
  - Rubber catheter
  - Knitting needle
  - Coat hanger
  - Pen
  - Air through a turkey baster
- Enemas
- Trauma

STAGES OF CARE AND REPRODUCTIVE HEALTH

Prenatal Care

Prenatal care includes the following measures, all of which are recommended by WHO (2010a):

- Information and counseling on self-care at home, including nutrition, safer sex, HIV prevention and care during pregnancy, breastfeeding, family planning, and the harmful effects of drugs, alcohol, and tobacco use during pregnancy
- Childbirth preparation and danger signs of pregnancy
- Support and care for women with HIV/AIDS
- Assessment and assistance with domestic violence
- Confirmation of pregnancy
- Monitoring of pregnancy progress, including maternal and fetal well-being
- Detection and treatment of pregnancy complications
- In some situations, antimalaria treatment, assessment of female genital mutilation, and deworming

Delivery and Newborn Care

Childbirth care increases safety and decreases complications for both mother and baby. It includes care from the onset of labor to at least 24 hours after childbirth, and can potentially reduce maternal mortality due to labor complications by as much as 95%, and asphyxia-related newborn complications by as much as 40%. Ideal childbirth situations should include the following:

- Skilled healthcare professionals
- Services accessible and available 24 hours a day for seven days a week
- Essential medicines and equipment available
- Care during labor and delivery:
  - Diagnosis and monitoring of progress of labor
  - Infection prevention and treatment
  - Pain relief
  - Detection and treatment of complications
  - Delivery and immediate newborn care
  - Newborn resuscitation
  - Initiation of breastfeeding
  - Referrals, counseling, and family support for complications and/or death of mother and/or baby
- A referral system for complications (WHO, 2010a).

Postpartum Care

Postpartum and immediate newborn care reduces maternal and newborn morbidity and mortality. These services should include the following (WHO, 2010a):

- Skilled healthcare professionals
- Early identification and treatment of complications of mother and baby

- Family planning counseling services
- Care for HIV/AIDS mothers
- Support for breastfeeding

MATERNAL MORTALITY AND MORBIDITY

Maternal mortality is a major global problem that affects families and society as a whole, as seen in Table 17-2.

Obstetrical complications are the leading cause of death for women of reproductive age in developing countries today. Ninety-nine percent of these deaths occur in developing countries, and most could be prevented. Maternal health services and maternal mortality rates are very specific indicators of the general functioning of healthcare systems of a country (UNFPA, 2011).

A maternal death is defined as the death of a woman while pregnant or within 42 days after the termination of a pregnancy, irrespective of the duration, site, cause, or management of the pregnancy. Direct maternal deaths may be caused by obstetrical complications during pregnancy, labor and delivery, or postpartum. They may be related to interventions, omissions, incorrect treatment, or other events; examples include sepsis, pregnancy-induced hypertension, or delivery complications. Indirect maternal deaths are due to a previous existing disease or a disease that developed during pregnancy, yet not directly due to obstetrical causes. The disease may have been exacerbated during pregnancy. Examples include malaria, HIV/AIDS, and cardiovascular disease (UNFPA, 2011).

TABLE 17-2 Global Rates of Death from Pregnancy or Childbirth

Region	Lifetime Risk of Dying from Pregnancy or Childbirth
Sub-Saharan Africa	1 in 13
South Asia	1 in 55
Middle East/North Africa	1 in 55
Latin America/Caribbean	1 in 150
East Asia/Pacific	1 in 280
Central and Eastern Europe and the Commonwealth of Independent States CEE/CIS	1 in 800
Least developed countries	in 16
Developing countries	1 in 60
Developed countries	1 in 4100
World	1 in 75

Data from USAID. (2008). *Child Survival and Maternal Health Program, 2008*. Retrieved from http://pdf.usaid.gov/pdf_docs/PDACL707.pdf

A common indicator of national health is the maternal mortality rate, which is the number of maternal deaths per 100,000 women of reproductive age for a specific period of time, usually one year. Obtaining accurate data on maternal mortality is problematic because many countries do not indicate on the death certificate that a woman was pregnant or recently pregnant. In addition, a significant amount of underreporting and misclassification of actual deaths occurs.

The causes of maternal mortality worldwide are ranked in the following list:

1. Hemorrhage
2. Sepsis
3. Hypertensive disorders
4. Abortion complications
5. Obstructive labor (UNFPA, 2011)

In addition to deaths, many women suffer pregnancy-related complications that have long-term effects. For example, a woman could develop an amniotic fluid embolism or a cerebrovascular disorder causing a chronic disability, or a hemorrhage necessitating a hysterectomy, resulting in early loss of fertility. Family planning, good nutrition, and prenatal care have been shown to reduce maternal mortality (UNFPA, 2011).

Skilled care has contributed to lowering of the maternal mortality rate, but in Sub-Saharan Africa the maternal mortality rate is not improving. Access to prenatal care and high-quality delivery and postpartum care are needed for all women who give birth. As mentioned, complications from pregnancy and childbirth remain the leading causes of death and disability for all women of reproductive age. The worldwide maternal mortality rate is 515,000 women per year. In addition, for each woman who dies, approximately 30 more experience injuries, infection, and disabilities (UNFPA, 2011; USAID, 2008).

In Sub-Saharan Africa, women face a 1 in 13 chance of dying during pregnancy, in childbirth, or during the postpartum period; this risk is 200 times greater than the corresponding risk in the United States. Indigenous women of southern Mexico have numerous health challenges during pregnancy and childbirth. Because of great poverty, poor education, and a shortage in medical staff, women die from childbirth in the state of Chiapas frequently from hemorrhage and lack of access to surgery when complications occur especially during childbirth. Mexico's national maternal mortality declined from 124 deaths per 1,000 live births in 1980 to 52 per 1,000 live births in 2008. In Mexico's three poorest states, Chiapas, Oaxaca, and Guerrero, health issues affecting women, particularly maternal mortality, are much worse than other parts of the country. In the state of Oaxaca, maternal and infant mortality is high because government services are inadequate to treat emergencies due to poor resources and inadequate numbers of professional staff. Oaxaca has only one bed per 1,000 people and needs more OB/GYN specialists. In Chiapas, there is only about one doctor per 3,000 people. Another problem is the lack of adequate transportation in isolated rural areas. In this region, the primary causes of maternal mortality are hypertension caused by pregnancy-induced hypertension (preeclampsia and eclampsia), hemorrhage, and infections. In addition, magnesium sulfate, which is often used to treat hypertension of pregnancy, is in short supply and not often used in this region. In addition, owing to cultural customs, pregnant indigenous women often find difficulty in having a male physician touch them in their "intimate" areas. Due to strong machismo in this culture, these women are also subject to male domestic violence. Poor nutrition as a result of poverty and lack of knowledge about making good food choices (health literacy) also contribute to malnutrition, including lack of folic acid, in turn, creates greater risks for hemorrhage, infection, and birth defects with poor infant and under-age child survival rates. In Chiapas approximately 25% of all children under five are malnourished (Lowenberg, 2010).

Efforts to Reduce Maternal Mortality and Morbidity

WHO estimates that more than 500,000 women die annually of pregnancy complications. Maternal mortality in Sub-Saharan African is very high, with an estimated 900 maternal deaths per 100,000 live births. Reasons for this high rate in Sub-Saharan Africa are due to delays in:

- Recognizing danger signs during pregnancy.
- Deciding to seek care.
- Reaching a healthcare facility.
- Receiving appropriate care when once at the healthcare facility.

Most complications of pregnancy can be prevented or well managed if the danger signs are well known and transportation is available. In the region of northern Tanzania, the Mwanza region, Care-Tanzania, along with the U.S. CDC and the local Ministry of Health and Social Welfare, implemented a community reproductive health project focused on improving the quality of maternal health care. Twenty-nine villages were involved in this project, which included intensive training of local healthcare providers; increasing the amount of hospital equipment and blood for transfusion; improving the water and electrical supply; administering HIV counseling, testing, and medical interventions; and establishing a community patient transport system. Specific educational programs addressed family planning, information about STDs, education about danger signs in pregnancy, and advice about labor and delivery and postpartum needs. These programs resulted in a decrease in maternal mortality from 2002 to 2005 in the Kwimba region (Ahluwalia, Robinson, Vallely, Gieseker, & Kabakama, 2010).

The need for culturally appropriate care with an increase in the cultural knowledge of the clients, as with any minority culture/ethnic group, was indicated by a study by Bar-Zeev, Barclay, Kruske, and Kildea (2014) of Aboriginal women of North Australia. The researchers found a significant gap in pregnancy and birth outcomes for the Torres Strait Islander women and their babies as compared to the other Australian women and their babies. Aboriginal women attended prenatal care and adhered to some of the prenatal care instructions, yet there was an increased prevalence of anemia, smoking, urinary tract infections, and STDs. Findings indicated that clients wanted more culturally relevant information performed by more Aboriginal healthcare providers. Aboriginal midwives and community health workers (cultural brokers) have recently been involved in studying and providing care for these women, This has been successful in respecting the women's knowledge and skills and increasing participation in health improvements.

Recently, Canada began a multibillion-dollar initiative on nutrition to help fight maternal and newborn mortality. The Canadian plan called for nations to adopt a Framework for Action on Nutrition, which was developed through the cooperative efforts of USAID, the World

Bank, the United Nations, and Bread for the World (an NGO). The Canadian International Development Agency, a food security program, states that nutrition is often overlooked as a high priority to promote maternal and newborn well-being. The plan called for government and international agencies to spend an additional $10.3 billion per year from public resources to benefit 360 million children in 36 countries in a campaign against malnutrition and prevent more than 1.1 million child deaths (Canadian Medical Association, 2010).

ACCESSING REPRODUCTIVE HEALTH CARE

Prenatal care reduces maternal and newborn complications through regular checkups by a trained nurse midwife or physician. This care includes risk assessment, treatment for medical conditions or risk reduction, and education. In the United States, access to prenatal care has increased through the availability of Medicaid coverage for pregnancy-related services. An important element in reducing health risks for mothers and children is increasing the numbers of births with assistance by medically qualified people. Proper medical attention and hygienic conditions during delivery can reduce the risk of complications and infections that cause serious illness or death to either mother or baby. Women who do not receive prenatal care are more likely to deliver at home without a medically qualified birth attendant.

The likelihood of mothers entering prenatal care increases with age and education, and decreases with number of children. The risk of poor birth outcomes is greatest in women ages 15 and younger. Prenatal care needs to begin with the initial pregnancy and continue throughout pregnancy. The American College of Obstetricians and Gynecologists recommends at least 13 visits for a full-term low-risk pregnancy. More frequent visits are needed for a high-risk pregnancy (a pregnancy with complications such as diabetes or hypertension). In the United States, more than three-fourths of women receive adequate prenatal care; however, this rate varies with race and ethnicity. In addition to the prenatal visits to a healthcare provider, women are encouraged to attend with their spouse/partner/friend a series of childbirth education classes.

INFANT HEALTH

The following is a list of terms useful for discussing infant mortality (Kochanek & Martin, 2005):[1]

- *Infant mortality rate*: Deaths of infants younger than 1 year per 1,000 or 100,000 live births. It is the sum of the neonatal and postneonatal mortality rates.
- *Neonatal mortality rate*: Deaths of infants age 0 to 27 days per 1,000 live births.
- *Early neonatal mortality rate*: Deaths of infants age 0 to 6 days per 1,000 live births.
- *Late neonatal mortality rate*: Deaths of infants age 7 to 27 days per 1,000 live births.
- *Late fetal mortality rate*: Fetal deaths of 28 or more weeks of gestation per 1,000 live births.
- *Perinatal mortality rate*: Late fetal deaths plus early neonatal deaths per 1,000 live births plus fetal deaths.
- *Low-birth-weight rate*: Births with weight at delivery of less than 2,500 grams per 100 live births.
- *Moderately low-birth-weight rate*: Births with weight at delivery of 1,500 grams to 2,499 grams per 100 live births.

---

[1]Copyright © 2005 by SAGE Publications, Inc. Reprinted by Permission of SAGE Publications, Inc.

- Very low-birth-weight rate: Births with a rate at delivery of 1,500 grams or less per 100 live births.
- *Term*: Births at 37 to 41 weeks of gestation.
- *Preterm*: Births at less than 37 completed weeks of gestation per 100 live births.

Infant mortality worldwide differs greatly between and within developing and developed countries. The highest rate areas are found in Sub-Saharan Africa. Table 17-3 identifies some of the unusually high infant mortality rates worldwide, defined as number of deaths per 100,000 live births. Compared to developing countries, developed countries have much lower infant mortality rates and higher life expectancies.

Table 17-3 compares maternal and infant mortality rates in various Latin American and Caribbean countries.

The United States does not have the lowest infant mortality rate in the world, despite the fact that more money per capita is spent on health care in the United States than anywhere else in the world. Within the United States, the infant mortality rates also differ greatly by state, depending on education, income, cultures, geography, and politics. The CDC established a wide range of programs to prevent infant mortality (2004a). These programs include efforts to improve access to prenatal and newborn care, such as Healthy Start, Medicaid, and State Children's Health Insurance (SCHIP). The possibility of mortality is greatest in the first 24 hours after birth (25–45%). Approximately 75% of all neonatal deaths worldwide occur during the first week of life. In developed nations that keep accurate statistics, the rate of neonatal death is less than 3%. In many developing countries, the vital statistics may come from verbal reports. Causes of neonatal deaths include the following:

- Preterm birth (low birth weight)
- Severe infection (sepsis, pneumonia, tetanus, and diarrhea)
- Asphyxia
- Congenital abnormalities

TABLE 17-3 Maternal and Infant Mortality in Latin America and Caribbean Countries

Country	Maternal Mortality per 1,000 Live Births	Infant Mortality per 1,000 Live Births	Under 5 Mortality per 1,000 Live Births
Bolivia	190	57.9	54
Dominican Republic	150	32.5	27
Guatemala	120	34.4	32
Haiti	350	69.9	165
Honduras	100	28.9	67
Nicaragua	95	33.2	27

Pablos-Mendez, A., Valdivieso, V., &Flynn-Saldaña, K. (2013). Ending Preventable Child and Maternal Deaths in Latin American and Caribbean Countries (LAC). *Perinatologia y Reproduccion Humana. 27*(3), 145–152, Table 1, p. 146.

In many developing countries, babies are not weighed at birth and often gestational age in unknown. Eighteen million babies worldwide are estimated to be low birth weight, with 50% of the low-birth-weight babies born in Southeast Asia (Lawn, Cousens, & Zupan, 2005; Lawn, Shibuya, & Stein, 2005).

PROGRESS TOWARD MILLENNIUM DEVELOPMENTAL GOALS 4 AND 5 IN BRAZIL

Global progress toward MDG 4 (reducing child mortality) has been inadequately accomplished, but MDG 5 (improving maternal health) has been the subject of the least progress worldwide. Diverse economic and political conditions have affected all nations worldwide, but have had a severe effect on many countries, including Brazil. Brazil's north and northeast regions are the least developed and poorest parts of the country. The northeast region has a population of 54 million, representing 28.2% of the total population. Significant health interventions implemented in these poorer regions of Brazil include the following: piped water to households; increased use of contraception; prenatal care; delivery attendance by a medically trained person; options for cesarean delivery; diphtheria–pertussis–tetanus (DPT) vaccinations; measles vaccinations; care for pneumonia; and oral rehydration. Results of a study in Brazil indicate that as a result of these interventions infant mortality dropped from 47.1 deaths per 1,000 live births in 1990 to 20.0 deaths per 1,000 live births in 2007. Neonatal mortality also dropped from 23.1 deaths per 1,000 live births in 1990 to 13.6 deaths per 1,000 live births in 2007. Overall progress was made in terms of infant and maternal health, with a significant reduction in the gap between the rich and poor regions of the country. Brazil has significantly met the issues of undernutrition (MDG 1), and is doing well in reducing child mortality (MDG 4), yet its progress toward improving maternal mortality (MDG 5) remains unclear (Barros et al., 2010).

INFANT ABANDONMENT IN CHINA

Research on the abandonment of children in China revealed that some of the country's population policies may lead to abandonment of "excess" daughters so that couples may have a son. Among 237 families who abandoned their daughters, most did so because of the gender of their child; 90% of the children affected were girls and 86% were healthy. In contrast, 60% of the abandoned boys were disabled or severely ill. Other couples who were infertile emerged spontaneously to adopt these abandoned girls. Those who already had a son were also willing to adopt an abandoned girl (Johnson, Huang, & Wang, 1998).

WATER, SANITATION, AND MATERNAL/CHILD HEALTH

Water and sanitation are known to be related to maternal, newborn, and child health. The World Health Organization found that almost one tenth of global disease could be prevented by improving water supply, sanitation, hygiene, and management of water resources.

Worldwide 1.4 million children die each year from preventable diarrheal diseases and 88% of these cases are related to unsafe water, inadequate sanitation, or insufficient hygiene. Pregnant women also are particularly vulnerable to anemia and vitamin deficiency. Fifteen percent of all maternal deaths are caused by infections in the first six weeks after childbirth and have been found mainly due to poor sanitation. Approximately 2.6 billion people in the world lack basic sanitation (Cheng, Schuster-Wallace, Newbold, & Mente, 2012).

SEXUALLY TRANSMITTED DISEASES

According to WHO (2014b), more than one million people acquire a sexually transmitted infection (STI) every day and each year; an estimated 500 million people become ill with one of four STIs: chlamydia, gonorrhea, syphilis, and trichomoniasis. More than 530 million people have the virus that causes genital herpes (HSV2), more than 290 million women have a human papillomavirus (HPV) infection, and the majority of STIs are present without symptoms. Some STIs can increase the risk of HIV acquisition threefold or more. STIs can have serious consequences beyond the immediate impact of the infection itself, through mother-to-child transmission of infections and chronic diseases. Drug resistance is a major threat to reducing the impact of STIs worldwide. The highest rates of STDs are found in urban populations among men and women between 15 and 35 years of age. Women generally become infected earlier than men. Of particular concern are adolescents who may have unplanned sexual relations without adequate information about these diseases, their treatment, and their prevention. Sexual intercourse prior to menarche, such as in the cases of child brides, causes even greater vulnerability. Rape and incest victims are especially vulnerable to STDs. Those who are most vulnerable are of childbearing age, live in poverty, abuse drugs, and are uneducated, institutionalized, or living within an unstable social environment. Although most of the 20 or more pathogens transmitted by sexual intercourse can be treated with antibiotics, STDs remain a large problem in developing as well as developed countries (WHO, 2014b).

Table 17-4 gives examples of classic STDs with a worldwide prevalence.

PREVENTION AND TREATMENT CARE

Prevention helps stop the spread of STDs by interrupting the transmission path, reducing the infection duration, and preventing complications. Primary prevention begins with sex education about the diseases and prevention methods related to safe sex behavior, such as abstinence and condom use. Treatment care involves access to healthcare practitioners, making an accurate diagnosis based on laboratory tests, and giving the appropriate medication and education. Lack of treatment can cause mortality and morbidity (WHO, 2014b).

According to WHO (2014c) safe and respectful childbirth is essential to maternal and newborn health. Many women experience abusive treatment during pregnancy and childbirth globally, which not only violates the rights of women to receive respectful care, but also can threaten their lives and health and that of their newborn. Access to safe, acceptable, good quality sexual and reproductive health care, particularly contraceptive access and maternal health care, can dramatically reduce global rates of maternal morbidity and mortality. Over recent decades, facility delivery rates have improved as women are increasingly incentivized to use

TABLE 17-4 Classic Sexually Transmitted Diseases, Bacterial and Viral

Disease (Classification)	Pathogen	Signs and Symptoms
Syphilis (bacterial)	*Treponema pallidum*	Anogenital ulcers, swelling, skin rash
Gonorrhea (bacterial)	*Neisseria gonorrhoea*	Urethral discharge, cervicitis, lower abdominal pain in women, newborn conjunctivitis, may be asymptomatic
Chlamydia (bacterial)	*Chlamydia trachomatis*	Urethral discharge, cervicitis, lower abdominal pain in women, neonatal conjunctivitis, may be asymptomatic
HIV/AIDS (viral)	Human immunodeficiency	Lymph node swelling, fever, weight loss, skin rash, may be asymptomatic
Herpes genitalis (viral)	Herpes simplex virus type 2 (HSV-2)	Anogenital vesicular (genital herpes) lesions and lacerations (HSV-2)
Genital warts (viral)	Human papillomavirus (HPV)	Anogenital warts, cervical warts, cervical cancer
Viral hepatitis (viral) H	Hepatitis B virus (HBV)	Nausea, malaise, fever, enlarged liver, jaundice, liver cancer, cirrhosis

Data from World Health Organization. (2014b). *Sexually transmitted infections*. Retrieved from http://www.who.int/topics/sexually_transmitted_infections/en/

facilities for childbirth. Many women across the globe experience disrespectful, abusive, or neglectful treatment during childbirth in facilities, which is a violation of trust between women and their healthcare providers and can also be a powerful disincentive for women to seek and use maternal healthcare services. While disrespectful and abusive treatment of women may occur throughout pregnancy, during childbirth and the postpartum period women are particularly vulnerable. Such practices may have direct adverse consequences for both the mother and infant.

HIV INFECTION AND REPRODUCTION

HIV-infected pregnant women are at an increased risk of having HIV-positive children, stillbirth, low-birth-weight neonates, and preterm babies. Children of HIV-positive mothers (irrespective of the child's HIV status) also have a higher mortality due to maternal ill health or death. Options for contraception are limited in many developing countries, which increase the risk of transmission of HIV to unborn children (CDC, 2014c).

In such countries as those in Sub-Saharan Africa, the social stigma of not having children may be equal to or greater than the stigma of having the HIV infection itself. Concerns about having an HIV-infected child and the stigma attached to the combination of HIV and pregnancy are also problematic. Artificial insemination is often used as a means of conception without fear of transfer of the disease to the partner or spouse. WHO recommends exclusive breastfeeding for infants from birth to six months. In the general population, exclusive breastfeeding for the first six months of life protects against infant morbidity and mortality from gastrointestinal and respiratory infections. Unfortunately, breastfeeding causes more transmission of the HIV virus from mother to child, and avoidance of breastfeeding by HIV-positive mothers has been recommended in developed countries. In contrast, in developing countries, infants who are breastfed and have the HIV virus are better off with breastfeeding alone than with mixed feedings. Antiretroviral medications have clearly reduced the rates of mother-to-child transmission of the HIV virus. In developing countries, however, children cannot be assured safe, feasible, affordable, and sustained breastmilk substitutes (CDC, 2014c).

FEMALE GENITAL MUTILATION

As provided by WHO (2014c) here are some key facts about the practice of female genital mutilation as it occurs today:

- Female genital mutilation includes procedures that intentionally alter or cause injury to the female genital organs for nonmedical reasons.
- The procedure has no health benefits for girls and women.
- The procedure can cause severe bleeding and problems urinating, and later cysts, infections, and infertility as well as complications in childbirth and increased risk of newborn deaths.
- More than 125 million girls and women alive today have been cut in the 29 countries in Africa and Middle East where the practice is concentrated
- The procedure is mostly carried out on young girls between infancy and 15.
- Female genital mutilation is a violation of the human rights of girls and women.

Female genital mutilation (also called female circumcision) is done to some girls and sometimes young women prior to marriage, as part of cultural practices conducted outside the medical system. This procedure involves the partial or complete removal of the external female genitalia or other injury to female genital organs. The majority of these procedures also include the removal of the clitoris and labia minora. The following list describes the different types of female mutilation:

- *Type I*: Excision of the prepuce, with or without excision of part or the entire clitoris.
- *Type II*: Excision of the clitoris with partial or total excision of the labia minora.
- *Type III*: Excision of part or all of the external genitalia and stitching/narrowing of the opening (infibulation).
- *Type IV*: Pricking, piercing, or incision of the clitoris and/or labia; stretching of the clitoris and labia; cauterization by burning of the clitoris and surrounding tissue; scraping of tissue surrounding the vaginal orifice or cutting of the vaginal cuts; introduction of corrosive substances or herbs into the vagina causing it to bleed, or tightening or narrowing the vaginal cavity.

The most common type of female genital mutilation is excision of the clitoris and the labia minora (80% of all cases); the most extreme form is infibulation (15% of all cases). The health consequences of these procedures vary according to the type and severity of the procedure. Long-term consequences include cysts, abscesses, keloid scars, damage to the urethra causing urinary incontinence, dyspareunia (painful sexual intercourse), sexual dysfunction, and painful childbirth.

In addition, women may suffer anxiety and depression. An estimated 100 to 140 million girls and women have undergone this procedure, and each year two million girls are subjected to it.

The reasons given for these procedures include the following:

- Reduce or eliminate sexual desire in the female.
- Maintain the girl's chastity or virginity before marriage and fidelity during marriage.
- Increase male sexual pleasure.
- Promote female hygiene and external sexual appeal (WHO, 2014c).

MALE REPRODUCTIVE HEALTH

The Alan Guttmacher Institute (2004) addresses global perspectives of male reproductive health needs and issues. Although most men in the world want intimate and sexual relationships and a stable family, their reproductive health needs have historically received little attention. Unplanned pregnancies, infertility, and STDs, including HIV, can all have a major impact on men's lives. The outlook for men who assume a traditional male role can be gloomy due to poverty and lack of job perspectives, which can make many men fatalistic about their futures. Presently, men in Sub-Saharan Africa are projected to have a significant reduction in lifespan, which may also decrease their motivation for adhering to preventive health measures. Fewer than half of these men aged 15 to 24 use any form of contraception, compared to 63 to 93% of their counterparts in developed countries. Urbanization may weaken support systems and also decrease the desire for large numbers of children. Many men are increasing their education, yet job opportunities are often not available, which leaves poor urban men with great frustrations (Alan Guttmacher Institute, 2004).

Men between the ages of 15 and 24 typically become more independent and begin to initiate sexual relationships. In most countries of the world, men have their first sexual encounter by age 20. Few men in their teens marry and/or have children; instead, most marry and become fathers in their late 20s and 30s and begin to settle down during that period of their lives. The more educated a man is, the more likely he will consider and use a method of family planning with his spouse or partner. Fifty percent of men in the world become fathers in their mid- to late 20s. Men in their 40s and 50s usually have had all the children they wish. Male and female sterilization is common in both males and females in developed countries, as well as in China (Alan Guttmacher Institute, 2004).

Reproductive hazards are substances that affect the ability to have healthy children. Males should learn more about specific exposures found to have reproductive effects in men and how they can lower their exposures. Some examples of reproductive hazards provided by the CDC (2014d) include:

- Radiation
- Pesticides
- Various chemicals and solvents
- Legal and illegal drugs
- Cigarettes
- Heat

CONCLUSION

This chapter has provided a worldwide perspective on male and female reproductive health issues, as well as cultural beliefs and practices related to pregnancy, childbirth, postpartum health, and infant health. Disparities in statistics demonstrate much of the perpetual inequality of health status, access to health care, available resources, research data collection, and health reporting worldwide. These health disparities exist not only between developing and developed nations, but also within both developed and developing nations, especially in those countries with populations that are heterogeneous in income, race, ethnicity, and socioeconomic status.

Study Questions

1. Explain the need for prenatal care and its relationship to better birth outcomes.
2. Relate causes of global maternal and infant mortality.
3. What is meant by "reproductive rights"?
4. Explain the relationship of skilled birth attendants, cleanliness at delivery, and better birth outcomes.
5. Give examples of cultural influences and reproductive health for men and women.
6. What are some causes of violence against women and what do you think can be done to decrease it?
7. Discuss the need for global male reproductive health.

Case Study 1: A Safe Motherhood Project in Nigeria

Nigeria has about 2% of the world's population yet accounts for 10% of the world's maternal deaths. The authors suggest that by providing pregnant women with cell phones as part of the Safe Motherhood Project their attendance to health clinics improved and they were thereby provided with necessary health information. This ultimately improved overall health care services to pregnant women and decreased maternal mortality rates in 10 participating health facilities. Pregnancy complications were lower (in the project area as compared to the controlled area without cell phones). The program's success was due to increased utilization of health care facilities for pregnant women with complications.

Case Study 1 Questions

1. How do you think access to cell phones improved attendance at prenatal clinics?
2. Why do you think that access to cell phones decreased maternal mortality rates?

Data from Oyeyemi, S., & Wynn, R. (2014). Giving free cell phones to pregnant women and improving services may increase primary health facility utilization: A case-control study of a Nigerian project. *Reproductive Health, 11*(8), 1–8.

Case Study 2: Obstetrical Fistula Crisis in Niger

An obstetrical fistula crisis in Sub-Saharan Africa in the country of Niger (and other nearby countries as well) is an ongoing struggle for many women. An obstetrical fistula is a structurally abnormal passageway from the vagina to the bladder and/or rectum, as a postpregnancy consequence of bearing a child at a very young age with an inadequately sized pelvis. This condition results from a cultural practice of very early marriage of young girls, ages 9 to 15, to older men to ensure a virgin bride and to financially help the girl's family through the dowry given to her family by the groom. The women involved are young and often malnourished, having incomplete growth of the pelvis at the time of their first pregnancy. This situation may result in a cephalo-pelvic disproportion leading to obstructed labor, and eventually causing maternal and/or infant morbidity or mortality. Frequently the young woman is left without a surviving infant as well as urinary and/or bowel incontinence. Her life without a surviving child, the constant incontinence of urine and feces, and an inability to obtain adequate clean water for personal hygiene often leaves her unable to maintain her hygiene, which in turn leaves her unable to meet the sexual expectations of her marriage. Such a woman may become a social outcast, having tremendous stigma and shame. She has a difficult time surviving in her community without bearing a live child, without keeping clean, and without being unable to have sexual relations with her spouse. If she is unable to produce more children, she may be divorced by her husband. In addition, she typically has difficulty finding and paying for a surgical repair of her fistula. This scenario results in "blaming the victim" because others believe that the cause of her dilemma is one or more of the following:

- Her own bad behavior
- Witchcraft
- Sexually transmitted disease
- Sexual promiscuity

Case Study 2 Questions

1. Explain the relationship between culture and obstetrical fistula.
2. How can education and financial assistance prevent this situation?
3. How can maternal and infant mortality be improved?
4. How does this situation affect the local community?

Data from Naracisi, L., Tieniber, A., Andriani, L., & McKinney, T. (2010). The fistula crisis in sub-Saharan Africa: An ongoing struggle in education and awareness. *Urologic Nursing, 30*(6), 341–346.

References

Ahluwalia, I., Robinson, D., Vallely, L., Gieseker, K., & Kabakama, A. (2010). Maternal health: Interagency youth working group. *Global Health Promotion, 17*(1), 39–49.

Alam, N., & Ashraf, H. (2003). Treatment of infectious diarrhea in children. *Therapy in Practice, 5*(3), 151–165.

Alan Guttmacher Institute. (2004). *In their own right: Addressing the sexual and reproductive health needs of men worldwide.* Retrieved from http://www.guttmacher.org

Alan Guttmacher Institute. (2014). *Reproductive health. Abortions.* Retrieved from http://www.who.int/ reproductivehealth/publications/unsafe_abortion/induced_abortion_2012.pdf?ua=1

Bar-Zeev, S., Barclay, L., Kruske, S., & Kildea, S. (2014). Factors affecting the quality of antenatal care provided to remote dwelling Aboriginal women in northern Australia. *Midwifery, 30*(3), 289–96. Retrieved from http://dx.doi.org/10.1016/j.midw.2013.04.009

Baculinao, E. (January 4, 2016). "China Braces for Baby Boom Under Two Child Rule." NBC News. Retrieved from: http://www.nbcnews.com/news/china/china-braces-baby-boom-under-new-two-child-rule-n489641

Barros, F., Barros, A., Villar, J., Matijasevich, A., Domingues, M., & Victora, C. (2010). *How many low birth weight babies in low- and middle-income countries are preterm?* Retrieved from http://www.scielo.br/pdf/ rsp/2011nahead/2289.pdf

Beamish, J., & Abderrazik. (2003, January). Adolescent and youth reproductive health in Morocco. *Policy Project,* 1–30.

Behboodi-Moghadam, Z., Salsali, M., Eftekhar-Ardabily, H., Vaismoradi, M., & Ramezanzadeh, F. (2013). Experiences of infertility through the lens of Iranian infertile women: A qualitative study. *Japanese Journal of Nursing Science,10*(1), 41–46. doi:10.1111/j.1742-7924.2012.00208.x

Boonstra, H., & Nash, E. (2014). A surge of state abortion restrictions puts providers—and the women they serve—in the crosshairs. *Guttmaker Policy Review, 17*(1). Retrieved from http://www.guttmacher.org/pubs/ gpr/17/1/gpr170109.html

Canadian Medical Association, (2010). Nutrition and integrated health care to highlight Canadian plan to fight child and maternal mortality, minister says. *Canadian Medical Association, 182*(9), E397–E398.

Canudas-Romo, V., Liu, L., Zimmerman, L., Ahmed, S., & Tsui, A. (2014). Potential gains in reproductive-aged life expectancy by eliminating maternal mortality: A demographic bonus of achieving MDG 5. *Plos One, 9*(2), e86694.

Centers for Disease Control and Protection. (2004a). *Healthy people 2010: Maternal, infant, and child health.* Retrieved from http://www.healthypeople.gov/Document/HTML/Volume2/16MICH.htm

Centers for Disease Control and Protection. (2004b). *Teen pregnancy.* Retrieved from http://www.cdc.gov/ teenpregnancy/

Centers for Disease Control and Protection. (2014a). *Infertility and public health.* Retrieved from http://www .cdc.gov/reproductivehealth/Infertility/PublicHealth.htm

Centers for Disease Control and Protection. (2014b). *Intimate partner violence: Data sources.* Retrieved from http://www.cdc.gov/violenceprevention/intimatepartnerviolence/datasources.html

Centers for Disease Control and Protection. (2014c). *HIV among pregnant women, infants, and children.* Retrieved from http://www.cdc.gov/hiv/risk/gender/pregnantwomen/facts/

Centers for Disease Control and Protection. (2014d). *Men's reproductive health in the workplace.* Retrieved from http://www.cdc.gov/niosh/topics/repro/mensWorkplace.html

Cheng, J., Schuster-Wallace, C., Watt, S., Newbold, B., & Mente, A. (2012). An ecological quantification of the relationships between water, sanitation and infant, child, and maternal mortality. *Environmental Health, 11*(4). doi:10.1186/1476-069X-11-4PMCID: PMC3293047

Childbirth by Choice Trust. (1999). *Abortion in law, history and religion.* Retrieved from http://www.cbctrust .com/abortion.html

Darmstadt, G. et al.·(2013). A strategy for reducing maternal and newborn deaths by 2015 and beyond. *BMC Pregnancy and Childbirth, 13*(216). doi:10.1186/1471-2393-13-216. Retrieved from http://www .biomedcentral.com/1471-2393/13/216

Gravett, C. (2012). Serious and life-threatening pregnancy-related infections: Opportunities to reduce the global burden. *PLOS Medicine.* Retrieved from http://www.sm2015.org/wmSfiles/products/sm2015/documents/ website/GRAVETT_PLoS_Medicine_Mater_al_Infections_2012.pdf

Grimes, D., et al. (2006). Unsafe abortion: The preventable pandemic. *Lancet, 368,* 1908–1919.

Gurmankin, A., & Caplan, A. (2004). Embryo disposal practices in IVF clinics in the United States. *Politics and the Life Sciences, 22*(2), 4–8.

Hasna, F. (2003). Islam, social traditions and family planning. *Social Policy and Administrative Issues. 37*(2).181–197.

Hirai, A., Sappenfield, W., Kogan, M., Barfield, W., Goodman, D., Ghandour, R., & Lu, M. (2014). Contributors to excess infant mortality in the U.S. South. *American Journal of Preventative Medicine, 46*(3), 219–227. doi:10.1016/j.amepre.2013.12.006

Infoplease. (2014). *Global abortion rates.* Retrieved from http://www.infoplease.com/science/health/global-abortion-rates.html#ixzz3BnAC3sFd

Johnson, K., Huang, B., & Wang, L. (1998). Infant adoption and abandonment in China. *Population and Development Review, 24*(3), 469–510.

Jones, R., & Boonstra, H. (2004). Confidential reproductive health services for minors: The potential impact of mandated parental involvement for contraception. *Perspectives on Sexual and Reproductive Health, 36*(5), 182–191.

Karlsen, S., Say, L., Souza, J., Hogue, C., Calles, D., Gülmezoglu, A., & Raine, R. (2011). The relationship between maternal education and mortality among women giving birth in health care institutions: Analysis of the cross-sectional WHO Global Survey on Maternal and Perinatal Health. *BMC Public Health, 11,* 606 doi:10.1186/1471-2458-11-606. Retrieved from http://www.biomedcentral.com/1471-2458/11/606

Kochanek, K., & Martin, J. (2005). Supplemental analysis of recent trends in infant mortality. *International Journal of Health Services, 35*(1), 101–115.

Komurembe, G. (2011). *The influence of cultural and gender practices on fertility rates in Ruhaama County, Ntungamo District.* Retrieved from http://hdl.handle.net/10570/2811

Kridli, S. (2002). Health beliefs and practices among Arab women. *Maternal and Child Nursing, 27*(3), 178–182.

Law of the People's Republic of China on maternal and infant care. (1995). *Population and family planning: Law on maternal and infant health care.* Retrieved from http://www.unescap.org/esid/psis/population/database/poplaws/law_china/ch_record006.htm

Lawn, J., Cousens, S., & Zupan, J. (2005). Four million neonatal deaths: When? Where? Why? *Lancet, 365*(9462), 89–900.

Lawn, J., Shibuya, K., & Stein, C. (2005). No cry at birth: Global estimates of intrapartum stillbirths and intrapartum-related neonatal deaths. *Bulletin of the World Health Organization, 83*(6), 409–417.

Levin, D. (2014, February 25). "Many in China can now have a second child, but say no," *New York Times.* Retrieved from http://www.nytimes.com/2014/02/26/world/asia/many-couples-in-china-will-pass-on-a-new-chance-for-a-second-child.html

Lowenberg, S. (2010). The plight of Mexico's indigenous women. *Lancet, 375* (9727), 1680–1682.

Mogilevkina, I., & Odlind, V. (2003). Contraceptive practices and intentions of Ukrainian women. *European Journal of Contraception and Reproductive Health Care, 8,* 185-196.

Murtagh, L., & Moulton, A. (2011). Working mothers, breastfeeding and the law. *American Journal of Public Health, 101*(2), 217–223.

Naracisi, L., Tieniber, A., Andriani, L., & McKinney, T. (2010). The fistula crisis in sub-Saharan Africa: An ongoing struggle in education and awareness. *Urologic Nursing, 30*(6), 341–346.

Oyeyemi, S., & Wynn, R. (2014). Giving free cell phones to pregnant women and improving services may increase primary health facility utilization: a case-control study of a Nigerian project. *Reproductive Health, 11*(8), 1–8.

Pablos-Mendez, A., Valdivieso, V., & Flynn-Saldaña, K. (2013). Ending preventable child and maternal deaths in Latin American and Caribbean countries (LAC). *Perinatologia Y Reproduccion Humana. 27*(3), 145–152.

Partnership for Safe Motherhood and Newborn Health. (2004, May). *An expanded initiative to promote the health and survival of women and newborns in the developing world.* Geneva, Switzerland: Author. Retrieved from http://www.safemotherhood.org

Purnell, L. D. and Paulanka, J. B., & (2005). *Transcultural Health Care: A Culturally Competent Approach.* Philadelphia: F. A. Davis Company.

Schenker, J. (2005). Assisted reproductive practice: Religious perspectives. *Reproductive BioMedicine Online.* Retrieved from http://www.rmonline.com

United Nations. (2004). *World Population Monitoring 2002: Reproductive Rights and Reproductive Health.* New York: Author.

United Nations Family Planning Association. (2011). *Stepping up efforts to save mothers' lives.* Retrieved from http://www.unfpa.org/public/mothers

U.S. Agency for International Development. (2008). *Child survival and maternal health programs.* Retrieved from http://www.usaid.gov/our_work/global_health/mch/publications/docs/mch08_overview.pdf

Vanderkruik, R., Tuncalp, O., Chou, D., & Say, L. (2013). Framing maternal morbidity: WHO scoping exercise. *BMC. Pregnancy and Childbirth. 13.* 213. . doi:10.1186/1471-2393-13-213

Vogel, J., Lee, A., & Souza, J. (2014). Maternal morbidity and preterm birth in 22 low- and middle-income countries: A secondary analysis of the WHO Global Survey dataset BMC Pregnancy and Childbirth, *14*(56). doi:10.1186/1471-2393-14-56. Retrieved from http://www.biomedcentral.com/1471-2393/14/56

World Health Organization. (2010a). *Packages of interventions for family planning, safe abortion care, maternal, newborn and child health.* Retrieved from http://www.who.int/maternal_child_adolescent/documents/fch_10_06/en/index.html

World Health Organization. (2010b). *Infertility.* Retrieved from http://www.who.int/reproductivehealth/publications/infertility/en/

World Health Organization. (2014a). *Adolescent pregnancy.* Retrieved from http://www.who.int/mediacentre/factsheets/fs364/en/

World Health Organization. (2014b). *Sexually transmitted infections.* Retrieved from http://www.who.int/topics/sexually_transmitted_infections/en/

World Health Organization. (2014c). *Female genital mutilation.* Retrieved from http://www.who.int/mediacentre/factsheets/fs241/en/

Zureick-Brown, S. et al. (2013). Understanding global trends in maternal mortality. *International Perspectives on Sexual and Reproductive Health*, *39*(1). Retrieved from https://www.guttmacher.org/pubs/journals/3903213.html

Zwillich, T. (2005). U.S. pharmacies vow to withhold emergency contraception. *Lancet, 365,* 1677–1688.

18

Global Health of Children

Kathie Aduddell

Objectives

After completing this chapter, the reader will be able to:

1. Define the most commonly used measures of children's health.
2. Describe the overall causes of death and illness in children in the world.
3. Examine specific strategies and interventions that may improve the global health of children.

INTRODUCTION

This chapter describes children's health in our world today as well as the strategies to alleviate specific health concerns for children. Included in the discussion is a historical perspective of how organizations such as the United Nations (UN) and the World Health Organization (WHO) began to call attention to children's health. In addition, the chapter provides current measurements of health and the leading causes of death in children. The final part of the chapter reviews the documented approaches and international strategies to alleviate these health concerns for children and addresses future challenges.

By 2050, there will be 2.6 billion children younger than 18 years of age in the world (UNICEF, 2014a). Currently, children and adolescents account for approximately 35% of the world's population (Population Reference Bureau, 2014). Although the world made a promise in 2000 to reduce the child mortality rate by two-thirds by 2015, this target will not be reached until 2026, even with the recent advances in improving child survival (UNICEF, 2014a). Nearly 5.9 million children under the age of five die each year, which translates to 16 children each day, or 11 children every minute (UNICEF, 2015; WHO, 2015d).

Children continue to bear an undue share of global disease as well as suffer disproportionately from the conditions that lead to disease and death. Because children are often the most vulnerable members of society, their health serves as a marker for the well-being of a society and its future potential. Children require not only the basic survival needs of food, water, adequate shelter, and appropriate hygienic requirements, but also basic social interactions, healthy play, and safe, supportive environments that allow for optimal growth and development. Foundations of health as well as healthy habits are established during childhood. These health habits, or lack thereof, then become part of an adult's methods to survive and flourish, leading to a healthy society and world.

BACKGROUND AND HISTORICAL PERSPECTIVE

According to Kotch (2013), understanding the health of the world's children is closely linked to the world's political history, the wars that occurred in our world, and economic conditions. For example, a focus on understanding diseases new to Europeans and the growth in world trade led to concerns about sanitation, hygiene, and disease outbreaks. In 1913, the Rockefeller Foundation established the International Health Commission, which focused on the control or elimination of specific diseases that affected trade and the productivity of workers. Other international agencies began and took the lead in providing programs and policy guidance in the area of global health. The United Nations was created after World War II as a vehicle for peace and conflict resolution among nations; specialized agencies of the UN were developed to focus on promotion and protection of health (Kotch, 2013; United Nations, 2011). Two such agencies that continue to have a major impact on children's health are the United Nations International Children's Emergency Fund (UNICEF), which was developed to assist the thousands of orphans and abandoned children that resulted from the war, and the World Health Organization, which began in 1948 as an intergovernmental institution to promote and protect global health.

Over the years WHO has called attention to the plight of children through such efforts as the World Summit of Children held in 1990, revision of the International Health Regulations in 2005, and *The World Health Report 2005: Make Every Mother and Child Count* (WHO, 2003). Although there have also been periods of stagnation or even reversal of trends since the World Summit, major gains have been achieved in reducing child mortality. For example, between 1970 and 1990, the under-five mortality rate dropped by 20% every decade, but between 1990 and 2000 it declined by only 12% (WHO, 2005). More recent reports such as *Child Survival: Call to Action* in 2012 and *Acting on the Call* in 2014 demonstrate the world is responding to ensuring the survival of our children (UNICEF, 2014a). Currently, the under-five mortality rate has declined faster than at any other time (UNICEF, 2014b). Ever-increasing globalization is associated with profound health implications, such as increased disease transfer and mobility risks, increased exchange of goods and information between countries in response to health problems, and changing roles of national governments and international organizations in the health field (Kotch, 2013; WHO, 2011a). As a result of the globalization trend and its profound implications for the health of the world, the UN unanimously adopted the *Millennium Declaration* in 2000. The Millennium Declaration Goals (MDGs) targeted issues, concerns, and problems

TABLE 18-1   United Nations Millennium Health Goals

Goal	Target Deadline
MDG 4: Reduce child mortality	By 2015, reduce the mortality rate by two-thirds among children
MDG 5: Improve maternal health	By 2015, reduce the ratio of women dying in childbirth by three-fourths
MDG 6: Combat HIV/AIDS, malaria, and other diseases	By 2015, halt and begin to reverse the spread of HIV/AIDS and lower incidences of malaria and other major diseases

Data from United Nations. (2004). *Millennium development goals.* Retrieved from http://www.un.org/millenniumgoals/poverty.shtml

related to the health and development of the world's population (United Nations, 2000, 2004, 2011). Three specific target objectives, displayed in Table 18-1, relate to the health of children (United Nations, 2004, 2011).

Other documents relevant to children's health have followed in the wake of the *Millennium Declaration*, such as the report from the UN's Special Session for Children (published in 2002), which recognized the growing need for a new social agenda for children and their families, and the report from the 2005 World Summit, which began to focus on the issue of inequity in our world (United Nations, 2002, 2011). In 2003, WHO's *Strategic Directions for Improving the Health and Development of Children and Adolescents* summarized seven priority areas for action and defined specific principles to guide their implementation. More recently, the Global Strategy for Women's and Children's Health established key areas where action is urgently required (WHO, 2010), and WHO's Six-Point Agenda outlined six strategies to respond to the increasingly complex and often blurred boundaries of public health (WHO, 2011b) The purpose of these documents, summits, and initiatives was to emphasize the importance of investing in children's and adolescents' health and development as a cost-effective strategy to secure future prosperity for countries and nations. Newer documents, such as WHO's *Health in 2015: From MDGs, Millennium Development Goals, to SDGs, Sustainable Development Goals* and UNICEF's *State of Children 2015: Reimagine the Future, Innovation for Every Child,* move toward a more integrated approach to seize opportunities to collaborate and exploit synergies in an effort to continue to improve the health of children in the world (UNICEF, 2014c; WHO, 2015d).

CHILDHOOD MORTALITY STATISTICS: MEASURING HEALTH IN CHILDREN

In general, an acceptable measure of the health of children is the mortality rate. Some authors have identified it as the ultimate indicator of poor child health outcomes as well as an indicator of the implementation of child survival interventions, and, more broadly, of social and economic development (You, Jones, & Wardlaw, 2011; You, Wardlaw, Salama, & Jones, 2009). The mortality rate is calculated as the number of deaths occurring in an age range divided by the number of children entering that particular age range in a given period of time. Because it captures the entire high-risk period in high-mortality settings, the under-five mortality rate is the most widely used and critical indicator to summarize child health from an international perspective (UNICEF, 2014c; WHO, 2015). This information is obtained through samples from vital registration systems in some countries; in others, it is gleaned from population-based surveys such as the Demographic and Health Survey (DHS) from the U.S. Agency for International Development and UNICEF's Multiple Indicator Cluster Surveys (UNICEF, 2014c; You, Jones, & Wardlaw, 2011).

Globally, child mortality declined by 53% from 1990 to 2015, though this decline remains insufficient to reach MDG 4 (Population Reference Bureau, 2014; UNICEF, 2015; WHO, 2015). Spectacular reductions in childhood mortality were achieved during the 1980s, reducing childhood mortality by one-third on a worldwide basis. The 1990 World Summit for Children set a goal of reducing childhood mortality by an additional one-third by the year 2000 (Global Health Council, 2006). Although the decline in the overall child mortality rate represents considerable progress, this progress is uneven across the regions of the world with substantial inequalities (WHO, 2015). Sub-Saharan Africa and southern Asia together account for four out of five under-five deaths globally (UNICEF, 2014a).

WHAT ARE THE HEALTH PROBLEMS FOR CHILDREN?

Globally, the major causes of death in children younger than five are pneumonia, diarrheal diseases, injuries, and malaria (UNICEF, 2014b; WHO, 2015d). Neonatal deaths still account for approximately 40% of all under-five deaths and document the vulnerability of the first 28 days of life (UNICEF, 2014b). Preterm birth complications, birth asphyxia, sepsis, and pneumonia cause the neonatal deaths (Black et al., 2010; WHO, 2015d; You, Jones, & Wardlaw, 2011). Other major causes leading to death in children include undernutrition/malnutrition, measles, and HIV/AIDS ((WHO, 2015; You, Jones, & Wardlaw, 2011). Specific diseases, however, cause more deaths in some regions—for example, malaria is the most significant cause of death in Sub-Saharan Africa, and AIDS is the leading cause of death for children in east and southern Africa. As the mortality rate for children declines in specific regions, the major causes of death tend to shift from diarrhea, pneumonia, and vaccine-preventable diseases such as measles to neonatal causes such as birth asphyxia and low birth weight (Black et al., 2010; Kotch, 2013). Generally, in regions with low child mortality rates, the leading cause of death comprises neonatal conditions such as congenital anomalies and injuries (Table 18-2).

Neonatal Deaths

The majority of newborn deaths in the world occur around the time of birth, typically within the first 24 hours after childbirth and are preventable (WHO, 2015c). The leading causes of death for these nearly 2.7 million neonates include severe infection, birth asphyxia, complications of prematurity and low birth weight, and congenital conditions (Global Health Council, 2015; You, Jones, & Wardlaw, 2010). The majority of these deaths occur in low resource settings without skilled birth attendants present and are linked to poor quality care (Global Health Council, 2015). According to the Global Health Council (2015), most of neonatal deaths occur in just four countries: India, China, Pakistan, and Nigeria. WHO indicates that malnutrition or undernutrition is the single largest contributor to premature death in children. When infants

TABLE 18-2   Causes of Child Mortality and Number of Deaths, 2008

Cause of Death	Share of All Child Mortality (%)	Number of Deaths (in millions)
Neonatal causes	41	3.575
Pneumonia	14	1.189
Diarrhea	14	1.257
Malaria	8	0.732
Other infections	9	0.753
Other noncommunicable diseases	4	0.228
Injury	3	0.279
AIDS	2	0.201
Pertussis	2	0.195
Meningitis	2	0.164
Measles	1	0.118
Congenital abnormalities	1	0.104

Reprinted from World Health Organization (WHO). (2015d). Health in 2015: from MDGs, Millennium Development Goals, to SDGs, Sustainable Development Goals. Retrieved from http://www.who.int/gho/publications/mdgs-sdgs/MDGs-SDGs2015_chapter4.pdf?ua=1, Chapter 4, p. 72, Copyright 2015.

are born weighing less than 2,500 grams (5.5 pounds), they are at a greater risk of death and disease than infants at normal and above-normal birth weights. Many times malnutrition results from the mother having poor nutrition and being deficient of essential minerals and vitamins such as vitamin A or zinc, which in turn increases the risk of her child dying from diarrhea, pneumonia, measles, or malaria (Global Health Council, 2006, 2011; Kotch, 2013; WHO, 2015c). In addition, children born to unhealthy mothers are at risk for being underweight, which can lead to difficulty combating illness.

Pneumonia

Acute respiratory infections, primarily pneumonia, killed approximately 1.6 million children in 2008 (Black et al., 2010; Global Health Council, 2011). Many of the deaths from pneumonia were the result of the child already being weakened by malnutrition or other diseases. Pneumonia is the leading cause of death for children younger than the age of five, with 95% of the infections in this age group occurring in developing countries (UNICEF, 2008, 2009). The development of such disease is also associated with indoor pollution resulting from the use of certain types of fuel combined with poor ventilation (Global Health Council, 2006). Pneumonia, although serious, can be effectively treated with the appropriate health care and availability of antibiotics, especially given that most fatal childhood pneumonia is of bacterial origin

(Global Health Council, 2006). The two main pathogens that cause pneumonia in children are *Streptococcus pneumoniae* and *Haemophilus influenzae* type b (Hib) (Global Health Council, 2011). Vaccines have been developed for both of these conditions, so prevention is possible. This fact raises serious questions about the availability of health resources in developing countries or nations—a dilemma that often acts to thwart the effectiveness of even important prevention tools.

Diarrheal Disease

Diarrheal diseases such as cholera, shigellosis, rotavirus, typhoid, dysentery, and other diarrheal diseases kill nearly 2 million children each year (Black et al., 2010; Global Health Council, 2011; WHO, 2009). Because children are more vulnerable to dehydration and electrolyte imbalances, diarrheal conditions may lead to death in children more quickly than in adults. Death can occur even more easily in children with preexisting vitamin deficiencies or nondiarrheal infections. When children are subject to poor sanitation conditions, such as unsafe drinking water or lack of proper food storage, food-borne and water-borne diarrheal infections can develop more easily, making prevention extremely difficult.

Death from diarrheal diseases is mostly preventable and can be avoided with the use of inexpensive oral rehydration solutions while the child has diarrhea. WHO and UNICEF have advocated zinc supplement tablets during diarrhea episodes to help prevent recurrences. Diarrhea can also be prevented through better nutritional practices in early childhood, particularly exclusive breastfeeding until the age of six months and the appropriate introduction of complementary foods during the weaning period (Global Health Council, 2006). Just through these two practices, child mortality can be reduced by 20%. Other interventions outside the health sector, such as the provision of safe drinking water and clean sanitation facilities, also play a major role in stopping needless diarrhea-related deaths in children. Children living in poor countries get diarrhea, on average, four times per year, with each episode being life-threatening (WHO, 2009).

Malaria and Measles

Approximately 732,000 children die each year from malaria, with 85% of these deaths occurring in children younger than age five (Black et al., 2010; WHO, 2008b). Malaria is the leading cause of hospitalization, mortality, and morbidity in children living in areas such as Sub-Saharan Africa. This illness can be prevented by using insecticide-treated bed netting and spraying with insecticides to decrease the infestation of mosquitoes. According to the Global Health Council (2006, 2011), both this intervention and the successful treatment of malaria with artemisinin derivatives are relatively affordable interventions. Unfortunately, resistance to these efforts has presented some barriers in eradicating this deadly disease.

Deaths from measles among children under five years of age fell from 482,000 in 2000 to 86,000 in 2012 due to improved immunization coverage (UNICEF, 2013). For example, in southern Africa, measles was almost eliminated as a cause of child death through an active vaccination campaign that cost only $1.10 per child (Levine & Kinder, 2004). Unfortunately, 95%

of deaths from measles, including complications from measles such as pneumonia and diarrhea, still occur in low-income or developing countries (Global Health Council, 2015).

HIV/AIDS

More than 2.1 million children younger than 15 are currently infected with the human immunodeficiency virus (HIV), and more than 200,000 children become infected with HIV each year (UNICEF, 2008). More than 95% of all HIV-infected infants acquired their infection before birth (in utero), during delivery, or through breastmilk, and approximately one-third of these infants die within one year of infection (Global Health Council, 2011). In 2008, the children younger than age five who died from AIDS-related causes resided primarily in Sub-Saharan Africa (Global Health Council, 2011; You, Wardlaw, Salama, & Jones, 2009). In addition, more than 12.1 million children, most living in Sub-Saharan Africa, have lost one or both parents to AIDS (Global Health Council, 2011). Other regions identified as having the potential for an emerging epidemics of HIV and its more serious sequela, acquired immunodeficiency syndrome (AIDS), include the Caribbean, China, India, central Asia, and Eastern Europe (Kotch, 2013).

Antiretroviral drugs (ARVs) can make a difference in saving children by substantially reducing the risk of transmitting HIV from a mother to her child. A single dose of an ARV can cut the risk of mother-to-child transmission of HIV by 50% (Global Health Council, 2011). Worldwide efforts to expand access to treatment for children with HIV have reached new milestones through various initiatives undertaken by the UN, WHO, and the U.S. President's Emergency Plan for AIDS Relief (Kotch, 2013; WHO, 2010). Most of these initiatives focus on four main strategies: primary prevention of HIV in young women; avoidance of unintended pregnancies among HIV-infected women; provision of ARVs targeted at preventing HIV transmission from HIV-infected women to their infants, safe delivery, counseling, and support for safer infant feeding practices; and provision of care and support for mothers and their families.

The treatment of children with AIDS has encountered barriers because of the lack of availability and accessibility of pediatric formulations of ARVs. The costs of these drugs are slightly higher for children than for adults, and the administration is more complicated to regulate in pediatric patients because children must have their medications adjusted as they grow (Dawson, 2006; Global Health Council, 2006). Thus, fewer children with HIV/AIDS in areas such as Sub-Saharan Africa get antiretroviral therapy because it is easier and cheaper to give the medicines to adults (Dawson, 2006). Another concern is the heavy emphasis on one single disease within severely resource-limited areas of the world, which could draw resources away from other health issues and concerns (Claeson, Gillespie, Mshinda, Troedsson, & Victora, 2003; Walker, Schwartlander, & Bryce, 2002).

Injuries

Approximately 3% of child deaths per year are due to injuries (Black et al., 2010; Global Health Council, 2011). Around the world, children are killed or hospitalized each year because of injuries caused by traffic accidents, fires, drownings, falls, and poisonings. Globally, the three major injury-related causes of death in children younger than five are drowning, road traffic accidents, and fire-related burns (UNICEF, 2008; WHO, 2008c). Most of these injuries and deaths can be prevented but occur in low- and middle-income countries and are more often associated with environmental conditions and outbreaks of armed conflict (Global Health Council, 2011). Over a 10-year period from 1999 to 2000, more than 20 million children were displaced by disasters (Torjesen & Olness, 2004). WHO attributes more than 1 million deaths of children and adolescents to injuries and violence. Injuries are also among the leading causes of mortality and lifelong disability for those who survive in higher-income countries.

Proven prevention measures have been developed that can result in major changes in injury risks for children. Some of these measures include laws on child-appropriate seat belts and helmets; hot tap-water temperature regulations; child-resistant closures on medicine bottles, lighters, and household product containers; draining of unnecessary water from baths and buckets; redesigning of nursery furniture, toys, and playground equipment; and strengthening of emergency medical care and rehabilitation services (WHO, 2008c).

Other Causes of Death in Children

Approximately 10% of all deaths of children younger than five years of age are due to other causes such as infectious diseases (other than those mentioned previously), childhood cluster diseases such as pertussis and tetanus, and other nutritional deficiencies (Global Health Council, 2006). Additional factors may lead to disease, disability, or chronic poor health. For example, malnutrition among pregnant women may lead to stunted growth and impaired learning in children. In 2015, one in four children were impacted by stunting and one in seven were underweight (WHO, 2015d). Good nutrition is the foundation for healthy development and prevention of illness. Children in developing countries who are not breastfed are six times more likely to die by the age of one month than are children who receive at least some breastmilk. Children are also particularly vulnerable from the age of six months onward, when breastfeeding is no longer sufficient to meet all nutritional requirements (WHO, 2003). In addition, many children around the world face the prospect of losing one or both parents to death from AIDS, which leads to more homeless children and children in poverty—a condition that has many health problems associated with it. Globalization has created an abundance of opportunities for many, yet resulted in a deepening of socioeconomic disparities in some regions of the world.

LARGER RAMIFICATIONS OF CHILDREN'S HEALTH PROBLEMS

The major determinants of childhood mortality can be traced to specific global issues such as poverty, lack of essential public health resources including safe water and proper sanitation, absence of prenatal care, inadequate diet, exposure to insect vectors of disease, and lack of basic health and preventive services (Global Health Council, 2006, 2011; Kotch, 2013). There is an equitable distribution of child deaths with the majority in low- and middle-income countries (WHO, 2015). These conditions and situations put children at a higher risk of death from numerous other conditions and diseases. More than 1.2 billion people still live on less than

$1.25 a day with disproportionately large numbers living in southern Asia and Sub-Saharan Africa (Population Reference Bureau, 2014). As another example, 39% of rural households in Niger have access to improved drinking water compared to 100% of urban households (WHO, 2014). These conditions also have larger ramifications, leading to unrealized human potential and negative effects on individuals, families, communities, and countries in terms of productivity, economics, and politics (Torjesen & Olness, 2004; WHO, 2008a, 2011a).

Impaired Learning and Other Disabilities

The effects of poor nutrition continue throughout a child's life by contributing to poor school performance, reduced productivity, and other measures of impaired intellectual and social development (Global Health Council, 2011; WHO, 2003). Children with undernutrition or malnutrition may drop out of school and have difficulty finding employment if they lack access to special education and training. Children who survive birth asphyxia may develop problems such as learning difficulties, cerebral palsy, and other disabilities (Global Health Council, 2011; WHO, 2005). Disabilities affect 1 in 10 children in developing countries, with the major causes of these disabilities being premature birth, malnutrition, infections, injuries, child neglect, and understimulation—all of which are preventable (WHO, 2003). These conditions can be prevented through early identification, early intervention, and rehabilitation for children who are either at risk of developing disabilities or already have them.

Disasters and Child Trafficking

Between 1999 and 2000, more than 20 million malnourished children were displaced by disasters (Torjesen & Olness, 2004). It is also vital to pay special attention to the rising numbers of orphans who have lost parents due to HIV infection, disasters, or violence. In 2000, more than 10 million children younger than 15 years had lost one or both parents to AIDS (Torjesen & Olness, 2004). Whether it is natural events such as the 2005 and 2010 tsunamis, industrial accidents such as the 1984 chemical disasters in Bhopal, or the world's many wars, including the ongoing Middle East conflict, children are greatly affected. Many of the children orphaned by these events live on the streets or are lost to institutionalization. Even if they have not lost their parents and other family members, they are still at risk for infectious diseases, malnutrition, and psychological trauma with the potential for lifelong damages. Children displaced from wars in Southeast Asia, central Africa, and Bosnia, for example, have shown a high prevalence of mental health problems that persist for years after resettlement (Torjesen & Olness, 2004).

Other problematic issues, such as trafficking, smuggling, physical and sexual exploitation, and economic exploitation, are realities for children in all regions of the world (WHO, 2003). It is estimated that more than 1 million children fall victim annually to child trafficking (Global Health Council, 2011; UNICEF, 2003). This problem occurs when children are exploited in agricultural and domestic service, as has been documented in Sub-Saharan Africa, or forced into prostitution, as seen in Southeast Asia, the Republic of Moldova, Romania, and Ukraine. In addition, WHO (2003) estimates that 300,000 children in Africa have been coerced into military service as soldiers, porters, messengers, and other positions.

Health Issues Later in Life

Many of these health conditions and issues become lifelong problems for children. For example, children may survive injuries but live with a long-term disability. Victims of interpersonal violence, such as children who were subjected to sexual abuse, are twice as likely to become depressed and four times as likely to attempt suicide (WHO, 2003). Child undernutrition is associated with shorter adult height, lower levels of academic achievement, reduced adult income, and low birth weight of their progeny (Victora et al., 2008). Once affected, a child's health and development are permanently altered.

Adolescents

Unfortunately, adolescents are often thought to be healthy simply because they survived any early childhood health issues. Until recently this premise has led to a lack of attention to adolescents' health and social needs. Although the adolescent birth rate has declined over the years, the declines were greater in the middle- and high-income countries; the vast majority of youths therefore continue to live in developing countries (UNICEF, 2011; WHO, 2015d). Deaths of adolescents are generally caused by injuries from unintentional causes, suicide, violence, pregnancy-related complications, and illnesses—all conditions that can be treated and prevented (UNICEF, 2011; WHO, 2015d).

This age group also has some unique health problems. For example, the highest rates of new sexually transmitted infections occur in youth 15 to 24 years of age. Adolescents are also vulnerable to the use of psychoactive substances such as amphetamines, opioids, and cocaine. Undernutrition and micronutrient deficiencies in girls in this age cohort may lead to adverse pregnancy outcomes. Finally, unhealthy diets and lack of physical activity in adolescents are leading to unprecedented increases in obesity and risk for chronic diseases such as diabetes, hypertension, and cardiovascular disease (UNICEF, 2011; WHO, 2003). The choices and habits established during this period of life will greatly influence the future health status of these up-and-coming adults.

Mental Health

Approximately 10 to 20% of children have one or more mental or behavioral problems (WHO, 2003). Mental health problems account for a large proportion of the disease burden among young people (UNICEF, 2011). Depression is the major contributor to mental illness in this group and often leads to suicide, which represents one of the leading causes of mortality among people aged 15 to 35 (UNICEF, 2011; WHO, 2015d). More than 70,000 adolescents commit suicide each year (UNICEF, 2011), and 10 to 20% of adolescents will experience a mental health problem such as depression or anxiety (WHO, 2015d).

Conflict, poverty, forced migration, and nutritional deficiencies may all affect the intellectual and social development of children. These factors present challenges and barriers that have consequences for the affected children's well-being and productivity as it relates to mental health.

Marginalized and Vulnerable Groups

Overt or implicit discrimination results in marginalized groups of children and adolescents, which, in turn, leads to vulnerability (WHO, 2003). Examples of these vulnerable groups include children who are permanently disabled or seriously injured by armed conflict, children displaced as refugees, street children, children suffering from natural and human-made disasters, children of migrant workers and other socially disadvantaged groups, and children who are victims of racial discrimination, xenophobia, and intolerance. Other disadvantaged groups include the orphans of the world and children who have been exploited economically, sexually, or physically. Even children who live in rural areas are approximately 1.7 times as likely to die as those who live in urban areas; children from the poorest areas of the world are twice as likely to die compared to those from wealthier areas (You, Jones, & Wardlaw, 2011).

One example of this marginalization involves refugees from ongoing military conflict, such as that taking place in Sudan. *The Nation's Health* report (2004) provides some staggering statistics and facts about the more than 1 million people who were refugees from the military conflict in Sudan. Malnutrition rates were up to 39% among these individuals, with 58% of children aged six months to five years having diarrhea and measles outbreaks. As many as 200 children died every month from violent acts, starvation, and disease. Many of these children worked the streets and would eventually return home—but not to a protective, nurturing family. In every country, children who live or spend most of their lives on the street are at greater risk for malnutrition, HIV infection, drug abuse, and violence (UNICEF, 2003).

STRATEGIES TO IMPROVE CHILD HEALTH AROUND THE WORLD

Widespread introduction of simple, inexpensive, "low-tech" interventions, successfully targeting major killers of children, can allow for a majority of the children in this world to survive and thrive. Two-thirds of children's deaths can be successfully averted by existing preventive and therapeutic strategies (Global Health Council, 2006; WHO, 2008c). Many of these proven prevention and treatment interventions used to improve child survival—such as exclusive breast-feeding; immunizations; micronutrient supplementation (particularly vitamin A and zinc); complementary feeding; antibiotics for pneumonia, dysentery, and sepsis; oral rehydration therapy for diarrhea; antimalarial drugs; and insecticide-treated bed netting—can be implemented even in resource-poor environments (Global Health Council, 2011; Kotch, 2013; Lopez, Mathers, Ezzati, Jamison, & Murray, 2006; WHO, 2011a). With only four years left to achieve the Millennium Development Goals, particularly MDG 4, the world and the various agencies and organizations concerned with global child health have much to do in a short time frame.

The WHO Expanded Program on Immunizations as well as the Diarrheal Disease Control Program are examples of effective programs with measurable impacts on child health (Bryce et al., 2003; Claeson, Gillespie, Mshinda, Troedsson, & Victora, 2003; WHO, 2011a). Launched in 1974, these programs focused on immunizing children against six major infectious diseases (diphtheria, pertussis, tetanus, tuberculosis, polio, and measles) before their first birthday. Great success was documented in various countries, but specific regions still lagged behind (Bryce et al., 2003; WHO, 2011a).

Broader approaches, such as the WHO Integrated Management of Childhood Illnesses (IMCI), were launched in the 1990s to improve case management skills of health staff, make improvements in the health systems to support effective management skills, and enhance family and community practices (Kotch, 2013). The IMCI was a positive step toward providing higher-quality, comprehensive care for children in developing countries. It used healthcare algorithms written at or slightly above the level of a village healthcare worker and targeted children younger than five years—the age group with the highest death rate from common childhood diseases (Torjesen & Olness, 2004). Complex analyses indicate that mortality from diarrheal diseases fell from 2.4 million deaths in 1990 to about 1.6 million deaths in 2001 as a result of efforts in diarrhea case management, including the use of oral rehydration therapy (Lopez, Mathers, Ezzati, Jamison, & Murray, 2006).

WHO (2003) called for addressing priority areas of action in its report entitled *Strategic Directions for Improving the Health and Development of Children and Adolescents.* These priority areas, as identified in Table 18-3, require focused attention because they affect the physical well-being as well as the psychosocial development of children and adolescents. In addition, the report includes three specific guiding principles to be used in implementing the strategic actions:

- Address inequities and facilitate the respect, protection, and fulfillment of human rights as outlined in the Convention on the Rights of the Child.
- Take a life-course approach that recognizes the continuum from birth through childhood, adolescence, and adulthood.
- Implement a public health approach by focusing on major health issues and applying a systematic development model to ensure the availability and accessibility of effective, relevant interventions.

In 2009, WHO, through the Partnership for Maternal, Newborn, and Child Health Strategy and Workplan, identified the need to build consensus and promote evidence-based, high-impact interventions with a focus on knowledge management systems and a core package of interventions and essential commodities, to strengthen human resources and advocacy for these populations, and to track progress and commitment toward the MDGs that affect these populations (WHO, 2009).

More recently, WHO's Six-Point Agenda has emphasized six strategies to continue a forward direction in achieving the MDGs:

- Promoting health development by focusing on equity
- Fostering health security through strengthened international health regulations
- Strengthening the world's health systems so services reach all populations, especially poor and underserved populations
- Harnessing research, information, and evidence to set priorities, define strategies, and measure results
- Enhancing partnerships with UN agencies and other international organizations, donors, civil society, and private sector to achieve results
- Improving performance by concentrating on efficiency and effectiveness (WHO, 2011b)

TABLE 18-3   Priority Areas for Actions Identified by WHO

Priority Area	Specified Action
Maternal and newborn health	Reduce neonatal mortality, provide skilled birth attendants with adequate facility support, promote prenatal care, and tackle the mother-to-child transmission challenge
Nutrition	Provide adequate nutrition to mothers and their children, promote breastfeeding, and implement the Global Strategy for Infant and Young Child Feeding
Communicable diseases	Avert more than 50% of childhood deaths by preventing communicable disease—specifically, pneumonia, diarrhea, malaria, measles, and HIV infection. Also prevent other diseases that pose a greater risk to children than to adults, such as syphilis, tuberculosis, meningitis, dengue, Japanese encephalitis, leishmaniasis, and trypanosomiasis. Move beyond addressing single diseases and toward integrated approaches for prevention and management of common diseases
Injury and violence	Draw attention to the prevention of injury and violence, which lead to death or lifelong disability in more than 1 million children and adolescents. Modify environments, change designs or structures, apply and reinforce regulatory measures, provide parent training and social support to families, and change unsafe behaviors through education. For the greatest success, combine the three strategies of regulatory measures, environmental changes, and education.
Physical environment	Use interventions to improve water supplies, sanitation, and hygiene, which can reduce child mortality by 65%. Also implement other interventions to improve indoor air pollution, prevent injuries, and minimize other environmental risk factors. Focus on WHO's six priority issues—household water security, hygiene and sanitation, air pollution, disease vectors, chemical hazards, and injuries and accidents
Adolescent health	Focus attention on support for mental, sexual, and reproductive health; the rights of adolescents to information, skills, services, and protection from exploitative relationships; and support to develop responsible behavior
Psychosocial development and mental health	Examine the long-term consequences for well-being to prevent these concerns. Implement early interventions in areas of feeding, play, and communication as appropriate

Data from World Health Organization (WHO). (2003). *Strategic directions for improving the health and development of children and adolescents*. Geneva, Switzerland: Author. Retrieved from http://www.who.int/maternal_child_adolescent/documents/9241591064/en/

By focusing on disease-specific interventions and broad community-based programs, marked advances in child survival and development have been achieved. When cost-effective interventions that aid the largest possible number of people are used, fewer children die. It is also understood that children who have educated mothers have a better survival and health outcome than children with noneducated mothers (You, Jones, & Wardlaw, 2011).

The obstacles to implementing general health strategies are similar to the obstacles associated with implementing child-survival strategies. They include high staff turnover, poor management and supervision, and inadequate funding, all of which continue to cause problems over and above

TABLE 18-4 Obstacles to Implementing Child Survival Strategies
• The highest rates of under-five mortality occur in a limited number of the poorest countries.
• Many of these countries have been involved in war or civil conflict.
• The government is unwilling to or incapable of providing health services effectively.
• The poor are marginalized and most difficult to reach.

the difficulty of acquiring adequate services in specific areas and regions (Kotch, 2013). The loss of children due to avoidable or treatable conditions is unnecessary, and the drastic decline in childhood mortality rates confirms that interventions can be successful, especially if the global health community, political leaders, governments, foundations, and private citizens make commitments to providing needed resources (Global Health Council, 2006; UNICEF, 2011). In 2006, four major obstacles were identified by the Global Health Council; these obstacles, which are shown in Table 18-4, remain challenges today. Although the current response to the needless deaths of children and the implementation of strategies to prevent these deaths are sometimes fragmented and uncoordinated, the Global Health Council has proposed four major actions to address the salient issues: effective leadership, strengthened health systems, evidence-based health delivery system guidelines, and evaluation systems to monitor progress toward improved survival.

Another important focus for eliminating health problems and issues for children and adolescents is to establish a developmental approach. WHO (2003) has outlined five developmental phases, accompanied by possible health outcomes and examples of interventions. Implementing this approach within a public health strategy that already targets the aforementioned obstacles could achieve the highest possible levels of health and well-being. For example, a study in Uttar Pradesh, India, demonstrated a 50% decline in neonatal mortality through raising awareness in the community with such simple survival strategies as cleaning, drying, and warming the newborn; skin-to-skin contact with the mother; and exclusive breastfeeding for the first six months of the infant's life (Darmstadt et al., 2005).

Some key strategies to consider include empowering women in developing countries, removing financial and social barriers to accessing basic services, increasing local health systems' accountability, and developing innovative approaches to deliver critical services in specific areas of the world (You, Jones, & Wardlaw, 2011).

FUTURE CHALLENGES

How can professional healthcare providers help children around the world? Which types of skills and systems are still needed by these individuals and institutions? Millions of children die each year from preventable causes. If they had appropriate and timely access to basic and inexpensive health prevention and therapeutic inventions such as rehydration, vaccines, vitamin A, and micronutrients, most of these children would survive (Rx for Child Survival, 2005).

The Global Health Council (2006) advocates these additional methods of improving children's chances of survival: (1) the continuance of breastfeeding through a child's first year,

(2) sanitation including clean water and waste disposal, (3) prevention of mother-to-child transmission of HIV in countries with a high prevalence of HIV through the use of antiretroviral drugs, and (4) the use of zinc therapy for diarrhea. These types of inventions are not expensive and could eliminate much unnecessary childhood deaths. If these interventions were available, there would be major decreases in child death for a fairly low cost (Global Health Council, 2006).

RESEARCH AND TECHNOLOGY

The United States has done an extraordinary job of documenting events surrounding perinatal health using the vital records system. This effort needs to continue to support the health of children on a population basis (Kotch, 2013). Some states monitor blood lead levels, hospitalizations, and injuries, as well as school physical examinations, but these efforts are not uniform across the country (Kotch, 2013). A more centralized database is needed so that these data can be used to effectively monitor and explore trends and issues that affect children's health, thereby allowing for advocacy of policies, initiatives, and programs to promote and maintain children's health care. On a global scale, more efforts need to continue in moving toward population-wide surveys and surveillance of child health parameters. Some authors suggest that one-third of all births in the developing world are not registered (Torjesen & Olness, 2004).

WHO (2003) recommends adoption of a public health model imbued with a strong research and technical implementation perspective. Priority should be given to research and development activities relevant to the needs of children and adolescents that would inform policy, lead to new technologies, and improve delivery strategies. For example, the Global Forum for Health Research's Child Health and Nutrition Research Initiative (CHNRI) has established a research priority-setting framework that takes into account an intervention's effectiveness, deliverability, affordability, sustainability, and potential to relieve the disease burden (Rudan, Arifeen, Black, & Campbell, 2007).

OTHER INFLUENCES ON CHILDREN'S HEALTH: POLITICS, ECONOMICS, AND CULTURE

Not only do health problems differ in various areas of the world, but communities and countries also set priorities and deal with children's health differently owing to local concerns, resources, and needs. Myriad factors influence children's health, ranging from political instability and violence in a country to the economic conditions and family resources that determine the healthcare decisions and resources provided for the children within a family. Children still must depend on their parents, advocates, and policymakers to articulate appropriate child healthcare policies and implement relevant programs (Akukwe, 2000). Most of the people living in poverty in this world are children, with the legacy of this condition being transmitted from one generation to the next (UNICEF, 2011). WHO (2005) estimates that poverty is directly responsible for the deaths of 12 million children younger than the age of five each year. For example, in Sub-Saharan Africa, most of the countries with stagnant or high child mortality rates also have the highest incidence of extreme poverty (WHO, 2005).

Many of the world's children come from diverse ethnic and cultural backgrounds that will need to be understood by their healthcare providers. Cultural and religious practices may limit or counteract the effectiveness of some medical and health practices (Torjesen & Olness, 2004). For example, the survival of an infant reflects more than just its health at birth; it is also dependent on the race and ethnic status of the mother, the socioeconomic status of the parents, the residence of the parents, the preconception health status of the mother, and the level of maternal education (Akukwe, 2000). In the United States, women with fewer than 12 years of education have higher rates of delayed prenatal care, infants with low birth weight, and neonatal deaths compared to the women with higher educational levels (Akukwe, 2000).

A recurrent theme that emerges in examining the health of children of the world is the inequality in health outcomes within and among countries worldwide. Although unfortunate health outcomes are seen in the poorer regions of the world, examination of data from the wealthiest countries also shows inequality within specific countries (Macinko, Shi, & Starfield, 2004). Numerous authors of national and international documents have identified three major factors that have significant salience for this inequality: socioeconomic status, gender, and education (Black et al., 2010; Kotch, 2013; Victora et al., 2003; WHO, 2003). Table 18-5 lists some of the conditions associated with each of these factors. Education of women and their children, higher socioeconomic status, and greater value and respect of women lead to more favorable health outcomes for children in countries and regions throughout the world (Black et al., 2010; Kotch, 2013; Victora et al., 2003). Poverty and health are inextricably linked, so the world must work toward eliminating poverty if it is to improve health.

UNICEF (2004) advocates four major goals to benefit children throughout the world. Accomplishing these goals would result in individual well-being and productivity for all children

TABLE 18-5 Three Major Factors Related to Inequality in Health Outcomes

Factor	Associated Conditions
Lower socioeconomic status	• Less use of antenatal and delivery care. • Exposure to poor sanitation, crowding, and undernutrition. • Less preventive health or appropriate and timely treatment for illness.
Gender	• Low status for women in various global areas leads to greater exposure to health risks such as gender-based violence and exposure to HIV (Blanc, 2001; Dunkle et al., 2004; Shiffman, 2000; WHO, 2003). • Stronger preference for sons leads to infanticide and neglect of female children in areas of the world such as northern India, China, and parts of east Asia (Victora et al., 2003; WHO, 2003).
Education	• Educated women and their children are less likely to die than their less educated counterparts (Kotch, 2005). • An increase in education leads to improved domestic health care and hygiene and increased use of health services.

and adolescents, with the overall result of healthy global communities. Today, fostering healthy families is a necessary global imperative. To continue to move beyond simple survival to ensure health, growth, and full development for all children, adolescents, and their families requires strong commitments from political leaders, clear identification of children's health as a priority, and strategic investments from nations' budgets, followed by investments in comprehensive and integrated efforts that have proved cost-effective and able to produce outcomes leading to improved child and adolescent health (Kotch, 2013; WHO, 2003).

CONCLUSION

Children are born into a world that has become more connected with lines between local and global problems often very blurred. Many children continue to die needless deaths because of missed opportunities and growing inequities in the provision of basic services. Although we have made tremendous progress over the last few years, serious issues continue to face children in the world today. The international *Sustainable Development Goals* can provide a clear strategy for improving children's health, with specific international organizations providing guidance and implementation tactics that can be used to achieve these goals (WHO, 2015d). If the world continues to seek creative, effective, and collaborative approaches to cross political, socioeconomic, and cultural barriers, all children will be adequately served, supported, and protected. Ideally, the value of the world's children will be elevated with an increased effort to guide and protect the world's future.

Study Questions

1. Discuss two UN children's organizations and relate how they promote global child health.
2. Compare and contrast the major childhood global diseases such as pneumonia, diarrheal disease, HIV/AIDS, malaria, and measles.
3. Why are child injuries a major global problem today?
4. Discuss the major issues in child trafficking.

Case Study for Caring for a Child from Bangladesh

Tanmayi was excited about studying abroad next year. As a four-year nursing student in a major university in the United States, she felt prepared and ready to provide nursing to the people of Bangladesh. It was very surprising to her when on her first day she became immediately immersed in the culture by trying to console a parent of a two-year-old child dying of pneumonia. When she wrote in her journal (a requirement for her course of study), she had to answer the following questions:

1. What is the leading cause of death in children younger than the age of five?
2. What is the difference between childhood mortality versus morbidity?
3. What would be the best practice for intervening to prevent further deaths in this area of the world?
4. Identify the interventions for the community, provider, and health system.

References

Akukwe, C. (2000). Maternal and child health services in the twenty-first century: Critical issues, challenges, and opportunities. *Health Care for Women International, 21,* 641–653.

Black, R., Allen, L., Bhutta, Z., Caulfield, L., de Onis, M., Ezzati, M., . . . Rivera, J. (2008). Maternal and child undernutrition: Global and regional exposures and health consequences. *Lancet, 371,* 243–260.

Black, R., Cousens, S., Johnson, H. L., Lawn, J. E., Rudan, I., Bassani, D. G., . . . Mathers, C. (2010). Global, regional, and national causes of child mortality in 2008: A systematic analysis. *Lancet, 375,* 1969–1987.

Blanc, A. K. (2001). The effect of power in sexual relationships on sexual and reproductive health: An examination of the evidence. *Studies in Family Planning, 32,* 189–213.

Bryce, J., el Arifeen, S., Pariyo, G., Lanata, C. F., Gwatkin, D., & Habicht, J. (2003). Reducing child mortality: Can public health deliver? *Lancet, 362,* 159–164.

Bryce, J., Boschi-Pinto, C., Shibuya, K., & Black, R. E. (2005). WHO estimates of the causes of death in children. *Lancet, 365,* 1147–1152.

Claeson, M., Gillespie, D., Mshinda, H., Troedsson, H., & Victora, C. (2003). Knowledge into action for child survival. *Lancet, 362,* 323–327.

Darmstadt, G., Kumar, V., Yadav, R., Singh, V., Singh, P., & Mohanty, S. (2005). *Community mobilization and behaviour change communication promote evidence-based essential newborn care practices and reduce neonatal mortality in Uttar Pradesh, India* [Poster]. Countdown to 2015: Tracking Progress in Child Survival, London.

Dawson, D. (2006). New hope for children with HIV/AIDS. *AIDMatters.* Retrieved from http://www.talcuk.org/aidmatters

Dunkle, K. L., Jewkes, R. K., Brown, H. C., Gray, G. E., McIntyre, J. A., & Harlow, S. D. (2004). Gender-based violence, relationship power, and risk of HIV infection in women attending antenatal clinics in South Africa. *Lancet, 363,* 1415–1421.

Global Health Council. (2006). *Child health.* Retrieved from http://www.globalhealth.org/view_top.php3?id=226

Global Health Council. (2011). *Annual report 2010.* Retrieved from http://www.globalhealth.org/Annual_Report.html

Global Health Council. (2015). *Annual report.* Retrieved from http://globalhealth.org/tag/global-health/

Grantham-McGregor, S., Cheung, Y. B., Cueto, S., Glewwe, P., Richter, L., & Strupp, B. (2007). Developmental potential in the first 5 years for children in developing countries. *Lancet, 369,* 60–70.

Hogan, M., Lopez, A., Lozan, R., Murray, C., Naghavi, M., & Rajaratnam, J. (2010). *Building momentum: Global progress toward reducing maternal and child mortality.* Seattle, WA: Institute for Health Metrics and Evaluation.

Jones, G., Steketee, R. W., Black, R. E., Bhutta, Z. A., & Morris, S. S. (2003). How many child deaths can we prevent this year? *Lancet, 363,* 65–71.

Kotch, J. B. (2013). *Maternal and Child Health: Programs, Problems, and Policy in Public Health* (3rd ed.). Sudbury, MA: Jones and Bartlett.

Levine, R., & Kinder, M. (2004). *Millions Saved: Proven Successes in Global Health.* Washington, DC: Center for Global Development.

Lopez, A. D., Mathers, C. D., Ezzati, M., Jamison, D. T., & Murray, C. J. L. (2006). Global and regional burden of diseases and risk factors, 2001: Systematic analysis of population health data. *Lancet, 367,* 1747–1757.

Macinko, J. A., Shi, L. Y., & Starfield, B. (2004). Wage inequality, the health system, and infant mortality in wealthy industrialized countries, 1970–1996. *Social Science and Medicine, 58,* 279–292.

The Nation's Health. (2004, October). Malnutrition, violence threaten Sudanese refugees. Retrieved from http://www.apha.org/NR/rdonlyres/67FD0431-3590-42FF-A7BE-CAA0570C59CF/0/TNHOct04full.pdf

Population Reference Bureau. (2014). *2014 World Population Data Sheet.* Washington, DC: PRB. Retrieved from http://www.prb.org

Rudan, I., Arifeen, S., Black, R. E., & Campbell, H. (2007). Childhood pneumonia and diarrhea: Setting our priorities right. *Lancet Infectious Diseases, 7,* 56–61.

Rx for Child Survival. (2005). *Rx for child survival campaign: A global health challenge.* Retrieved from http://www.pbs.org/wgbh/rxforsurvival/about-project.html

Shiffman, J. (2000). Can poor countries surmount high maternal mortality? *Studies in Family Planning, 31,* 274–289.

Torjesen, K., & Olness, K. (2004). Child health in the developing world. In R. E. Behrman, R. M. Kliegman, & H. B. Jenson, *Nelson Textbook of Pediatrics* (17th ed., pp. 12–14). Philadelphia: Saunders.

United Nations Children's Fund. (2003). *State of the World's Children.* Geneva, Switzerland: United Nations.

United Nations Children's Fund. (2004). *End of the decade databases.* Retrieved from http://www.childinfo.org/index2.htm

United Nations Children's Fund. (2008). *United Nations, Department of Economic and Social Affairs, Population Division: World population prospects: The 2008 revision.* Retrieved from http://www.un.org/esa/population/publications/wpp2008/wpp2008_highlights.pdf

United Nations Children's Fund. (2009). *The State of the World's Children 2009.* New York: United Nations.

United Nations Children's Fund. (2011). *The State of the World's Children 2011.* New York: United Nations.

United Nations Children's Fund. (2013). *The State of the World's Children 2013.* New York: United Nations.

United Nations Children's Fund. (2014a). *Committing to Child Survival: A Promise Renewed.* New York: United Nations.

United Nations Children's Fund. (2014b). *State of the World's Children 2015: Reimagine the Future, Innovation for Every Child.* New York: United Nations.

United Nations Children's Fund. (2014c). *Every Child Counts: Revealing Disparities, Advancing Children's Rights.* New York: United Nations.

United Nations Children's Fund. (2015). *Current status and progress.* New York: United Nations. Retrieved from http://www.data.unicef.org/child-mortality/under-five.html.

United Nations. (2000). *The millennium declaration.* Retrieved from http://www.un.org/millennium/declaration/ares552e.htm

United Nations. (2002). *Special session on children.* Retrieved from http://www.un.org/documents

United Nations. (2004). *Millennium development goals.* Retrieved from http://www.un.org/millenniumgoals/poverty.shtml

United Nations. (2011). *Update on millennium goals.* Retrieved from http://www.un.org

Victora, C., Adair, L., Fall, C., Hallal, P., Martorell, R., Richter, L., & Sachdev, H. S. (2008). Maternal and child undernutrition: Consequences for adult health and human capital. *Lancet, 371,* 340–357.

Victora, C. G., Wagstaff, A., Schellenberg, J. A., Gwatkin, D., Claeson, M., & Habicht, J. P. (2003). Applying an equity lens to child health and mortality: More of the same is not enough. *Lancet, 362,* 233–241.

Walker, N., Schwartlander, B., & Bryce, J. (2002). Meeting international goals in child survival and HIV/AIDS. *Lancet, 360,* 284–289.

World Health Organization. (2003). *Strategic Directions for Improving the Health and Development of Children and Adolescents.* Geneva, Switzerland: Author. Retrieved from http://www.who.int/maternal_child_adolescent/documents/9241591064/en/

World Health Organization. (2005). *The World Health Report, 2005: Make Every Mother and Child Count.* Geneva, Switzerland: Author.

World Health Organization. (2008a). *Children and AIDS: Third Stocking Report, 2008.* Geneva, Switzerland: Author & UNICEF.

World Health Organization. (2008b). *World Malaria Report 2008.* Geneva, Switzerland: Author.

World Health Organization. (2008c). *World Report on Child Injury Prevention.* Geneva, Switzerland: WHO & UNICEF.

World Health Organization. (2009). *The Partnership for Maternal, Newborn, and Child Health Strategy and Workplan 2009–2011.* Geneva, Switzerland: Author.

World Health Organization. (2010). *WHO Agenda.* Retrieved from http://www.who.int/about/agenda/en/index.html

World Health Organization. (2011a). *Fact sheet: 10 facts—October 2007*. Retrieved from http://www.who.int/features/factfiles/child_health2/en/index.html

World Health Organization. (2011b). *General page*. Retrieved from http://www.who.int

World Health Organization. (2014). *Water Sanitation Health*. Retrieved from http://www.who.int/water_sanitation_health/publications/2014/jmp-report/en/

World Health Organization. (2015a). *Estimates of Child Causes of Death 2000–2015*. Geneva, Switzerland: Author.

World Health Organization. (2015b). *Progress on Sanitation and Drinking Water: 2015 Update and MDG Assessment*. Geneva, Switzerland: Author.

World Health Organization. (2015c). *Maternal, Newborn, Child and Adolescent Health*. Retrieved from http://www.who.int/maternal_child_adolescent/epidemiology/en/

World Health Organization. (2015d). *Health in 2015: From MDGs, Millennium Development Goals, to SDGs, Sustainable Development Goals*. Geneva, Switzerland: Author.

World Health Organization. (2015e). *WHO checklist targets major causes of maternal and newborn deaths in health facilities*. Retrieved from http://www.who.int/medicenter/news/releases/2015/maternal-newborn.

You, D., Jones, G., & Wardlaw, T. (2010). *Levels and Trends in Child Mortality: Estimates Developed by the UN Inter-agency Group for Child Mortality Estimation*. United Nations Inter-agency Group for Child Mortality Estimation. New York: UNICEF.

You, D., Jones, G., & Wardlaw, T. (2011). *Levels and Trends in Child Mortality: Report 2011*. United Nations Inter-agency Group for Child Mortality Estimation. New York: UNICEF.

You, D., Wardlaw, T., Salama, P., & Jones, G. (2009). Levels and trends in under-5 mortality, 1990–2008. *Lancet, 9*, 61601–61609.

19

Global Health of the Older Adult

David B. Mitchell*

Objectives

After reading this chapter, the reader will be able to:

1. Define gerontology.
2. Compare and contrast the health concerns of the older adult in a developed vs. developing country.
3. Explain the influences of culture and geographic location on aging in various parts of the world.
4. Discuss gender differences in aging.
5. Relate legal and ethical issues related to global aging.

INTRODUCTION

Who is the older adult? Is it a person who is elderly? When does one become old or—to put it another way—when does aging begin? Under normal circumstances, a newborn baby begins its life with the same biological and psychological apparatus regardless of where in the world it is born. However, older individuals are clearly not all equally equipped. Although it is often said that all generalizations are false—including this one—a major hallmark of aging is that there are a variety of life span developmental trajectories (Nesselroade, 2001). A key concept to understanding the older adult is an appreciation of individual differences in patterns of aging, because there is no prototypical older adult. For example, one 79-year-old may be frail, suffering from osteoporosis, and experiencing significant deficits in strength and hearing. Another older person—of the same chronological age—might be in peak physical and mental condition

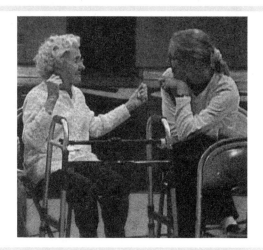 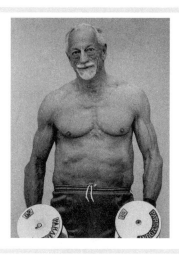

FIGURE 19-1 Two Individuals of the Same Chronological Age (79) with Significantly Different Aging Experiences
Photo on left is Courtesy of Dr. Angela Baldwin Lanier. Photo on right is Reproduced from Clark, E. (1995).
Growing old is not for sissies II: Portraits of senior athletes. Rohnert Park, CA: Pomegranate Artbooks.

(see Figure 19-1). How do aging and the experiences of elderly individuals vary around the world, as a function of different environments, cultures, religions, and political landscapes? We will attempt to answer some of these questions in this chapter.

Gerontology (from *geron,* the Greek word for "old man") is most commonly defined as the scientific study of aging. The term was introduced by Élie Metchnikoff in 1903. A broader definition of gerontology also includes the following aspects: studies of the processes associated with aging; studies of mature and aged adults; studies of aging scholarship from the perspective of art, philosophy, history and literature; and applications for the benefit of older adults (Kastenbaum, 2006).

Not to be confused with gerontology, *geriatrics* is a subfield of gerontology concerned specifically with the medical aspects of aging. The American Geriatrics Society was established in 1942 (Rockwood, 2006).

In the field of gerontology, studies of older populations typically use the index of chronological age, starting at age 65. However, the passage of time per se does not cause the biological changes associated with age (Arking, 2006, p. 4). Because most biologists believe that aging begins at conception (Carnes, Olshansky, & Hayflick, 2013; Hayflick, 1996), the selection of the age of 65 is arbitrary and certainly not biologically precise. Further, even though normative ages may be used to define specific stages of maturation, including adolescence and menopause, there is no such thing as a normative age at which a person "turns old." The historical reason for the use of 65 years as a cutoff is based on a story about German chancellor Otto von Bismarck, who lived from 1815 to 1898. Bismarck noted that his major political rivals were federal employees older than the age of 65. He succeeded in pushing through legislation that required retirement at age 65, and then "ascended to power with ease" when he was 56 years old (Hayflick, 1996, p. 108). Ironically, he held his position as chancellor until age 75!

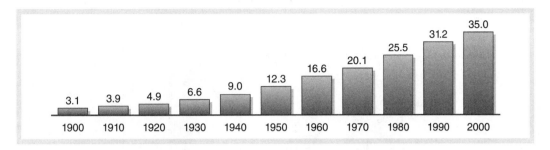

FIGURE 19-2 Number of Older Adults in the United States in the 20th Century (in millions)
Reproduced from He, W., Sengupta, M., Velkoff, V. A., & DeBarros, K. A. (2005). U.S. Census Bureau, Current Population Reports, P23-209, *65+ in the United States: 2005*. Washington, DC: U.S. Government Printing Office.

The 65-plus criterion has long been the standard in most European and American aging research (He, Sengupta, Velkoff, & DeBarros, 2005; Howden & Meyer, 2011; West, Cole, Goodkind, & He, 2014), and is also used in studies of global aging (Haub & Kent, 2008; Kinsella & Phillips, 2005). However, this particular chronological milestone may not serve equally well for research conducted in developing countries, because, as we discuss in the next section, a relatively smaller proportion of people in less developed countries survive past age 65 years.[1] Nevertheless, with a few exceptions (Lutz, Sanderson, & Scherbov, 2008; United Nations Programme on Aging, 2001; World Health Organization [WHO], 2015) who prefer to use age 60-plus (the "second half of life"), the 65-plus criterion is the most commonly used index for defining the older adult category.

Chronological age is still the best marker available for making global comparisons of aging phenomena. We will start with data from the U.S. Census Bureau to describe the increase in the older portion of the population over the past century; we will then examine the same phenomenon across the globe. As Figure 19-2 illustrates, the number of older people in the United States increased greatly during the past century (not shown are the data for 2010, where 40.2 million were over 65). The population as a whole also grew substantially (from 76 million in 1900 to 309 million in the 2010 census), so a simple count—even in millions—could be misleading. Perhaps the growth in the number of older people simply parallels the overall growth of the country as a whole. That is, as 3.1 million older adults represented 4.1% of the population in 1900, we might expect a similar percentage in 2010 (i.e., 4.1% of 309 million, or 12.7 million). However, this is not the case. A more informative perspective is provided in Figure 19-3, where the percentage increase of older adults in America is compared to the percentage increase of those under age 65. It is clear from this graph that the size of the older population has grown disproportionately, increasing at a much faster rate than the younger population. In other words, while the younger population increased 3.7 times (368%), the older adult population increased more than 13 times (from 3.1 to 40.2 million, or 13.0% in 2010, up a whopping 1,307%). This phenomenon is called *population aging*, defined as "the disproportionate growth of older age groups" (West, Cole, Goodkind, & He, 2014) (p. 5). It is "one of the most distinctive demographic events in the world today" (Chakraborti, 2004, p. 33), and global population

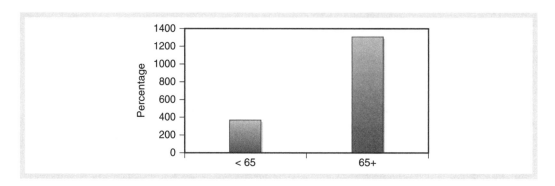

FIGURE 19-3 Increased Growth Percentages of Adults Age 65 and Older Compared to those Under Age 65 in the U.S. Population, 1900–2010
Data from He, W., Sengupta, M., Velkoff, V. A., & DeBarros, K. A. (2005). U.S. Census Bureau, Current Population Reports, P23-209, *65+ in the United States: 2005*. Washington, DC: U.S. Government Printing Office.

aging is accelerating (Lutz, Sanderson, & Scherbov, 2008; Phillipson, 2013; WHO, 2015). Indeed, 50 countries already have a higher proportion of older adults than the United States does, and this phenomenon is projected for 98 countries (nearly half the world) by 2050 (West, Cole, Goodkind, & He, 2014).

The aforementioned demographic facts have led to an increased interest in the field of gerontology. Prior to 1974, the United States did not have a national health institute dedicated to aging; today, the National Institute on Aging has a budget of more than $1 billion and sponsors a number of important research projects aimed at increasing our understanding of aging and improving the lives of older Americans. The increased interest in gerontology is apparent on a global basis as well, as evidenced by the convening of the Second World Assembly on Aging in Madrid in 2002, 20 years after the United Nations convened the First World Assembly on Aging in Vienna in 1982. The International Association of Gerontology and Geriatrics held its 20th World Congress in 2013 in Seoul. In Figure 19-4, it is clear that although the percentage of older adults worldwide increased only slightly (2%) from 1950 to 2000, it is projected to increase dramatically (Lutz, Sanderson, & Scherbov, 2008), possibly doubling, by 2050 (WHO, 2015).

MORTALITY AND MORBIDITY STATISTICS

Before we consider life expectancy and mortality rates around the world, it is crucial to understand the distinction between two widely used measures: life expectancy and maximum life span (Hayflick, 1996). Life expectancy involves taking a statistical snapshot of a population during a particular year and calculating an arithmetic mean based on those persons' age at death. Although it is most commonly calculated from the time of birth, life expectancy can be calculated from any age. Maximum lifespan, in contrast, is simply the longest lifespan

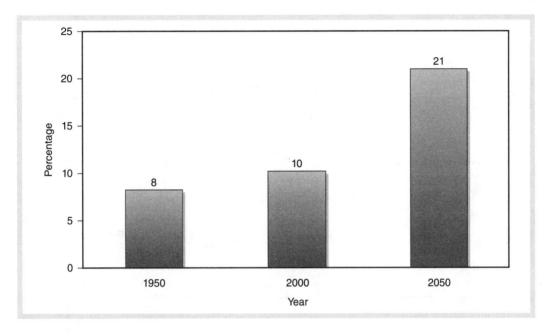

FIGURE 19-4   Older Adults (60+) as a Percentage of Total World Population
Data from United Nations. (2002). *World Populations Ageing: 1950–2050.* United Nations publication, Sales
No. E.02. XIII.3; World Health Organization. (2015). *World Report on Ageing and Health.* Luxembourg.

(or longevity) recorded. Although biologists typically place the maximum at 120 (Carnes, Olshansky, & Hayflick, 2013), the human record is currently 122 years.

As before, we will start with data from the U.S. Census to describe how life expectancy has changed in the United States over the past century, and then we will examine the same phenomenon across the globe. Figure 19-5 reveals the astonishing fact that the average life expectancy from birth has increased dramatically in the United States, from only 47 years in 1900 to 77 years in 2000, and up to 78.7 in 2010. However, this increase in life expectancy is often misinterpreted. For example, one headline proclaimed, "New Health Statistics Show Americans *Living Longer*" ("New Health Statistics," 2011; emphasis added). Journalists such as *New York Times* columnist William Safire also make this mistake, saying, "When you look back over the last 50 or 75 years . . . you see these enormous advances in science where you are actually extending the life of a human being from 47 in 1900 to 77 today" (Morgan, 2006, p. 24). Although less sensational, a more accurate headline stated, "Life Expectancy in the USA Hits a Record High" (*USA Today*, 9 October 2014). In other words, individuals are not setting new longevity records, but more people are surviving into the stage of old age, defined as older than 65 years.

Unlike life expectancy, the most compelling fact about the maximum life span is that it has not changed. That is, since these data have been recorded over the last few thousand years of human history, there have always been a few people who live to be older than 100 years, close

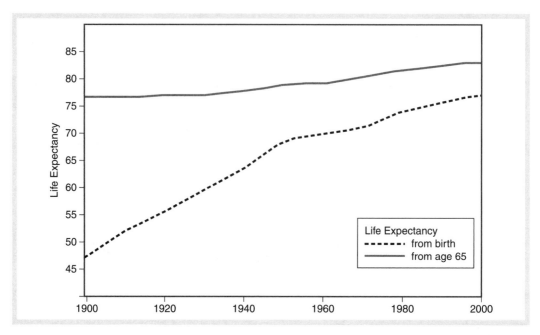

FIGURE 19-5 Changes in Mean Life Expectancy, United States, 1900–2000
Note the dramatic change in life expectancy from birth, contrasted with much less change in remaining life expectancy for those who reached age 65.
Data from He, W., Sengupta, M., Velkoff, V. A. & DeBarros, K. A. (2005). U.S. Census Bureau, Current Population Reports, P23-209, *65+ in the United States: 2005*. Washington, DC: U.S. Government Printing Office; Hayflick, L. (1996). *How and Why We Age*. New York: Ballantine Books.

to the maximum of approximately 120 years of age. One prominent biologist went so far as to say that "there is no evidence that the maximum human life span has changed from what it was about a hundred thousand years ago" (Hayflick, 1996, p. 66). According to more recent history, the prophet Moses lived to exactly 120 years old, dying on his birthday in 1273 BC. More than 1,600 years ago (according to Athanasius, patriarch of Alexandria), Saint Anthony died in AD 356 at the age of 105 (Perls & Silver, 1999). In 1899, Geert Boomgaard of the Netherlands died at the age of 110. In England, Ann Pouder died in 1917 at the age of 110, and in the United States, Louisa Tiers lived to be 111, when she died in 1926.[2] In 1906, the biologist Metchnikoff (1912) interviewed Mme. Robineau at 106, and included her photograph in his book. Most recently, Jeanne Calment (Figure 19-6) died in 1997 at age 122 (Allard, Lèbre, & Robine, 1998). Even though Calment's life span may set a new record, a two-year increase over the past 3,280+ years of recorded human history is not nearly as impressive as the changes seen in average life expectancy.

In addition, if life expectancy is calculated from ages beyond birth, very little change has occurred. As far back as 1693, Edmund Halley (famous for the comet bearing his name) reported that although life expectancy was only 33 years as calculated from birth (in the city of Breslau), those persons who made it to 80 years old, however, could expect to live an average of

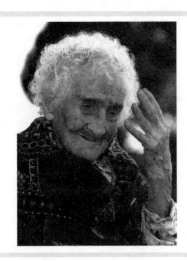

FIGURE 19-6 Madame Jeanne Calment (Arles, France), Photographed in 1995 at the Age of 120
She died in 1997 at the age of 122.
Photo by Jean-Paul Pelissier, REUTERS, October 17, 1995. Retrieved from http://pictures.reuters.com/archive/-RP1DRIDAGVAC.html

six more years (Hayflick, 1996). In the United States, life expectancy at age 65 increased only six years from 1900 to 2000 (from 11.9 to 17.9 years beyond 65, for a total of 76.9 to 82.9 years; see the top line in Figure 19-5). In the same time period, life expectancy increased only 1.7 years for those persons who reached age 85.

Yet another way to understand the changes in life expectancy is to plot the percentage of people surviving to a given age, according to calendar years. For example, in the United States in 1900, only 88% of newborn babies reached their first birthday; by 2000, that percentage was up to 99% (He, Sengupta, Velkoff, & DeBarros, 2005). These changes are plotted on the left side of Figure 19-7. As more people survive into older age ranges, the survival curve starts to approximate the shape of a rectangle. If all of us survived to the maximum life span, the survival curve would become "rectangularized." As is illustrated in Figure 19-7, the U.S. population is moving in that direction. The same phenomenon is happening globally, albeit at a much lower rate and slower pace.

Another type of rectangularization can be seen in the *population pyramids* in Figure 19-8. In 1900, these data did exhibit a pyramidal shape, but by 2010, this demographic structure had grown fatter in the middle (a "midriff bulge"), and now the upper tip is widening as well. (The projections for 2030 and 2050 are resolutely rectangular; the pyramid metaphor may have to be dropped in the not-too-distant future.)

It is estimated that there were more than 616 million people worldwide older than the age of 65 in 2015 (*International Data Base*, U.S. Census Bureau), which represents 8.5% of the world's population. Paradoxically, because developed countries tend to have more elderly residents than developing countries, 59% of these older adults live in developing countries (He,

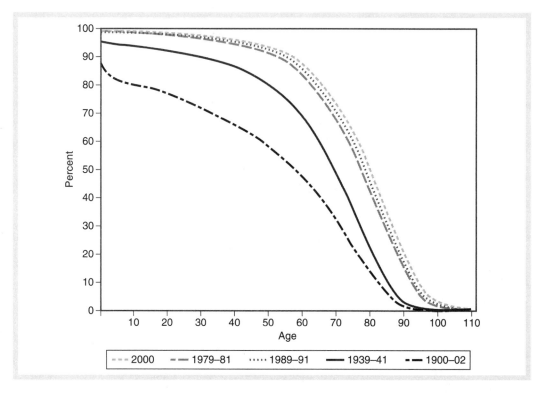

FIGURE 19-7 Percent of People Surviving to Certain Ages for Selected Years in the United States
Reproduced from He, W., Sengupta, M., Velko , V. A., & DeBarros, K. A. (2005). U.S. Census Bureau, Current
Population Reports, P23-209, *65+ in the United States: 2005*. Washington, DC: U.S. Government Printing Office.

Sengupta, Velkoff, & DeBarros, 2005). These figures reveal a lopsided proportion of older adults
in Africa, Asia, Central America, the Caribbean, and Oceania. As for the shape of the worldwide
population structure, developing countries are still much more pyramidal, but in due course,
the statistical prediction is that their population pyramids will also become rectangularized.
This phenomenon is shown graphically in Figure 19-9, which compares more developed countries with less developed countries, with data from 1950 and 1990, and projections for 2030.
The percentages of people 65 years of age and older are shown for different regions of the world
in Figure 19-10. Africa is expected to experience the smallest increase over the next 30 years,
due in large part to the HIV/AIDS epidemic. Of the 18.8 million people who died of AIDS by
2001, 79% resided in Africa (Kinsella & Phillips, 2005). Countries with the highest percentages
of adults (65+, as of 2005) are plotted in Figure 19-11. (Remember that the U.S. elderly population grew to 13% in 2010.) Using the criterion of 60+, the World Health Organization reported
that Japan had more than 30% in 2015. Based on 2010 census data, the populations with the
longest life expectancies are females in Japan (86.9 years) and males in Singapore (81.1 years)
(West, Cole, Goodkind, & He, 2014). The populations with the shortest life expectancies, only
33 years, are females in Botswana and males in Swaziland (Haub, 2006).

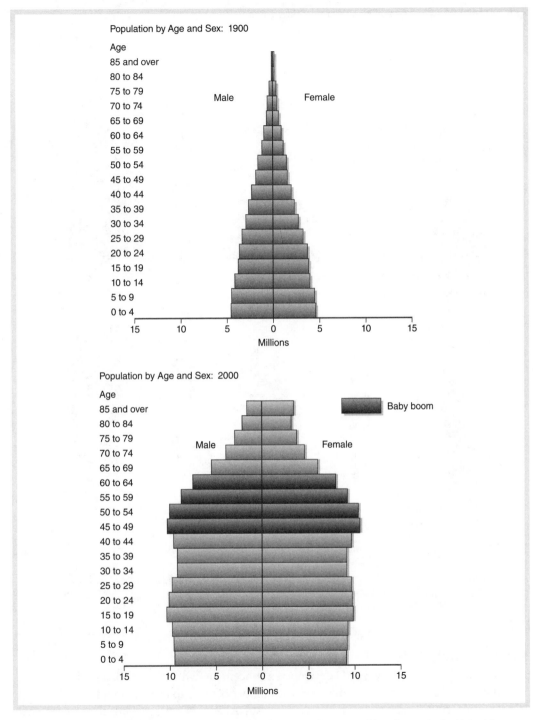

FIGURE 19-8 Population Pyramids Demonstrating the Changes in Structure of Age Groups in the United States, 1900–2010

Reproduced from West, L., Cole, S., Goodkind, D., & He, H. (2014). U.S. Census Bureau, Current Population Reports, P23-212, *65+ in the United States: 2010*. Washington, DC: U.S. Government Printing Office.

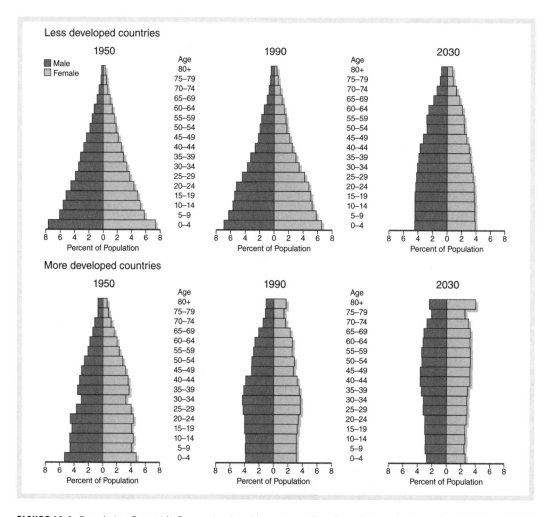

FIGURE 19-9 Population Pyramids Comparing Less Versus More Developed Countries (Data from 1950 and 1990 with Projections for 2030)

Reproduced from Kinsella, K., & Phillips, D. R. (2005). Global aging: The challenge of success. *Population Bulletin, 60*(1), 3–42, p. 14, Figure 2 (UN Population Division, World Population Prospects: The 2002 Revision (http://esa .un.org/unpp, accessed Dec. 9, 2004).)

Disability-Adjusted Life Expectancy

Beyond basic life expectancy, WHO developed a concept known as the disability-adjusted life expectancy (DALE), meaning the expected number of years to be lived in full health (Chakraborti, 2004). In 2000, Japan had the highest DALE of 74.5 years, while Sierra Leone had the lowest DALE of less than 26 years. In subsequent years, global health agencies and epidemiological researchers have changed to a different positive index, HALE (healthy life expectancy), as well as the negative index of DALYs. A recent study of 188 countries found that overall

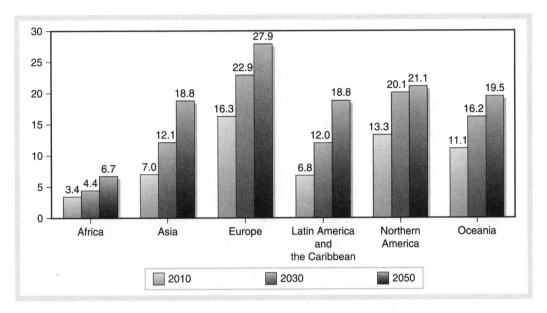

FIGURE 19-10 Percent of the Population Aged 65 and Older in Various Regions (2010, Projected for Years 2030 and 2050)
Reproduced from West, L., Cole, S., Goodkind, D., & He, H. (2014). U.S. Census Bureau, Current Population Reports, P23-212, *65+ in the United States: 2010*. Washington, DC: U.S. Government Printing Office.

"global health is improving" (Murray et al., 2015). Based on the Global Burden of Disease Study data (2013), average life expectancy from birth rose to 71.5 years. The highest expectancy was in Andorra (83.9), and the lowest was in Lesotho (48.3), which also had the lowest HALE (42.0). The average HALE index rose to 62.3 years, with Japan reporting the highest (73.4). In contrast, DALYs went up or down (down is better), based on disease category: Communicable diseases have decreased, but noncommunicable diseases (e.g., heart disease, lower respiratory infections, and cerebrovascular disease, due primarily to aging) have risen. Finally, there is "tremendous variation" across sociodemographic status and countries. Indeed, a parallel study by Murray and colleagues reported that India has no national data on the cause of death estimates.

The Oldest-Old, Centenarians, and Supercentenarians
Among those persons older than 65 years, further distinctions are now recognized: young-old, oldest-old (more than 85 years old), and centenarians (100 years and older) (He, Sengupta, Velkoff, & DeBarros, 2005). Centenarians account for the fastest-growing segment of the oldest-old. Surprisingly—given the age-related functional decline of people in their sixth, seventh, eighth, and ninth decades of life—approximately 25% of centenarians are in very good health (Perls, 2004). There are two centenarian research centers located in the United States, one in Massachusetts and the other in Georgia. The New England Centenarian Project, directed by Dr. Thomas Perls, was founded in 1995 and is still active in 2015. The Georgia Centenarian Study, founded and directed

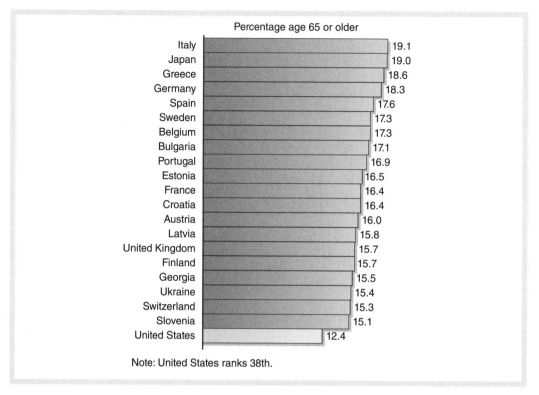

Note: United States ranks 38th.

FIGURE 19-11 Countries with the Greatest Percent of Older Population
The United States now ranks 26th, according to West, Cole, Goodkind, & He, 2014.
Reproduced from Kinsella, K., & Phillips, D. R. (2005). Global aging: The challenge of success. *Population Bulletin, 60*(1), 3–42, p. 7, Figure 1 (U.S. Census Bureau, International Data Base (www.census.gov/ipc/www/idbnew.html, accessed Dec. 12, 2004).)

by Dr. Leonard Poon, ran from 1988 to 2009. In 2010, the U.S. Census counted over 53,400 centenarians (West, Cole, Goodkind, & He, 2014). Regarding the prevalence of centenarians around the world, Vaupel and Jeune (1995) estimated that there were approximately 8,800 people of age 100 and older in Japan and the Western European countries combined. More recently, Goodman (2014) reported that the worldwide estimate is now 450,000.

Supercentenarians (age 110 and older) are a much smaller and even more elite group. According to the Gerontology Research Group (www.grg.org), there are 49 validated supercentenarians alive in the world today (October 2015), only one of whom is male. The current oldest person is 116, a woman living in New York. We discuss this gender gap in the next section.

Gender Differences

Although males outnumber females at birth, by midlife this gender ratio is reversed. The relative proportion of females to males becomes even more exaggerated as age increases. This

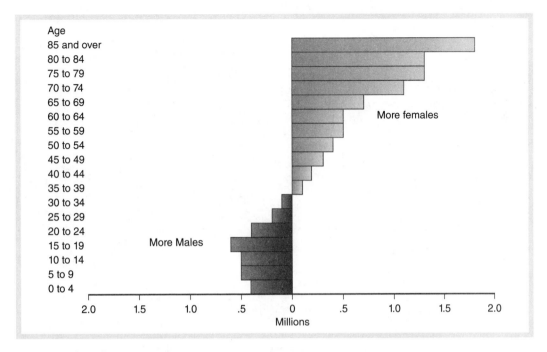

FIGURE 19-12 Different Numbers of Males and Females as a Function of Age
Reproduced from He, W., Sengupta, M., Velkoff, V. A., & DeBarros, K. A. (2005). U.S. Census Bureau, Current Population Reports, P23-209, *65+ in the United States: 2005*. Washington, DC: U.S. Government Printing Office.

dramatic life span change is depicted graphically in Figure 19-12. The gender differential in life expectancy shown in the figure is especially noticeable in more developed countries, where the average gender gap is about seven years. Gender differences are typically smaller in less developed countries, and are even reversed in some south Asian and Middle Eastern countries. In some of these cultures, women have a lower social status, which, combined with a societal preference for male children, has a negative impact on female life expectancy. Table 19-1 presents a sample of gender ratios in 20 countries. Some researchers have labeled this phenomenon the "feminization of the elderly" (Chakraborti, 2004, p. 58). As we have mentioned, although the percentage of females increases with age, gender ratios are less favorable for women living in developing countries. For example, among those persons 80 and older, women account for 71% of this group in Europe versus 59% in Africa.

RESEARCH AND TECHNOLOGY

In speaking of modern gerontology research, "It is more beneficial to opt for a healthy and vigorous, albeit finite, life than to search in vain for the elixir of immortality" (Arking, 2006, p. 5). As some gerontologists have suggested, we need to focus more on adding life to years, and less on adding years to life (Maddox, 1994). In both theory and practice, most current

TABLE 19-1 Gender Ratios Among People Aged 65 and Older			
More Developed Countries		**Less Developed Countries**	
Australia	79	Bangladesh	117
Bulgaria	72	Brazil	70
France	69	Ethiopia	84
Germany	68	Fiji	85
Italy	71	Ghana	89
Poland	62	Honduras	90
Russia	46	India	103
Ukraine	51	Iran	98
United Kingdom	74	Mexico	84
United States	71	Zambia	79

Note: Ratios are number of men per 100 women.
Reproduced from Kinsella, K., & Phillips, D. R. (2005). Global aging: The challenge of success. *Population Bulletin, 60*(1), 3–42, p. 24, Table 4 (U.S. Census Bureau, International Data Base (www.census.gov/ipc/www/idbnew.html, accessed Dec. 12, 2004).)

gerontological research and policy are committed to the goal of "successful aging" (e.g., Fernández-Ballesteros et al., 2010). The seminal concept of successful aging was introduced by Rowe and Kahn in 1987, in a bid to replace gerontology's fixation on loss with an emphasis on "heterogeneity and the potential for growth" (Pruchno, 2015, p. 4; see the special issue on successful aging in *The Gerontologist*, February 2015). Biologists have emphasized that "gerontology is committed not to a search for immortality but to the elimination of premature disability and death" (Arking, 2006, p. 5). Nowhere is this more true than in the arena of global aging, because life spans for the majority of people, at least in developing nations, fall far short of what can and should be expected.

The advances in communication and computer technologies "offer a promising future for older adults" (Mundorf, Mundorf, & Brownell, 2006, p. 242). More and more older adults are logging on to the Internet to use such sites as www.SeniorNet.org, which celebrated its 25th anniversary in 2011, and to use the worldwide Web for e-mail, purchases, and medical information. U.S. Census Bureau data in 2005 revealed that 35% of older adults had a home computer, and 29% had Internet access (Greenberg, 2005). In 2009, home computer use was reported by 45% of older adults and use of the Internet by 41% (Greenberg, 2010; Keenan, 2009). By 2013, Internet usage among the older population was up to 61.7% (File, 2013). New technologies are also playing a key role in new employment opportunities for older workers, at least in the United States (Riggs, 2004). Although no data were found, it is likely this trend is occurring in other developed countries (e.g., Japan and Europe) as well.

A significant portion of the research effort is to develop strategies and technology to help older adults age in place (Rogers & Fisk, 2010). Some of these initiatives involve providing good old-fashioned, low-tech social support. Sending out birthday cards to older clients is one option being explored by faculty of the University of Auckland in New Zealand ("Helping Elderly Stay at Home," 2006). Other countries, such as Korea, have more ambitious plans involving robot maids for their elderly (Tae-gyu, 2006).

Work by Dr. Wendy Rogers and her colleagues (an interdisciplinary team of psychologists, engineers, and computer programmers at the Georgia Institute of Technology) has resulted in the creation of an "aware home," in which communication and control systems (involving cameras, sensors, and computers) maximize the independence of older adults living alone by monitoring many of their daily activities, ranging from providing recipe reminders during cooking to assisting in more complex tasks such as measuring insulin accurately (Rogers & Fisk, 2010; see awarehome .imtc.gatech.edu). The advantage of such a house is that the older person can function without requiring around-the-clock help from a nurse or other live-in assistant. Of course, expense is a serious obstacle, making this concept entirely impractical in developing countries at this time.

Following are some vignettes of vibrant centenarians, taken from data gathered by volunteers at the Georgia Centenarian Study (University of Georgia, 2006):

- Mary Sims Elliott writes poetry and works on social issues at her church. At 105, she published her autobiography, cleverly titled *My First One Hundred Years.*
- Geneva McDaniel (107) teaches aerobics at a senior citizens center, and also recruits retirement community residents to exercise as well.
- Jessie Champion (107) was a sharecropper married to a younger woman (86 years old). After his wife passed away, he moved in with his daughter, where he enjoys gardening.

The researchers at the Georgia Centenarian Study (1988-2009) generally agree that the secret of longevity is still a mystery. First, according to former director Leonard Poon, no two centenarians are the same: "For as many optimistic people, we find as many who are grumpy." Furthermore, "centenarians are far more different than they are alike," according to Dr. Peter Martin, who codirected the centenarian study, "There are many paths to longevity, and each situation is very different." As for a family history of longevity, Dr. Poon says: "People aren't likely to live long just because their parents did. It seems the genetic contribution is important for some centenarians who come from a long line of long-lived people. But we have as many people who do not come from long-lived families" (University of Georgia, 2006). In contrast, other researchers have found a select group of centenarians living in Nova Scotia (Duenwald, 2003). This province has approximately 21 centenarians per 100,000 people, compared to a rate of 18 per 100,000 people in the United States and only 3 per 100,000 people worldwide. In Nova Scotia, it appears that longevity does run in families. For more centenarian stories, visit the National Centenarian Awareness Project at www.adlercentenarians.org.

Family medicine physicians are also rediscovering the advantages of home care: "in light of the aging population, advances in portable medical technology, and changes in Medicare reimbursement" (Landers, 2006, p. 366). A smartphone "app" was investigated to assist with rheumatoid arthritis self-management (Azevedo, Bernardes, Fonseca, & Lima, 2015); one finding was that the majority of the patients willing to use the app were younger. This is in line with studies that have underscored the crucial need for the successful adoption of technology for the functional independence of older adults (Czaja et al., 2006; Lee & Coughlin, 2015; Tsai, Shillair,

Cotten, Winstead, & Yost, 2015). Again, the implementation of these technologies in developing countries will be dependent on significant increases in per capita income. In addition, compensations for age and individual differences in cognitive/motor/perceptual abilities, and literacy and numeracy, are necessary for health self-management (Mitzner, McBride, Barg-Warlow, & Rogers, 2013).

LEGAL AND ETHICAL ISSUES

Ethics of Aging Research

In the United States, the institutional review board (IRB) of any research institution considers all research on older adults to involve a vulnerable group, comparable to doing research with children or pregnant women. The IRB has to review all research done with older adults, such as basic cognitive aging research involving memory differences between young and older adults (Bruss & Mitchell, 2009). However, in practice, IRBs routinely grant permission to use the same consent forms used for younger adults with healthy older adults. When research participants have some degree of cognitive impairment, such as Alzheimer's disease (e.g., Mitchell & Schmitt, 2006), the participant's ability to understand and sign an informed consent form can be a significant issue (High & Doole, 1995). If the research participant is too cognitively impaired, the IRB will usually require a consent form signed by the participant's spouse (or other legal guardian or caregiver), as well as an assent provided verbally by the participant (cf. Fazio & Mitchell, 2015).

IRBs were created through legislature in 1974 in the United States via the National Research Act, which established a National Commission for the Protection of Human Subjects of Biomedical and Behavioral Research. This act was based on the Declaration of Helsinki, made at the 18th World Medical Assembly in Helsinki, Finland, in 1964, which was in turn based on the Nuremberg Code. The latter was an outcome of the Nuremberg war crimes trials in 1947, in which 23 Nazi German physicians were found guilty of "performing medical experiments upon concentration camp inmates and other living human subjects, without their consent, in the course of which the defendants committed murders, brutalities, cruelties, tortures, atrocities, and other inhuman acts." The court prescribed guidelines for permissible medical experiments, including voluntary consent, benefits outweighing risks, and the ability of subjects to terminate participation. The 1996 revision of the Helsinki declaration from the 48th General Assembly states: "Concern for the interests of the subject must always prevail over the interests of science and society."

WHO established an international Research Ethics Review Committee and stated that "all research involving human participants must be conducted in an ethical manner that respects the dignity, safety and rights of research participants" (WHO, 2006). Most of the current ethical concerns revolve around vaccines, cloning, and HIV. Although WHO singles out children, adolescents, and women as vulnerable populations, it has said little about research ethics specific to older adults. At the UN-sponsored World Conference on Human Rights in Vienna in 1993, it was determined that "neither ageing as a process, nor older persons as a group, are specifically mentioned in the text of the Convention" (Loza, 2001, p. 72). Clearly, different cultural and political systems and values affect the ethics of research procedures (and related legislation) followed in specific countries. At the same time, there is a growing interest in the establishment of universal standards for the concept of international elder law (Doron, 2005).

In "smart house" environments, "Big Brother" issues are raised, because the elderly person is being monitored 24 hours a day, seven days a week. Rogers and Fisk (2010) asked their aware home participants how they felt about the compromise of their privacy by the technology in their home. Among the nearly 3,000 replies were the following comments (p. 650):

- "If this [monitoring system] would keep me independent longer, I wouldn't mind as much."
- "If it's only my daughter who monitors me, it's alright."
- "If you really need it, privacy becomes secondary."

Only 19% of the comments were about intrusiveness. (Incidentally, note that residents in nursing homes and even assisted-living arrangements already sacrifice a great deal of privacy.)

Euthanasia

Euthanasia is not specifically an aging issue, but it is often addressed in a death and dying unit at the end of gerontology courses and textbooks. Assisted suicide is still illegal in most of the United States. Indeed, the American Medical Association's (AMA's) Code of Medical Ethics says that "[p]hysician-assisted suicide is fundamentally incompatible with the physician's role as healer" (Freedman, 2015). However, since the second edition of this book was published, four states—Washington, Montana, Vermont, and California—have legalized physician-assisted suicide. In 2009, Washington reported 36 such incidents of suicides. Assisted suicide has also been legalized in some countries. In the Netherlands, in 1995 alone, 3,600 patients died via assisted suicide or euthanasia (Stern, 1998). In the field of bioethics, many view this trend as a slippery slope (Foley & Hendin, 2002). The most notorious proponent and conductor of assisted suicide, Jack Kevorkian, served a prison sentence from 1999 to 2007 for second-degree murder in the poisoning death of a 52-year-old man in Michigan. Dr. Kevorkian claimed to have assisted in the suicides of at least 130 other individuals. (Kevorkian himself died of thrombosis in 2011 at age 83.) Obviously, different countries, cultures, and religions have vastly differing views on euthanasia, but that is beyond the scope of this chapter.

INFLUENCES OF POLITICS, ECONOMICS, CULTURE, AND RELIGION

Ageism

Among the myriad topics covered in this book, one issue unique to the field of aging is *ageism*. Ageism is defined as "a process of systematic stereotyping and discrimination against people because they are old, just as racism and sexism accomplish this for skin color and gender" (Butler, 2006, p. 41). An entire *Encyclopedia of Ageism* (Palmore, Branch, & Harris, 2005) exists, with coverage of topics ranging from abuse to voice quality. For the purposes of this chapter, we consider whether ageism varies as a function of culture. Other than the United States, the encyclopedia entries cover only Japan. However, at least one study found ageism to be prevalent among British physicians (Young, 2006). Given that the awareness of ageism is relatively new in progressive countries (Butler, 1969; Palmore, 1990), it is likely to be widespread around the globe. Indeed, WHO claims that "[n]egative ageist attitudes are widely held across societies. . . . Research suggests that ageism may now be even more pervasive than sexism and racism. [Ageism] may also seriously impact the quality of health and social care that older people receive" (WHO, 2015, p. 11).

Elder Abuse

Elder abuse is an extreme version of ageism, involving both attitude and behavior. In the late 1970s, the issue of elder abuse and neglect began to receive more attention in the United States (Lantz, 2006). In 1999, the U.S. Administration on Aging published a report entitled the "National Elder Abuse Incidence Study," which "identified more than 550,000 elderly persons who experienced abuse or neglect in community or institutional settings." Such abuse is thought to be "an extremely underreported crime" (Lantz, 2006, pp. 352–353). Elder abuse in other cultures has also begun to receive more attention both from researchers and from government policy makers. For example, Chakraborti (2004) reported that widows, in particular, constitute a disproportionately large number of the elderly in Asia, because women in those cultures tend to marry men who are 10 to 15 years older than themselves. As a result, they "have to endure longer periods of widowhood. Their conditions are worsened by the fact that they are unable to fend for themselves." Even worse, "abandonment of elderly widows, even from educated families, is on the rise" (Chakraborti, 2004, pp. 26–27). WHO (2015) reported that "the prevalence of elder abuse in high- or middle-income countries ranged from 2.2% to 14%" (p. 74). The most common types of abuse were physical, sexual, psychological, financial, and neglect.

Culture

The experiences of older adults vary widely around the world, not only because of individual differences in biological and psychological aging, but also because the "frameworks of social beliefs and values" (Wilson, 2000, p. 17) vary dramatically across different cultures.

Research in many non-Western cultures is lacking. For example, regarding Asia:

> Although aging research has been well developed and well documented in Europe and other developed countries, including Japan, it has yet to take shape in most other parts of Asia. To a great extent the lack of interest in aging research in Asia owes its origin to the belief that the family support system is and will continue to be foolproof insurance against all the problems faced during old age. (Chakraborti, 2004, pp. 25–26)

Family Support for the Elderly

A long-standing American myth is that *The Waltons* (a 1970's television show in which an extended family, including parents, children, and grandparents, live under one roof) was once the norm, and that older adults are now relegated to a lonely incarceration in nursing homes.

In fact, only 3.1% of those aged 65 or older were residents of nursing homes in 2010 (West, Cole, Goodkind, & He, 2014). On the other hand, frequent feelings of loneliness are reported in roughly 10% of older adults—especially those who live alone (Hughes, 2006). In 2010, 28.3% of older adults lived alone, and due to higher widowhood, the ratio of women to men was almost 3 to 1 (West, Cole, Goodkind, & He, 2014).

Outside of America, "the family is an effective provider of old-age support in India and most other Asian countries" (Chakraborti, 2004, p. 26). In contrast to most countries in the Western world, where many programs have been developed specifically to support the needs of older adults, "many Asian countries have barely begun to think about their elderly; and given the pace of population aging in Asia and the corresponding lack of adjustment mechanisms, a 'time bomb' or 'age quake' may not be very far" (Chakraborti, 2004, p. 27). Chakraborti goes on to say that glaciers might provide a more appropriate metaphor for rapid aging, "since a glacier moves at a slow pace but with enormous effects wherever it goes and with a long-term momentum that is unstoppable" (p. 29).

Developed countries, mostly in Europe and North America, have established institutions for dealing with older adults' health needs, in contrast to Asian countries, where family-based support of the elderly is the norm. Between these two extreme scenarios, Australia provides an interesting comparison, having the distinction of "a European tradition and an Asian future" (Kendig & Quine, 2006, p. 431). Ninety percent of the Australian population is concentrated in coastal urban areas. (For an interesting analysis of growing old in cities, specifically New York, London, Paris, and Tokyo, see Rodwin & Gusmano, 2006.) Australia's population aging profile is similar to that of the United States, in which older adults are projected to constitute 18% of the total population by 2021. Also similar to the United States, more than 90% of older adults live in private households, with the remainder living in nursing homes or boarding houses in 1998 (Kendig & Quine, 2006). Among older adults with disabilities, 77% have "some informal support from family or friends," and 53% receive some "formal support" in the form of community or private services (Kendig & Quine, 2006, p. 433). Although Australia—unlike most Asian countries—has formal community services available, "children have strong values of family obligation for frail older parents who wish to remain independent" (Kendig & Quine, 2006, p. 434). Thus, Australia continues to provide a fascinating microcosm of the phenomenon of world population aging in the 21st century.

Respect and Status

Modernization theory—"a paradigm . . . to explain the diffusion of Western styles of individual, economic, and cultural development" (Achenbaum, 2006, p. 792)—has been applied to population aging. This theory predicts that "the status of elders . . . decline[s] with the degree of modernization" (Luborsky & McMullen, 1999, p. 83). Cowgill and Holmes (1972) found support for their modernization hypothesis by looking across 15 societies varying from preliterate to peasant to industrial. However, the relationship between cultural changes and the position of the elderly is quite complex, as revealed by a summary of 10 key propositions listed in Box 19-1.

BOX 19-1 Proposed Relationships Between Modernization and Aging

1. The concept of old age itself appears to be relative to the degree of modernization.

2. Longevity is directly and significantly related to the degree of modernization.

3. Modernized societies have a relatively high proportion of older people in their populations.

4. The aged are the recipients of greater respect in societies where they constitute a low proportion of the total population.

5. Societies that are in the process of modernizing tend to favor the young, while the aged are at an advantage in more stable, sedentary societies.

6. Respect for the aged tends to be greater in societies in which the extended family is prevalent, particularly if it functions as if they are part of the household unit. (The implication here is that modernization breaks down the extended family.)

7. In nonindustrial (developing) societies, the family is the basic social group providing economic security for dependent aged; in industrial societies, the responsibility tends to be partly or totally that of the state.

8. The proportion of aged who retain leadership roles in modern societies is lower than in industrial (developed) ones.

9. Religious leadership is more likely to be a continuing role of the aged in preindustrial societies than in modern societies.

10. Retirement is a modern invention found only in modernized, high-productivity societies.

Data from Holmes, E. R., & Holmes, L. (1995). *Other Cultures, Elder Years.* Thousand Oaks, CA: Sage.; Luborsky, M. R., & McMullen, C. K. (1999). Culture and aging. In J. C. Cavanaugh & S. K. Whitbourne (Eds.), *Gerontology: An Interdisciplinary Perspective* (pp. 65–90). New York, NY: Oxford University Press.

In the Jewish religion, there is great respect for older adults, regardless of the culture where the Jews are living. Instead of 65, the operational definition of elder (*zaken* in Hebrew, which also means "wise") is age 70 and older. For example, Jewish law specifies that one should stand up when anyone 70 years old enters a room. In practice, children in religiously observant homes (i.e., Orthodox Jewish) stand up when either their parents or any other older person enters a room. In Israel, children and teenagers have been observed to leap to their feet to offer their seat on the bus to an older adult. This kind of respect is also true of many other religions and cultures, but even when this tenet is observed, does it translate into a lack of prejudice and discrimination in milieus such as the workplace, or treatment of patients? Unfortunately, respect for elders is not a characteristic of all cultures. For example, in India, it is not uncommon for older widows to be abandoned by their families (Chakraborti, 2004).

Cognitive Neuroscience and Aging

Cognitive neuroscience issues in aging and culture have begun to receive some attention (Han et al., 2013; Park & Gutchess, 2006). Although the basic neurological and psychological mechanisms of perception, memory, and cognition—which by and large are affected negatively by normal aging—would not be expected to vary across cultures, some unusual phenomena (e.g., picture naming as a measure of semantic memory [Mitchell, 1989]) have been explored across different languages and cultures (Yoon, Feinberg, & Gutchess, 2006). Indeed, one study found a positive correlation between attitude toward aging and explicit memory performance; older Chinese persons had both a more positive attitude and higher memory scores compared to a group of older Americans (Levy & Langer, 1994). Even something as fundamental as hearing loss (a ubiquitous aging phenomenon) has been found to be correlated with negative attitudes about hearing held by older adults ages 70 to 96 themselves (Levy, Slade, & Gill, 2006).

Aging Phenomena in South America

In South American countries, more attention is being focused on the lives of older women (Loza, 2001) who have disproportionate illiteracy rates and suffer from poverty and loneliness (Gragnolati, Jorgensen, Rocha, & Fruttero, 2011). In Brazil, researchers have documented dramatic differences in aging cultures as a function of socioeconomic status, meaning those who are marginalized versus the well-to-do "self-sufficient" (Leibing & Py, 2005). Leibing (2005) examined historical changes in Brazilian culture and attitudes spanning from 1967 to 2002. Her investigation revealed a shift from an emphasis on old age to a "third age" label. Leibing describes third age as a phase between adulthood and old age, in which successful aging involves the "empowerment of elderly persons by fighting against aging stereotypes and for better living conditions" (2005, p. 18). This phenomenon was epitomized by Fernanda Montenegro, considered by many to be Brazil's most talented actress, who was nominated for an Academy Award at age 70. Although Montenegro called herself "the old lady from Ipanema" (Tom Jobim & Vinicius de Morae's song, "Garota de Ipanema") and did not try to conceal the visible effects of aging ("prominent wrinkles"), Leibing's analysis still portrays a class of people who use fame and financial power to transcend a more traditional life course (i.e., avoiding superficial signs of aging). Although positive aging stereotypes are welcome, in Brazil, it is only the rich and the famous who can afford to continue fighting and spending in the "struggle against becoming old" (Leibing, 2005, p. 22). In a country with significant poverty, the beautiful old lady is the exception, not the rule.

Religious Lifestyle in Israel

Bnei Brak, Israel's most religious city (Rosenblum, 2001), was found to have the highest global life expectancy in 2001: 81.1 years for women and 77.4 years for men (up to 83.9 and 80.3 in 2012). What is most interesting about this small city's longevity record is that life is long in spite of other demographics: Bnei Brak is also Israel's poorest city, confounding the normal correlation between poverty and poor health (Rosenblum, 2001). In addition, the Orthodox Jewish residents are known neither for engaging in exercise nor for maintaining a low-fat diet. The most likely formula for long life in this community appears to be a highly engaged level of religious enthusiasm. Although the conclusions are not unequivocal, a majority of studies investigating the relationship between religious practice/spirituality and health and psychological well-being have discovered a positive correlation (Lawler-Row & Elliott, 2009; Schaie, Krause, & Booth, 2004).

In Israel, a very exhaustive study ($N = 3,900$ over a 16-year period) compared 11 religious versus 11 secular *kibbutzim* (best translated as egalitarian collectives). It was found that the mortality rate in the religious groups (3.9%) was less than of that in the secular groups (9.1%) (Kark et al., 1996). The authors ruled out potential confounds due to a variety of sociodemographic variables, including education, ethnic origin, and social support. The only explanation remaining was an "embracing protective effect of religious observance" (p. 346).

It will be interesting to see future studies of this relationship in other cultures around the world. To date, very few international or cross-national studies have been published (Schaie, Krause, & Booth, 2004). In one notable exception (Musick, Traphagan, Koenig, & Larson, 2000), researchers compared religious and spiritual practices in the United States with those in Japan and found a very different perspective on the relationship between spirituality and health. Older religious Japanese "employ religious activity in an attempt to avoid a decline into poor health as they grow older," including visits to *pokkuridera* (sudden death temples), "at which they pray for a sudden, peaceful, death devoid of excessive suffering" (p. 84).

Forecast: "The Crossing"

Demographers and gerontologists are projecting that an "unprecedented shift will occur between 2015 and 2020, when the percentage of older people . . . in the global population will surpass the percentage of the very young" (children under 5) for the first time in history (see Figure 19-13). This "crossing" occurred in the United States in the late 1960s (West, Cole, Goodkind, & He, 2014, p. 20).

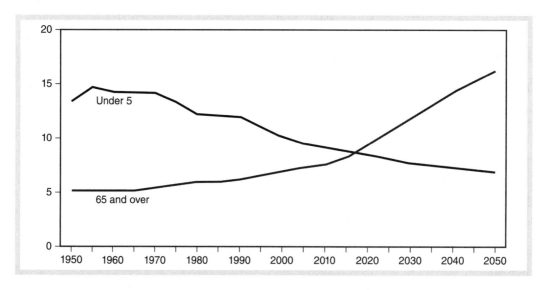

FIGURE 19-13 Percentage of World Population under Age 5 and 65 and Over: 1950 to 2050
From World Population Prospects: The 2010 Revision, Medium Fertility Variant (Updated: 28 June 2011). United Nations, Department of Economic and Social Affairs, Population Division, Population Estimates and Projections Section, © 2011 United Nations. Reprinted with the permission of the United Nations.

CONCLUSION

Biologist Élie Metchnikoff said, "Old age is not a disease and cannot be cured." Although Metchnikoff published his insights over a century ago(1912), only a few biologists and even fewer gerontologists have grasped this message (Hayflick, 2006). According to Hayflick (2007), the best strategy at our disposal for slowing the rate of aging is to promote good health. Or, as many gerontologists have said—in light of some of the medical advances that can keep a person alive longer via artificial means—our goal should not be to add years to life, but rather, to add "life to years" (i.e., to improve people's health and decrease the proportion of old age spent in morbidity). James Fries (2006) has called for health policy promoting the compression of morbidity by shortening the period "between an increasing average age of the onset of disability and the age of death" (p. 257). This is certainly a worthwhile goal to pursue globally, particularly in developing countries.

Study Questions

1. Describe and give examples of ageism worldwide. How does ageism affect the life of older adults?
2. Describe the unique characteristics of the oldest-old.
3. Compare and contrast the influences of religion, politics, and culture on the aging adult worldwide.
4. Give examples of legal and ethical issues related to the older adult.

Case Study: Ageism

Dr. Robert Butler, a physician who founded the National Institute on Aging in the United States, related the following incident involving a centenarian friend. His 100-year-old friend had a pain in his left knee, so he went to see his internist about it. After examining the patient, the doctor concluded that it was just "old age." Dr. Butler's friend retorted, "But doc, my right knee is also 100 years old, and it doesn't hurt!" In this case, the physician's lack of knowledge (or at least inadequate diagnosis) resulted in a fairly benign outcome, although the patient's left knee did not receive treatment. However, it is difficult to imagine a 25-year-old being told that an ailment was the result of "youth."

Dr. Kevin Hendler specializes in geriatric dentistry at Emory Healthcare in Atlanta, Georgia, and related the following incident (Hendler, 2005). A 97-year-old woman presented with the need for some dental work. The patient and her family were not very enthusiastic about dental work, assuming that the older lady did not have much longer to live anyway, given her age. Dr. Hendler convinced her to go ahead with the dental work, and the lady went on to live to the age of 108. Imagine how different the last 11 years of her life would have been without the ability to chew food. If this dentist had succumbed to ageism, his patient would have lost many years of normal eating. At the other end of the life span, no one would suggest depriving a growing child of 11 years of normal life. As Dr. Hendler emphasizes, "Treatment decisions by patients or family members should not be based solely on the number that represents age, but rather on health and quality of life" (personal communication, September 22, 2006). Older patients who decided not to have recommended dental work have subsequently told him that had they known they would live so long, they would have done things differently. Sometimes patients tell Dr. Hendler, "I don't know how much longer I have," and he replies, "That's right, you don't know, so you should be comfortable because it may be a while" (personal communication, September 22, 2006). Sometimes patients in their 70s will say they do not want better treatment because they will not need it for very long; Dr. Hendler's reply is, "How do you know?"

Another Atlanta dentist related a similar experience. Dr. Edward Berger treated Iva for more than 30 years. Iva taught Dr. Berger a lesson in avoiding ageism.

> At the age of 91½, she presented with a lower premolar sheared off to the gum line. I explained that the tooth was hopeless and needed to be extracted. She asked what else needed to be done. I examined her bite and watched her talk, and explained that nothing needed to be done. The teeth would not shift dramatically, and her bite would not change significantly. The missing tooth was hardly noticeable when she talked. I felt that if the missing tooth showed a bit to others . . . who should really care at her age. She said "Wow that sounds great," but then, "Wait Dr. Berger—what would you do if the same thing happened to your exact tooth in your mouth?" I replied that I would have a dental implant and a crown. "Really Dr. Berger," she replied. "You do realize that you did not present that option to me? Do you think that I have one foot stuck in the ground?" I apologized and admitted that I took her age into consideration. She replied to X-ray her teeth but never ever X-ray her age or desire to be whole. "Now Dr. Berger," she continued, "you have just established that I have a very limited time on the planet Earth. I must be seen today by your oral surgeon."
>
> I called one of my favorite oral surgeons, and explained that I had just stepped into mud with a patient and needed a huge favor. I asked him what was the oldest patient that he had placed a dental implant in their jaw bone. He had recently placed one in a 67-year-old. I asked "how about a 91-year- old?" He asked if this was joke. I said no, and that she needed to be seen today. He offered 2 pm and she took it. He removed the old root and placed an artificial tooth root (a dental implant). After seeing her, he told me that she was a "spitfire,"and predicted that she would live to be 100. When she was 92, I finished the job by placing a crown on her implant. Iva did indeed live another 8 years until the age of 100. I have never X-rayed another patient's age or desire again.

(Edward Berger, personal communication, August 23, 2015).

These cases provide only a few concrete examples of how attitudes toward the elderly can make an enormous difference. Unfortunately, hundreds of studies (684 citations in a 2015 MEDLINE search) reveal that ageism is alive and well among health professionals. Dr. John Young (2006), head of the Academic Unit of Elderly Care and Rehabilitation at St. Luke's Hospital in England, writes that institutionalized ageism in his country is endemic, based on a number of recent medical studies. For example, a population-based study found that patients older than the age of 80 with minor stroke and transient ischemic attacks were under-referred and undertreated (Fairhead & Rothwell, 2006). "Institutional ageism" has also been reported in the realm of anesthesia (White, 2014). Nevertheless, Dr. Young expresses hope for the future, as the "UK government has recently been embarrassed into action" (Young, 2006, p. 509). Mortality rates from heart disease and cancer declined in the United Kingdom after a policy initiative called the National Service Framework for Older People was established. Perhaps other governments around the world will follow suit in the 21st century.

Case Study Questions

1. Give three reasons why physicians and dentists may lack the motivation to do an intervention based on the advanced age of the patient.
2. If a physician or dentist declined giving an elderly relative of yours an intervention based on the patient's age, what could you do to help reverse that decision?

References

Achenbaum, W. A. (2006). Modernization theory. In R. Schulz (Ed.), *The Encyclopedia of Aging* (4th ed., Vol. II, pp. 792–794). New York: Springer.

Allard, M., Lèbre, V., & Robine, J.-M. (1998). *Jeanne Calment: From Van Gogh's Time to Ours: 122 Extraordinary Years* (B. Coupland, Trans.). New York: W. H. Freeman.

Arking, R. (2006). *The Biology of Aging: Observations and Principles* (3rd ed.). New York: Oxford University Press.

Azevedo, R, Bernardes, M., Fonseca, J., & Lima, A. (2015). Smartphone application for rheumatoid arthritis self-management: Cross-sectional study revealed the usefulness, willingness to use and patients' needs. *Rheumatology International, 35*, 1675–1685.

Browning, R. (1942). Rabbi Ben Ezra. In P. Loving (Ed.). *The Selected Poems of Robert Browning* (pp. 260–266). Roslyn, NY: Walter J. Black.

Bruss, P., & Mitchell, D. (2009). Memory systems, processes, and tasks: Taxonomic clarification via factor analysis. *American Journal of Psychology, 122*, 175–189.

Butler, R. N. (1969). Ageism: Another form of bigotry. *Gerontologist, 9*, 243–246.

Butler, R. N. (2006). Ageism. In R. Schulz (Ed.), *The Encyclopedia of Aging* (4th ed., Vol. I, pp. 41–42). New York: Springer.

Carnes, B., Olshansky, S., & Hayflick, L. (2013). Can human biology allow most of us to become centenarians? *Journals of Gerontology: Biological Sciences, 68*(2), 136–142. doi:10.1093/gerona/gls142

Chakraborty, R. D. (2004). *The Greying of India: Population Ageing in the Context of Asia*. New Delhi: Sage.

Clark, E. (1995). *Growing Old Is Not for Sissies II: Portraits of Senior Athletes*. Rohnert Park, CA: Pomegranate Artbooks.

Cowgill, D. O., & Holmes, L. D. (1972). *Aging and Modernization*. New York: Appleton-Century-Crofts.

Czaja, S. J., Charness, N., Fisk, A. D., Hertzog, C., Nair, S. N., Rogers, W. A., & Sharit, J. (2006). Factors predicting the use of technology: Findings from the Center for Research and Education on Aging and Technology Enhancement (CREATE). *Psychology and Aging, 21*, 333–352.

Doron, I. (2005). From national to international elder law. *Journal of International Aging, Law, & Policy, 1*, 43–67.

Duenwald, M. (2003, January). Puzzle of the century. *Smithsonian*, 73–80.

Fairhead, J. F., & Rothwell, P. M. (2006). Underinvestigation and treatment of carotid disease in elderly patients with transient ischaemic attack and stroke: Comparative population based study. *British Medical Journal, 333*, 525–534.

Fazio, S., & Mitchell, D. B. (2015). Self-preservation in individuals with Alzheimer's disease: Empirical evidence and the role of the social environment. In C. Dick-Muehlke, R. Li, & M. Orleans (Eds.), *Psychosocial Studies of the Individual's Changing Perspective in Alzheimer's Disease* (pp. 183–207). Hershey, PA: IGI Global.

Fernández-Ballesteros, R., Garcia, L. F., Abarca, D., Blanc, E., Efklides, A., Moraitou, D., . . . Patricia, S. (2010). The concept of "ageing well" in ten Latin American and European countries. *Ageing & Society, 30,* 41–56.

File, T. (2013). Computer and Internet use in the United States. *Current Population Survey Reports,* P20-568. Washington, D.C.: U.S. Census Bureau.

Foley, K., & Hendin, H. (Eds.). (2002). *The Case Against Assisted Suicide: For the Right to End-of-Life Care.* Baltimore, MD: Johns Hopkins University Press.

Freedman, J. L. (2015). *Death with dignity?* Retrieved from http:// www.aish.com/ci/sam/Death-with-Dignity .html?s=mm.

Fries, J. F. (2006). Compression of morbidity. In R. Schulz (Ed.), *The Encyclopedia of Aging* (4th ed., Vol. I, pp. 257–259). New York: Springer.

Goodman, S. (2014, December 6). How many people live to 100 across the globe? *The Centenarian.* Retrieved from http://www.thecentenarian.co.uk/how-many-people-live-to-hundred-across-the-globe.html

Gragnolati, M., Jorgensen, O. H., Rocha, R., & Fruttero, A. (2011). *Growing Old in Older Brazil.* Washington, DC: The World Bank.

Greenberg, S. (2005). *A profile of older Americans 2005.* Retrieved from http://www.aoa.gov/AoAroot/Aging_ Statistics/Profile/2005/index.aspx

Greenberg, S. (2010). *A profile of older Americans: 2010.* Retrieved from http://www.aoa.gov/aoaroot/aging_ statistics/Profile/2010/docs/2010profile.pdf

Han, S., Northoff, G., Vogeley, K., Wexler, B., Kitayama, S., & Varnum, M. (2013). A cultural neuroscience approach to the biosocial nature of the human brain. *Annual Review of Psychology, 64,* 335–359. doi:10.1146/ annurev-psych-071112-054629

Haub, C. (2006). *2006 world population data sheet.* Retrieved from http://www.prb.org

Haub, C., & Kent, M. M. (2008). The 2008 world population data sheet. Washington, DC: PRB.

Hayflick, L. (1996). *How and Why We Age.* New York: Ballantine Books.

Hayflick, L. (2006). La dolce vita versus la vita sobria. *The Gerontologist, 46,* 413–416.

Hayflick, L. (2007). Biological aging is no longer an unsolved problem. *Annals of New York Academy of Science, 1100,* 1–13.

He, W., Sengupta, M., Velkoff, V. A., & DeBarros, K. A. (2005). *65+ in the United States: 2005.* Washington, DC: U.S. Census Bureau.

Helping elderly stay at home. (2006, November 6). *Howick and Pakuranga Times* (New Zealand).

Hendler, K. (2005, June). *The relationship between oral health and general health: New research in health maintenance and promotion.* Paper presented at the Consortium on Active Retirement and Aging, Kennesaw State University, Kennesaw, GA.

High, D., & Doole, M. (1995). Ethical and legal issues in conducting research involving elderly subjects. *Behavioral Sciences and the Law, 13,* 319–335.

Holmes, E. R., & Holmes, L. (1995). *Other Cultures, Elder Years.* Thousand Oaks, CA: Sage.

Howden, L. M., & Meyer, J. A. (2011). *Age and Sex Composition: 2010.* Washington, DC: U.S. Census Bureau.

Hughes, M. E. (2006). Loneliness. In R. Schulz (Ed.), *The Encyclopedia of Aging* (4th ed., Vol. II, pp. 674–675). New York: Springer.

Kark, J. D., Shemi, G., Friedlander, Y., Martin, O., Manor, O., & Blondheim, S. H. (1996). Does religious observance promote health? Mortality in secular vs. religious kibbutzim in Israel. *American Journal of Public Health, 86,* 341–346.

Kastenbaum, R. (2006). Gerontology. In R. Schulz (Ed.), *The Encyclopedia of Aging* (4th ed., Vol. I, pp. 460–461). New York: Springer.

Keenan, T. A. (2009). *Internet use among midlife and older adults.* Retrieved from http://assets.aarp.org/rgcenter/ general/bulletin_internet_09.pdf

Kendig, H., & Quine, S. (2006). Community services for older people in Australia. In H. Yoon & J. Hendricks (Eds.), *Handbook of Asian Aging* (pp. 431–451). Amityville, NY: Baywood.

Kinsella, K., & Phillips, D. R. (2005). Global aging: The challenge of success. *Population Bulletin, 60*(1), 3–42.

Landers, S. H. (2006). Home care: A key to the future of family medicine? *Annals of Family Medicine, 4,* 366–368.

Lantz, M. S. (2006). Elder abuse and neglect. In R. Schulz (Ed.), *The Encyclopedia of Aging* (4th ed., Vol. I, pp. 352–355). New York: Springer.

Lawler-Row, K. A. & Elliott, J. (2009). The role of religious activity and spirituality in the health and well-being of older adults. *Journal of Health Psychology, 14,* 43–52.

Lee, C., & Coughlin, J. F. (2015). Older adults' adoption of technology: An integrated approach to identifying determinants and barriers. *Journal of Product Innovation Management, 32,* 747–759.

Leibing, A. (2005). The old lady from Ipanema: Changing notions of old age in Brasil. *Journal of Aging Studies, 19,* 15–31.

Leibing, A., & Py, L. (2005). The new old: Aging and gerontology in Brasil. *AGHExchange, 28*(3), 1–19.

Levy, B., & Langer, E. (1994). Aging free from negative stereotypes: Successful memory in China and among the American deaf. *Journal of Personality and Social Psychology, 66,* 989–997.

Levy, B. R., Slade, M. D., & Gill, T. M. (2006). Hearing decline predicted by elders' stereotypes. *Journal of Gerontology: Psychological Sciences, 61B,* P82–P87.

Loza, M. D. (2001). Ageing in transition: Situation of older women in Latin America region. In United Nations Programme on Aging (Ed.), *The World Ageing Situation: Exploring a Society for All Ages* (pp. 70–98). New York: United Nations.

Luborsky, M. R., & McMullen, C. K. (1999). Culture and aging. In J. C. Cavanaugh & S. K. Whitbourne (Eds.), *Gerontology: An Interdisciplinary Perspective* (pp. 65–90). New York: Oxford University Press.

Lutz, W., Sanderson, W., & Scherbov, S. (2008). The coming acceleration of global population ageing. *Nature, 451,* 716–719.

Maddox, G. L. (1994). Social and behavioural research on ageing: An agenda for the United States. *Ageing and Society, 14,* 97–107.

Metchnikoff, É. (1912). *The Prolongation of Life: Optimistic Studies* (P. C. Mitchell, Trans.). New York: G. P. Putnam's Sons & Knickerbocker Press.

Mitchell, D. B. (1989). How many memory systems? Evidence from aging. *Journal of Experimental Psychology: Learning, Memory, and Cognition, 15,* 31–49.

Mitchell, D. B., & Schmitt, F. A. (2006). Short- and long-term implicit memory in aging and Alzheimer's disease. *Aging, Neuropsychology, and Cognition, 13,* 611–635.

Mitzner, T. L., McBride, S. E., Barg-Warlow, L., & Rogers, W. A. (2013). Self-management of wellness and illness in an aging population. *Reviews of Human Factors and Ergonomics, 8,* 277–333.

Morgan, R. (2006, August). The medium is still the message. *Observer, 19,* 21–24.

Mundorf, N., Mundorf, J., & Brownell, W. (2006). Communication technologies and older adults. In R. Schulz (Ed.), *The Encyclopedia of Aging* (4th ed., Vol. I, pp. 242–247). New York: Springer.

Murray, C. J. et al. (2015, August 27). Global, regional, and national disability-adjusted life years (DALYs) for 306 diseases and injuries and healthy life expectancy (HALE) for 188 countries, 1990–2013: Quantifying the epidemiological transition. *Lancet.* doi 10.1016/S0140-6736(15)61340-X

Musick, M. A., Traphagan, J. W., Koenig, H. G., & Larson, D. B. (2000). Spirituality in physical health and aging. *Journal of Adult Development, 7,* 73–86.

National Centenarians Project. (2014). Retrieved from: http://www.adlercentenarians.org/

National Institute on Aging. (2011). *Global health and aging.* Retrieved from https://www.nia.nih.gov/research/publication/global-health-and-aging/

Nesselroade, J. R. (2001). Individual differences. In G. L. Maddox (Ed.), *The Encyclopedia of Aging* (3rd ed., Vol. I, pp. 532–533). New York: Springer.

New health statistics show Americans living longer. (2011, March 17). Retrieved from http://uk.reuters.com/article/2011/03/17/us-statistics-idUKTRE72G00P20110317

Palmore, E. (1990). *Ageism*. New York: Springer.

Palmore, E. (1998). *The Facts on Aging Quiz* (2nd ed.). New York: Springer.

Palmore, E., Branch, L., & Harris, D. K. (Eds.). (2005). *Encyclopedia of Ageism*. Binghamton, NY: Haworth Pastoral Press.

Park, D., & Gutchess, A. (2006). The cognitive neuroscience of aging and culture. *Current Directions in Psychological Science, 15*, 105–108.

Perls, T. T. (2004). The oldest old. *Scientific American Special Edition, 14*(3), 6–11.

Perls, T. T., & Silver, M. H. (1999). *Living to 100: Lessons in Living to Your Maximum Potential at Any Age.* New York: Basic Books.

Phillipson, C. (2013). *Ageing*. Cambridge, UK: Polity Press.

Pruchno, R. (2015). Successful aging: Contentious past, productive future. *Gerontologist, 55*, 1–4.

Riggs, K. E. (2004). *Granny@work: Aging and New Technology on the Job in America.* New York: Routledge.

Rockwood, K. (2006). Geriatric medicine. In R. Schulz (Ed.), *The Encyclopedia of Aging* (4th ed., Vol. I, pp. 452–455). New York: Springer.

Rodwin, V. G., & Gusmano, M. K. (2006). *Growing Older In World Cities: New York, London, Paris, and Tokyo.* Nashville, TN: Vanderbilt University Press.

Rogers, W. A., & Fisk, A. D. (2010). Toward a psychological science of advanced technology design for older adults. *Journal of Gerontology: Psychological Sciences, 65B*, 645–653.

Rosenblum, J. (2001, February 16). L'chaim in BneiBrak. *Jerusalem Post*.

Rowe, J. W., & Kahn, R. L. (1987). Human aging: Usual and successful. *Science, 237*, 143–149.

Schaie, K. W., Krause, N., & Booth, A. (Eds.).(2004). *Religious Influences on Health and Well-being in the Elderly.* New York: Springer.

Stern, Y. (1998, March). Hospice care: Can it have a Jewish heart? *Jewish Observer*, 21–25.

Tae-gyu, K. (2006, November 6). Robot maids for elderly to make debut in 2013. *Korea Times*.

Tsai, H. Y. S., Shillair, R., Cotten, S. R., Winstead, V., & Yost, E. (2015). Getting grandma online: Are tablets the answer for increasing digital inclusion for older adults in the U.S.? *Educational Gerontology, 41*, 695–709.

United Nations. (2002). *World Populations Ageing: 1950–2050*: United Nations publication, Sales No. E.02. XIII.3.

United Nations Programme on Aging. (2001). A society for all ages: Evolution and exploration. In United Nations Programme on Aging (Ed.), *The World Ageing Situation: Exploring a Society for All Ages* (pp. 1–12). New York: United Nations.

University of Georgia, Institute of Gerontology, College of Public Health. (2006). *Georgia centenarian study*. Retrieved from http://www.publichealth.uga.edu/geron/research/centenarian-study

U.S. life expectancy up to 77.6. (2005, March 1). *Boston Globe*, p. 1.

Vaupel, J. W., & Jeune, B. (1995). The emergence and proliferation of centenarians. In B. Jeune & J. Vaupel (Eds.), *Exceptional Longevity: From Prehistory to the Present.* Odense, Denmark: Odense University Press.

West, L., Cole, S., Goodkind, D., & He, H. (2014). *65+ in the United States: 2010.* Washington, DC: U.S. Government Printing Office.

White, S. M. (2014). Ethical and legal aspects of anaesthesia for the elderly. *ANAESTHESIA, 69*, 45–53.

Wilson, G. (2000). *Understanding Old Age: Critical and Global Perspectives.* London: Sage.

World Health Organization. (2006). *Research ethics review committee.* Retrieved from http://www.who.int/rpc/research_ethics/en

World Health Organization. (2015). *World Report on Ageing and Health.* Luxembourg.

Yoon, C., Feinberg, F., & Gutchess, A. H. (2006). Pictorial naming specificity across ages and cultures: A latent class analysis of picture norms for younger and older Americans and Chinese. *Gerontology, 52*, 295–305.

Young, J. (2006). Ageism in services for transient ischaemic attack and stroke. *British Medical Journal, 333*, 507–508.

Footnotes

* Support for the preparation and writing of this chapter was provided by a grant from the WellStar College of Health and Human Services and a Fulbright Award. Thanks to Deborah Garfin for her unswerving logistical support.

1. Various terms are used to differentiate national developments. In the United Nations usage, "more developed," "developed," and "industrialized" refer to countries in Europe and North America, and to Australia, New Zealand, and Japan. All other countries are referred to as "less developed," "developing," and "nonindustrialized" (Kinsella & Phillips, 2005). The terms "less developed" and "more developed" are used in this chapter.

2. The Gerontological Research Group, which includes Dr. Thomas Perls, director of the New England Centenarian Study (Perls, 2004), maintains a carefully validated list of supercentenarians, defined as anyone who has lived to be 110 years old or older. Boomgaard, Pouder, and Thiers top this list, which includes supercentenarians born in 29 different countries.

SECTION **IV**

WORLDWIDE HEALTH ISSUES AND TRENDS BY SPECIFIC COUNTRY

20

A Unique Perspective on Health Care in Panama

Larry Purnell

Objectives

After reading this chapter, the reader will be able to:

1. Compare and contrast the cultural background, history, economics, and geography of the people of the Republic of Panama and their relationships to health and health care.
2. Relate the status of technology and transportation to health care in Panama.
3. Compare and contrast the significant infectious diseases within Panama, such as hantavirus pulmonary syndrome (HPS), malaria, Chagas disease, chikungunya fever, dengue fever, leishmaniasis, filariasis, and yellow fever.
4. Describe the traditional practitioners and the use of herbal medicine among the indigenous people of Panama.
5. Describe ethical issues in health care in Panama.

OVERVIEW

To understand the healthcare system and health care in the Republic of Panama, one must be knowledgeable about (1) the people and their heritages, (2) the unique topography and biocultural ecology of the country, (3) the history of the Panama Canal, and (4) the relationship of Panama with the United States and other countries. The republic is a mixture of cosmopolitanism and traditionalism, wealth and poverty, advanced allopathic medicine and traditional medicine, biodiversity, and multiculturalism.

The Republic of Panama (Panama means "plenty of fish") is located on the narrowest and lowest part of the S-shaped Isthmus of Panama that links North America and South America. Panama is slightly smaller than South Carolina, approximately 77,082 kilometers^2 (km^2

[29,761 miles^2 or mi^2]). The country's two coastlines are the Caribbean on the north and the Pacific on the south. To the east is Colombia and to the west is Costa Rica. The highest point in the country, Volcán Barú near the Costa Rican border, rises to almost 3,500 meters (m [11,483 feet or ft]). The lowest elevation is in the middle of the country where the Panama Canal crosses. The estimated 2014 population of 3.6 million has a growth rate of 1.35%. The capital, Panama City, is home to one-third of the population. Overall, 75% of the population is considered urban. The unit of currency is the balboa, which is equal to the U.S. dollar. Balboas are available only in coins; otherwise, Panama uses the U.S. dollar. Spanish is the official language, although the U.S. influence in the Canal Zone reinforces the use of English as a second language by 14% of the population. November 3 is celebrated as the official date of independence from Colombia; the country's independence was won from Spain in 1821.

Panama is divided into nine provinces and three provincial-level *comarcas,* which are similar to reserves. Each province is somewhat unique in its history, culture, and lifestyle. The more than 350 San Blas Islands, located near Colombia, are strung out for more than 160 km along the sheltered Caribbean coastline. Other principal islands are those of the Archipiélago de las Perlas in the middle of the Gulf of Panama, the penal colony on the Isla de Coiba in the Gulf of Chiriquí, and the decorative island of Taboga, a tourist attraction that can be seen from Panama City. In all, some 1,000 islands are found off the Pacific coast of Panama. Many of the islands have little if any modern services in terms of health care and technology.

Panama has a tropical climate. Temperatures are uniformly high, as is the relative humidity, with little seasonal variation. Diurnal ranges are low; on a typical day during the dry season in the capital city, the early morning minimum may be 24°C (75°F) and the afternoon maximum 29°C (84°F). The temperature seldom exceeds 32°C (90°F) for more than a short time. Temperatures are markedly cooler in the mountain ranges in western Panama, where frosts occur. Panama's tropical environment supports an abundance of plants. Forests dominate, interrupted by grasslands, scrub, and crops. Although nearly 40% of Panama is still wooded, deforestation is a continuing threat to the rain-drenched woodlands.

Almost 500 rivers traverse Panama, with many originating as highland streams. The Río Chagres, one of the longest rivers, was dammed to create Gatun Lake, which forms a major part of the transit route between the locks near each end of the Panama Canal.

TRANSPORTATION

The only fully functioning railroad has been restored and runs from Colon to Panama City. More than 9,535 km (5,925 mi) of roads twine through Panama. The Pan-American Highway, running from Costa Rica through Panama, ends in Darien. Existing roads do not connect from Darien into Colombia. Sixty percent of the roadways are unpaved and not passable during parts of the rainy season. Of 107 airports, only 57 are paved. One international airport, Tocumen, is sited near Panama City. Buses are available between all major cities throughout Panama. Inexpensive intracity bus lines are available but are not yet sufficient to meet the needs of outlying areas.

PEOPLE OF PANAMA

Panama has long enjoyed a measure of ethnic diversity, which has given rise to a number of distinct subcultures. Most Panamanians view their society as composed of three principal groups: the Spanish-speaking Roman Catholic mestizo majority, the English-speaking Protestant Antillean blacks, and indigenous Indians. The racial and ethnic divisions are 70% mestizo (mixed Amerindian and white), 14% West Indian (Amerindian and mixed), 10% white Spanish, and 6% Amerindian. Included in these groups are Chinese, Middle Easterners, Swiss, Yugoslavian, and North American immigrants; all have contributed to the multiculturalism of Panama. Only 7.6% of the population is older than 65 years and 27.4% is younger than 14 years. Panama has a young population, with a median age of 27.2 years.

Panama is increasingly becoming a country for retirees, especially U.S. citizens who are mostly former Canal Zone employees. Small groups of Hispanic blacks (*playeros*) and Hispanic Indians (*cholos*) live along the Atlantic coast lowlands and in Darién. Their settlements date from the colonial era and are concentrated along waterways. They rely on farming and raising livestock that have adapted to the tropical forest environment.

The Cuna, also referred to as the Kuna, are concentrated mainly along the Caribbean coast, on the San Blas Islands, which are small coral islands. The largest of these islands, Aligandí, is only 32 acres (13 hectares). Only native Kuna are allowed on the island overnight and only with prior permission from their independent government. Kuna homes are made with cane walls and guava-thatched roofs. Bathroom facilities are a short walk to the end of piers where outdoor toilets have the Atlantic Ocean as their automatic flushing system. Fresh water is piped from the mainland. In addition, a small number of Kuna are scattered in the remote mountains of western Panama and the interior of Darién.

The Bribri, part of the Talamanca tribe of Costa Rica, have substantial contact with outsiders. Many are employed on banana plantations. The Bókatá live in eastern Bocas del Toro and have little exposure to outsiders. Since the early 1980s, a small dirt road has served the area, though it is passable only in dry weather. The Chocó (or Embera) occupy the southeastern portion of Darién along the border with Colombia. Most are bilingual in Spanish and Chocó.

All tribes are under the jurisdiction of both the provincial and national governments. The indigenous policy section of the Ministry of Government and Justice bears primary responsibility for coordinating programs that affect Indians. The 1972 constitution required the government to establish reserves (*comarcas*) for indigenous tribes, but the extent to which this mandate had been implemented varies. Most settlements of any size have a primary school; a few also have secondary schools. With a stress on education for all people, secondary schools are increasing.

Urban society includes virtually all members of the elite. Centered mainly in Panama City, this group comprises old families of Spanish descent and newer families of immigrants. More established families think of themselves as aristocracy from birth. Newer families have less prestige and social status. Until the dominance of General Omar Torrijos, whose power base was the National Guard, an oligarchy of older elite families virtually controlled the country's politics under the auspices of the Liberal Party. Politics is considered the quintessential career for a young man of elite background. The old, aristocratic families have long provided the republic's presidents, cabinet ministers, and members of the legislature. Older elite families are closely interrelated and in the past were careful to avoid racially mixed unions.

Antillean blacks have had little success in attaining elite status, even when wealthy; however, Spanish-speaking Roman Catholic blacks are able to gain acceptance. An increasing degree of admixture with mestizo and more recent immigrants has been occurring in recent years, as many such families enter the elite and intermarry with members of the older families. Commercial success has become a substitute for an illustrious family background—a phenomenon acknowledged in the popular saying "Money whitens everyone."

Panama's middle socioeconomic class is predominantly mestizo. Like the elite, the middle class is largely urban, although many small cities and towns of the interior have their own middle-class families. Middle-class parents make great sacrifices to send their children to the best schools possible. Young men are encouraged to acquire a profession, and young women are steered toward office jobs in government or business. In contrast with the elite, the middle class views teaching and nursing as respected occupations for a young woman.

Ethnically, the lower socioeconomic classes have three principal components: mestizo migrants from the countryside, children and grandchildren of Antillean blacks, and Hispanicized blacks who are descendants of former slaves. The split between blacks and the rest of the populace is particularly marked. Although some social mixing and intermarriage occurs, religious and cultural differences tend to isolate Panama's black population. As a group, they are gradually becoming more Hispanicized, but the first generation usually remains oriented toward its Caribbean origins. The second and third generations are under North American influence through exposure to U.S. citizens in the Canal Zone, where most blacks are employed.

Because the majority of rural migrants to metropolitan regions are women, women outnumber men in many larger urban areas. Many come in search of work as domestics. Young, single mothers constitute a significant proportion of the urban population.

ETHICAL ISSUE

The Guaymí, a vulnerable group related to the Nahatlan and Mayan nations of Mexico and Central America, are concentrated in the western provinces. In the 1980s, the government began developing a copper mine, a highway, a pipeline, and a hydroelectric plant on Guaymiland in the province of Chiriquí. The Guaymí have continued to attempt to protect their land and publicize their misgivings about the projects because of the impact on their lands and the effect of dam construction on fishing and water supplies.

An ethical principle of distributive justice is that basic goods should be distributed so that the least advantaged members of society are benefited. Distributive justice also means that the rights of one group are balanced against another. What is your opinion about the Panamanian government developing copper mines, traversing roads, and building pipelines through Guaymí Indian territory?

HISTORY, POLITICS, AND GOVERNMENT

As early as 8000 BC, people used the Isthmus of Panama to continue their southward migration and settle in South America. Whether they used land routes or sea routes or a combination of both to make their journeys is not known, but long before the arrival of Europeans, the Indians of North and South America established ocean routes for trade and cultural commerce along the Pacific coast. The Caribbean coast may also have had some maritime commerce among the Indians.

Columbus landed in Panama on his fourth voyage in 1502. In 1510, Vasco de Balboa crossed the isthmus and was the first European to see the Pacific Ocean. Pizarro used the isthmus for his subjugation of the Incas. Charles V ordered the first survey for a proposed canal in 1534. Although no construction was undertaken, a cobblestone mule trail, called Las Cruses, was built to support the conquest of South America's Pacific coast and to carry tons of gold being shipped to Spain from Peru. Parts of that trail are still visible today. Subsequently, the indigenous population of Panama was greatly reduced and Spanish control over the area was established. In 1821, under the leadership of Simon Bolivar, the Spanish colonies revolted against Spain; in the aftermath, Panama became a province of New Granada, which included Colombia, Ecuador, and Venezuela.

In 1882, the French began work on the Panama Canal; however, financial troubles, yellow fever, malaria, tuberculosis, cholera, diphtheria, smallpox, and bubonic plague among the workers ended the project. In 1885, the Republic of Colombia was formed with Panama as a Colombian province. Only in 1903, after Colombia's first civil war had killed nearly 100,000 people, did Panama gain independence with U.S. support. When Panama declared independence from Colombia, the new country and the United States entered into a treaty by which the United States undertook the construction of an interoceanic canal across the isthmus. Before any work could begin, indigenous Indians were relocated. The United States appointed an American physician, William Gorgas, to examine the area. Gorgas and his medical team eradicated yellow fever and brought malaria under control, making it possible to build a canal with international benefit.

ETHICAL ISSUE

The ethical principle respecting autonomy means that individuals are free to decide how they live their lives as long as their decisions do not negatively affect the lives of others. This principle is balanced with distributive justice. What are your thoughts and concerns about the forced relocation of people that has international implications?

The 1904 Panamanian constitution gave the United States the right to intervene in any part of Panama and to reestablish public peace and constitutional order. This provision gave the United States the right to add more territory to the Canal Zone whenever it believed this step was necessary for defensive purposes. Later in the 20th century, these grants of power to the United States caused increasing discontent in Panama, particularly in the 1950s and 1960s.

The 51-mile canal, completed in 1914, was originally operated exclusively by the United States. A 1977 agreement transferred the canal from the United States to Panama at the end of the century. The canal is to remain a neutral zone, and the United States is legally entitled to intervene to maintain its neutrality. Because many of today's ships are larger than the original construction of the canal was designed to handle, the Panama Canal Commission is widening it to allow larger container vessels to pass through. This expansion is expected to be completed in April 2015 and ready for operation in early 2016 (Canal de Panama, 2014).

The Panamanian government is divided into three branches: the executive, the legislative, and the judiciary. The executive branch has one president and two vice presidents, all elected by popular vote for five-year terms. The legislative branch is the Unicameral National Assembly; its members are also elected by popular vote and serve five-year terms. In the judiciary branch, the Supreme Court of Justice has nine appointed judges who serve 10-year terms.

In 1990, the Panamanian military was abolished and replaced with the Panamanian Public Forces. Four years later, the legislative assembly approved a constitutional amendment prohibiting the creation of a standing military force but allowed for the temporary establishment of special police units to counter acts of "external aggression." *Personalism*—giving one's political loyalties to an individual rather than to a party—has influenced the political scene of Panama since its independence. Whereas government officials giving special privileges and positions to a family member is not unique to Panama, a high rate of nepotism continues to occur in Panama.

ETHICAL ISSUE

Balancing the rights of one individual against another is the ethical principle of justice. What concerns do you have with appointing and promoting family members over others who may be more qualified for a position?

ECONOMICS

Panama has one of the fastest growing economies in Latin America and dedicates substantial funding to social programs, yet poverty and inequality remain prevalent. The indigenous population accounts for a growing share of Panama's poor and extreme poor, while the nonindigenous rural poor have been more successful at rising out of poverty through rural-to-urban labor migration. The government's large expenditures on untargeted, indirect subsidies for water, electricity, and fuel have been less than effective, but its conditional cash transfer program has shown some promise in helping to decrease extreme poverty among the indigenous population.

With an estimated 2013 per capita income of $16,500 (up from $2,509 in 1999), 26% of Panamanians still live in poverty, which is more prevalent in rural areas than in urban areas. The 2013 unemployment rate of 4.5% was significantly lower than it was in the early 1990s.

Panama's main crops are bananas, sugarcane, rice, corn, coffee, beans, tobacco, melons, and flowers. Livestock, forestry, and fishing are major commercial enterprises. Natural resources include copper, mahogany forests, shrimp, and hydropower. Major industries include construction, petroleum refining, brewing, manufacturing cement and other construction materials, and sugar milling. The country has an oversupply of nonskilled workers. International banking is also big business, as Panama operates as an offshore financial center.

Its extensive shoreline is responsible for Panama being a major transshipment point and primary laundering center for narcotic and money-laundering activities, especially in the Colon free trade zone. Most of the country's exports go to the United States and China, followed by Costa Rica, Germany, Belgium, the Netherlands, and Italy.

In addition to the substantial income generated by the Panama Canal, ecotourism is another major source of income. A land full of history, art, and culture, Panama's privileged geographical position shelters a rich and abundant natural flora and fauna, resulting in one of the most important natural areas of the world. More than 50% of the world's floral species can be found in Panama, consisting of vascular plant flowers, moss, lichens, algae, and fungi. Panama is also a destination for bird-watchers, as it is home to 940 species of birds; of these, 127 are migratory and 23 are endemic. The national bird of Panama, the harpy eagle, is considered the most powerful bird of prey in the world. Panama also claims 214 species of reptiles, 143 species of amphibians, 225 species of mammals, and 1,500 species of butterflies. The maritime wealth is also fascinating, and includes 207 species of fish, algae, cetaceans, and coral reefs. Overall, Panama has 15 national parks that are major tourist attractions.

Scientists have discovered a new frog in Panama in el Valle de Anton. The news of a new species of frog in Panama comes on the heels of news that a deadly, amphibian-killing fungus has been found on the East side of the Panama Canal. The discovery is so new that scientists have not yet picked a name for the new species of frog. The finding of a surviving frog species when other species of frog are dying is attributed to conservation efforts. The new frog species was discovered during a nature survey carried out by the Smithsonian Tropical Research Institute in conjunction with the Amphibian Center at El Valle de Anton, the University of Miami, the Atlanta Zoo, and Utah State University.

A pygmy sloth, only described scientifically in 2001, lives only on Isla Escudo de Veraguas, a tiny island northeast of Bocas del Toro in Panama. They are critically endangered; current data suggest that there are fewer than 500 pygmy sloths left on the island, but the figure could be smaller than 100 animals.

TECHNOLOGY

Until the early 2000s, Panama had only one telephone company, Cable and Wireless Panama, and it took Panamanians in some areas as long as six months to get telephone services. The impetus for improved services and competition started with the introduction of Radio Shack, where one could purchase a telephone and get immediate telephone service. Now the government has awarded new concessions for fixed-line and mobile services and rapidly improving Internet communication throughout most urban areas.

In 2000, the Global Academy Institute for Integrative Medicine convened a conference called Health Today: Realities, Obstacles and Perspectives to offer the medical community and other constituencies of the healthcare sector of Panama a variety of health and medical perspectives. Cosponsors were the Foreign Ministry of Panama, the Health Ministry of Panama, the Global Academy Genome Institute, the Pan-American Health Organization, and the United Nations Development Program. The presentations and dialogues focused on two themes: (1) integrative medicine and its relevance in terms of the traditional healing systems of the Americas and its potential for low-cost medical services and (2) genetic technology and its impact on the future of health care. This conference demonstrated the importance Panamanians see for technology and health care in their future.

In 2003, Panama hosted Info Com 2003, a trade event aimed at promoting e-business and information technology in Panama and the Latin American region. Info Com 2003, an initiative of American Chamber of Commerce and Industries of Panama, stimulated executives to find the most effective and efficient ways to administer resources and increase the use of technological options. Info Com 2003 had three major aims: (1) promoting the concept of the new Panama Canal; (2) offering technological solutions related to information systems, management, client relations, telecommunications, Internet access, electronic commerce, and network infrastructure; and (3) identifying new business opportunities that arise from technology.

EDUCATION

Overview of Education

Public education began in Panama soon after independence from Colombia but presented an extremely paternalistic view of education. For example, a 1913 meeting of the First Panamanian Educational Assembly stated, "The cultural heritage given to the child should be determined by the social position he or she should occupy. For this reason, education should be different in accordance with the social class to which the student should be related" (Library of Congress, n.d.). This elitist focus changed under U.S. influence. Now, education has been recognized as a mark of status. Most people of elite status receive a university education, attend private schools either at home or abroad, and typically study a profession, with law and medicine being the most favored. Having a profession is viewed not as a means of livelihood but as a status symbol and as an adjunct to a political career.

Since the 1920s, successive Panamanian governments have given high priority to developing a system of universal primary education. Adult literacy, which was only 30% in 1923, rose to 50% in less than a decade. By the early 1950s, adult literacy had increased to more than 70%, then to 87% in 1980, and is currently more than 94%. Men and women are almost equally represented among the literate, with more women than men attending college. The most notable disparity in education is between urban and rural Panamanians.

School attendance is compulsory for children from ages 6 to 15 years, or until the completion of primary school. However, some isolated areas of Panama still do not have a secondary school.

ETHICAL ISSUE

The principle of justice requires meaningful equality among individuals for those positions in society that bring greater economic and social rewards. What are your thoughts about the government not providing facilities for secondary education in some rural areas of Panama?

Secondary school programs follow an academic-oriented program or a vocational-type program. The academic program, which is followed by nearly three-fourths of all secondary school enrollments, features a standard curriculum that includes Spanish, social studies, religion, art, and music. The upper cycle consists of two academic courses of study: arts and sciences, leading up to entrance to the university, or a less rigorous course of study, representing the end of a student's formal education.

Vocational secondary-school programs offer professional or technical courses aimed specifically at giving students the technical skills for employment following graduation. Like the more academic-oriented secondary school programs, the vocational-type programs are divided into two cycles. Students can choose their studies from a variety of specializations, including agriculture, art, commerce, and industrial trades.

The oldest, largest, and most highly regarded institution of higher education, the University of Panama, has produced many public figures—hence its nickname "the nest of eagles." Most of its student body comes from upwardly mobile rather than long-established elements of the elite; students are well known for their political activism. Nearly three-fourths of all university students in the country attend the University of Panama. In addition to its main campus, the university operates regional centers and extensions. Other universities include the University of Santa Maria la Antigua, a private Roman Catholic institution established in 1965; Technical University, founded in 1981; and the Autonomous University of Chiriquí, which is rapidly expanding after separating from the University of Panama in 2000. In addition, some small, private universities with English as the language of instruction are located in Panama City.

Education for the Health Professions

Panama has one public medical school, which is located at the University of Panama, and two private ones. The university also has a master's program in health promotion geared toward multidisciplinary needs, which is located in the School of Public Health. Paramedic programs are provided at the baccalaureate level. Nurse–midwives work in many rural areas and inner-city clinics. The government finances higher education in public universities, but housing and books are not included in these subsidies.

Only baccalaureate nursing programs exist in Panama; there is one public program at the University of Panama, which affiliates with the University of South Florida in the United States, and one at the Autonomous University of Chiriquí in David. Baccalaureate nursing programs include 144 semester credits, which is equivalent to many master's degree programs in the United States. In their senior year, students provide health care to a community, sometimes in extremely remote areas where the student may travel two to three days on horseback to get to the destination, and then be the only healthcare provider in the area; their living arrangements may be in an elementary schoolhouse without heat or air conditioning. All nursing students complete a senior research thesis.

Panama has a master's degree program in nursing administration in which the author of this chapter consulted and taught for several years. As of 2011, the University of Panama has a doctoral program, the first in Panama. Many nursing faculty have obtained their master's degrees and doctorates from U.S. universities. Others have master's degrees in nursing from Colombia, Costa Rica, and Mexico. The role of advanced practice nurses is being developed but has not been widely accepted to date.

COMMUNICATION

The official language of Panama is Spanish, but many members of the population are bilingual in Spanish and English. Some speak a third language, such as Chinese, Japanese, Portuguese, or Italian. Most of the indigenous populations are bilingual in their native languages and Spanish.

Contextual speech patterns among Panamanians can include a high-pitched, loud voice and a rate that seems extremely fast to the untrained ear. The language uses apocopation, which accounts for this rapid speech pattern. An apocopation occurs when one word ends with a vowel, and the next word begins with a vowel. This creates a tendency to drop the vowel ending of the first word and results in an abbreviated rapid-sounding form. For example, the Spanish phrase for "How are you?," *¿Cómo está usted?*, may become *¿Comestusted?* The last word, *usted*, is frequently dropped. Some may find this fast speech difficult to understand. However, if one asks the individual to enunciate slowly, the effect of the apocopation or truncation is less pronounced. For the first three days of each trip to Panama, this author has a mantra, *Habla mas despacio, por favor* ("Speak more slowly, please"), until becoming accustomed to the rapid speech patterns.

Using Spanish to communicate with Panamanian clients is important. The healthcare provider who assumes a total understanding of Panamanian Spanish, however, may negatively affect his or her interactions with these clients. Attempt speaking Spanish, but do not be overly confident; the idiomatic expressions are numerous and change from country to country.

Respect (*respeto*) is extremely important, especially when meeting a Panamanian for the first time. Always greet the person formally, unless told to do otherwise. Greeting the person with *Señorita* (Miss), *Señora* (Mrs.), *Señor* (Mister), *Doña* (Madam), *Don* (Sir), and *Doctor* or *Doctora* sets the stage for formal communication. Familism—the value of family—is also an important concept. For health teaching to be effective, the provider must engage the entire family.

Approaching the Panamanian client with *personalismo*, being friendly, and directing questions to the family spokesperson (usually the male) may help to facilitate more open communication. However, one must remember that the spokesperson is not necessarily the decision maker. The woman may make the decision, but the culturally prescribed role is for the man to transmit the message. *Personalismo* emphasizes people and family orientation and is essential for building confidence, promoting health, and establishing a cultural connection. On repeat visits, polite conversation includes briefly asking about family members. The concept of *personalismo* may be difficult for some healthcare professionals because many are socialized to create rigid boundaries between the caregiver and the client and family.

Cultural Communication Patterns

While some topics such as income, salary, and investments are taboo, Panamanians generally like to express their inner beliefs, feelings, and emotions once they get to know and trust a person. Meaningful conversations are important, often becoming loud and seemingly disorganized. To the outsider, the situation may seem stressful or hostile, but this intense emotion means that the participants in the conversation are having a good time and enjoying one another's company.

Panamanians place great value on closeness and togetherness, including when they are in an inpatient facility. They frequently touch and embrace others and like to see relatives and significant others. Touch between a man and a woman, between two men, and between two women is acceptable. To demonstrate respect, compassion, and understanding, healthcare providers should greet the Panamanian client with a handshake, but a man should wait until the woman extends her hand. On establishing rapport, providers may further demonstrate approval and respect through backslapping, smiling, and affirmative nods of the head.

Many Panamanians consider sustained eye contact when speaking directly to an older person to be rude. Direct eye contact with teachers, physicians, nurses, and superiors may be interpreted as insolence. Avoiding sustained and direct eye contact with superiors is a sign of respect. This practice may or may not be seen among the more educated and in the younger generation, but it is imperative that healthcare providers take cues from the client and family. Many among the indigenous Indian populations do not maintain eye contact with persons older than themselves or people in hierarchical positions.

Out of respect for the healthcare provider, many Panamanians may avoid disagreeing, expressing doubts, or asking questions. Certainly, any negative feelings about the healthcare encounter would not be expressed. Nevertheless, encouraging patients to ask questions, even if it is through an interpreter, is considered polite behavior.

Temporal Relationships

Many Panamanians, especially those from lower socioeconomic groups, are focused on the present, out of choice and necessity. Many individuals do not consider it important or do not have the income to plan ahead financially. The trend is to live in the "more important" here and now, because *mañana* (tomorrow) cannot be predicted. With this emphasis on living in the present, preventive health care and immunizations may not be a priority. *Mañana* may or may not really mean tomorrow, but rather often means "not today" or "later."

Some Panamanians perceive time as relative, rather than as categorically imperative. Deadlines and commitments are flexible, not firm. Punctuality is generally relaxed, especially in social situations. Because of their more relaxed concept of time, Panamanians may arrive late for appointments, although the current trend is toward greater punctuality, especially when meeting with someone in a hierarchical position. Healthcare facilities that use an appointment system for clients may need to make special provisions to see clients whenever they arrive. Healthcare providers must listen carefully for subtle cues when discussing appointments. Disagreeing with healthcare providers who set the appointment may be viewed as rude or impolite. Therefore, some Panamanians will not tell healthcare providers directly that they cannot make an appointment. In the context of the discussion, they may say something like, "My husband goes to work at 8:00 a.m. and the children are off to school, then I have to do the dishes . . ." The healthcare professional should ask: "Is 8:30 a.m. on Thursday okay for you?" The person might say yes, but the healthcare professional must still intently listen to the conversation and then possibly negotiate a new time for the appointment. Many Panamanians consider it rude to openly disagree in social situations. Because it might be seen as rude to directly say no, the Panamanian may say yes. In reality, "yes" may mean "I hear you, but I am not going to follow your instructions," "I hear you, and I do not agree," "I will think about it," "I am not sure what you mean, but I do not want to embarrass myself or you to explain it more," or "I understand you, agree with you, and will follow your instructions and advice."

Format for Names

Names in most Spanish-speaking populations seem complex to those unfamiliar with the culture. A typical name is La Señorita Olga Gaborra y Rodriguez. Gaborra is the name of this individual's father, and Rodriguez is her mother's surname. When she marries a man with the surname name of Guiterrez, she becomes La Señora (denotes a married woman) Olga de Guiterrez y Gaborra y Rodriguez. The word *de* is used to express possession, and the father's name, which is considered more important than the mother's name, comes first. However, this full name is rarely used except on formal documents and for recording the name in the family Bible. Out of respect, most Panamanians are more formal when addressing nonfamily members. Thus the best way to address Olga is not by her first name, but rather as Señora de Guiterrez. Use of titles such as *Don* and *Doña* for older respected members of the community and family is also common.

Healthcare providers must understand the role of older adults when providing care to people of Panamanian culture. To develop confidence and *personalismo*, an element of formality must exist between healthcare providers and older adults. Becoming overly familiar by using physical touch or using first names may not be appreciated early in a relationship. As the healthcare professional develops confidence in the relationship, becoming familiar may be less of a concern. However, using the first name of an older adult client might never be appropriate.

SPIRITUALITY AND RELIGION

The religious affiliations of Panamanians are 85% Roman Catholic and 15% Protestant. Small groups exist of Latter Day Saints, Seventh Day Adventists, Jehovah's Witnesses, Episcopalians,

Buddhists, Muslims, Jews, and Baha'i. Purnell's research (1999) reported a number of participants who self-identified as atheists. The Panamanian constitution prescribes that there shall be no prejudice with respect to religious freedom, and the practice of all forms of worship is authorized. At the same time, the constitution recognizes that the Roman Catholic faith is the country's predominant religion and contains a provision that it be taught in the public schools. Such instruction or other religious activity is not compulsory, however. The constitution does not specifically provide for the separation of church and state, but it implies the independent functioning of each entity.

Members of the clergy may not hold civil or military public office, excepting the posts that may be concerned with social welfare or public instruction. The constitution stipulates that senior officials of the church hierarchy in Panama must be native-born citizens.

ETHICAL ISSUE

Respecting autonomy is an ethical principle that allows groups to make decisions about their lives and organization as long as they do not have a negative effect on the decisions of other groups. Do you think that requiring church officials in hierarchal positions to be native-born Panamanians violates this principle?

Devout Panamanians regard church attendance and the observance of religious duties as regular features of everyday life, and even the most casual or nominal Roman Catholics adjust their daily lives to the prevailing norms of the religious calendar. Although some sacraments are observed more scrupulously than others, baptism is almost universal; in fact, baptism is generally considered the most significant religious rite. Throughout the country, births and deaths are marked by religious rites observed by all but a very few individuals.

Virtually every town has its own Roman Catholic Church, but many do not have a priest in residence. Many rural inhabitants receive only an occasional visit from a busy priest who travels among a number of isolated villages. In rural areas, families often have to travel some distance to the nearest parish center. This trip is important and people willingly undertake it to practice religious rites.

The Antillean black community is largely Protestant. Indians follow their own indigenous belief systems, although both Protestant and Catholic missionaries are active among the various tribes. However, Roman Catholicism permeates the social environment culturally as well as religiously. Religious attitudes, customs, and beliefs differ between urban and rural areas, although many members of the urban working class and recent migrants from rural regions usually retain their folk beliefs.

Panamanians, regardless of their religious affiliation, take their religion seriously. Purnell's study (1999) reported that 81% of participants prayed for good health; however, the most important thing in their lives was family, followed by religion. If healthcare delivery is to be effective for Panamanians, care and health teaching must be delivered in the family context.

RESEARCH AND DEMONSTRATION PROJECTS

The National Geographic research station near Panama City and the American Institute of Biological Sciences conduct research on marine issues, fungal infections in frogs, and other environmental concerns. A cagelike steel gondola on top of a crane gives researchers a bird's-eye view of the jungle canopy where research studies are conducted. A number of archeological and anthropological sites are also being studied.

The Institute of Nutrition of Central America and Panama at the University of Panama sponsors an ongoing research project on breastfeeding among diverse populations in Panama. One finding is a widespread belief that maternal milk plays a definite role in the etiology of diarrheal diseases. One of the explanatory models of diarrheal disease in children is the hot–cold theory of illness and disease causation: If the mother is too hot or too cold at the time of breastfeeding, the child will get diarrhea. Examples of this belief were explained to this author while teaching and taking nursing and dietetic students to Panama: (1) if ironing (a hot activity), wait a while before breastfeeding; (2) if the mother has been in the hot sun, she should cool off before breastfeeding, (3) if exposed to cold wind, the mother should wait until she gets warm before breastfeeding, and (4) she should not immediately breastfeed if she has consumed cold liquids or been exposed to the open door of a cold refrigerator.

The City of Knowledge created in 1995 and governed by a private nonprofit organization, is an international complex for education, research, and innovation located at the former Fort Clayton military base in the Panama Canal Zone. The City of Knowledge offers facilities and support for establishing programs in education, research, and technological development and helps develop and strengthen the relationship between the academic, scientific, and business worlds with an international orientation. Current researchers at this complex come from the University of South Florida, University of Delaware, Purdue University, and Iowa State University, to name a few.

Partners of the Americas: Delaware–Panama Partners of the Americas

Partners of the Americas have had a significant, sustained, and positive influence on people's lives in Panama as has the state of Delaware through Delaware–Panama Partners of the Americas. In 1963, President John F. Kennedy launched the Alliance for Progress, a program of government-to-government economic cooperation across the Western Hemisphere. At the same time, he called for a parallel people-to-people initiative, one that would allow private citizens to work together for the good of the Americas. These initiatives were established as part of the U.S. Agency for International Development.

The Delaware-Panama partnership developed because both Delaware and Panama are international banking centers, each has only one major university, both have a canal (Delaware Canal and the Panama Canal), and both have shared interests in farmer-to-farmer programs. Beekeeping for the production of honey and research on bee venom for allergies are also shared interests. Student exchanges from high school through university settings have been accomplished. Although Delaware–Panama Partners is not strictly a research-oriented organization, it has produced many noteworthy research projects. On the research side, faculty from the

University of Delaware and the University of Panama has completed the following research studies and projects:

1. Young women's attitudes and involvement toward future needs of older adults for caregiving.
2. Panamanian health beliefs and the meaning of respect afforded them by healthcare providers.
3. Folic acid project financed by the March of Dimes to increase the awareness of the importance of folic acid in the diet of women of childbearing age in Panama and in Delaware, and the development of bilingual materials because of the increased risk of Hispanic populations for spina bifida and other neural tube defects that are related to folic acid deficiency.
4. Culturally congruent material for tobacco use prevention geared toward a variety of age groups as well as material to aid teachers, physicians, and other health personnel with new approaches.
5. Environmental impact and cleanup of the Panama Canal Zone because of the effect that contamination has had on the environment and health of the people living in the Canal Zone.
6. Graduate student and faculty exchanges in pediatric oncology, disabilities studies, and disaster management. The U.S. Center for Disaster Management is located at the University of Delaware.
7. A family-life project to develop reproductive health education materials suitable for use in Panama and the Latin American community in Delaware.
8. Culturally relevant health information for emergency preparedness.
9. Higher education linkages to develop ongoing, self-sustaining programs in higher education.
10. Promotion of knowledge of women's rights to build awareness of the revised code of family law as it affects women's rights.
11. A service-learning program to promote and train participants in school and community leadership.

ETHICAL ISSUE

The ethical principle of nonmaleficence means that we as individuals, groups, or organizations should not engage in activities that run the risk of harming others. The U.S. military used the Panama Canal Zone as a dumping ground for biohazardous waste. What responsibility do you think the United States should have in cleaning up the Canal Zone, even though it is now under the control of the Panamanian government?

HEALTH AND HEALTHCARE PRACTICES

Overview of the Healthcare System

Panama has high-quality health care and modern hospitals in metropolitan areas. For example, the Johns Hopkins–affiliated Punta Pacifica Hospital is the most technologically advanced medical center in Latin America. Other private hospitals are affiliated with Tulane in Louisiana and the Cleveland Clinic in Ohio. In the city of David, in the Chiriquí Province in the western region of Panama, there are two medical centers with modern facilities, the latest being a specialty hospital where Indigenous Indians who come from great distances can stay in accommodations on the hospital grounds. Towns including Boquete, Chiriquí, and Coronado, and Province of Panama have new medical centers. Many Panamanian physicians are U.S. trained and board certified while others come from high-quality medical schools in Panama, Spain, Cuba, and Mexico. The standards at the top city hospitals compare very favorably with those in the United States, Canada, and Europe. However, smaller hospitals in outlying areas do not favor as well, mostly due to lack of resources.

Private health insurance is available and much less expensive than insurance in the United States, because physician's fees and hospital visits are much cheaper. In addition, health insurance in Panama is affordable; malpractice insurance is very low because the laws do not allow for frivolous lawsuits. Prices for prescription drugs are low as well, because manufacturers price them for the market. Some drugs that require a prescription elsewhere are available over the counter in Panama.

A few of the hospitals are accredited by Joint Commission International. These international standards for patient safety and quality have led to a rapid increase in medical tourism in Panama. Most medical travelers come from the United States and Canada. While cosmetic procedures are the most requested services in Panama, dental procedures, laser eye surgery, and many other medical treatments are also offered.

The Panamanian constitution guarantees the right to medical and health care throughout the nation's territories. The public health sector comprises the Ministry of Health, which covers 60% of the population, and the Social Security Fund, which covers 40% of the population. The overall hospital bed capacity is 2.4 beds per 1,000 population. This number should significantly increase in the near future with a new hospital being built outside Panama City. The current government's health objectives are to offer universal access to comprehensive health programs, to improve the quality of the services, and to reduce gaps through a decentralized model of care that emphasizes primary health care. The Social Security Institute and the Ministry of Health have attempted, with limited success, to coordinate what in essence are two separate public healthcare systems in an effort to eliminate redundancy. Public hospitals may have a long wait for patients to be seen or to have nonurgent care provided. Private health insurance is available for those who can afford it.

The Department of Environmental Health is charged with administering rural health programs and maintaining a safe water supply for communities with fewer than 500 inhabitants, communities that make up roughly one-third of the total Panamanian population. The National Water and Sewage Institute and the Ministry of Public Works share responsibility for urban water supplies. Public health efforts are aimed at changing the emphasis from curative, hospital-based medical care to community-based preventive medicine. The Ministry of Health bears primary responsibility for public health programs.

The Ministry of Health and the Social Security Institute of Panama have cooperative agreements to strengthen their coordination in the management of emergencies and disasters. The agreements are part of the Safe Hospitals global strategy and prioritize a shared agenda to achieve the goal of keeping hospitals safe from disasters.

ETHICAL ISSUE

Which ethical principles have been violated with poor distribution of healthcare services in Panama? How is this different from the United States and other more or less developed countries?

Healthcare Workforce

The most recent data on the healthcare workforce are from 2004, so there may be questions about their accuracy. In 2004, there were 11.7 physicians, 2.4 dentists, and 10.7 nurses per 10,000 population. The number of nurses is inadequate to meet Panama's needs, and the supply is unevenly distributed between urban and rural areas. Nurses who are willing to practice in remote areas receive as much as a 50% increase in pay. The country is also short on laboratory technicians. All health professionals in the public sector are protected by union contracts, which set their pay scales.

ETHICAL ISSUE

Higher education is free in Panama. The health-sector distribution and statistics are not what one expects for a developing country. What do you suggest to address the ethical principles of justice, beneficence, autonomy, and nonmaleficence?

The birth rate of 18.61 births per 1,000 population has been gradually decreasing over the past three decades. Infant mortality for males is 10.7 deaths per 1,000 live births; for maternal mortality, it is 9.2 deaths per 1,000 live births. Most infant mortality is attributable to congenital abnormalities, pneumonia, intestinal infections, protein-calorie malnutrition, and accidental injuries. Rural Panama has disproportionately high infant and maternal mortality rates. Rural babies are roughly 20% more likely to die than their urban counterparts; childbearing is five times more likely to be fatal in rural Panama than in cities. The infant mortality rate of Panama Province is one-third that of Bocas del Toro and one-fourth that of Darién.

Overall longevity for Panamanians is 78.3 years; for women it is 81.22 years, and for men it is 75.51 years. Overall health expenditure for Panama as a percentage of the gross national product is 8.2%, significantly lower than that of the United States and is comparable to more developed countries worldwide.

ETHICAL ISSUE

Which ethical principles are involved with health disparities in Panama? Can you make suggestions for addressing these disproportionate health disparities? How are these disparities different from or similar to wealthier nations?

The overall fertility rate of 2.48 per woman varies significantly from urban to rural areas. In his research, Purnell (1999) reported that nonuse of family planning services might be due in part to indigenous Indians' strong cultural values related to family. In 2012, Panama legislation updated the law on male and female sterilization as a method of birth control. The new legislation clarifies that sterilization is a personal right and is voluntary on the part of the woman, although it does not specify the age at which to apply sterilization, only that the woman be an adult (18). The bill also encompasses male sterilization with consent and provided information is given on the risks of a surgical procedure and the consequences of a vasectomy. To proceed with sterilization, the woman must present a voluntary petition and medical recommendation, as well as a test to prove she is not pregnant. The procedure will be stopped if the woman expresses before the end of medical intervention that she was not presented with information about alternative methods of contraception.

The legislation also ensured the health and education of pregnant adolescents and created lactation rooms in schools where teenage mothers can attend to their children, in order not to interrupt their education and to encourage measures to reduce the number of teenage pregnancies and abortions (Panama Guide, 2014).

The crude death rate is 4.6%, with a maternal mortality rate of 6.4%. The life expectancy is 80.5 years for women and 74.85 years for men.

Service Facilities and Quality of Services

Panama has 22 hospitals, some of which are privately owned. The province of Panama has 12 hospitals, many of which are specialty specific, such as those geared toward psychiatry, maternal–child, pediatrics, or medical and surgical services. Chiriquí Province has three hospitals. The western provinces have only one hospital, and Bocas del Toro, Cocle, and Darien do not have any hospitals but do have clinics. Medical facilities, including nearly all laboratory and special-care facilities, are concentrated in the capital city. Roughly 87% of the hospital beds are in publicly owned facilities and are mostly located in Panama City. Hospital Punta Pacifica, which is affiliated with Johns Hopkins University, and Clinica Hospital San Fernando, which is affiliated with Miami Children's Hospital, Tulane University, and Miami Baptist Health Center, has English-trained and English-speaking physicians and staff.

Medical facilities and personnel are concentrated beyond what might reasonably be expected, even given the capital city's share of the country's total population. Panama City has roughly two and a half times the national average of hospital beds and doctors per capita and nearly three times the number of nurses per capita. The effect of this distribution is seen in continued regional disparities in health indicators.

ETHICAL ISSUE

Which ethical principles are involved with the maldistribution of healthcare facilities in Panama?

Most hospitals have active infection-control programs. Specialty women's hospitals have active milk banks. In public hospitals that cater to the indigenous rural populations, facilities are available where one family member can stay in the hospital with the patient, while the rest of the family lives in adjacent facilities on hospital property.

ILLNESS, DISEASE, AND INJURY PROFILE

The illness, disease, and injury profile of Panama is changing from one of infectious diseases to one similar to the more developed nations. Nevertheless, some infectious diseases that were almost eliminated in the past are reemerging, and newer ones are arising. The leading causes of death are (1) malignant neoplasms; (2) accidents, self-inflicted injuries, assaults, and other acts of violence; (3) cerebrovascular diseases; (4) ischemic heart disease; (5) chronic diseases of the lower respiratory tract; and (6) diabetes mellitus.

Children are immunized for various diseases including diphtheria, tetanus, polio, and measles, and incidences of these illnesses are now at an all-time low. The Panamanian authorities have banned smoking in all public places: You cannot have a cigarette in any place where people gather. The number of smokers is still high, but this number is gradually decreasing as people are discouraged from the practice.

The rate for communicable diseases has decreased significantly over the last 15 years. Tuberculosis is on the rise; however, HIV has decreased to 0.7% present which is equivalent to that of the United States at 0.6%. All but one resident in the San Blas Islands have type B+ blood; testing for HIV does not exist in these islands. HIV in the rest of the country is on the rise, with 44% of such infections transmitted through heterosexual activity, 40% through homosexual or bisexual activity, 10% through intravenous drug use, 1% through blood transfusions, and 5% perinatally.

The leading causes of morbidity treated at public health facilities are influenza, diarrhea and gastroenteritis, rhinopharyngitis, the common cold, and malnutrition. Health workers, nurses in urban areas, and either nurses or community health promoters in rural areas are trained to provide follow-through on mental health programs, control of vector-borne diseases, tuberculosis, and cervical cancer. The leading discharge diagnoses in public health hospitals are problems related to childbirth and the puerperium, diseases of the respiratory tract, multiple trauma, infectious parasitic diseases, and problems with the newborn and the perinatal process.

Although the country supposedly has an adequate blood supply, places in remote areas such as the San Blas Islands do not have storage facilities. When someone on these islands needs a transfusion, the donor and the recipient lie side by side on tables while the transfusion occurs.

A wide variety of medicines are available on an over-the-counter basis in Panama, as are herbal and traditional remedies. Family members may go to the pharmacy and purchase drugs, such as injectable diazepam, and then administer it to a relative or friend in the hospital.

Drug abuse is considered a priority health problem for younger groups and constitutes the leading cause of violence and crime in the country. Alcohol is the drug of choice for the population as a whole. Men are more likely to abuse illicit drugs and women are more likely to abuse less powerful tranquilizers. Cocaine use is on the rise, mainly in the young-adult population. Illegal narcotic operations in Colombia continue to operate within the remote border region of panama. Money laundering is especially heavy in the Colon Free Zone where corruption remains high.

Panama is a source, transit, and destination country for women and children trafficked for the purpose of commercial sexual exploitation. Some Panamanian women are trafficked to Jamaica, Europe, and Israel for commercial sexual exploitation, but most victims are trafficked to and within the country into Panama's sex trade. Nongovernmental organizations (NGOs) report that some Panamanian children, mostly young girls, are trafficked into domestic servitude. Government agencies indicate that indigenous girls may be trafficked by their parents into prostitution in Darien province. Most foreign sex-trafficking victims are adult women from Colombia, the Dominican Republic, and neighboring Central American countries; some victims migrate voluntarily to Panama to work but are subsequently forced into prostitution. Weak controls along Panama's borders make the nation an easy transit point for trafficked persons (Human Trafficking & Modern-day Slavery, 2009).

Infectious Diseases

The Gorgas Memorial Institute of Tropical and Preventive Medicine, founded in 1921, was named after William C. Gorgas, a U.S. Surgeon General known throughout the world as the conqueror of malaria and yellow fever. His pioneering efforts in halting an epidemic of yellow fever enabled the United States to complete the Panama Canal. The institute, which moved in 2002 to the University of Alabama, continues to focus on tropical and preventive medicine. After decades of healthcare and research projects, the hospital is now a specialty oncology hospital financed by Japanese investors.

Because of the Gorgas hospital, much research on infectious disease has been completed in Panama. Despite the progress made in eliminating many tropical and infectious diseases, Panama has recently seen a reemergence of cholera, classical dengue, and dengue hemorrhagic fever, malaria, tuberculosis, and Venezuelan equine encephalitis.

Hantavirus pulmonary syndrome (HPS), transmitted by rodents, made its debut in Panama in 1999. HPS is an infectious disease typically characterized by fever, myalgia, and headache, followed by dyspnea, noncardiogenic pulmonary edema, hypotension, and shock. Common laboratory findings include elevated hematocrit, leukocytosis with the presence of immunoblasts, and thrombocytopenia. The case-fatality rate can be as high as 52%. Hantaviruses are most often transmitted to humans through the inhalation of infectious rodent feces, urine, or saliva. However, strain-specific virus transmission may occur from person-to-person contact. HPS was first recognized in 1993 in the Four Corners region of the United States. Since then, 363 cases of HPS have been confirmed in the United States. An outbreak of hantavirus pulmonary syndrome occurred in the province of Los Santos, Panama, in late 1999 and early 2000. Eleven cases were identified, three of which were fatal.

Arthropod-borne Diseases

Arthropod-borne diseases common in Panama include malaria, Chagas disease, dengue fever, leishmaniasis, filariasis, and yellow fever. A brief description of these diseases follows:

- Malaria, an infectious disease characterized by cycles of chills, fever, and sweating, is caused by a protozoan of the genus *Plasmodium* that takes up residence in red blood cells; the pathogen is transmitted to humans by the bite of an infected female anopheles mosquito. The period between the mosquito bite and the onset of malarial illness is usually one to three weeks. Prevention and treatment are frequently the same: Chloroquine phosphate and primaquine are the most commonly used medications, but other drugs are also used, such as artemether, artesunate, quinidine, doxycycline, mefloquine, and sulfa preparations.
- Chagas disease, also called trypanosomiasis, is caused by the parasite *Trypanosoma cruzi* and is transmitted by reduviid bugs (kissing bugs), which are primarily found in cracks and holes in substandard housing. Infection is spread to humans when an infected bug deposits feces on a person's skin, usually while the person is sleeping. The person may then accidentally rub the feces into the bite wound, in an open cut, the eyes, or mouth. An infected mother can pass infection to her baby during pregnancy, at delivery, or while breastfeeding. Chagas disease is characterized by fever and enlargement of spleen and lymph nodes. Acute symptoms occur only approximately 1% of the time; most people do not seek medical treatment.
- Dengue fever, a tropical disease transmitted by *Aedes aegypti* mosquitoes, is characterized by high fever, rash, headache, and severe muscle and joint pain. The disease usually occurs in five-year cycles and strikes people who have low levels of immunity. The mosquito flourishes in rainy seasons and can breed year-round in water-filled flowerpots, plastic bags, and cans. The incubation period ranges from 3 to 15 days. Only supportive therapy is available, in the form of treating or preventing dehydration.
- Leishmaniasis, which is caused by a flagellate protozoan, is transmitted to humans by blood-sucking sand flies. The parasites, which can live in animals or in humans, affect white blood cells. The more serious type of infection affects internal organs, causing fever, anemia, splenomegaly, and discoloration of the skin. If left untreated, it can become fatal. Treatment relies on amphotericin B, drugs containing antimony, or the newest drug available, miltefosine, which had a 95% effectiveness in clinical trials in 2003.
- Yellow fever, a tropical disease caused by a bite from the female *Aede saegypti* and *haemagogus* mosquitoes, is characterized by high fever, jaundice, and gastrointestinal hemorrhaging. In severe cases, prostration and renal failure may occur. Because there is no specific

treatment for this infection, vaccination is important. Symptoms appear suddenly after an incubation period of three to five days.

- Filariasis, also called lymphatic filiariasis or elephantiasis, is caused by threadlike parasitic round worms (nematodes) and their larvae and is transmitted by mosquitoes. Acute episodes of local inflammation involving skin, lymph nodes and lymphatic vessels often accompany the chronic lymphedema or elephantiasis. Some of these symptoms are caused by the body's immune response to the parasite, but most are the result of bacterial infection of skin where normal defenses have been partially lost due to underlying lymphatic damage. In endemic communities, some 10% to 50% of men suffer from genital damage, especially hydrocele, and elephantiasis of the penis and scrotum. Elephantiasis of the entire leg, the entire arm, the vulva, or the breast swelling up to several times normal size affects as many as 10% of men and women with filariasis. The worst symptoms of the chronic disease generally appear in adults, and in men more often than in women. Treatment consists of albendazole and diethylcarbamazine.

The following are recommendations to help prevent arthropod-borne diseases.

- Wear a long-sleeved shirt and long pants while outside to prevent illnesses carried by insects.
- Use insect repellent containing DEET (diethylmethyltoluamide) in 30–35% strength for adults and 6–10% strength for children.
- Use a bed net impregnated with the insecticide permethrin.
- Properly dispose of household trash.
- Do not leave water-filled flowerpots with standing water.
- Eliminate other sources of standing water.
- Chikungunya fever, first identified in the Americas in 2013, is a viral disease transmitted by the bite of infected mosquitoes such as Aedes aegypti and Aedes albopictus. It can cause high fever, joint and muscle pain, and headache. Chikungunya does not often result in death, but the joint pain may last for months or years and may become a cause of chronic pain and disability. There is no specific treatment for chikungunya infection, nor any vaccine to prevent it. Pending the development of a new vaccine, the only effective means of prevention is to protect individuals against mosquito bites. Persistent joint pain after chikungunya virus infections can be hard to distinguish from the symptoms of rheumatoid arthritis.

Chikungunya fever affects all age groups and both genders. Following an incubation period of three to seven days (range: 1–12 days) from the mosquito bite, the chikungunya virus causes a febrile illness usually associated with arthralgia/arthritis, backache, and headache. The joint pain tends to be worse in the morning, relieved by mild exercise, and exacerbated by aggressive movements. Ankles, wrists, and small joints of the hand tended to be the worst affected. Larger joints like knee and shoulder and spine were also involved. Migratory polyarthritis with effusions may been seen in around 70% of the cases

In a majority of the patients, symptoms resolve in one to three weeks. However, some patients might have a relapse of rheumatologic symptoms (e.g., polyarthralgia, polyarthritis, tenosynovitis) in the months following acute illness. Variable proportions of patients report persistent joint pains for months to years. Neurological, emotional, and dermatologic sequelae are also described. Older individuals and those with underlying rheumatic and traumatic joint disorders seem to be more vulnerable to develop the chronic joint symptoms. Mortality is rare and occurs mostly in older adults.

Food-borne and Waterborne Illnesses

Waterborne and food-borne diseases commonly identified in Panama include amoebiasis, brucellosis, cholera, hepatitis A, and typhoid fever. Other diseases include rabies and hepatitis B. Myiasis, a condition caused by a botfly, is endemic in Central America. A brief description of these illnesses follows:

- Amoebiasis, an infection caused by pathogenic amoebas, especially *Entamoeba histolytica,* is usually contracted by ingesting water or food contaminated by amoebic cysts. Symptoms include diarrhea, abdominal pain or discomfort, and fever. Symptoms take from a few days to a few weeks to develop and manifest themselves in approximately two to four weeks. This pattern is analogous to that seen with cardiovascular disease: It may take five years for cardiovascular disease to develop, but symptoms do not become evident until many years later. Most infected people are asymptomatic, but amoebiasis has the potential to make the sufferer dangerously ill, especially if the individual is immunocompromised.
- Brucellosis, a bacterial disease caused by the *Brucella* pathogen, is transmitted by contact with infected animals or through contaminated milk or milk products. The disease is also called undulant fever because of the rising and falling of fevers, sweats, malaise, weakness, anorexia, headache, and muscle and back pain.
- Cholera, an infectious disease caused by the bacterium *Vibrio cholerae,* is characterized by profuse watery diarrhea, vomiting, muscle cramps, and severe dehydration. Some persons experience a mild version of cholera, with few to no symptoms.
- Hepatitis A, also called infectious hepatitis, is an infection of the liver caused by an RNA virus that is transmitted by ingesting infected food and water or through contact with infected feces. Symptoms range from flulike symptoms to more severe symptoms such as nausea, poor appetite, abdominal pain, fatigue, jaundice, and dark urine. Recovery can be complete in a few weeks to months. Very few cases progress to death. Treatment is symptomatic and includes rest and fluids.
- Typhoid fever, a highly infectious disease caused by *Salmonella typhi,* is transmitted by contaminated food or water and is characterized by fever, headache, coughing, intestinal hemorrhaging, and rose-colored spots on the skin. Treatment includes antibiotics such as ampicillin, chloramphenicol, trimethoprim–sulfamethoxazole, or ciprofloxacin.
- Myiasis, the condition caused by botfly, is endemic in Central America. It is caused by parasitic dipterous fly larvae feeding on the host's necrotic or living tissue. With this infection, botflies lay their larvae in open wounds. The larvae stage appears as maggots, which then live off the tissue. Treatment entails removing larvae through pressure or the maggots with forceps and then cleaning and disinfecting the wound.

The following are recommendations to prevent food-borne and waterborne illnesses:

- Vaccinations for hepatitis A or immune globulin (IG)
- Hepatitis B or immune globulin vaccination
- Rabies vaccination, if you might be exposed to wild or domestic animals through your work or recreation
- Typhoid vaccination—particularly important because of the presence of S. *typhi* strains resistant to multiple antibiotics in Panama
- A booster for tetanus and diphtheria—if not vaccinated within the last 10 years
- Yellow fever vaccination

Also helpful is this overall general advice for staying healthy:

- Wash your hands often with soap and water.
- Drink only boiled water or water and carbonated (bubbly) drinks in cans.
- Avoid tap water, fountain drinks, and ice cubes.
- Eat only thoroughly cooked food or fruits and vegetables you have peeled yourself.
- Do not eat fruit purchased from street vendors. Boil it, cook it, peel it, or forget it.

Other Health Concerns

Other illnesses commonly found in Panama include contact dermatitis caused by pesticides and fungicides; it is observed among banana plantation workers, especially in the western provinces where Chiquita Banana and United Fruit Banana are major employers (Penagos, 2002). Efforts to teach workers how to protect themselves are being made, along with translating written materials into indigenous languages for those for whom Spanish and English are a second language.

In addition, drowning as a result of strong currents and undertows are common throughout Panama. One should always check with local authorities before attempting to swim in coastal areas. The problem is not the surf per se, but rather the unusual undertows from the surf.

TRADITIONAL PRACTITIONERS AND HERBAL MEDICINE

Traditional Practitioners

Panamanians from all socioeconomic levels rely on traditional care providers. Healers include *curanderos(as), sobadores(as), espiritistas, brujos(as), masajistas, and (y)jerberos(as).* Traditional practitioners, who are usually well known by the family, are often consulted before and during biomedical treatment. Although usually no contradictions or contraindications to traditional remedies arise, healthcare providers must always consider the client's use of these practitioners to prevent prescription of conflicting treatment regimens.

Curanderos receive their talents from God or serve an apprenticeship with an established practitioner. *Curanderos* are regarded with great respect by the community, accept no monetary

TABLE 20-1 Herbal Teas and Conditions for Use

Herbal Tea	Conditions for Use
Aguacate (avocado)	Hypertension, aphrodisiac
Ajo (garlic)	Bronchitis, respiratory conditions, hypertension, anti-inflammatory, infections, lower cholesterol
Canella con aniz (cinnamon)	Toothache, flu, coughs, pain, ulcers
Cebola (onion)	Bronchitis, respiratory conditions, flu
Cipres (cypress)	Whooping cough
Eucalyptus	Colds, coughs, allergies
Ginseng	Aphrodisiac, anemia, heart problems, diabetes, depression, hypertension, ulcers
Guanabano	Diarrhea, vomiting
Guava	Colds, diarrhea
Limon (lemon)	Colds, flu, calms nerves, sleep, headache, stomachache
Llanten (plantain)	Liver problems, stomachache
Malazana (tuberlike yam)	Colic
Manzanilla (chamomile)	Nerves, calms children, antispasmodic, diaphoretic, ulcers, aids digestion
Marano (mangrove)	Inflammation, edema
Mastranto	Colds, headache, stomachache, nerves, stress in children
Naranjo (orange)	Colds, flu, stomachache
Sabila (aloe)	Colds, gives strength, headache
Salvia (sage)	Worms, diabetes, ulcers, stomachache, headache, gives strength, strengthens nerves, stops sweating
Tilo (lime)	Colic, quiets nerves, flu, stomachache, ulcers
Toronjo (grapefruit)	Stomachache
Valleriana	Sleep, sedation, hypertension

payment (but may accept gifts), are usually a member of the extended family, and treat many traditional illnesses. These healers do not usually treat illnesses caused by witchcraft. Currently, *curanderos* prescribe drugs, a practice that allopathic physicians are trying to stop. However, because *curanderos* can prescribe only over-the-counter medicines, this practice is likely to continue. In Panama, one can purchase a wide variety of antibiotics and other medicines without a prescription.

Yerberos (also spelled *jerberos*) are folk healers with specialized training in growing herbs, teas, and roots, who prescribe these remedies for the prevention and cure of illnesses. A *yerbero* may suggest that the person go to a *botanica* (herb shop) for specific herbs. In addition, these traditional practitioners frequently prescribe the use of laxatives.

Sobadores subscribe to treatment methods similar to those of a chiropractor in the Western medicine tradition. The *sobador* treats illnesses that primarily affect the joints and musculoskeletal system by using massage and manipulation.

Brujos (witches) treat illnesses and conditions caused by witchcraft. Specific rituals are performed to eliminate the evils from the body.

Espiritistas, or spiritualists, work with clients in terms of their spiritual connections, including religious connections. They do not usually prescribe medications but might prescribe herbal remedies and religious icons.

Herbal Medicine

Multiple studies on herbal remedies have been completed on Mexican and Mexican American patients. However, the only research study found in the literature on herbal medicine of Panamanians was conducted by Purnell (1999). In this study, 61% of Panamanians reported that they regularly used herbs and herbal teas to maintain their health. Moreover, 74% used herbs and teas when they were ill. Many people grow such herbs in their yards. In the home in which this author stays when in Panama, the middle-class family grows a number of herbs. If they have an overabundance of herbs, they are sold to the local pharmacist, who dries and prepares them for sale to the general public. For some of the preparations, leaves are used; for others, the roots are used. Table 20-1 lists these teas and their uses.

Study Questions

1. Identify strategies for integrating allopathic healthcare providers and practices with traditional healthcare practices and providers.
2. How might churches and religious leaders assist healthcare providers in educating communities for health promotion and wellness, as well as illness, disease, and injury prevention?
3. What are some key elements that nurses should include in delivering educational programs to vulnerable populations in Panama with low literacy and with Spanish as a second language?
4. What are some positive and negative influences that the United States has had on the health of Panamanians?
5. What are the underlying cultural beliefs, values, and practices of Panamanians that have helped shape the country's healthcare delivery system?
6. What are the advantages and disadvantages of the Panamanian healthcare delivery system versus the healthcare delivery system of the United States (or another country) in meeting the healthcare needs of the population?

Case Study 1: Cross-Cultural Learning

McDowell Memorial Medical Center and a state university have joined forces to sponsor sending 10 nursing students and 10 nursing staff to Panama for a two-week cross-cultural learning experience. Students and staff come from maternal–child, pediatric, medical–surgical, community, and psychiatric nursing. All students and staff identify with the dominant American culture. Only one student and two staff nurses have traveled outside the United States; their travel experiences were in Rio de Janeiro, Brazil; Ontario, Canada; and London, England. Three of the participants have limited experience with the Spanish language from high school; the remainder knows only a few expressions in Spanish.

Brenda Polek, a nurse manager from the Medical Center, and Alan Hardy, a faculty member from the university, will accompany the group. Both feel they have a "fair" understanding of the Spanish language. The main reason for students to participate in this experience is to complete an elective course on international nursing. Multidisciplinary staff nurses are participating in the trip to specifically learn about the Panamanian culture because the medical center has increasing numbers of Panamanians on maternal–child, pediatric, and medical–surgical inpatient units and outpatient departments. All students and staff will be housed with Panamanian families throughout their travels.

All students in this cultural immersion experience will be able to attend classes in the nursing programs while in Panama. When in the clinical areas, staff and students will be accompanied with staff nurses in outpatient clinics and on inpatient units. Not all students and staff will get the same clinical rotations. They will be in formal learning experiences four days each week and have three days each week for traveling and sightseeing. Journaling, in which students and staff record their observations and experiences, will be a large part of this program.

Brenda Polek and Alan Hardy, in conjunction with faculty and staff in Panama, will arrange housing and clinical experiences; some of them will be with indigenous Indian groups. The students and staff nurses will plan any other details before they leave for Panama.

Case Study 1 Questions

1. How would you feel about staying with a family in Panama if you do not speak the Spanish language well?
2. How might you prepare to improve your Spanish language skills before you depart from home?
3. What are the passport and visa requirements for traveling to Panama? (These requirements will change depending on your country of origin.)
4. Which vaccinations or medications will you take before you leave home? Where will you go to find out what is currently recommended for traveling to Panama?
5. What do you need to know about verbal communication practices of Panamanians so as not to violate social taboos?
6. What do you need to know about nonverbal communication practices of Panamanians so as not to violate social taboos?
7. How might you go about visiting a traditional healer while in Panama?
8. A few Panamanians, especially the younger generation, are anti-American because of U.S. influence in the Canal Zone, the environmental concerns left by the military in the Canal Zone, and the Manuel Noriega experience. How might you handle negative comments from Panamanian students about Americans?

9. What do you need to know about arthropod-borne diseases and food-borne and waterborne illnesses you may encounter on your trip?

10. Make a list of at least 10 strategies to maintain your health, your personal safety, and the safety of your group while traveling in Panama.

Case Study 2: Panamanian Challenges to Care

Leticia Maria de Isaacs Blancas y Chamorro, age 35, is married, with four children, ages 15, 12, 10, and 6. Her husband, Omedo, works on a banana plantation distant from their small orange and banana farm in rural Panama; he makes it home only every other weekend. Leticia has been over-weight since the birth of their first child and has never seen it as a problem. Approximately three months ago, she began losing weight, even though she was eating her usual diet and drinking a lot of carbonated beverages. She also has a rash on her arms and legs for which she has been using a poultice made from eucalyptus that helps the itching but does not clear up the rash.

Because going to the bathroom several times during the night was interfering with her sleep, Leticia sought advice from her mother. Her mother suggested a trip to the local botanica for herbs that a cousin used several years ago for the same condition. After trying the herbs for two weeks without improvement, she sought advice from a local curandera, who recommended guanabano and ginseng because Leticia was also having frequent bowel movements that she attributed to parasites. The curandera also recommended an antibiotic that did not require a prescription. Leticia obtained the antibiotic from the *farmacia*(pharmacist) and took it for five days, with no apparent improvement. In fact, her diarrhea and thirst worsened.

Leticia left her children with her younger sister and mother and took a bus 42 miles to a city with a physician. The physician wanted to admit Leticia to the hospital for a few days for a more complete health workup for diabetes mellitus. However, Leticia refused, saying that she needed to return home to her children. The physician reluctantly gave her an oral hypoglycemic prescription and an instruction for a weight-reduction diabetic diet and encouraged her to re-turn in one week. Leticia agreed to return if her husband came home that weekend with money so she could afford a second bus trip to the city. She also stated that if she could not return the following week, the curandera, whom she has known since she was an infant, would help her.

You are a public health nurse (health worker) who lives in the same town as Leticia and have heard of her health problems being discussed at local stores. You plan to make a visit to Leticia and offer advice if she will see you.

Case Study 2 Questions

1. Leticia has a rather long name. What is her married name? What is the family name of her father? What is the family name of her mother?

2. What might you do to build a trusting relationship with Leticia before giving her health advice?

3. Which advantages might there be in visiting Leticia in her home?

4. Which disadvantages might there be in visiting Leticia in her home?

5. What do you think has caused the rashes on Leticia's arms and legs?
6. Would you encourage or discourage Leticia from using eucalyptus on the rashes?
7. Would you encourage her to take antibiotic and herbal medicine recommended by the *curandera* along with the hypoglycemic prescription?
8. What do you think might happen if you advised Leticia to refrain from taking the antibiotic and herbal medicine recommended by the *curandera* along with the hypoglycemic prescription?
9. How might you help Leticia integrate the care recommended by the physician and *curandera*?
10. Would you discourage Leticia from seeing the *curandera* completely?
11. Leticia tells you that she does not want to lose any more weight because her husband likes her being "stout." She eats a "traditional" Panamanian diet, which is high in fat but replete with fresh fruits and vegetables. Which dietary recommendations would you make to negotiate an acceptable weight and still maintain control of her diabetes?
12. If Leticia agrees to be admitted to a hospital for treatment, would she be admitted to a Social Security hospital or a Ministry of Health hospital?

References

American Society of Tropical Medicine and Hygiene: The Gorges Memorial Institute. (2014). Retrieved from http://www.astmh.org/Gorgas_Memorial_Institute_Research_Award.htm

Business Panama. (2014). *Panama at a glance.* Retrieved from http://www.businesspanama.com/about_panama/glance.php

Centers for Disease Control and Prevention. (2014). *Chikunguna Virus. ta.* (2014). Retrieved from http://www.cdc.gov/chikungunya/

Canal de Panama. (2014). Retrieved from https//www.pancanal.com/eng/expansion/rpts/compenen

Central American Data. (2014). Retrieved from http://centralamericadata.com/en/search?q1=content_en_le:%22Information+Technology+Development%22

Central Intelligence Agency. (2014). *World factbook: Panama country profile.* Retrieved from https://www.cia.gov/library/publications/the-world-factbook/geos/pm.html

El Ciudad del Saber. (n.d.). *The city of knowledge.* Retrieved from http://ciudaddelsaber.org/en

GlobalSecurity.Org. (2014). *Fort Sherman.* Retrieved from http://www.globalsecurity.org/military/facility/fort-sherman.htm

Hospital Punta Pacifica: Panama. (2014). Retrieved from http://panamamedicalvacations.com/index/panama-medical-tourism/johns-hopkins-affiliate

Human Trafficking & Modern-day Slavery; Panama. (2009). Retrieved from http://www.gvnet.com/humantrafficking/Panama.htm

Hurtado, E. (1989). Breastfeeding in the etiology of diarrhea. *Archives of Latin American Nutrition, 39*(3), 278–291.

Library of Congress.(n.d.). *Cuna.* Retrieved from http://countrystudies.us/panama/29.htm

Library of Congress.(n.d.). *Panama. Education.* Retrieved from http://countrystudies.us/panama/39.htm

Native American tribes of Panama. (2009). Retrieved from http://www.native-languages.org/panama.htm

Outbreak of hantavirus pulmonary syndrome, Los Santos, Panama, 1999–2000. (2000, March). *Mortality and Morbidity Weekly Review, 17*(49), 205–207.

Panama. (2014). *Pictures of Panama.* Retrieved from http://www.info-panama.com/panama-gallery/index.php?lang=english

Panama Guide. (2014). http://www.panama-guide.com/article.php/20120126133900656

Panama Canal Authority. (2014). *Welcome to the Panama Canal.* Retrieved from http://www.pancanal.com/eng/index.html

Panama: Major infectious diseases. (2014). *Index Mundi.* Retrieved from http://www.indexmundi.com/panama/major_infectious_diseases.html

Pan-American Health Organization. (2004). *Profile of the health services system of Panama.* Washington, DC: Author.

Pan-American Health Organization. (2005). *Information on health: Panama.* Retrieved from http://www.paho.org/English/D/P39.pdf

Partners of the Americas. (2014). Retrieved from http://www.partners.net/partners/default.asp

Penagos, H. G. (2002). Contact dermatitis caused by pesticides among banana plantation workers in Panama. *International Journal of Occupational and Environmental Health, 8*(1), 14–18.

Purnell, L. (1999). Panamanian health beliefs and the meaning of respect afforded them by healthcare providers. *Journal of Transcultural Nursing, 14*(4), 331–340.

University of Panama. (2014). Retrieved from http://www.up.ac.pa

Universities in Panama. (2014). Retrieved from http://www.4icu.org/pa/

University of South Florida, Office of International Programs. (2010). Retrieved from http://health.usf.edu/intprog/panama/About_the_International_Foundation.htm

Warren, C. W., Monteith, R. S., Johnson, J. T., Santiso, E., Guerra, F., & Oberle, M. W. (1987). Use of maternal–child health services and contraception in Guatemala and Panama. *Journal of Biosocial Sciences, 19*(2), 229–243.

World Bank. (2014). *Health Inequities in Panama.* Retrieved from http://www.worldbank.org/en/news/feature/2013/09/11/mother-child-healthcare-inequalities-latin-america

World Health Organization. (2014). *Panama.* Retrieved from http://www.who.int/countryfocus.

21

Health and Health Care in Mexico

Rick D. Zoucha and Anelise Zamarripa-Zoucha

Objectives

After completing this chapter, the reader will be able to:

1. Relate a brief history of Mexico.
2. Discuss major health issues of the people of Mexico.
3. Compare and contrast the backgrounds and cultures of the people of Mexico.
4. Compare and contrast the Mexican healthcare system, including health facilities, to those of other developing nations.

INTRODUCTION

This chapter addresses health and health care in Mexico. The information presented here will be beneficial to healthcare professionals who may be interested in caring for people in Mexico, or to those who may be caring for people who are either temporary residents of other countries or migrants from Mexico who cross between countries frequently. Appreciation of the health and health system in Mexico can provide a clearer understanding of the context for health, illness, and care for people from Mexico. Specific information is presented about the history of Mexico, along with a description of the country's people, including their cultural values and beliefs. Additional information about the health of the people in Mexico as well as the health system (professional and folk) and workforce is provided as well.

MEXICO AND ITS PEOPLE

Mexico is a country located on the North American continent, situated south of the United States and northwest of Guatemala. The land area occupied by Mexico is approximately

1,964,375 km² (761,600 mi²), or roughly three times the size of Texas. The topography of the country includes coastal lowlands, mountains, and central-high plateaus, which have climates ranging from tropical to desert (U.S. Department of State, 2015).

The official name of the country is United Mexican States. Contemporary Mexico consists of 31 states and one federal district. Its capital, Mexico City, is located in the Federal district. The type of government is a federal republic comprising three branches: executive (the president is the chief of state and head of government), legislative (Senate and a Chamber of Deputies), and judicial (federal and state court systems). Several major political parties operate in Mexico, including the Institutional Revolutionary Party (PRI), National Action Party (PAN), Party of the Democratic Revolution (PRD), Green Ecological Party (PVEM), Labor Party (PT), and several small parties (U.S. Department of State, 2015).

BRIEF HISTORY OF MEXICO

The history and people of Mexico have been intertwined with the country's rich and diverse landscape dating back centuries before the Spanish conquest of Mexico in 1519. Prior to the Europeans' arrival, the land now described as Mexico was inhabited by several highly developed and organized cultures such as the Mayas, Toltecs, Aztecs, and Olmecs. After the conquest Spain established a colony that spanned three centuries. In many cases, the Spanish conquest resulted in the destruction of people and their cultures. However, remnants of the culture can still be seen as the people culturally mixed over the centuries, resulting in what is known as modern-day Mexico.

On September 16, 1810, independence was declared through the efforts of Father Migel Hidalgo, who is known as the "Father of Mexican Independence." The struggle for independence lasted more than 10 years, until 1821. A treaty finally recognized the country's independence from Spain with the planned establishment of a constitutional monarchy. The attempt to proceed with this plan failed, however, and in 1822 a republic was proclaimed; it was firmly established in 1824.

The political context of Mexico was again challenged in 1862, when French forces invaded Mexico. The French invaders instituted a monarchy, with Hapsburg Archduke Ferdinand Maximilian of Austria serving as emperor of Mexico from 1864 to 1867. His reign came to an end in 1867 when liberal forces in Mexico overthrew and executed the emperor. Mexico then remained independent from foreign rule until the revolution of 1910. Severe social and economic problems led to a 10-year revolution and establishment of the new constitution in 1917. The new constitution set the stage for the present federal republic with three separate forms of power structure: executive, legislative, and judicial branches of the government (U.S. Department of State, 2015).

During the Mexican Revolution of the early 20th century, many Mexicans left Mexico for its northern neighbor, the United States, to seek political, religious, and economic freedoms (Casa Historia, 2015). Following the Mexican Revolution, strict limits were placed on the activities of the Catholic Church; for example, until recently clerics were not allowed to wear their church garb in public. For many residents, such rules restricted the expression of their faith and represented a minor factor in their immigration north to the United States (Meyer & Beezley, 2010). In the years since the "Great Migration," limited employment opportunities in Mexico, especially in rural areas, have encouraged Mexicans to migrate to the United States as immigrants or with undocumented status; the latter are often derogatorily referred to as "wetbacks" (*majodos*) by the white and Mexican American populations.

The People

The population of Mexico is estimated at 121,736,809. The ethnic makeup of the people of Mexico includes Indian Spanish (mestizo), who represent 62% of the total population; Indian (Native American), 28%; Caucasian, 9%; and other, 1% (Central Intelligence Agency [CIA], 2015). The blend of Spanish white, Native American, Middle Eastern, and African heritage can be traced to descendants of Spanish and other European whites; Aztec, Mayan, and other Central American Indians; Inca and other South American Indians; and people from Africa (Schmal, 2014). Lesser-known ethnic groups whose members have historically immigrated to Mexico include Chinese and Jewish populations. Traditions and values of these cultures can still be seen in contemporary Mexico in music, food, and celebrations (Schmal, 2014).

Religion and Faith

The predominant religion in Mexico is Catholicism. The major religions in Mexico are Roman Catholic, 76.5%; Protestant, 6.3%; unspecified, 13.8%; and identified with no religion, 3.1%. Since the mid-1980s, religious groups such as Mormons, Jehovah's Witnesses, Seventh Day Adventists, Presbyterians, and Baptists have been gaining in popularity in Mexico (CIA, 2015). Although many Mexicans may not appear to be practicing their faith on a daily basis, they may still consider themselves devout Catholics, and their religion has a major influence on daily living and beliefs. It is common to see religious symbols on public buses and taxis as well as in public squares.

Migration to Urban Areas

Historically, there has been consistent migration from the rural areas of Mexico to the urban areas due to lack of jobs and opportunities in underdeveloped sections of the country. It is estimated that 76% of the Mexican population resides in urban areas of the country. The population of Mexico City alone is estimated to exceed 22 million people, with sharp increases in population also occurring in other cities such as Guadalajara, Puebla, and Monterrey (U.S. Department of State, 2015).

Communication

Mexico is considered the most populous Spanish-speaking country in the world, with more than 80 million residents who speak the language. Although the dominant language of Mexicans is Spanish, the country also has 54 indigenous languages and more than 500 different dialects (Lewis, Simons, & Fennig, 2015). For example, major indigenous languages include Nahuatl and Otami, spoken in central Mexico; Mayan, in the Yucatan peninsula; Maya-Quiche, in the state of Chiapas; Zapotec and Mixtec, in the valley of Oaxaca; Tarascan, in the state of Michoacan; and Totonaco, in the state of Veracruz. Many of the Spanish dialects spoken by Mexicans have similar word meanings, but the dialects of Spanish spoken by other groups may not have the same meanings. Because of the rural nature of many ethnic groups and the influence of native indigenous languages, the dialects are so diverse in some regions that it may be difficult to understand the language, regardless of the degree of fluency in Spanish (Lewis, Simons, & Fennig, 2015).

Education

The mean educational level in Mexico is five years. Until 1992, Mexican children were required to attend school through the sixth grade, but since the Mexican School Reform Act of 1992, a ninth-grade education has been required. In recent years, great strides have been made in improving educational standards in Mexico, which now reports a 95.1% literacy rate among its population (CIA, 2015). A common practice among parents in poor rural villages is to educate their children in what they need to know related to the immediate context of their lives. People from rural areas often find immigration to the United States to be a good option for both the individual and the family in terms of obtaining education. For many Mexicans, high school and a university education are unavailable and, in many cases, unattainable (Zoucha & Zamarripa, 2013).

Economy

The economy of Mexico is considered a free-market economy in the trillion-dollar class. It is based on a mixture of modern and outmoded industry and agriculture, which is becoming more dominated by the private sector. In recent years, there has been an expansion of competition in seaports, railroads, telecommunications, electricity generation, natural gas distribution, and airports. Overall, per capita income is roughly one-third of that found in the United States, and overall income distribution remains highly unequal. Since the advent and implementation of the North American Free Trade Agreement (NAFTA) in 1994, Mexico's share of U.S. imports has increased from 7% to 12%, and its share of Canadian imports has doubled to 5% (U.S. Department of State, 2015).

Mexico is rich in natural resources such as petroleum, silver, copper, gold, lead, zinc, natural gas, and timber. Agriculture accounts for 5% of the country's gross domestic product (GDP), including such products as corn, wheat, soybeans, rice, beans, cotton, coffee, fruit, tomatoes, beef, poultry, dairy products, and wood products. Approximately 31% of the country's GDP is attributable to industrial production, including manufacture of such items as food and beverages, tobacco, chemicals, iron and steel, petroleum, mining, textiles, clothing, motor vehicles, and consumer durables. Services such as commerce and tourism, financial services, transportation, and communications provide 64% of the GDP (U.S. Department of State, 2015).

Family and Kinship

Historically and in contemporary society, family is an all-encompassing value among Mexicans, for whom the traditional family remains the foundation of the culture. Family takes precedence over work and all other aspects of life. In many Mexican families, it is often said, "God first, family, then self." The family is of foremost importance to most Mexicans, and individuals get strength from family ties and relationships. Individuals may speak in terms of a person's soul or spirit (*alma or espiritu*) when they refer to his or her inner qualities. These inner qualities represent the person's dignity and must be protected at all costs in times of both wellness and illness.

In addition, Mexicans derive great pride and strength from their nationality, which embraces a long and rich history of traditions (Zoucha & Zamarripa, 2013).

In the Mexican culture, the concept of family moves beyond the nuclear family to incorporate a system of kinship that connects people as family without blood ties. In the Catholic faith, it is common to have godparents for an infant at baptism. Members of the Mexican culture may invite friends and family to be godparents (*padrinos*) for other sacraments in the faith in addition to baptism, including *padrinos* for communion, confirmation, and marriage. When individuals are asked to be *padrinos,* then they become *compadres* or family. It is a great honor and responsibility to be invited to be a *padrino* in the Mexican culture (Zamarripa, personal communication, 2015).

Other important events in which people are invited to be a *padrino* include the *quinceañera*, a very special event in which the 15-year-old girl is presented as a young woman. The *quinceañera* celebration begins with a thanksgiving mass, which is followed by a dinner and dance. These events symbolically represent the movement from childhood to young adulthood. The *quinceañera* is a family and community celebration in which the young woman, wearing a ball gown, is presented at church by her parents and *padrinos* and accompanied by a court of honor. The young women in the court, called *damas,* are accompanied by young men called *chambelanes* (Zamarripa, personal communication, 2015).

Because family is the first priority for most Mexicans, activities that involve family members usually take priority over work and other issues. Putting up a tough business front may be seen as a weakness in the Mexican culture. Most Mexicans tend to shun confrontation for fear of losing face. Many are very sensitive to differences of opinion, which are perceived as disrupting harmony in the workplace. Mexicans find it important to keep peace in relationships in the workplace and family (Zoucha & Zamarripa, 2013).

For many Mexicans, truth is tempered by diplomacy and tact. When a service is promised for tomorrow, even when they know the service will not be completed tomorrow, the promise is intended to please, not to deceive. Thus, for many Mexicans, truth is seen as a relative concept. These conflicting perspectives about truth can complicate communication with non-Mexicans (Zoucha & Zamarripa, 2013).

For most Mexicans, work is viewed as necessary for survival and may not be highly valued in itself, whereas money is for enjoying life. Many Mexicans place a higher value on other life activities. Material objects are usually necessities, rather than ends in themselves. The concept of responsibility is based on values related to attending to the immediate needs of family and friends rather than on the work ethic. For most Mexicans, titles and positions may be more important than money (Zoucha & Zamarripa, 2013).

Many Mexicans believe that time is relative and fluid, so they set flexible deadlines rather than stressing punctuality. In Mexico, shop hours may be posted but not rigidly respected. A business that is supposed to open at 8:00 a.m. may open when the owner arrives; a posted time of 8:30 a.m. may mean the business will open at 9:00 a.m., later, or not at all. The same attitude toward time is evidenced in reporting to work and in keeping social engagements and medical appointments. In some cases, if people believe that an exact time is truly important, such as the time a bus leaves, then they may keep to a schedule (Zoucha & Zamarripa, 2013).

Foods and Celebration

Mexicans often celebrate with food. Mexican foods are rich in color, flavor, texture, and spiciness depending on the state and region of the country. Any occasion—including births, birthdays, Sundays, religious holidays, official and unofficial holidays, and anniversaries of deaths—is seen as a time to celebrate with food and enjoy the togetherness of family and friends. Because food is a primary form of socialization in the Mexican culture, many Mexicans, from a health perspective, have difficulty adhering to a prescribed diet for illnesses such as diabetes mellitus and cardiovascular disease (Zoucha & Zamarripa, 2013).

The Mexican diet is varied, and its content may depend on the specific region of Mexico. The staples of the Mexican American diet are rice (*arroz*), beans, and tortillas, which are made from corn (*maíz*) treated with calcium carbonate. Popular Mexican American foods are eggs (*huevos*), pork (*puerco*), chicken (*pollo*), sausage (*chorizo*), lard (*lardo*), mint (*menta*), chili peppers (*chile*), onions (*cebollas*), tomatoes (*tomates*), squash (*calabaza*), canned fruit (*fruta de lata*), mint tea (*hierbabuena*), chamomile tea (*té de camomile* or *manzanilla*), carbonated beverages (*bebidas de gaseosa*), beer (*cerveza*), cola-favored soft drinks, sweetened packaged drink mixes (*agua fresa*) that are high in sugar (*azucar*), sweetened breakfast cereals (*cereales de desayuno*), potatoes (*papas*), bread (*pan*), corn (*maíz*), gelatin (*gelatina*), custard (*flan*), and other sweets (*dulces*). Other commonly eaten dishes include chili, enchiladas, tamales, tostadas, chicken mole, arroz con pollo, refried beans, tacos, tripe soup (*menudo*), and other soups (*caldos*). Soups are varied in nature and may include chicken, beef, and pork with vegetables (Zoucha & Zamarripa, 2013).

Alcohol plays an important part in the Mexican culture, and many celebrations include alcohol consumption. Men overall may drink in greater proportion than women, but this trend is changing. Today, Mexican women are consuming more alcohol than their mothers or grandmothers did (Bunting, personal communication, 2015). Because of these drinking patterns, alcoholism represents a crucial health problem for many Mexicans.

Health of the People

Many variables, ranging from violence to air pollution, affect the health and well-being of the people of Mexico. The life expectancy at birth is 75.5 years for males and 80.2 years for females (*World Health Statistics*, 2015). In recent years, certain regions of Mexico have been plagued by extreme incidents of violence and death as the result of drug wars. The areas affected most are the northern states of Chihuahua, Coahuila, Nuevo Leon, and Tamaulipas, with recent spikes occurring in the Gulf state of Veracruz. According to a *Frontline* report, 164,345 drug-related deaths have been reported in Mexico between 2007 and 2014 (and a total of more than 50,000 drug-related deaths have been reported since 2006 (*Frontline*, 2015).

In addition to violence related to drugs wars, a large number of people in Mexico are killed in road accidents. According to the Ministry of Health, 16,714 people were killed as a result of road traffic crashes in 2014 and an additional 603,541 were injured. Most of those injured or killed on Mexico's roads are between the ages of 15 and 29 years—this group makes up 48% of the total population. Road traffic crashes are the leading cause of death for the group aged 10 to 29 (World Health Organization [WHO], 2016). Table 21-1 lists leading health issues in Mexico, including the ages, causes of mortality, and mortality rates.

TABLE 21-1 Specific Health Problems in Mexico: Analysis by Population Group

Age	Mortality Rate	Leading Causes	Other Health Problems
0–4 years	15 per 1,000 live births (lb.)	Conditions originating from the perinatal period Congenital malformations Infections from influenza and pneumonia	
5–14 years	34 per 100,000	Accidents (11 per 100,000) Malignant tumors (5 per 100,000) Congenital malformations (2 per 100,000)	
15–24 years		Accidents (31 per 100,000) Homicide (14 per 100,000) Malignant neoplasms (6 per 100,000) Intentional self-harm (6 per 100,000)	Male versus female mortality rates by gender: Males: 135 per 1,000 Females: 75 per 1,000 (all ages) Fertility rate: 70 per 1,000 women (aged 15–44)
20–59 years	283 per 100,000	Malignant neoplasms (40 per 100,000) Accidents (39 per 100,000) Diabetes mellitus (31 per 100,000) Heart diseases (29 per 100,000)	Hospitalizations related to: • Pregnancy, childbirth, and the puerperium (67%) • Disorders of the digestive system (6%) • Trauma from accidents (6%)
60 years and older	4,763 per 100,000	Heart disease (1,106 per 100,000) Ischemic heart disease (706 per 100,000) Malignant neoplasms (612 per 100,000): • Trachea, bronchia, and lung (91 per 100,000) • Prostate (72 per 100,000) • Stomach (63 per 100,000) Diabetes mellitus (584 per 100,000) Cerebrovascular diseases (417 per 100,000)	

Data from Pan American Health Organization (PAHO). (2010). *PAHO basic health indicators on Mexico*. Retrieved from www.paho.org/English/DD/AIS/cp_484.htm.

In addition to the list of health concerns previously mentioned, there are major problems regarding the health of Mexicans owing to the consistent increase in number of HIV/AIDS cases in Mexico. The estimated number of adults and children (aged 15 and older) living with HIV/AIDS ranged from 140,000 to 270,000 in 2014 (WHO & UNAIDS, 2014). However, the rate of increase in HIV/AIDS in Mexico is relatively low in comparison to other countries in Central America and the United States. In the past, the Mexican government acted quickly and formed an effective response to the epidemic through the creation of CONAIDA, a national AIDS council. In addition, the council created an effective surveillance system to track the spread of the virus. A series of interventions decreased the spread of the virus, including bans on private blood clinics, mandatory testing of blood donations, and regulation of sex workers across the country. The AIDS council also promoted education on the use of condoms across Mexico as prevention for HIV/AIDS (Smallman, 2007). The threat of HIV/AIDS continues to be of great concern for Mexican health, however, and efforts aimed at decreasing the spread of the virus continue.

THE MEXICAN HEALTHCARE SYSTEM

The modern Mexican health system traces its origins to 1943, with the creation of three significant institutions: the Ministry of Health (MoH), the Mexican Institute for Social Security (IMSS), and Mexico's Children Hospital. These institutions were established to provide care to a variety of people. For example, the IMSS cared for the industrial workforce and the Ministry of Health was concerned with care for the urban and rural poor (Gomez-Dantes, 2010).

Between the inception of the Mexican health system in the 1940s and the 1980s, many changes occurred to bring about healthcare reform in Mexico. Because health care was delivered primarily in hospitals, its cost increased dramatically over the years. In addition, the incidence of common infections and illness showed a sharp decline, while the incidence of noncommunicable diseases and overall injuries showed dramatic increases.

In the mid-1980s, healthcare reform was launched to promote more efficiency in the system and decentralization of health services for the uninsured. The government built health centers and district hospitals to better serve the population. By the 1990s, however, at least 50% of the population was paying for health care out of pocket and lacked health insurance. The recognition of this problem prompted the Mexican legislature to enact reforms in 2003 that established the Social Protection in Health program (Gomez-Dantes, 2010). As a result of these historical struggles and evolution, Mexico's current health system includes care delivered by both the public and private sectors. The public sector encompasses the social security systems of Instituto de Seguridad y Servicios Sociales de los Trabajadores del Estado (IMSS), which is a state health insurance system for workers of social service, the Mexican State Institute for Social Security Services (ISSTE), Petroleos Mexicanos (PEMEX), the social security institution for oil workers, Secretaría de la Defensa Nacional (Sedena), the insurance for people in the army armed services, SEDENA, Mexican Navy employees' insurance, SEMAR, and Seguro Popular, the healthcare services to the uninsured population in Mexico. The last institution includes services provided by the Ministry of Health, State Health Services (SESA), and IMSS–Oportunidades Program (Jaff, 2010).

The social security institutions are financed with contributions from employees, employers, and the government. The Ministry of Health and SESA are financed by the federal and state government as well as through a small fee charged to users when receiving care. The IMSS–Oportunidades Program is financed by the federal government and administered by the IMSS. Federal and state funding and family contributions fund the Seguro Popular, although families at the bottom 20% of the income levels are exempt from this contribution (Gomez-Dantes, 2010).

The private sector of the health system in Mexico includes hospitals, health centers, clinics, and health providers such as physicians and nurses who provide services mostly on a for-profit basis. Such services are financed mostly with out-of-pocket payments, with a small allocation coming from people who pay for private insurance (Gomez-Dantes, 2010).

Healthcare Facilities

The Mexican healthcare system consists of a total of 23,269 facilities. The majority of facilities comprise ambulatory clinics and 4,466 hospitals. Of the total number of hospitals, 1,121 are public; 628 are social security institutions, and the remainder care for people who lack social security. Private hospitals in Mexico account for 3,082 of the total number of hospitals in the system. In Mexico overall, there are 1.1 hospitals per 100,000 population. This ratio varies regionally, however. For example, Baja California has 3.2 hospitals per 100,000 population, whereas there is only 0.5 hospital per 100,000 population in the state of Mexico (Secretaria de Salud, 2015).

On a per capita basis, the healthcare workforce in Mexico is below the average of many South American countries. It is estimated that there were 2.1 doctors per 1,000 population and 2.5 nurses per 1,000 population in Mexico in 2011, although these ratios are expected to increase over the next 10 years (World Bank, 2016). At the present time, Mexico has a total of 82 medical schools and 593 nursing schools (Gomez-Dantes, 2010). There has been a movement in Mexico over the last 20 years to educate nurses in university-based settings and to increase the level of education for Mexican nurses. In the last 10 years, Mexico opened the first PhD program in nursing to promote education and research at an advanced level (Becerril Cardenas, Gandara Sanchez, Mejia Carmona, & Gomez Arana, 2009).

Mexican Folk Practices

In addition to following Western systems of health, many people in Mexico engage in folk medicine practices and use a variety of prayers, herbal teas, and poultices to promote health and treat illnesses. The folk beliefs and practices noted in Mexico vary according to the region of the country, as well as between and among families.

One such folk belief and practice focuses on the hot and cold theory, which suggests that many diseases and illness are caused by a disruption in the hot-and-cold balance of the body. The belief is that eating foods that have the opposite effect (i.e., if cold, eat hot food; if hot, eat cold food) may either cure or prevent specific hot and cold illnesses. Likewise, physical or mental illness may be perceived as being due to an imbalance between the person and the environment.

Cold diseases may be characterized by lower metabolic rate and may include menstrual cramps, *frio de la matriz*, rhinitis (*coryza*), pneumonia, *empacho*, cancer, malaria, earaches, arthritis, pneumonia and other pulmonary conditions, headaches, musculoskeletal conditions, and colic. Common hot foods used to treat cold diseases and conditions include cheeses, liquor, beef, pork, spicy foods, eggs, grains other than barley, vitamins, tobacco, and onions (Neff, 2011).

Hot diseases may be characterized by vasodilation and a higher metabolic rate and may include pregnancy, hypertension, diabetes, acid indigestion, *susto*, *mal de ojo* (bad eye or evil eye), *bilis* (imbalance of bile, which runs into the bloodstream), infection, diarrhea, sore throat, stomach ulcers, liver conditions, kidney problems, and fever. Cold foods used to treat hot diseases may include fresh fruits and vegetables, dairy products, barley water, fish, chicken, goat meat, and dried fruits (Neff, 2011).

A variety of folk healers are incorporated within Mexican culture, including *curanderos* (believed to be empowered by God), *yerberos* (herbalists), and *parteras* (lay midwives). At times families may consult a folk healer to cure illness or promote health. Folk healers in Mexico may also be called to treat a variety of illnesses commonly found in the culture—that is, culture-bound disorders. For example, the ailment known as *mal de ojo* may occur when one person looks at another in an admiring fashion; its result may be fever, anorexia, and vomiting to irritability. This evil spell can be broken if the person doing the admiring touches the person admired while it is happening. Children seem to be more susceptible to this condition than women, and women are more susceptible than men. To prevent *mal de ojo*, the child may wear a bracelet with a seed (*ojo de venado*) or a bag of seeds pinned to the clothes (Kemp, 2001).

Susto (soul loss) is associated with epilepsy, tuberculosis, and other infectious diseases and is believed to be caused by a fright or by the soul being frightened out of the person. This culture-bound disorder may be psychological, physical, or physiological in nature. Symptoms can include anxiety, depression, loss of appetite, excessive sleep, bad dreams, feelings of sadness, and lack of motivation. Treatment sometimes includes elaborate ceremonies at a crossroads with herbs and holy water to return the spirit to the body (Zamarripa, personal communication, 2015).

Empacho (blocked intestines) is an illness that may be caused by a lump of food that sticks to the gastrointestinal tract. The healer may place a fresh egg on the abdomen to assess the problem. If the egg appears to stick to a particular area, this finding confirms the diagnosis. The folk healer treats the illness by administering herbal teas and by massaging the abdomen and back to dislodge the food and promote its passage through the body (Zoucha & Zamarripa, 2013).

Many other folk beliefs and practices contribute to the health and well-being of the people of Mexico. In some cases, specific folk healers are called upon to perform healing rituals, provide herbal medicines, and treat a variety of illness as well as promote health. In many communities, certain family members and neighbors are viewed as knowledgeable about healing and may perform the folk care locally.

CONCLUSION

Mexico is a country with a long and rich history dating back centuries. Its population is composed of a mixture of many cultures, including indigenous people with cultural roots connected to the Mayas, Toltecs, Aztecs, Olmecs, Spanish, French, and Africans, to name a few sources. The historical roots of these rich cultures come together to form the contemporary Mexican culture and people. Mexico is a rapidly developing country with a fairly stable economy, whose growth is linked to both industry and petroleum.

The health of the Mexican people is in constant flux due to economic changes and ongoing violence in some parts of the country. Drug-related violence and homicides related to "turf wars" have resulted in record increases in the overall rate of violence and murder in Mexico. The potential for violence and actual violence has affected the health and well-being of the Mexican people. In addition, the incidence of HIV/AIDS in Mexico continues to increase, despite early efforts to monitor and control the spread of the virus.

The health system in Mexico has undergone several reforms since the 1940s, as the Mexican government has sought to provide health care to all its citizens. Most Mexican citizens are provided with health care through several institutions run by the state and federal governments as well as by private insurance and institutions. Regardless of the individual's financial situation, some form of health care is provided through cooperation between the government, employer, employee, and social security and, in some cases, through private insurance.

Study Questions

1. Discuss the major health issues in Mexico. How do these problems compare to health concerns in other Central American countries and in other developed nations?
2. Compare and contrast strengths and weaknesses in the Mexican healthcare system.
3. What are the major areas needed for improvement in the healthcare system? What do you suggest that can be accomplished within the economical constraints?
4. How do you think politics, economics, geography, and education affect the health of residents and the healthcare system of Mexico?

Case Study: Health Care in Guanajuato, Mexico

Dr. Loretta Scott, a nursing professor at a local university, has accepted an invitation from a nurse colleague to assist with the health needs of people at a small urban clinic in Guanajuato, Mexico. She has gathered a total of six healthcare professionals, including two nursing students, one family nurse practitioner, one physician, and two public health nurses, to assist at the clinic. The visiting healthcare professionals will be working in the clinic for about three weeks.

Guanajuato is a city of 100,000 people located in the center of Mexico, in a relatively high elevation surrounded by mountains. The climate is dry, with warm days and cool evenings. The health clinic serves an area of the city located near its outskirts. The clinic is funded by the government and is considered an IMSS institution.

Upon the group's arrival to the city and clinic, the nurse tells the team that the number one concern is health education regarding diabetes, followed by HIV/AIDS prevention. Other concerns include education about injury prevention, such as auto accidents and treatment for influenza and pneumonia.

Case Study Questions

1. As a healthcare provider in Mexico, why is it important to know whether the people who come to the clinic for services will pay out of pocket based on the type of institution?
2. What will the visiting healthcare provider need to know historically about HIV/AIDS prevention in Mexico? Will the interventions and education be the same as or different from the interventions and education delivered in the United States?
3. What does the visiting healthcare provider need to know about diabetic education and nutrition in Mexico?

References

Becerril Cardenas, L., Gandara Sanchez, M., Mejia Carmona, B., & Gomez Arana, B. (2009). Nursing in Mexico. In K. Breda Lucas (Ed.), *Nursing and Globalization in the Americas: A Critical Perspective* (p. 185). Amityville, NY: Baywood.

Casa Historia. (2015, April 26). *Mexican revolution and beyond.* Retrieved from http://www.casahistoria.net/mexicorevolution.htm

Central Intelligence Agency. (2015). *The world factbook: North America: Mexico.* Retrieved from https://www.cia.gov/library/publications/the-world-factbook/geos/mx.html

Frontline. (2015). Instituto Nacional de Estadistica, Geografia Informatica (Mexico). WGBH Educational Foundation. Retrieved from http://www.pbs.org/wgbh/frontline/article/the-staggering-death-toll-of-mexicos-drug-war/

Gomez-Dantes, O. (2010). Mexico. In J. A. Johnson & C. H. Stoskopf (Eds.), *Comparative Health Systems: Global Perspectives* (p. 337). Sudbury, MA: Jones & Bartlett Learning.

Jaff, H. (2010, March 27). The right to health in Mexico: Seguro Popular. *World Poverty and Human Rights Online.*

Kemp, C. (2001). *Hispanic health beliefs and practices: Mexican and Mexican-Americans (clinical notes).* Retrieved from http://www.nursingworld.org/MainMenuCategories/ANAMarketplace/ANAPeriodicals/OJIN/TableofContents/Volume112006/No3Sept06/ArticlePreviousTopics/CulturallyCompetentNursingCare.html

Lewis, M. P., Simons, G. F., & Fennig, C. D. (Eds.). (2015). *Ethnologue: Languages of the World* (18th ed.). Dallas, TX: SIL International. Retrieved from http://www.ethnologue.com/

Meyer, M., & Beezley, W. (2010). *The Oxford History of Mexico.* Oxford, UK: Oxford University Press.

Neff, N. (2011). *Folk medicine in Hispanics in the Southwestern United States.* Retrieved from http://www.rice.edu/projects/HispanicHealth/Courses/mod7/mod7.html

Pan American Health Organization. (2010). *PAHO basic health indicators on Mexico.* Retrieved from www.paho.org/English/DD/AIS/cp_484.htm

Schmal, J. (2014). *Essays and research on indigenous Mexico.* Retrieved from http://www.somosprimos.com/schmal/schmal.htm

Secretaria de Salud. (2015). *Programa nacional de salud 2007–2012.* Mexico City: Author.

Smallman, S. (2007). *The AIDS Pandemic in Latin America.* Chapel Hill, NC: University of North Carolina Press.

Stanley Bunting, J. (2011). Chemical dependency within the Hispanic population: Considerations for diagnosis and treatment. In G. Lawson & A. Lawson (Eds.), *Alcoholism and Substance Abuse in Diverse Populations* (2nd ed., pp. 227–242). Austin, TX: Pro-Ed.

U.S. Department of State. (2015). *Background notes: Mexico*. Retrieved from http://www.state.gov/r/pa/ei/bgn/35749.htm

The World Bank. (2002). Retrieved from http://web.worldbank.org/WBSITE/EXTERNAL/NEWS/0,contentMDK:20052226~menuPK:141310~pagePK:34370~piPK:34424~theSitePK:4607,00.html

The World Bank. (2016). Retrieved from http://data.worldbank.org/indicator/SH.MED.PHYS.ZS and http://data.worldbank.org/indicator/SH.MED.NUMW.P3

World Health Organization. (2016). *Mexico Road Safety: Report on Ten Countries*. Geneva, Switzerland: WHO Department of Injuries and Violence Prevention and Disability.

World Health Organization & UNAIDS. (2014). *Epidemiological Fact Sheet on HIV and AIDS, Core Data on Epidemiology and Response: Mexico 2015 Update* (Update No. 089-735). Geneva, Switzerland: Author.

World Health Statistics. (2015). Geneva, Switzerland: WHO Press.

Zoucha, R., & Zamarripa, C. (2013). People of Mexican heritage. In Larry D. Purnell (Ed.). *Transcultural Health Care: A Culturally Competent Approach* (4th ed., pp. 374–390). Philadelphia, PA: F. A. Davis.

22

Health and Health Care in Israel

Orly Toren and Michal Lipschuetz

Objectives

By the end of this chapter the reader will be able to:

1. Relate a brief history of the establishment of the State of Israel, and its healthcare system.
2. Compare and contrast population statistics.
3. Compare and contrast the healthcare system of previous to current times.
4. Discuss the application of healthcare laws to the health of the population groups.
5. Relate current healthcare goals.
6. Relate the state of nursing and medicine in Israel today.

INTRODUCTION

This chapter will address the health and healthcare issues of Israel from a historical perspective as well as a current view. Numerous health and healthcare issues will be examined within the cultural, economic, and legal systems. A unique focus will include an examination of the stress of anticipation and actual war and the impact it has on the health of the population. The professions of nursing, medicine, and other healthcare professionals will also be reviewed.

HISTORY

Israel, the land of Jewish and other ethnic groups, is located in the Middle East, in the midpoint of three continents (Asia, Europe, and Africa) and two seas (the Mediterranean and the Red sea). The many groups in addition to Jewish peoples include religious and secular groups: Christians, Muslims, Arabs, Druze, Bedouins, Cherkassys, and Samaritans.

During the last centuries, the strategic geographic location of Israel has attracted many states to invest in Israel (creating communication lines, missionaries' organizations, absorbing new immigrants, etc.) which has promoted it to a leading position. This was the basis for its occupation by Great Britain in 1917, at the end of the First World War.

Israel gained its independence in 1948 and was established as a Jewish democratic state. By its establishment, the founders declared that it would be open to all Jewish members around the world, would focus on the development of the country for the advantage of its members, and would be based on the principles of freedom, justice, and peace. It would provide freedom to practice any religion and allow for residents to follow their conscience language and culture, and also preserve the holy places for all religions.

POPULATION AND DEMOGRAPHY

The Israeli population includes 8.345 million people. The most important characteristic is its population diversity (Table 22-1). The majority of the population consists of Jews (74.9%) and Arabs (20.7%), and there are many other smaller ethnic and religious groups, such as the Samaritans and the Cherkassy (Israel Central Bureau of Statistics, 2014).

Israel is a fairly young country when compared to the other Organisation for Economic Co-operation and Development (OECD) countries, with a young population (median age 28.3 years), and has a low infant mortality rate (4.5 per 1,000 deliveries). Israel also has a long life expectancy: males, 80.3 years, females, 83.9 years (Israel Central Bureau Statistics, 2015).

Elderly persons aged 65 and over account for 10.6% of the population. The proportion of persons aged 75 and over among the Israeli population has grown moderately over the

TABLE 22-1 Statistics of Israeli Demography and Economics

	Israel	OECD
Health expenditure per capita	2,303	3,484
Fertility rate (for women 15–49 years)	3	3
Dependency ratio*	62.5	53.6
% population >65 years**	10.3	15.4
Life expectancy (Men)	79. 9 years	77.7 years
Life expectancy (Women)	83.6 years	80.2 years
No. of general beds per 1,000 population	3.1	4.8
Occupancy rate (general beds)	96.6%	75.1%
Out-of-pocket money for health services (from total healthcare expenditure)	25.9%	19.0%
Physician rate (per 1,000 population)	3.3	3.2
Nurses rate (per 1,000 population)	4.8	8.8

Data from Israel Central Bureau of Statistics. (2014). Selected data from the *Statistical Abstract of Israel No.65*. Retrieved from http://www.cbs.gov.il/reader/newhodaot/hodaa_template.html?hodaa=201411257; *The World Bank. (2015). *Age dependency ratio*. Retrieved from http://data.worldbank.org/indicator/SP.POP.DPND/countries?display=graph; **Israel Ministry of Health. (2014a). *Health 2013*. Retrieved from http://www.health.gov.il/PublicationsFiles/health2013.pdf.

years: 3.8% at the beginning of the 1990s compared to 4.9% in 2013. Predictions are that the population will continue to get older due to the decrease in the percent of children being born and the increase of the older group within the general population. The number of residents aged 65 and over is expected to grow more than other age groups. It is estimated that at the end of 2035, this segment of the population will number approximately 1.7 million as compared to 763,000 people at the end of 2010, representing an increase of 117%. The relative share of the older adult population will increase from 10 to 14.6%, respectively (Israel Central Bureau of Statistics, 2013a, 2014).

Since Israel's establishment, its population size is almost 10 times larger. The annual rate of population growth was 1.9% in 2014. Part of the reason for Israel's rapid growth is the major waves of immigration into the country. As an immigration country, the population grew by 16% between 2000 and 2008. The highest growth rate was for persons aged 55 to 64 (50% higher) and persons aged 75 and older (25% higher).

The percentage of children aged 14 and under in the population has been stable at 28% in the last decade (Israel Central Bureau of Statistics, 2014).

HEALTHCARE SYSTEM IN ISRAEL

History
Since the establishment of the State of Israel in 1948, health care has always been an important issue of the public agenda. The pluralistic nature of the healthcare system and its current organization have deep roots in the preestablished state period (Bin Nun, Berlovitz, & Shani, 2010). Many historical events, such as the waves of immigration since the 19th century and polio and malaria epidemics, have led the state to seek financial backing, particularly from wealthy Jewish barons, to establish a basis for social healthcare aid.

Prior to its establishment, Israel was under Ottoman occupation, a period in which missionary organizations treated the healthcare needs of the population entering and leaving Israel. The first hospital was built in 1854 by the Rothschild family; later many hospitals were established, mainly in Jerusalem, but also in Jaffa, Tiberias, and Zfat. With the first wave of immigration at the end of the 19th century, many healthcare services were established to serve the healthcare needs of the newcomers, mainly farmers. The end of World War I brought many diseases to the people in the country, a situation that inspired Hadassah: The Women's Zionist Organization, an organization of volunteers, to build the Hadassah Organization in Israel in order to organize health services. This organization provided health aid to the community, primarily to treat infectious diseases and provide preventive medicine services to children. These services included first aid treatment and hospitalization services.

From 1917 to 1948, Israel was occupied by the United Kingdom. During this period, the healthcare trend was to transfer the health services to other authorities such as local municipalities and other sick funds (health maintenance organizations [HMOs]). These organizations provided both preventive and first aid treatment, and at the same time built hospitalization services. The sick funds served as organizations for mutual aid, providing health care to their members:

TABLE 22-2 Number of Hospital Beds by Ownership, 1948–1970

Ownership	1948	1950	1960	1970
Government	689	2,996	5,785	10,063
Municipal	451	583	793	195
Kupat Holim Klalit	649	997	2,636	3,744
Hadassah	431	541	477	590
Private	1,367	1,449	3,394	5,606
Other	1,039	461	2,528	3,529
Summary	5,626	7,627	15,613	23,727

Reproduced from Bin Nun, G., Berlovitz, Y., & Shani, M. (2010). *The healthcare system in Israel.* Tel Aviv: Am Oved Pub.

seven HMOs were operating by the evening of the declaration of the state. The largest with the most insured population (805,000) was Kupat Holim Clalit, and the remainder of the population was served by several smaller sick funds. By the end of 1948, only 53% of the Jewish population was insured (Bin Nun, Berlovitz, & Shani, 2010; Israel Ministry of Foreign Affairs, 1995).

The first two years after its establishment, the population of the State of Israel doubled to 1.2 million people due to the mass immigration of Holocaust survivors from Europe and Jewish refugees from Arab countries. Within a decade, the population reached 2.1 million. The percentage of those insured increased dramatically during those years. Both the Ministry of Health and Kupat Holim Clalit expanded their medical facilities to cope with the increasing demand for health services.

In 1953 all military hospital facilities were transferred to the Ministry of Health to enhance financial and management efficiency, and the ministry became the major provider of hospitalization services. Kupat Holim Clalit also took steps to expand its services, building more hospitals and community clinics. Smaller sick funds attempted to follow Kupat Holim Clalit's example and compete by opening more clinics in the community. Table 22-2 contains data about the number of hospital beds by ownership. The major trend during this period is the growth in the number of government beds, from 12% of total hospital beds in 1948 to 42% in 1970 (Bin Nun, Berlovitz, & Shani, 2010).

PRESENT HEALTHCARE SYSTEM

Healthcare Coverage
With the establishment of the country in 1948, official institutions were formulated, including governmental offices and the Ministry of Health (MOH). The MOH is responsible for the Israeli healthcare system, including hospitals, clinics, and other medical institutions (Israel Ministry of Health, 2010).

Other roles of the Israeli Ministry of Health include the following:

- Responsibility for all activities in the health sector in Israel, including among other things, preventive medicine, public health, environmental health, health of students and employees, and health promotion.
- Responsibility for licensing and supervising health professionals. Professionals include, among others, physicians, nurses, midwives, dentists, pharmacists, dietitians, occupational therapists, physiotherapists, psychologists, and others.
- Responsibility for supervising the activities of funds according to the National Health Insurance Law.
- Responsibility for such matters as clinical trials in humans and animals, monitoring the activities of Magen David Adom (Israel National Rescue Organization), partnership overseeing the environmental issues along with the Environmental Protection Agency, and supervising the production and importation of food, medicines, and the like.

At the beginning of 1995, the year in which Israel's National Health Insurance Law came into effect, approximately 5.2 million persons were insured in HMOs, whereas at the end of 2013, 7.93 million persons were insured (Israel Ministry of Health, 2014b).

The four sick funds are Kupat Holim Clalit (52.5% of market share), Maccabi (24.8%), Meuchedet (13.6%), and Leumit (9%). Under this law, residents have the right to choose their preferred sick fund, as well as the right to transfer between the four. Health care should be provided to all insured citizens with no discrimination based upon age, state of health, or other potential risk factors.

About 53% of the cost of the medical services basket is covered by revenues from the health insurance fee and 41% is paid for out of the state budget. The remainder of the funding is paid by copays collected from the public as a progressive income tax. In the past two years, the state's share in the funding of the basket costs has increased (Arieli, Horev, & Keidar, 2014).

Laws Affecting the Healthcare System

Two primary laws were issued toward the end of the last century: the National Health Insurance Act and the Patient's Right Act.

The National Health Insurance Act

The National Health Insurance Act is a legal framework that enables and facilitates basic, compulsory universal health care. The law was put into effect by the Knesset (Parliament) on January 1, 1995. It was issued on the basis of the recommendations of a National Committee of Inquiry, which examined the need for restructuring the healthcare system in Israel in the late 1980s. Prior to the issue of the law, several problems had been recognized. These are as follows:

- Membership in the largest fund (Kupat Holim Calalit) required a member to belong to the Histadrut labor organization, even if a person did not wish to (or could not).
- Selection based on age and health status was used by some sick funds for acceptance of new members.

- Different funds provided different levels of benefit coverage or services to their members.
- Although small, a certain percentage of the population did not have health insurance coverage at all.

The law ensured that *all* citizens would have health coverage and determined a uniform benefits package for all citizens—a list of medical services and treatments that each of the sick funds are required to fund for its members. The state is responsible for providing health services to all residents of the country, who can register with one of the four health sick funds. To be eligible, a citizen must pay a health insurance tax. Coverage includes medical diagnosis and treatment, preventive medicine, hospitalization (general, maternity, psychiatric, and chronic), surgery and transplants, preventive dental care for children, first aid and transportation to a hospital or clinic, medical services at the workplace, treatment for drug abuse and alcoholism, medical equipment and appliances, obstetrics and fertility treatment, medication, treatment of chronic diseases, and paramedical services such as physiotherapy and occupational therapy.

The law sets out a system of public funding for healthcare services by means of a progressive health tax, administered by Israel's Social Security organization, which transfers funding to the sick funds according to a certain formula based on the number of members in each fund, the age distribution of members, and a number of other indices. The sick funds also receive direct financing from the states. Although most of the services are covered by the law, certain services are administered and covered directly by the state; these include geriatrics, public health, and until recently, mental health.

In addition to the uniform benefits package provided to all citizens, each sick fund provides its members with supplementary services and treatments usually covered with a private insurance that may be a "supplementary insurance" of the sick fund, or a private insurance from any insurance company.

While membership in one of the funds is compulsory, there is a free choice to transfer from one sick fund to another, making the various sick funds equal for all members among the populace. Annually, a committee appointed by the minister of health publishes a "basket" or uniform package of medical services and prescription formulary that all funds must provide as a minimum service to all their members. Achieving this level of equality ensures that all citizens are guaranteed to receive basic health care regardless of their fund affiliation, which was one of the principal aims of the law. An appeals process was put in place to handle rejection of treatments and procedures by the funds and evaluating cases falling outside the basket of services or prescription formulary.

The law is generally considered a success and Israeli citizens enjoy a high standard of medical care. Despite more competition being introduced into the field of health care in the country, the law has some limitations, as listed below:

- Some say that the basket is not large enough to provide coverage to every medical situation.
- Another criticism is that in order to provide universal coverage to all, the tax income base amount (the maximum amount of yearly earnings that are subject to the tax) was set rather high, causing many high-income taxpayers to see the amount they pay for their health premiums (now health tax) skyrocket.
- After 20 years of issuing the law, some say that the constantly rising costs of copayments for certain services are a leading problem of health care.

The Patient's Right Act

The Patient's Right Act of 1996 aims to establish the rights of every person who requests medical care or who is in receipt of medical care, to protect his or her dignity and privacy (Israel Ministry of Health, 1996). This act contains several parts:

- *The Right to Acquire Care.* A major part of the act is the way that it outlines rights to medical care in Israel. Medical facilities and clinicians are not allowed to discriminate against patients on the basis of race, gender, religion, nationality, country of birth. or other similar grounds. Patients are required to get proper care, and everyone visiting an emergency medical facility is allowed to have an examination.
- *Privacy Rights.* Physicians and other medical staff are required to maintain medical confidentiality; they are not to disclose any information about patients' medical conditions and treatments.
- *Informed Consent Rights.* Informed consent is required prior to any medical intervention. Physicians must explain treatment and other medical information to patients, including diagnosis, prognosis, risks of treatment, risks of nontreatment, information about alternative treatments, and likelihood of treatment success. If an ethics committee determines that medical information might cause a severe threat to a patient's mental or physical health, physicians may withhold information from the patient. Informed consent can be given verbally, in writing, or through another behavioral demonstration to the patient. Some situations are exceptional for informed consent, such as when patients are not in a mental state that allows them to understand medical information. In these cases, an appointed legal guardian can make the medical decisions for them.
- *Medical Records.* Physicians and medical staff are required to keep detailed medical records for patients. Patients may have access to their own medical records. Physicians can only disclose medical information to other medical members for treatment or when an ethics committee decides that disclosure of medical information is necessary for the health of the general public.

In many respects, Israel's Patient's Rights Act differs little from the policy and practice of other nations (Gross, 2005). Patients enjoy a wide range of rights including national health care, the right of informed consent, privacy, confidentially, and respect for dignity. Meaningful informed consent facilitates healthcare professionals to provide a wealth of information about risks, benefits, and alternative treatments.

Ministry of Health Policy to Promote Population Health

The "pillars of fire" is a strategic plan introduced in 2011 that was implemented as a policy to reach the goals of the Ministry of Health. Professor Gamzu, the former CEO of the Ministry of Health, stated that the

> Israeli Health Care System is one of the most advanced in the Western world. It contains many different health care indicators. The strongest points of the system are public infrastructures with sick funds and other health care organizations caring for the citizens' health. However, the weakest point of the system is the low investment for health, growing private expenditure for

health care, health discrepancies between populations and geographical areas, and the lack of a national infrastructure to measure outcome quality. (Israel Ministry of Health, 2010)

The plan contains five main goals:

1. *Promote public health.* This goal is intended to decrease hazardous behaviors, limiting the population exposure to external influences (mainly food and environment) and the ability to prevent diseases. To achieve this goal officials use promotion campaigns to elevate public awareness to recommended nutrition, health activity, active legislation against smoking, and improving treatment of children by immunizations and monitoring child development.
2. *Decrease inequalities in health (geographically and socially).* This goal will focus on the reduction of economic inequalities to purchase health services, the reduction of the cultural influence on healthcare services consumption, promote adequate personnel and infrastructures in the periphery of the country, and give incentives to the HMOs to invest in reducing inequalities.
3. *Strengthen the public nature of the healthcare system in Israel.* The focus is to expand the public "healthcare basket" and reduce private financing of the system.
4. *Ensure the quality of health and the quality the healthcare system.* The goal is to build a national database to measure quality healthcare indicators for the different population groups in the system (hospitals and community healthcare services).
5. *Accommodate healthcare services to future healthcare developments.* This is to be done by creating a national strategic plan to prepare the system to address the healthcare needs in the medium and long run, to reduce the gaps of professional healthcare providers and infrastructures to meet their healthcare needs. This goal will require creating an organizational structure for future policy planning.

Most of these goals are still relevant to date. Other aspects of emphasis are related to the following:

- *Quality improvement.* This entails monitoring clinical quality indicators and setting clear targets for clinical excellence in congruence with international standards (OECD, Joint Commission Israel (JCI]).
- *Improving service to the public.* Improvements are to be made while setting clear goals and monitoring the service indicators in all healthcare facilities.
- *Personnel planning.* This can be accomplished by increasing the supply of physicians and nurses; regulating the interfaces between healthcare professionals and the population needs; preparing the health system for the population aging; constructing more effective continuity of care by strengthening ties between hospitals and community settings.
- *Promoting online and computer-based health services.* This will be achieved by improving access to public service on the basis of advanced technology and developing a national infrastructure for managing medical information (State of Israel, 2014).

Another major trend in promoting the population's health is to focus on mental health. Although the legislation of the National Health Insurance Law ensured universal access to an extensive basket of benefits, the mental health system was not covered. Mental health functioned separately as reflected in its funding, planning organization, and operating frameworks.

Reforms in mental health effective July 2015 transfer insurance liability for mental health services from the Ministry of Health to the HMOs. The reform applies only to funding the services, which means that mental health services, like any other general medical service, are provided by the HMOs.

The intent behind this reform is to increase the quality, availability, and accessibility of mental health services for the citizens of Israel. Dozens of mental health clinics will be opened across the country, which will bring more treatment options by different professionals, expansion of clinics hours of service, and reduction of waiting lists. Because eligibility for mental health treatment is included in the health basket, these services will be provided to all citizens at the minimal cost of their deductibles (as in other areas general medicine).

The reform is expected to contribute significantly to quality service by reducing the social stigma against mental disorders, reinforcing the public awareness to mental health issues, and facilitating community integration of those suffering mental difficulties (Israel Ministry of Health, 2015a).

HEALTH IN ISRAEL: STATISTICS AND TRENDS

Israel has its own unique healthcare characteristics. Life expectancy at birth is increasing. In 2013 it was 83.9 years for females and 80.3 years for males, 84.3 and 81 for Jews and others respectively, and 80.9 (females) and 78 (males) for Arabs (Averbuch & Anvi, 2014).

Maternal age for first childbirth is also increasing. In 2013, the median age was 27.5 compared with 25.1 in 1994. Differences also varied within ethnic groups: The maternal age for Jewish mothers was 25.8 years, as compared to 23.6 years for Arab mothers (Israel Central Bureau of Statistics, 2014).

Israel's death rate is decreasing. General mortality rate, standardized by age per 1,000 residents in 2012, was 6.0 in men and 4.4 for women. Stratified by population group mortality rate in this year among Jewish men, was 5.8 and for Jewish women 4.3. In the Arab population in the same year, the mortality rate was 7.6 among men and 5.7 among women (Averbuch & Anvi, 2014).

The infant mortality rate is decreasing and is similar to the median for OECD countries. In 2013, the rate was 3.4 per 1,000 live births; 2.5 among Jews and 6.3 among Moslems. The main causes of infant death among the Jews were perinatal and among the Moslems were congenital anomalies (Averbuch & Anvi, 2014). The percentage of infants born weighing less than 2,500 grams was stable in the last decade at 8.1% in 2012 (Keidar, Plotnik, Nakmoli Levi, & Horev, 2014).

The crude mortality rate decreased in 2012 with a rate of 532 per 100,000 population compared to 599 per 100,000 residents in 2000, reflecting a 11% decrease. The adjusted death rate is lower than OECD average. The adjusted death rate in Israel was in the lowest sixth out of 33 OECD countries in 2011. The age-adjusted suicide rate in Israel is lower than in most OECD countries (OECD average 12.4 per 100,000) with 7.3 per 100,000 persons aged 15 and older. In 2011, 409 suicide cases were reported in Israel: 322 men and 87 women.

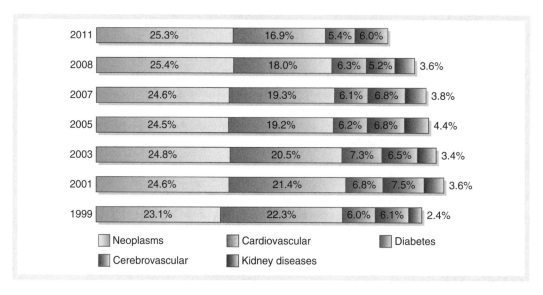

FIGURE 22-1 Leading Causes of Death in Israel (%)
Data from Israel Ministry of Health. (2014a). *Health 2013*. Retrieved July 12, 2015, from http://www.health.gov.il/
PublicationsFiles/health2013.pdf

Malignant neoplasms have been the leading causes of death in Israel since the end of the 1990s. In 2011, the leading causes of death were malignant neoplasms (25.3%), heart diseases (16.9%), cerebrovascular diseases (6%), and diabetes (5.4%). The leading cause of death among people aged 15 to 44 was accident. At age 75 and over, the leading cause was heart disease. Malignant neoplasm was the leading cause for males aged 45 to 74 and females aged 25 to 74 (Israel Ministry of Health, 2014a).

PREPARING FOR EMERGENCY SITUATIONS AND MASS CASUALTY EVENTS

Part of the responsibility of the Ministry of Health is to deploy and prepare the system for emergency situations. Israel created the Department of Emergency Situations and Mass Casualty Events, which is very active in preparing hospitals, HMOs, the Israeli ambulance services (MDA, similar to the Red Cross), and the general population for all kinds of attacks (conventional, chemical, biological, radiological, and atomic attacks). The goal of this department is to prepare hospitals and community healthcare services to treat patients injured from conventional and unconventional emergency situations and mass casualty events (State of Israel, 2002). In addition, this department is working closely with other emergency services such as the fire department, police. and the army. Because the frequency of mass casualty events is particularly high in Israel, the healthcare system must be prepared for any scenario (Rassin et al., 2007).

The Department for Emergency Situations and Mass Casualty Event is responsible for writing standards and protocols for all kinds of situations, controlling and preparing for these situations, the education of staff members for all levels of care, the development of technological infrastructures, adopting and verifying for the right equipment in the adequate amount, performing life and simulated drills, and adjusting workers and equipment among healthcare organizations as needed.

As a result of the many mass casualty events that have occurred in the nation, Israeli teams have gathered extensive experience in handling the crises. They share it globally in different situations, from educating and preparing teams to deal with all kinds of mass casualty events, to real situations of life-saving, as occurred in the recent earthquakes in Haiti and Japan.

HEALTHCARE PROFESSIONALS IN ISRAEL

In 2009, of the 170,000 total people employed in the Israeli healthcare system, 94,000 were healthcare professionals: of these, 34% were physicians and nurses, 24% were allied healthcare professionals, and the rest were from other occupations (Israel Ministry of Health, 2010). From 2000 to 2008, the number of nurses decreased by 5%, the rate of the other healthcare professionals increased by 5%, and physicians increased by 1%. More than half of the physicians (58%) and nurses (77%) work in hospitals, a stable rate during the past decade.

Medicine

The number of physicians in Israel at the end of 2011 was 34,657, of which 26,065 were under 65 years old (Israel Central Bureau of Statistics, 2013b). The rate of physicians per 1,000 population is still high compared to most of the OECD countries (3.3 per 1,000 in Israel, and 3.2 per 1,000 in the OECD), although it has decreased in the last decade and the country is at risk for a shortage of physicians (OECD Health Statistics, 2014).

Until recently, the Israeli physician supply relied heavily on physicians trained in other countries, primarily immigrants from the former Soviet Union and Eastern Europe. However, the massive immigration of the early 1990s has dramatically decreased, and the sources of new immigrant physicians are decreasing. The rate of new graduates from Israeli medical schools was 3.8 to 100,000 in 2012, compared with the average of the OECD rate of 11.2 (Israel Central Bureau of Statistics, 2013b).

To address this shortage, Israel has opened another medical school in the north to join the other four existing medical schools (Rosen & Merkur, 2009). The number of registrations has risen in the years after the decline in the late 1990s. In 2013, 1,011 new licenses were issued, up from 547 in 2007, of which 42% were from Israeli graduates (Israel Ministry of Health, 2015b).

The majority of the physicians (62%) are employed by the sick funds or governmental institutions, mainly hospitals (Shemesh, Rotem, Haklai, Georgi, & Horev, 2012). An increase in the rate of older physicians (age 55 and over) is noted during the last decade (28% in 2000 and 49% in 2008). The percentage of female physicians is rising; women comprise 46% of all physicians (Israel Ministry of Health, 2015b).

The percentage of specialty experts among the total number of physicians is rising (56% in 2013 compared to 44% in 2000). In this group, the percentage of men is higher than that of women (58 and 49%) (Bin Nun, Berlovitz, & Shani, 2010).

Nursing

Nursing in Israel is regulated by the Division of Nursing, a part of the Ministry of Health. Its roles are to originate the policy of nursing on the national level. The manager of the nursing division (National Chief Nurse) is a registered nurse, who serves both as a member of the Ministry of Health Management and as a consultant to the Minister of Health for all aspects of nursing and nurses. Part of the National Chief Nurse's responsibilities include nursing education, registration, nursing standards, and development. In addition, he or she monitors patients and the healthcare system's needs to accommodate the role of healthcare trends and society needs.

In Israel, there are three levels of nurses—practical nurses (LPNs), registered nurses (diploma graduates), and nurses with academic degree (academic graduates). On a national level, it was decided to upgrade the level of the nursing profession's education level; a BSN (Bachelor of Sciences in Nursing) became the entry-level requirement for admission into the profession (Toren & Picker, 2009). This level of training exists in Israel's five universities and several colleges (Israel Ministry of Health, 2015b). The rate of registered nurses per 1,000 population in Israel, has always been low and among the lowest of OECD countries (4.8 nurses per 1,000 population in 2012 as compared with the OECD average of 8.8), and still continues to decline, despite governmental efforts to change this trend (OECD Health Statistics, 2014).

Because of the severe nursing shortage in the 1980s, nursing in Israel has been recognized as a "preferential profession," offering remunerations and benefits. The worker shortage may have been even larger, but the large wave of immigration in the early 1990s brought with it many new immigrants and among them nurses who were recognized in Israel as practical nurses (Figure 22-2). Special training tracts to a diploma-registered nurse level were opened for them, as well as second-career retraining tracts for university graduates. The many graduates of these programs have integrated into the country's healthcare system. On the one hand, due to the aforementioned statistics, the global nursing shortage was only evident in Israel in recent years. On the other hand, despite the increasing number of nurses under the age of 60, the

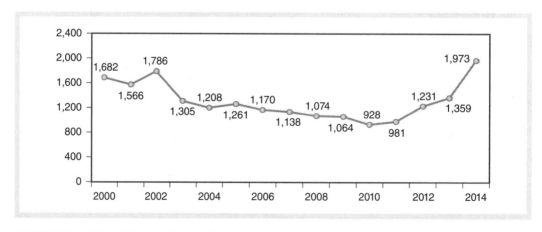

FIGURE 22-2 Additional Registered Nurses by the Year They Are Licensed
Reproduced from Israel Ministry of Health, Nursing Division. (2014c). *Activity report and work goals for 2015, 109/15*. Retrieved July 12, 2015, from http://www.health.gov.il/hozer/ND109_2015.pdf

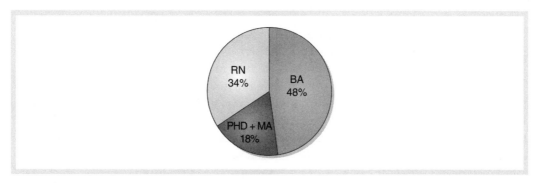

FIGURE 22-3 Distribution of Academic Degrees in Nursing
Data from Nirel N., Yair, Y., Riba, S., Reicher, S., Toren, O. (2010). *Registered Nurses in Israel: workforce supply—pattern and trends*. Jerusalem: Myers, JDC, Brookdale institute (ed).

population growth was slightly greater than the rate of increase in the number of nurses, resulting in a decreased rate of nurses per 1,000 population. In recent years, the waves of immigration have stopped and with it the special training programs for this specific population, resulting in a greater shortage of nurses.

The majority of the nurses in Israel have academic degrees: 48% have baccalaureate and 18% have graduate degrees. Fewer than one-third of the nurses hold a diploma to practice nursing (Figure 22-3) (Nirel, Yair, Riba, Reicher, & Toren, 2010).

Nursing Development in Israel

There is a growing trend toward accepting nursing students into academic schools and opening more colleges to educate students toward earning a BSN degree. In 2014, 34 education programs for registered nurses were opened, along with other academic programs, resulting in a total of 2,850 new nursing students enrolled at the beginning of the academic year (Israel Ministry of Health, 2014c). In addition, in 2014/2015, three more colleges were licensed to educate nursing at the baccalaureate level, resulting in the addition of 150 academic graduates.

Academic nursing schools are also responsible for teaching clinical courses in post-basic clinical practice. The courses in special clinical fields are mandatory for nurses who work in special clinical practices, providing them with the knowledge and authority for specific clinical interventions. The courses are under the rubric of Post-Basic Education (PBE), are license-based training. Fifteen courses are offered to nurses, targeting education to specific clinical fields. The curriculum is designed by the Nursing Division in the Ministry of Health (MOH) for the theoretical part as well as the clinical practice. Examples of PBE courses are pediatric intensive care, gerontology, psychiatry, oncology, neonatal intensive care, operating room (OR) nursing, community health, infection control, nephrology, and midwifery. A prerequisite for acceptance to these courses is a baccalaureate degree in nursing, and passing a general nursing test with the grade of 70.

A PBE program lasts about 1 year, with a range of 300 to 600 academic hours. About 50% of the courses are theoretical and the rest are clinical practice courses. The students are required to take a national qualifying examination to acquire certification. Success in this examination endows a license to perform a series of nursing care interventions for which only the program's graduates are qualified (Toren, Kerzman, Kigli-shemes, & Kagan, 2011).

Nursing specialization was in its preliminary stages in 2009, with the recognition of palliative care as the first area for nursing specialization. This trend was developed, and more programs for nurse practitioner training evolved in areas such as geriatrics, neonatology, and surgery. At the end of 2014, 62 new specialists joined the nursing force. The satisfaction from the graduates is high, and in light of this, it was decided to expand this policy into other areas of practice. In the next few years, plans include the areas of primary care, medical care, pain and rehabilitation for nursing specialization (Israel Ministry of Health, 2014c).

The quality of nursing care and patient safety are primary goals of nursing in Israel. Many activities are being embedded and monitored related to nursing quality care. Such activities include standardization, implementation, and monitoring of many activities. Examples for these activities are the determination of the unique role of nurses in the roles within the hospital and community; the impact of nursing prevention on patients' falls and bed sores (decubitus); and the role of nursing in providing breastfeeding counseling and guidance given by lactation nursing consultants.

Allied Healthcare Professionals

In addition to nurses and physicians, other healthcare professionals work in the system. Some of the professions, such as dentists, work primarily in the private sector (most dental care is not covered by national healthcare insurance).

The rate of dentists employed in Israel is 0.68 per 1,000 population. The number of graduates of dental schools is lower in Israel (0.77) than the average OECD (2.45). The ratio of physicians age 65 and under has decreased to 1.00 in 2013, compared to 1.05 in 2000, a decrease of 5%. The rate per 1,000 population of other healthcare professionals such as pharmacists, psychologists, physiotherapists, dietitians, speech therapists, and occupational therapists has been rising since 2000.

In addition, the Act to Regulate the Health Professions (physiotherapists, dietitians, speech therapists, and occupational therapists) to ensure a qualified level of care was issued in 2008. This law joins other laws governing the professions of medicine, psychology, and social work. Nursing still has no unique law regulating the profession, and it operates under the regulation of the medical profession and public health acts.

CONCLUSION

As a relatively young modern democratic country, Israel has gained many accomplishments in the healthcare system. It has had a national healthcare system with universal healthcare coverage for more than 15 years, which is predominantly publicly financed and government regulated, with competition among providers (both health plans and hospitals). The healthcare system is based on health plans that benefit the population as a whole. It succeeded in achieving above-average levels of health status despite the below-average level of resources the country is allocated (Rosen & Merkur, 2009).

Israel's small geographic size with good access to high-quality care services throughout the country enables it to give a considerably high level of care both in the preventive as well as curative and palliative care. This quality care relies, in part, on the strong academic training for most of the healthcare professionals. The decreased number of physicians and the shortage of nurses impede this trend of success. In addition, as a country that has absorbed immigrants from all around the world, the largest wave from the former Soviet Union and Ethiopia, Israel faces the challenge of closing both cultural and health gaps among the different groups of immigrant patients.

Study Questions

1. Discuss the influences of religion and ethnic background to the health issues of the people in Israel.
2. What are Israel's greatest challenges and assets regarding health and health care for all its residents?
3. Relate how Israel is prepared for emergency health crisis situations.

Case Study: Prehospital Use of Hemostatic Dressings by the Israel Defense Forces Medical Corps

Hemostatic dressings are advanced topical dressings designed to control hemorrhage by enhancing clot formation, called "quickclot combat gauze." A study was conducted between 2009–2014 and found that these new dressings were an effective tool for controlling hemorrhage.

Data from Shina, Lipsky, Nadler, Levi, Benov, Ran, Yitzhak, & Glassberg (2015). Prehospital use of homostatic dressings by the Israel Defense Forces Medical Corps: A case series of 122 patients. *Journal of Trauma Acute Care Surgery, 79*(4 Supplement 2), S2094-9.

Case Study Questions

1. What do you think is the motivation for development of hemostatic dressings in Israel?
2. What beneficial use can this development bring to other trauma situations in Israel and worldwide?

References

Arieli, D., Horev, T., & Keidar, N. (2014). *The National Health Insurance Law statistical data—19 years of the National Health Insurance Law*. Retrieved August 10, 2015 from http://www.health.gov.il/PublicationsFiles/Stat1995_2013.pdf

Averbuch, E., & Anvi, S. (2014). *Coping with health inequalities*. Retrieved August 10, 2015 from http://www.health.gov.il/PublicationsFiles/inequality-2014.pdf

Bin Nun, G., Berlovitz, Y., & Shani, M. (2010). *The Health Care System in Israel*. Tel Aviv: Am Oved Publishing.

Gross, M. L. (2005). Treating competent patients by force: The limits and lessons of Israel's Patient's Rights Act. *Journal of Medical Ethics, 31*, 29–34.

Israel Central Bureau of Statistics. (2013a). *Projections of Israel population until 2035.* Retrieved from http://www1.cbs.gov.il/reader/newhodaot/hodaa_template.html?hodaa=201301170

Israel Central Bureau of Statistics. (2013b). *Israel health: From where and where to?* Retrieved from http://www.cbs.gov.il/publications13/rep_06/pdf/part05_h.pdf

Israel Central Bureau of Statistics. (2014). Selected data from the *Statistical Abstract of Israel No.65.* Retrieved from http://www.cbs.gov.il/reader/newhodaot/hodaa_template.html?hodaa=201411257

Israel Central Bureau of Statistics. (2015). *Mortality and life expectancy.* Retrieved from http://www.cbs.gov.il/reader/cw_usr_view_SHTML?ID=591

Israel Ministry of Foreign Affairs. (1995). *National health insurance.* Retrieved from http://www.mfa.gov.il/MFA/MFAArchive/1990_1999/1998/7/National+Health+Insurance.htm

Israel Ministry of Health. (1996). *The Patient's Right Act.* Retrieved from http://www.health.gov.il/LegislationLibrary/Zchuyot_01.pdf

Israel Ministry of Health. (2010). *Manpower.* Retrieved from http://www.health.gov.il/PublicationsFiles/mp_june2010.pdf

Israel Ministry of Health. (2014a). *Health 2013.* Retrieved from http://www.health.gov.il/PublicationsFiles/health2013.pdf

Israel Ministry of Health. (2014b). *Nineteen years of the National Health Insurance Law.* Retrieved from http://www.health.gov.il/English/News_and_Events/Spokespersons_Messages/Pages/03112014_1.aspx

Israel Ministry of Health. (2014c). *Activity report and work goals for 2015,109/15.* Retrieved from http://www.health.gov.il/hozer/ND109_2015.pdf

Israel Ministry of Health. (2015a). *Mental health reform.* Retrieved from http://health.gov.il/Subjects/mental_health/reform/Pages/default.aspx

Israel Ministry of Health. (2015b). *Health professions workforce in 2013.* Retrieved from http://www.health.gov.il/PublicationsFiles/manpower2013.pdf

Keidar, N., Plotnik, R., Nakmoli Levi, D., & Horev, T. (2014). *Health care comparison between Israel and OECD countries.* Retrieved from http://www.health.gov.il/PublicationsFiles/OECD_2012.pdf

Nirel, N., Yair, Y., Riba, S., Reicher, S., & Toren, O. (2010). *Registered nurses in Israel: workforce supply—pattern and trends.* Jerusalem: Myers, JDC, Brookdale Institute.

OECD Health Statistics. (2014). *How does Israel compare?* Retrieved from http://www.oecd.org/els/health-systems/Briefing-Note-ISRAEL-2014.pdf

Rassin, M., Avraham, M., Nasi-Bashari, A., Idelman, S., Peretz, Y., Morag, S., Silner, D., & Weiss, G. (2007). Emergency department staff preparedness for mass casualty events involving children. *Disaster Management Response, 5*(2), 36–44.

Rosen, B., & Merkur, S. (2009). Israel: Health system review health systems in transition. *European Observatory on Health Systems and Policies, 11*(2), 1–226.

Shemesh, A., Rotem, N., Haklai, T., Georgi, M., & Horev, T. (2012). *Occupational characteristics of Israel physicians.* Retrieved from www.health.gov.il/PublicationsFiles/Econ_Doctors_2012.pdf

Shina, A., Lipsky, A.M., Nadler, R., Levi, M., Benov, A., Ran, Y., Yitzhak, A. & Glassberg, E. (2015). Prehospital use of homostatic dressings by the Israel Defense Forces Medical·Corps: A case series of 122 patients. *Journal of Trauma Acute Care Surgery, 79*(4 Supplement 2), S2094-9.

State of Israel. (2002). *Emergency department.* Retrieved from http://www.health.gov.il/emergency/yehud.htm

State of Israel. (2014). *The ministries' work plans for 2014.* Retrieved from http://plans.gov.il/Plan2012/Documents/Yearplan2014LR.pdf

The World Bank. (2015). *Age dependency ratio.* Retrieved from http://data.worldbank.org/indicator/SP.POP.DPND/countries?display=graph

Toren, O., Kerzman, H., Kigli-shemes, R., & Kagan, I. (2011). The difference between professional image and job satisfaction of nurses who studied in a post basic education program and nurses with generic education: A questionnaire survey. *Journal of Professional Nursing, 27,* 28–34.

Toren, O., & Picker, O. (2009). Staff development in the national level. In O. Toren & O. Picker (Eds.), *Nursing Leadership and Management in Israeli Hospitals* (pp. 27–41). Jerusalem: Magness.

Index

Page numbers followed by b, f, or t indicate material in boxes, figures, or tables, respectively.